Behavioral Medicine:
Theory and Practice

Behavioral
Theory and

Medicine:
Practice

Edited By

OVIDE F. POMERLEAU, Ph.D.

Associate Professor of Psychology in Psychiatry
and Director, Center for Behavioral Medicine
Department of Psychiatry
University of Pennsylvania School of Medicine
Philadelphia, Pennsylvania

and

JOHN PAUL BRADY, M.D.

Kenneth E. Appel Professor and Chairman,
Department of Psychiatry
University of Pennsylvania School of Medicine
Philadelphia, Pennsylvania

THE WILLIAMS & WILKINS COMPANY
Baltimore

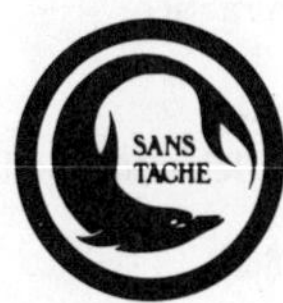

Made in the United States of America

Library of Congress Cataloging in Publication Data

Main entry under title:

Behavioral medicine, theory and practice.

Includes bibliographies and index.
1. Medicine and psychology. 2. Behavior modification. I. Pomerleau, Ovide F. II. Brady, John Paul.
R726.5.B426 616.8'9 78-11866
ISBN 0-683-06956-X

Composed and printed at the
Waverly Press, Inc.
Mt. Royal and Guilford Aves.
Baltimore, Md. 21202, U.S.A.

Preface

This volume represents an attempt to define behavioral medicine by reviewing the methodology and technology on which it is based and by presenting representative applications.

At present there is no source book that provides—within one cover—a systematic and comprehensive discussion of the historical, methodological, experimental, and clinical issues that face this burgeoning new field. Reviews on biofeedback (Birk, 1973), psychosomatic medicine (Lipowski, 1977), self-management (Mahoney and Thoresen, 1974), weight control (Stunkard, 1975), and preventive medicine (Pomerleau, Bass, and Crown, 1975) have been helpful, but because they have been directed to specialized audiences, the general implications of the approach have yet to be communicated to the many scientists and physicians whose qualifications and interests make them likely contributors to research and practice in behavioral medicine. A number of excellent books have dealt with behavioral medicine indirectly as part of a general survey of behavior therapy (Leitenberg, 1976), or directly in a compendium of reprinted articles (Katz and Zlutnick, 1975) or published papers from a conference (Williams and Gentry, 1977). In contrast, the present volume is an integrated text with original critical evaluations by leading clinicians and researchers which treats both basic concepts and clinical applications.

Given the recent rapid development of the field, there is a need for a well-elaborated introduction to behavioral medicine—one which allows the medical practitioner to grasp the potential benefits of the scientific analysis of behavior and which also allows the behavioral scientist to recognize the medical significance of various health habits. We hope that *Behavioral Medicine: Theory and Practice* will serve as a stimulus for increased interaction and collaboration between professionals with service orientation—physicians, nurses, clinical psychologists, specialists in preventive medicine and public health—and basic scientists and methodologists—epidemiologists, experimental psychologists, and physiologists.

The book is divided into two main sections: basic concepts and clinical applications. In the basic concepts section (chapters 1–4), research findings in behavioral epidemiology, learning and conditioning, biofeedback, and self-management are presented. The techniques and methods which characterize the field are given, along with examples relating to applications described in later chapters and suggestions for further research. For the non-specialist, extensive bibliographies facilitate access to the various disciplines represented; for the specialist, critical reviews of current contributions to the field are provided to improve and to stimulate basic research.

In the clinical sections (chapters 5–12), representative applications are described and discussed. Where appropriate, relevant medical or physiological background is presented in the context of reviewing etiology, assessment, treatment, and outcome for the particular problem. Sufficient detail is given to illustrate clinical principles, pointing out various therapeutic and experimental difficulties as well as suggesting directions for future inquiry. As in the methodology section, the needs of both the specialist and non-specialist are taken into account.

The rationale for the order of chapters is as follows. Epidemiology was chosen as the first chapter because, historically and conceptually, observations concerning relationships between behavior and disease have preceded behavioral intervention on medical problems. A discussion of learning and conditioning concepts follows, because the experimental analysis of behavior—more than any other discipline—has made possible the active-intervention technology which characterizes behavioral medicine. The section on basic concepts is completed by chapters on biofeedback and self-management—the two principal forms of intervention in clinical behavioral medicine. The section on applications begins with chapters which emphasize exteroceptive control and direct manipulation of the environment by the therapist, of which behavioral pediatrics and the management of chronic pain provide excellent examples. The section ends with chapters in which self-management procedures predominate—techniques in which the patient or client modifies his or her own environment to engender more adaptive behavior, as illustrated by the chapters on smoking, problem drinking, and obesity. The middle chapters—musculoskeletal disorders, sexual dysfunction, and hypertension—are characterized by a mixture of direct and indirect environmental modification techniques.

There are numerous interrelationships among the sections and various topics. Thus, epidemiological findings have contributed to interest in dietary management, hypertension, smoking, and problem drinking. As has been mentioned, learning and conditioning concepts apply to all topics presented. Biofeedback methods have played an important role in the treatment of musculoskeletal disorders and hypertension as well as the management of chronic pain, whereas self-management principles have been used extensively in obesity, smoking, and problem drinking. Compliance, as a general theme, is emphasized in the chapters on chronic pain, obesity, hypertension, smoking, problem drinking, and behavioral pediatrics, while prevention of disease is an important consideration in the chapters on dietary managment, hypertension, smoking, and problem drinking. Finally, while the clinical chapters clearly represent the interests of psychiatry, family medicine, and internal medicine, the volume as a whole may be regarded broadly as the application of psychology to problems in medicine.

We have attempted to obtain more than the usual degree of integration in an edited book. Each contributor was sent a preliminary draft of the introduction, and the information in the introduction was taken into account by the authors before writing each chapter. The authors then modified the introduction to reflect their opinions as to the scope and promise of behavioral medicine and then returned the revision to the editors. The resulting introductory section is thus an expression of the editors' view of behavioral medicine influenced by the authors' added perceptions.

The authors for the present volume are basic researchers and clinical investigators who have gained recognition for their contributions to behavioral medicine. In most cases, they have written major reviews of their area for a more specialized context. Since it is clearly impossible to present all the topics which come under the rubric of behavioral medicine, we have arbitrarily limited selection to those areas which have important clinical and research implications and which are sufficiently well developed to be subjected to stringent critical evaluation. The existence of an articulate spokesperson for a given area also influenced our choices. We do not claim that the list of topics is exhaustive, but rather offer it as a preview of future developments.

The present volume represents interests in the Department of Psychiatry of the University of Pennsylvania that go back nearly a decade, beginning with research on obesity by Albert J. Stunkard. Nearly six years ago, we began to extend some of the innovative techniques used in weight control to smoking cessation and problem drinking. This led to a conceptual shift, from disorders of self-control to disorders of self-management, a change which emphasized a more general context for treatment—namely, *prevention* of disease through risk-factor modification and *adherence* to treatment through contingency management. Accordingly, in 1973, a new clinical unit—the first of its kind—was formally organized and took the name, "Center for Behavioral Medicine." Since that time, our colleagues have introduced relaxation procedures, biofeedback, health evaluation, and several new clinical areas to the original Center activities. It is with gratitude that we acknowledge the help and assistance provided by our various colleagues at the University and by the staff of the Center in this promising venture called behavioral medicine.

Ovide F. Pomerleau, Ph.D.
John Paul Brady, M.D.

References

BIRK, L. (Ed.). *Biofeedback: Behavioral medicine.* New York: Grune & Stratton, 1973.

KATZ, R. C., AND ZLUTNICK, S. *Behavior therapy and health care.* Elmsford, N.Y.: Pergamon Press, 1975.

LEITENBERG, H. (Ed.). *Handbook of behavior modification and behavior therapy.* Englewood Cliffs, N.J.: Prentice Hall, Inc., 1976.

LIPOWSKI, Z. J. Psychosomatic medicine in the seventies: An overview. *Am. J. Psychiatry,* 1977, *134,* 233–244.

MAHONEY, M., AND THORESEN, C. *Self control: Power to the person.* Monterey, Calif.: Brooks/Cole, 1974.

POMERLEAU, O. F., BASS, F., AND CROWN, V. The role of behavior modification in preventive medicine. *N. Engl. J. Med.,* 1975, *292,* 1277–1282.

STUNKARD, A. J. From explanation to action in psychosomatic medicine: The case of obesity. *Psychosomatic Med.,* 1975, *37,* 195–236.

WILLIAMS, R. B., JR., AND GENTRY, W. D. (Eds.). *Behavioral approaches to medical treatment.* Cambridge, Mass.: Ballinger Publishing Company, 1977.

Contents

CLINICAL APPLICATIONS

Introduction: The Scope and Promise of Behavioral Medicine

OVIDE F. POMERLEAU, PH.D.
Associate Professor of Psychology in Psychiatry
Director, Center for Behavioral Medicine
Department of Psychiatry
University of Pennsylvania School of Medicine
Philadelphia, Pennsylvania

JOHN PAUL BRADY, M.D.
Kenneth E. Appel Professor
Chairman, Department of Psychiatry
University of Pennsylvania School of Medicine
Philadelphia, Pennsylvania

What is Behavioral Medicine?

The term "behavioral medicine" is being used with increasing frequency to describe certain kinds of intervention and research in psychophysiological and medical problems. Behavioral medicine is still in the process of evolving conceptually and, although any definition promulgated at present must be seen as tentative, a working definition should be attempted as this volume's first order of business.

Although interest in the interactions between behavior and disease is as old as the practice of medicine, systematic behavioral medicine is a relatively recent development. A brief discussion of the relationship between behavioral medicine and related areas may be helpful in understanding the approach.

Psychosomatic medicine, for example, is concerned with the interplay between psychosocial and physiological variables in disease, although it constitutes a broad area of interest rather than a particular methodological approach. In its most recent forms, it has been seen as comprising a "biopsychosocial" model which encompasses all health and disease (Weiner, 1977). Historically, the field has drawn heavily from the psychoanalytic theories of Freud and Alexander and, more recently, has been characterized by considerable psychophysiological research in medical and psychiatric contexts; the emphasis has been primarily on etiology and the pathogenesis of physical disease (Schwartz and Weiss, 1977). Medical psychology has been employed to describe the use of psychological principles and techniques in the diagnosis and assessment of physical illness and the use of certain research strategies in the evaluation of treatment. The term medical psychology also refers to a broad field of activity, one in which psychometric assessment, projective testing, and personality theory have played major roles. The emphasis in medical psychology has been on the understanding of medical illness in its psychological and social context rather than on therapy.

Behavior modification and behavior therapy are more specific terms, conveying a particular type of intervention as well as a strategy for diagnosis and a specific research methodology. Behavior modification has used experimentally derived principles of learning and conditioning in a wide variety of situations to modify maladaptive behavior or to inculcate more adaptive patterns (e.g., Risley and Baer, 1973). While the procedures for intervention are clearly delineated, the term behavior modification does not limit applications to any particular area—although historically, it has been associated with behavior change in educational and rehabilitative settings. Similarly, behavior therapy indicates a method of treatment. While its clinical purpose corresponds more closely to behavioral medicine, in that it implies a contractual agreement between therapist and patient or client to modify or treat a designated problem behavior (e.g., Wolpe, 1969), historically, behavior therapy has remained the province of the clinical psychologist and psychiatrist, being concerned less with physical disease and more with neurosis and affective disorders.

Behavioral medicine as a clinical activity is an outgrowth of behavior modification and therapy, borrowing procedures and techniques as well as assessment and research strategies. While some definitions have been attempted, not all have emphasized its origins in modern behaviorism (Skinner, 1953). For example, Schwartz and Weiss (1977) have characterized behavioral medicine as the "field concerned with the development of behavioral-science knowledge and techniques relevant to the understanding of physical health and illness and its application . . . to prevention, diagnosis, treatment, and rehabilitation." The definition is useful because it specifies a sphere of interest, delineates problem areas, and designates both research and clinical activity as relevant. A major drawback to the definition, however, is the implication that behavioral medicine owes its existence equally to the variety of specialties and disciplines subsumed under the term "behavioral sciences": It thus becomes an amalgam of elements from personality theory, medical sociology, and cultural anthropology, as well as an application of social learning theory to the health field. While there have been numerous important contributions from the social as well as the biological sciences—particularly epidemiology and physiology—these and related disciplines have constituted a *necessary but not sufficient* condition for the development of behavioral medicine (Pomerleau, 1978).

This issue was anticipated clearly by Agras (1975) in his introduction to *Behavior therapy and health care*:

> The fact that behavior affects both disease and the maintenance of health has long been known, and for just as long has been minimized or overlooked both by medical research workers and clinicians. One reason for this minimization of the importance of behavior and even the behavioral sciences in medicine has been the lack of procedures derived from these sciences which change behavior in a clinically useful way. The development of behavior therapy has begun to alter this undesirable state of affairs. First, by introducing innovative and effective treatment procedures, and second, by acting as a vehicle for the application of the research methods and findings of experimental psychology to the health field (p. xi).*

We propose that the initial definition of behavioral medicine give adequate emphasis to the experimental analysis of behavior, as the inspiration and the source for much of the current activity. We recognize that the delimitation of a new field poses a special challenge—if the initial definition is too narrow, future activity may be misguided or stifled; if it is too broad, there may be insufficient identity to stimulate directed movement. Therefore, we suggest the following definition as a compromise:

> *Behavioral medicine* can be defined as (a) the clinical use of techniques derived from the experimental analysis of behavior—behavior therapy and behavior modification—for the evaluation, prevention, management, or treatment of physical disease or physiological dysfunction; and (b) the conduct of research contributing to the functional analysis and understanding of behavior associated with medical disorders and problems in health care.

Ultimately, a field is defined by what it does; if conditions change, then the definition of behavioral medicine should be modified accordingly.

* Reprinted by permission from R. C. Katz and S. Zlutnick (Eds.). *Behavior therapy and health care*. Elmsford, New York: Pergamon Press, 1975.

Basic Concepts

Behavioral medicine as a technology is an outgrowth of developments in certain basic sciences. The contribution of the descriptive sciences to behavioral medicine is illustrated by work in epidemiology and the contribution of the experimental sciences, by psychology.

Epidemiology. Epidemiology can be defined as the study of health and disease of populations and of groups in relation to their environment and ways of living. While the clinician usually deals with individual cases, the epidemiologist is concerned with cases as they occur in the population. An example of the kind of inferences that have been drawn from epidemiological research is provided by statistics on mortality from all causes, for middle-aged men and women in England and Wales, as described by Morris (1957). From the turn of the century to the 1920's, death rates for both sexes began to fall in response to sanitary reform. From the 1920's to the 1950's, however, female mortality kept its downward course, but males failed to show a corresponding decrease. Males show a decrease in death rate during this time only when pulmonary cancer and coronary heart disease are partitioned out of the samples. This suggests that, for men, improvements in mortality from prophylaxis and more effective treatment of infectious diseases were offset by the increasing incidence of certain chronic degenerative diseases. This general observation has been replicated with various populations in Western industrial nations over the years (Pomerleau, Bass, and Crown, 1975).

Both retrospective and prospective studies are representative of the epidemiological method. Retrospective observation has the advantage of focusing on the phenomenon of interest (e.g., the onset of a given disease or condition) after it occurs, in an attempt to determine contributory variables. However, there is often great difficulty in ascertaining all of the key events which lead to disease after the fact. For this reason, prospective, longitudinal methodologies are receiving increased attention. Among their particular advantages is that information can be obtained in a similar fashion for both future cases and their controls, thus reducing potential sources of bias or error. The incidence and circumstances of new cases can be obtained more accurately, which is important in conditions like coronary heart disease where sudden death is the first clinical manifestation for a substantial percentage of cases. Moreover, the forward-looking study may be the only way to investigate the natural history of a complex disease process.

Epidemiological research has played an important role in demonstrating the relationships between certain behavioral variables and morbidity and mortality. The correlational relationships have provided pre-morbid predictors for certain disease states and have, of late, resulted in useful recommendations for the prevention and management of chronic degenerative diseases. For example, the Framingham Study (Kannel, Castelli, and McNamara, 1968) showed how the presence of certain patterns of behavior such as cigarette smoking was associated with increased incidence of coronary heart disease. Thus, cigarette smoking and its pathophysiological sequelae constitute a risk factor for heart disease. Other demonstrated or suggested risk factors for heart disease are obesity, hyperlipidemia, lack of exercise, type A behavior pattern, hypertension, diabetes, and family history of heart disease. It is interesting to note that behavior or behavioral management is involved in the modification of each of these risk factors—even family history can be seen as having a behavioral component, for it reflects in part, traditions and preferences which increase risk.

The correlational relationships carry certain implications. If cigarette smoking, in the above example, is associated with increased risk of heart disease, then quitting smoking is likely to decrease the probability of such disease. Studies of morbidity and mortality in former smokers bear this out (Hammond, 1962). What has not been done in any systematic way, however, is to test whether former smokers assume a lower risk as a result of quitting or if their "spontaneous" quitting reflects a common variable which also puts them at decreased risk. The best way to study this relationship is to treat current smokers and to compare the incidence of smoking-related diseases in those who quit and those who do not quit. Beyond the time and expense involved in conducting such a study, the chief limiting factor has been the lack of potent intervention techniques. Promising trends in behavioral smoking cessation treatment, however, may resolve this difficulty.

Just as epidemiology has provided basic observations which make possible risk-factor modification in the prevention of heart disease, descriptive methodology from other sciences has contributed in like fashion to the understanding of various medical conditions and disorders. For example, Kinsey, Pomeroy, and Martin (1948, 1953) studied normal sexual behavior and frequency and severity of sexual disorders, and Masters and Johnson (1966) studied the physiology of the sexual response. Similarly, cross-cultural studies of pain, longitudinal studies on the course of essential hypertension, and prospective studies of pre-morbid characteristics of alcoholics have all influenced treatment practice.

Psychology. Experimentation on learning and conditioning provides the foundation for treatment in behavioral medicine. The development of a technology for modifying maladaptive behavior effectively is relatively new, representing an extension of basic research on animal learning by Pavlov (1927) and Skinner (1938) to problems in human behavior. Learning and conditioning approaches are referred to as "behavioral" in keeping with the emphasis on relating measurable activity (behavioral responses) to antecedent and subsequent environmental events (stimuli).

Two of the concepts growing out of this approach—contingency management and stimulus control—have been particularly useful. Contingency management is based on the experimental observation that consequences of behavior (reinforcing stimuli) determine the pattern of subsequent behavior; thus, a reinforcer is a behavioral consequence that has the effect of making the behavior that preceded it or produced it more likely to be repeated (Rachlin, 1970). A reward such as praise or money given for a designated behavior is an example of a reinforcer. Frequently employed consequences which increase the frequency of behavior are presentation of reward (positive reinforcement) and interruption of aversive stimulation (negative reinforcement); consequences which decrease the frequency of behavior are interruption of rewarded activity (time out) and presentation of aversive stimulation (punishment). Thus, a major aspect of behavior modification is the deliberate scheduling of response-contingencies to increase adaptive behavior and to decrease maladaptive behavior.

A second important concept is stimulus control, which refers to the influence of environmental events (including stimuli both internal and external to the organism) in providing the context for on-going behavior (Terrace, 1966). A stimulus can affect behavior because it has been associated with a reinforcer (e.g., respondent conditioning) or because the stimulus signals a situation in which the behavior has been associated with a reinforcer (e.g., operant conditioning). A stimulus control analysis is used in many behavioral applications to specify how the environment determines the problem behavior. Typically, a detailed analysis is carried out on the target behavior and on the social and physical events within the environment which are temporally related to the behavior. Behavioral management is then sought through manipulation of these environmental stimuli. A stimulus control analysis can thus be seen to serve a similar function to traditional clinical assessment.

Shaping and modeling represent techniques which are also frequently utilized in behavioral treatment (Bandura, 1969). When a desired behavior does not occur, or occurs with an extremely low frequency, the behavior most closely approximating the desired terminal behavior is selected for reinforcement. Then, reinforcement is made contingent upon successively closer approximations to the desired behavior, thus "shaping" the response gradually in the new direction. Modeling is a technique for modifying behavior through observation and imitation. Typically, the model emits the desired behavior and the subject is rewarded for imitating or approximating it.

Representative Interventions

Biofeedback. Biofeedback, an important tool for understanding and treating psychophysiological disorders, may be regarded as a special application of operant-reinforcement procedures. Traditionally, the shaping of behavior by arranging its consequences has been thought to apply to "voluntary" responses, i.e., skeletal-muscle behavior. The key notion in biofeedback is that operant-reinforcement techniques may also be used to modify responses which are traditionally regarded as "involuntary," i.e., responses of smooth muscles and glands.

Miller (1969) and his colleagues and, more recently, investigators such as Thornton and Van Toller (1973) and Gliner, Horvath, and Wolpe (1975) have demonstrated that animals can learn to modify autonomic physiological responses in highly specific ways if immediate, rewarding consequences are provided for small incremental changes. In the earliest experiments, the animals were paralyzed with curare in an attempt to ensure that the organism's learned control of heart rate, blood pressure, or other physiological variables was not simply a matter of inducing a change indirectly by means of skeletal-muscle responses. Typically, avoidance of aversive shock or the direct stimulation of positive reinforcement centers in the brain were used as reinforcers. Even more convincing demonstrations have been carried out with human subjects who have been taught to alter physiological variables in highly specific ways not generally regarded as being under voluntary control (e.g., Shapiro, 1977; Taub and Emurian, 1976). In human experiments, feedback is usually provided by transforming the physiological variables of interest into electrical signals which are then used to control visual or auditory stimuli, thereby providing information to the subject on his or her own physiological state. Changing the physiological variable in the desired direction is usually sufficient reinforcement, although other consequences, such as monetary rewards, can be attached to successful learning. An important characteristic of the approach is that, with appropriate transducers, it is possible to add the specificity and discriminability of exteroceptive stimulation (such as light and sound) to less well-defined information provided by the usual interoceptive cues (proprioception, kinesthesis, etc.).

The elegance of these experimental demonstrations notwithstanding, the capability of human beings to gain control over physiological variables has been known in other contexts for a long time. The celebrated Indian Yoga is an example of a person who has learned to control many physiological variables by techniques which may be similar. A very dramatic demonstration of learned control over certain physiological variables, presumably without the mediation of skeletal-muscle responses, was provided by Lapides, Sweet, and Lewis (1957). After administering curare and related drugs to eliminate skeletal-muscle responses in 16 volunteer subjects, Lapides et al. demonstrated that normal adults were still able to initiate and terminate micturition on request. The experiment was performed to demonstrate that, in keeping with anatomical studies, only smooth muscles are essential for micturition, but also, in the normal course of development, humans learn to control voluntarily a complex series of smooth-muscle responses.

In addition to its theoretical implications, biofeedback is of interest as a method of treatment and as a tool for the study of pathophysiological mechanisms. However, as is often the case with a new mode of treatment, the number of disorders for which biofeedback has been shown to be specific and clinically useful is fewer than some uncritical and overly enthusiastic reports would suggest. Well designed, controlled studies are needed with extended follow-up to demonstrate that the beneficial changes produced by biofeedback are not the result of suggestion or other nonspecific factors and that they generalize to the natural environment, are of sufficient magnitude to be clinically useful, and persist for a significant period of time to represent a therapeutic advance. The potential of these methods for the treatment of medical disorders is discussed in the chapters on biofeedback, musculoskeletal disorders, and hypertension.

Of equal promise is the use of biofeedback techniques as an investigational tool. An example of this use is provided by Weiss (1977) in his studies on the treatment of premature ventricular contractions and other cardiac arrhythmias using heart rate biofeedback training. By blocking specific neuromechanisms in the regulation of heart rate using pharmacological agents such as atropine and propanolol, Weiss has identified some of the mechanisms involved in learned heart rate alterations.

Self-management. The recent emergence of specialized behavioral techniques for enhancing self-control and self-management

(Mahoney and Thoresen, 1974) has important implications for the application of behavioral principles to medical problems. In much of the earlier work on behavior modification, change was brought about directly through environmental manipulations that modified the behavior of the person with the problem. With self-management procedures, however, the therapist teaches the person with the problem to change aspects of his or her environment which in turn modify the problem behavior. Thus, with self-management methods, the passive role of patient is transformed into the active one of participant; the role of the therapist becomes one of devising effective behavior change techniques and of motivating participants to carry them out. (The degree to which self-management versus clinician-controlled intervention is used varies widely, as can be seen in the various clinical application chapters.)

As discussed by Pomerleau et al. (1975), using an alarm clock to wake up in the morning is an example of a simple, but effective self-management strategy:

> The strategy is based on the observation that before the subject goes to sleep the night before, the reinforcing value of getting up on time in the morning is greater than that of sleeping late, whereas the next morning the values reverse (Rachlin and Green, 1972). Setting an alarm clock thus serves as a commitment strategy to enhance adaptive patterns of behavior—in this case rising early—that maximize certain long-range positive consequences such as arriving at work on time. In like manner, strategies can be devised to modify maladaptive habits so as to minimize long-range negative consequences; for example, self-control tactics may be used to increase control over drinking behavior, thereby avoiding alcoholism as an ultimate aversive consequence. Self-control procedures in which people change their own behavior to achieve certain long-range advantages seem more likely to succeed than those that attempt to modify behavior by simply trying to control or remove misused substances from the environment, as is demonstrated by the lack of success in legislating self-control by raising the price of cigarettes through taxation (Bernstein, 1969) or by prohibiting the sale of alcoholic beverages (p. 1278).†

† Reprinted by permission from *N. Engl. J. Med.*, 1975, *292*, 1277–1282.

While derived from learning and conditioning concepts and sharing many techniques and strategies with traditional behavior modification and therapy, behavioral self-management has several characteristics which set it apart. Before examining them, however, it is useful to distinguish between self-control or self-management and willpower. Although sometimes used synonymously, willpower refers to a hypothetical inner force which purports to account for self-regulatory behavior. Thus, as Mahoney and Thoresen (1974) point out, if a heavy smoker quits "cold turkey," he is sometimes described as having willpower. How do we know he has willpower?—because he quite smoking. In addition to being a tautology which provides no real information beyond a rephrasing of the original behavioral observation, willpower has the additional disadvantage of discouraging further inquiries into the controlling conditions for the behavior.

Self-management techniques come under three main headings: observation, modification of environmental variables, and alteration of behavioral consequences. A knowledge of controlling variables is crucial to successful behavior change. Typically, this is accomplished by having the subject record his or her behavior and the conditions under which it occurs. Thus, the smoker trying to quit can record each day the time, the place, the social circumstances as well as mood, cigarette-by-cigarette (Pomerleau, Adkins, and Pertschuk, 1978). The individual who self-monitors behavior becomes more aware of his or her own actions and receives immediate feedback on the status of the problem behavior. In addition, specific information (stimulus control analysis) concerning the variables controlling the problem behavior is provided for the therapist. An example is smoking after each meal, or being with a certain friend, or feeling tense socially. While self-monitoring is usually not sufficient in itself to change maladaptive behavior completely, it does constitute a first and critical step toward successful self-management.

As in standard behavior modification or therapy, self-management techniques are concerned with changing those antecedent stimuli which set the occasion for maladaptive behavior. A key difference is that the participant or client rather than the therapist changes the controlling environment. In weight control programs, for example, participants are told not to stockpile fattening foods—"If it isn't there, you can't eat it." In the reduction phase of smoking programs, participants are asked to carry only the exact number of cigarettes authorized in their daily quota. Restricting prepotent environmental variables constitutes an important second step toward effective self-management.

The third step involves altering the consequences of behavior—contingency management. Again, the participant or client provides the actual modification, with suggestions provided by the therapist. Thus, the person trying to lose weight might persuade a few friends to form a jogging group, thus obtaining social reinforcement for exercising. The smoker alters reinforcement contingencies for smoking by increasing the intervals between craving and lighting up, thus weakening the habit. Finally, contracts involving money can serve as useful tools by setting up a schedule of extrinsic reinforcement: For example, in a program for problem drinking (Pomerleau, Pertschuk, Adkins, et al., 1978), a prepaid "commitment fee" of up to $300 can be earned back contingent on keeping daily records of drinking or craving, on attending treatment sessions without detectable breath alcohol, on carrying out designated monitored non-drinking activities, and on attending follow-up sessions; the money is forfeited if the participant drops out of treatment.

Obesity, smoking, and problem drinking are examples of common self-management disorders. Although each disorder has its own clinical tradition, the behavioral approach makes it possible to place them in a common conceptual framework. Since the behavioral treatment of obesity has a well documented record of effectiveness, this disorder will be used as an example.

The work of Ferster, Hurnberger, and Levitt (1962) has been most influential among the early attempts to treat obesity with behavioral methods. The developments that grew out of their work included stimulus control analysis, specification and disruption of reinforcers for overeating, and the identification of the "ultimate aversive consequences" of overeating to provide a rationale and motivation for attempting behavior change. Subsequently, Stuart (1967) adopted Ferster's approach for use in a small group setting. Among his innovations was a stimulus control analysis based on a written record of daily eating behavior and assessment of progress by monitoring weight gained or lost on a weekly basis; in addition, total caloric intake was reduced by limiting the number of situations in which eating was authorized (e.g., eating in only one location and engaging in no other activities during eating) and by developing new techniques to enhance behavioral control (e.g., shopping for food after a meal rather than before). One year after the end of treatment in an initial group of 10, Stuart's procedure had resulted in weight losses of more than 18 kg (each) in three participants and more than 14 kg in six others. The work was extended to additional groups, with comparable success (Stuart and Davis, 1971). These findings have since been replicated by Stunkard and his co-workers (Penick, Filion, Fox, et al., 1971; Stunkard, 1972), and the general method has been shown to be more effective than non-behavioral approaches (Stunkard, 1975).

Among the current trends in self-management research is a shift in emphasis from short-term intervention to long-term maintenance. The chapters on smoking, problem drinking, and obesity take up the issue at some length. Another, particularly promising development is the possibility that research on underlying mechanisms may eventually generate a truly rational therapy for some of the more common self-management disorders. The potential of the approach is discussed in recent reviews of psychobiological research on obesity (Rodin, 1978) and smoking (Pomerleau, 1979).

Major Themes in Current Practice

There are four principal lines of development in behavioral medicine at present. The first involves intervention to modify a behavior which in itself constitutes a problem. Examples are behavior modification with children, self-management training, behavior therapy for sexual disorders, or biofeedback for a psychophysiological disorder that is not part of another disease process. As numerous illustrations are provided throughout the book, this area will not be discussed further here.

In a second area of development, the focus of intervention is on the behavior of a health-care provider, in order to improve delivery of service to a patient or client. Although less work has been done, the area shows much promise for the future (e.g., Berni and Fordyce, 1973). A study by Pomerleau, Bobrove, and Smith (1973) on psychiatric aides illustrates the general approach. The behavior of aides was considered a limiting factor in the treatment of highly disruptive state hopsital psychotics. Baseline observations showed that aides typically ignored their patients unless they caused trouble. Special contingencies of reinforcement were introduced to increase the number and quality of therapeutic interactions between aides and patients—in particular to encourage attention for more appropriate social behavior by patients. Under the "aide incentive plan," a small number of patients was (randomly) assigned to each aide. In a given week, the aide's performance was ranked by comparing the comportment of his or her assigned patients (rated on a standardized scale, the *Ward Behavior Inventory*). The aide whose patients improved more than those of the other aides was designated "aide of the week" and received attention and praise. In various conditions, the "aide of the week" received no award, or $10, $20, or $30 awards. The amount of disruptive or inappropriate behavior by patients on the ward as a whole was found to decrease in direct proportion to the amount of monetary incentive given to the aide of the week. Performance feedback and contingent choice of days off have also been shown to produce beneficial effects on staff behavior in institutional settings (Quilitch, 1975; Iwata, Bailey, Brown, et al., 1976).

Similar work has been carried out on medical wards. In research which is particularly timely, several investigators have studied overutilization of laboratory tests (redundant or unnecessary tests). Dixon and Laszlo (1974) limited house officers to eight tests per inpatient per day and reported decreased use of the laboratory by 25%, while increasing the clinical utility of the average test. Griner and Liptzin (1971) showed that laboratory utilization at a teaching hospital remained constant rather than continuing to increase, after guidelines were issued on the proper use of the laboratory. Eisenberg, Williams, Garner, et al. (1977) developed a computer-based medical audit to screen out patients who received unnecessary laboratory tests and provided feedback to the responsible physician; they found that mean weekly use of designated tests decreased during the feedback condition compared with baseline. Systematic research on this and related problems has great potential for making medical care more cost-effective.

A third area of development is concerned with the use of behavioral techniques to improve the patient's adherence to the treatment regimen. The behavior to be modified is important to the extent that it limits the effectiveness of treatment, whether medical or behavioral. Patient compliance has been a particularly frustrating and difficult problem in medical practice, as case histories in the treatment of diabetes, hypertension, chronic pain, and physical rehabilitation illustrate dramatically. Because the problem constitutes a major theme which recurs in several of the clinical chapters in the present volume, adherence to the therapeutic regimen will be reviewed in some detail below in a separate section.

The fourth line of inquiry has to do with prevention of disease. Here, the behavior to be changed is important because it leads to or exacerbates a medical condition or disease. Coronary artery disease, cancers, and cerebrovascular accidents constitute the leading causes of morbidity and mortality in adults at the present time. The prevention and management of these chronic degenerative diseases presents a tremendous challenge for medical and behavioral technology. Because of its importance and the fact that it is a theme which cuts across most of the clinical chapters of the book, prevention of disease through behavior change will also be discussed below.

Adherence. In recent years there has been a growing awareness that the failure of patients to adhere to prescribed medical regimens is probably the single greatest problem in bringing effective medical care to the individual patient. Although the degree of adherence varies with the nature of the regimen, the patient population, and many other variables, it is not uncommon for studies to disclose an adherence rate as low as 50% in many situations. It is, par excellence, a behavioral problem since the task is to alter the patient's health-related behaviors, such as taking prescribed medications in the proper dosage and schedule, adhering to prescribed diets to control diabetes or reduce hyperlipidemia, or modifying life-styles to reduce the risk of cardiovascular disorders.

The issue of adherence is sometimes referred to as compliance in the medical literature. As Stimson (1974) has argued, however, the term compliance is value-laden and suggests a defect or limitation in the patient—a kind of personality characteristic in which the patient "fails to comply with" his doctor's orders. Adherence is the preferable term because it is free of these connotations. Clearly, we must look to the social context in which the patient lives and in which he or she is treated, to identify the environmental variables which will influence adherence behavior.

Central to the study of the problem of adherence is devising reliable methods for assessing and measuring the phenomenon. Numerous studies have shown that the patient interview, the most commonly used method in clinical settings, is notoriously unreliable. There is a general tendency for adherence to be overstated and non-adherence understated by the patient (Dunbar and Stunkard, 1977). Equally invalid are clinical judgments by the prescribing physician. In regimens that consist mainly of taking medications, determining the percentage of pills taken out of the total prescribed is a commonly used measure. Although more valid than interviews and clinical ratings, pill counts are of limited value because the patient may fail to return some of the pills not taken and the procedure does not detect erratic patterns of pill taking.

A more ambitious and sophisticated approach consists of biochemical assessment of markers placed in the medication or of the metabolic by-products of the therapeutic substance itself in serum or urine. These more direct measures of adherence also have limitations. Generally one cannot determine the exact degree of adherence since they do not usually yield quantitative measures. Also these procedures are only sensitive to recent doses of prescribed medications. Another promising approach consists of having patients maintain daily records of pill taking or other behaviors which constitute the therapeutic regimen. This procedure was first developed in behavioral weight-reduction programs and has been extended, at the University of Pennsylvania, to programs for alcohol abuse, cigarette smoking, and the treatment of hyperlipidemia by dietary programs. It has been used little in programs consisting only of taking medications. Self-monitoring of this sort is a reactive measure in the sense that the recording of desirable activities, such as adhering to a medical regimen, tends to increase these behaviors. Self-monitoring also has its limitations, however: the patient may not comply with the monitoring instructions and there is also the problem of the accuracy of his or her self-reporting.

Finally, some authors have suggested using treatment outcome as a measure of adherence, such as reduction in blood pressure for patients on antihypertensive medications. However, this procedure contaminates two variables—adherence and response to a treatment regimen. It is well known that many patients will respond with a drop in blood pressure to placebo medication because of expectation or other factors. In fact, some studies have shown a rather poor correlation between adherence to antihypertensive regimens and response to treatment (Sackett, Haynes, Gibson, et al., 1975). Nevertheless, this approach may have some clinical usefulness. One may focus on the non-responders to treatment to identify for more intensive study those patients who are not adhering to the treatment regimen, in distinction to those who adhere but fail to respond to the particular drugs prescribed.

A good deal of attention has been focused on demonstrating factors which influence or predict adherence. Surprisingly, common demographic variables such as age, sex, marital status, and socioeconomic status have little independent influence on adherence. (Dunbar and Stunkard, 1977; Matthews and Hingson, 1977). Comprehension and ability to recall the details of the treatment regimen does contribute to adherence as does satisfaction with the care and the caretakers. Not surprisingly the characteristics of the clinician-patient relationship and the ambiance of the clinic are important factors. Seeing the same clinician on each visit, having a clinician who is warm and empathic, and receiving treatment in a clinical setting which is positive and accepting, all facilitate adherence. However, the greatest contribution to adherence comes from the nature of the treatment regimen itself. The greater the complexity of the treatment regimen, the poorer the adherence; the presence of alarming or unexpected side effects from medications also decreases cooperation with treatment.

Enhancing adherence to the treatment regimen is of great clinical importance. Matthews and Hingson (1977) recommend that the medical history itself be compliance-oriented so that patients who are likely to have problems in adherence can be identified and ways of enhancing cooperation instituted. As in other behavioral approaches to medical problems, a functional analysis of the behaviors which constitute the treatment regimen is essential. That is, it is important to identify those environmental cues which elicit or set the occasion for performing elements of the treatment regimen and also behavioral consequences for following treatment.

In an insightful and scholarly review of the relevant literature, Dunbar and Stunkard (1977) outline some of the behavioral techniques useful in increasing adherence. The whole range of behavior modification techniques has application here. Important are educating the patient concerning the regimen and its rationale, making use of self-monitoring techniques, and tailoring the regimen so that the specific behaviors required fit into the patient's daily routine. Other procedures include shaping the desired performance (as may be necessary in more complex dietary regimens) and contingency contracting between patient and clinician. A very promising innovation consists of conducting treatment at the patient's place of work. This has been done recently with some large populations of patients with essential hypertension (Alderman, 1976). The advantages include eliminating the number of broken appointments almost entirely, reducing costs by having unions cosponsor treatment, and increasing adherence to treatment through social reinforcement provided by co-workers. A common element in many of these procedures is the use of positive reinforcement contingent on carrying out the treatment regimen, as well as on the more remote but critical variable, improvement or favorable response to treatment. Consistent with the above research, numerous studies have documented the enormous importance of social support from the patient's family, co-workers, employers, and other associates in facilitating adherence to treatment regimens.

Prevention. For many years, various experts in the field of health have proposed that specific aspects of life-style, such as diet, physical activity, cigarette smoking, and consumption of alcohol, have an important influence on morbidity and mortality (Pomerleau, et al., 1975). Recent research underscores these observations. Excessive consumption of saturated fats has been shown to raise blood lipids, thereby increasing the risk of cardiovascular disease (Friedman, 1969; Paffenbarger, 1972) and shortening life expectancy (Metropolitan Life, 1960; Walker, 1968). Physical activity, through mechanisms still not well understood, is also associated with increased risk of coronary artery disease (Belloc and Breslow, 1972; Morris and Crawford, 1958). Cigarette smoking, sustained over a number of years, not only raises the rate of pulmonary disease, such as lung cancer, bronchitis, and emphysema (National Center for Health Statistics, 1973; Weir and Dunn, 1970), but also contributes to a substantial increase in death from coronary heart disease (Jenkins, Rosenman, and Zyzanski, 1968; United States Department of Health, Education, and Welfare, 1973). Finally, chronic excessive consumption of alcohol is associated with a number of serious illnesses, of which the principal one is cirrhosis of the liver (Rubin and Lieber, 1974; Schmidt and de Lint, 1969), as well as increased risk of accidental death (Lalonde, 1974; Hauser, 1974).

The leading causes of death among adults in Western industrial nations are coronary artery disease, cerebrovascular disease, chronic obstructive pulmonary disease, lung cancer, and accidents (United States Department of Health, Education, and Welfare, 1973; Ministry of Health and Welfare, Canada, 1974; Lalonde, 1974). To the extent that health practices can be modified, the prevalence of such diseases can be greatly reduced (Belloc and Breslow, 1972; Turner and Ball, 1973). *Thus, a major task for preventive medicine in Western society has become changing the patterns of behavior that increase the risk of chronic disease in the population.*

Impetus for prevention is also derived from economic considerations. Kristein, Arnold, and Wynder (1977) have argued that the American health-care system is becoming progressively less cost effective. They suggest that the problem is the result of an emphasis on disease care rather than health care and on a lack of effective market controls to check rising costs. They point out that in 1950, Americans spent 4.6% of their gross national product (GNP) on health and in 1975, 8.3%—nearly twice as much. Medical care is now the second largest industry in the nation. Abelson (1976) has predicted that even doubling expenditures for the present system of medical care would have little impact on longevity.

Various solutions to the problem have been suggested. Mechanic (1974) has proposed revision of the third party medical insurance system, to build in safeguards against increased utilization of services and to provide incentives for physicians to economize on treatment components. Health maintenance organizations (HMOs), establishing peer review, and regulating occupational safety, all represent formal attempts to legislate such changes. The main emphasis at present has been on restraining present practices, but clearly what is called for in the future is the identification of those environmental and behavioral variables which constitute risk factors for chronic disease in susceptible individuals and the development of effective prevention and management through life-style and environmental modification (United States Public Health Service, 1976). In short, in national health planning, prevention is being emphasized and crisis intervention de-emphasized.

The kind of radical departure suggested above has been considered at some length in a Canadian Government Working Document entitled, *A new perspective on the health of Canadians* (Lalonde, 1974). The report was prompted by a retrospective examination of various measures intended to promote health in Canada which indicated that, in spite of a rapid improvement in the quality and accessibility of health services over 20 years, there had been little measurable improvement in the overall health of the nation. The development of prepaid health insurance over the years, culminating in the introduction of national universal Medicare in 1967, brought health services to all Canadians without cost but had virtually no impact or mortality rates. An analysis of the principal causes of morbidity and mortality revealed that environmental factors and life-style contributed so greatly as to constitute the key to effective control. On the basis of these findings, the Health Planning Branch proposed that methods for dealing with life-style and environmental influences on health be elevated to the same prominence in the health field as hospitals, clinics, and private physicians.

A recent study by Meyer and Henderson (1974) of the Stanford Heart Disease Prevention Program illustrates some of the possibilities for using behavioral techniques in preventive medicine, in this case on risk factor modification for cardiovascular disease in an industrial population. Out of 240 employees volunteering for the study, 36 were identified as being at risk of cardiovascular disease and were assigned randomly to one of the following treatments: twelve behavior-modification sessions using self-control techniques lasting for 2 to 3 hours in a group setting, nine 15-minute individual-counseling sessions with a health educator, or one 20-minute counseling session with a physician. Treatment lasted for 11 weeks and was followed by a post-treatment evaluation at the end of 3 months. For each group the goal of treatment was to decrease the consumption of saturated fats and carbohydrates, to lower overall caloric intake, to increase the level of physical activity, and to terminate or reduce the amount of cigarette smoking.

The results indicated that behavior modification produced greater changes in health habits than the other procedure and that the improvements observed were more lasting. Although individual counseling with a health educator was less effective than behavior modification, it was clearly superior to a single consultation with a physician. All three procedures produced improvements in the physiological measures of risk—blood cholesterol and triglyceride levels.

While the study represents a major first step in evaluating the use of behavioral technology to prevent disease, the work is far from complete. An important issue that is still not settled is whether the behavior modification and individual counseling procedures used were sufficiently maximized to allow a proper comparison: adding techniques to improve the education approach might well affect the magnitude of the differences observed and thus the conclusions drawn about relative efficacy. The duration of treatment represents another dimension that must be explored before firm conclusions can be drawn about effectiveness. It should be remembered also that, while the various changes reported may be statistically significant, they are not necessarily clinically significant—cigarette smoking, for example, was greatly reduced but still above zero.

An important replication and extension has been provided on a community-wide basis by the same group (Farquhar, Maccoby, Wood, et al., 1977; Maccoby, Farquhar, Wood, et al., 1977). Three California towns, matched on relevant demographic variables, were studied. Two towns were subjected to a multimedia campaign on cardiovascular disease risk factors over 2 years and a third town served as a control, receiving no information; in addition, in one of the towns receiving information, high-risk subjects were given access to a behavior modification program to change their life style. The decrease in cardiovascular risk factors was greatest in the town receiving information plus behavior modification, intermediate in the town receiving information only, and least in the control town. The trends have been sustained in follow-ups 3 years from the onset of intervention.

Conclusion

The extent to which learning is a factor in illness and disease has yet to be fully elucidated, but there are suggestions that it is considerable. A recent study by Ader and Cohen (1975) makes this point in a dramatic way. Using a Pavlovian conditioning paradigm in rats, they demonstrated conditioned suppression of the antibody response to a foreign protein (injected sheep red blood cells). With cyclophosphamide, an immunosuppressant, as the unconditional stimulus, they were able to elicit immunosuppression to the previously neutral conditional stimulus, saccharin. Appropriate control groups did not exhibit this phenomenon. As Schneiderman, Weiss, and Engel (1978) point out "the demonstration of psychological influences on the immune system illustrates the ubiquity of neurally mediated effects on biological systems, and supports the value of a broad concept of psychosomatic processes. Furthermore, data such as these indicate the power of conditioning procedures, and they support strongly the notion that whenever one can specify a neurally mediated response which is pathognomonic, there is a strong possibility that this response can be brought under stimulus control."

In addition to pointing out the relevance of behavioral intervention in the treatment of a number of functional physiological disorders and medical conditions, some additional considerations are worth noting. In particular, behavioral technology seems especially well-suited to the management of the chronic disease state, in that its side effects are relatively benign compared with most drugs and surgery. For this reason, behavioral procedures can be sustained indefinitely—over the lifetime of the individual if necessary. The principal limitations are degree of therapeutic effectiveness, generalizability across situations and over time, and adherence to the therapeutic regimen. Although the problems are far from solved, behavioral technology has made sufficient advances of late to justify vigorous further exploration.

There have been serious reservations concerning behavioral treatment in the past. The issue of symptom substitution was considered a major theoretical difficulty from a psychodynamic point of view. Under this formulation, maladaptive behavior was seen as a "symptom" of unresolved emotional conflicts which, if not removed, led to the development of new symptoms or to relapse. Under conditions in which behavioral assessment and treatment have focused on an appropriately comprehensive clinical entity (rather than on the most superficial maladaptive response), numerous problem behaviors have been successfully modified without generating new difficulties (Yates, 1970). While the above concerns were primarily directed toward the behavioral treatment of neuroses, they were also held to apply in other clinical areas such as self-management. Stunkard (1972) has shown that the behavioral treatment of obesity is more effective than psychotherapy in inducing weight loss and produces fewer adverse psychological side effects than dieting. Similarly, with enuretic children, research has shown that behavioral treatment is more effective than psychotherapy (Yates, 1975) and, in addition, resolution of the problem is associated with *favorable* rather than unfavorable personality changes (Baker, 1969).

There has also been concern from various quarters over the potential misuse of behavioral technology for purposes which are not in the best interests of the individual whose behavior is being modified. As pointed out by Yates (1970) the control of human behavior—whether deliberate or not—is a fact of daily life, and in this sense, behavioral technology involves nothing new. Indeed, the raison d'etre of any psychotherapeutic procedure, whether psychodynamic or behavioral in orientation, is the expectation that behavior will change in some manner (Brady, 1977). Increasing the power to control through scientific research and application, however, does raise the issue of who shall control and for what purpose (Rogers and Skinner, 1956; Ulrich, 1967).

In their broadest social context, these issues are not straightforward (Krasner, 1976). In the more restricted technical domain of behavioral medicine, however, some resolution is possible. First, the objective of any effective treatment method is prediction and control over the phenomenon of interest and, from that standpoint, there is little difference between the goals of behavioral medicine or those of surgery or other organic therapies. Second, it is important to distinguish between proper and improper applications. Thus, psychosurgery on involuntary subjects is a questionable activity if the goal is simply to produce a more docile or tractable patient. Moreover, despite the classification of such techniques as "behavioral" in the popular press, they are no more so than any approach which has the side effect of affecting behavior, whether it be surgery, a drug, or religion. *To qualify as a behavior modification therapy technique, a procedure should be based on the laws of conditioning and learning or on its methodology.*

While the problems concerning life-style modification to prevent disease on a societal basis are complicated, previous experience provides some useful guidelines (Lalonde, 1974). Legislation which attempts to ban smoking in public places has clear precedent in the prohibition of spitting in public as an attempt to control the spread of tuberculosis (Bass, 1976). In similar fashion, providing lower health insurance rates to the individual who is at decreased risk of cardiovascular disease or who undergoes risk factor modification, is not materially different than selling automobile insurance at lower cost to drivers who have had fewer accidents. Finally, the use of self-management methodology in the area of prevention alleviates many difficulties, in that the patient performs the treatment on himself or herself, using the therapist as an advisor and teacher.

Despite our evident enthusiasm over behavioral medicine, we do not want to minimize some of the problems the approach faces. While behavioral medicine follows the traditions of scientific medicine in emphasizing testable hypotheses as well as theory and practice based on empirical evidence, some of the implications of research in behavioral medicine may run counter to established procedures, such as, for example, modifying doctor-patient interactions to enhance compliance or changing the health care delivery system to increase efficiency—areas which have been notoriously resistant to change.

Some cautionary statements are in order, also. Schneiderman, Weiss, and Engel (1978) have urged great care in the extension of behavioral technology to serious medical problems:

> When behavioral techniques are used to treat aberrant behavior, contemporary theorists make no assumptions about underlying "diseases" which "cause" the atypical behavior (Yates,

1975). When one is dealing with medical problems where often a great deal is known about antecedent pathophysiological events, such a formulation is inappropriate. When one attempts to change behavior in a phobic patient, the explicit treatment goal is to change that behavior. However, if one is dealing with a patient who has a history of myocardial disease, the treatment goal is to modify the aberrrant response (sometimes within the heart itself) *to the extent possible within the limitations set by the pathology.*

The dictum, "primum, no nocere," applies as much to behavioral medicine as to general medicine.

A final consideration, as Agras (1975) has ably pointed out, is that in any new endeavor there is always the danger of "oversell." "Nothing is so promising as beginnings" goes an old saying. Behavioral medicine is no exception. By way of concluding, we wish to stress that a new treatment approach is only as valid as its supporting data show it to be and only as useful as its applications. To date, the most important contribution made by behavioral medicine is not its specific recommendations for treatment but its emphasis on the rigor of scientific methodology for dealing with problems in medical care which involve behavior.

References

ABELSON, P. H. Cost effective health care. *Science*, 1976, *192*, 619.

ADER, R., AND COHEN, N. Behaviorally conditioned immunosuppression. *Psychosom. Med.* 1975, *37*, 333–340.

AGRAS, S. Foreword. In R. C. Katz and S. Zlutnick (Eds.), *Behavior therapy and health care.* Elmsford, N.Y.: Pergamon Press, 1975.

ALDERMAN, M. H. Organization for long-term management of hypertension. *Bull. N.Y. Acad. Med.*, 1976, *52*, 697–717.

BANDURA, A. *Principles of behavior modification.* New York: Holt, Rinehart, and Winston, 1969.

BAKER, B. L. Symptom treatment and symptom substitution in eneuresis. *J Abnormal Psychol.*, 1969, *74*, 42–49.

BASS, F. A public-health approach to illness producing behavior, the example of tuberculosis control applied to cigarette smoking. In *Preventive medicine U.S.A.: Health promotion and consumer health education,* A task force report by the John E. Fogarty International Center for Advanced Study in the Health Sciences, National Institutes of Health, and the American College of Preventive Medicine. New York: Prodist, 1976.

BELLOC, N. B., AND BRESLOW, L. Relationship of physical health status and health practice. *Prev. Med.*, 1972, *1*, 409–421.

BERNI, R., AND FORDYCE, W. *Behavior modification and the nursing process.* St. Louis: C. V. Mosby, 1973.

BERNSTEIN, D. A. Modification of smoking behavior: An evaluative review. *Psychol. Bull.*, 1969, *71*, 418–440.

BRADY, J. P. Psychiatry as the behaviorist views it. In J. P. Brady, J. Mendels, M. T. Orne and W. Rieger (Eds.), *Psychiatry: Areas of promise and advancement.* New York: Spectrum Publications, 1977, pp. 89–102.

DIXON, R., AND LASZLO, J. Utilization of clinical chemistry services by medical housestaff. *Arch. Int. Med.*, 1974, *134*, 1064.

DUNBAR, J., AND STUNKARD, A. J. Adherence to diet and drug regimen. In R. Levey, B. Rifkind, B. Dennis and N. Ernst (Eds.), *Nutrition, lipids, and coronary heart disease.* New York: Raven Press, 1977.

EISENBERG, J. M., WILLIAMS, S., GARNER, L., VIALE, R., AND SMITS, H. Computer-based audit to detect and correct overutilization of laboratory tests. *Med. Care*, 1977, *15*, 915–921.

FARQUHAR, J. W., MACCOBY, N., WOOD, P., ALEXANDER, J., BREITROSE, H., BROWN, B., HASKELL, W., MCALISTER, A., MEYER, A., NASH, J., AND STERN, M. Community education for cardiovascular health. *Lancet*, 1977, *1*, 1192–1195.

FERSTER, C. B., NURNBERGER, J. I., AND LEVITT, E. E. The control of eating. *J. Mathetics*, 1962, *1*, 87–109.

FRIEDMAN, M. *Pathogenesis of coronary heart disease.* New York: McGraw-Hill, 1969.

GLINER, J. A., HORVATH, S. M., AND WOLPE, R. R. Operant conditioning of heart rate in curarized rats: Hemodynamic changes. *Am. J. Physiol.*, 1975, *228*, 870–874.

GRINER, P., AND LIPTZIN, B. Use of the laboratory in a teaching hospital: Implications for patient care, education, and hospital costs. *Ann. Int. Med.*, 1971, *75*, 157.

HAMMOND, E. C. The effects of smoking. *Sci. Am.*, 1962, *207*, 39–51.

HAUSER, D. J. Seat belts: Is freedom of choice worth 800 deaths a year? *Can. Med. Assoc. J.*, 1974, *110*, 1418–1426.

IWATA, B., BAILEY, J., BROWN, K., FOSHEE, T., AND ALPERN, M. A performance based battery to improve residential care and training by institutional staff. *J. Appl. Behav. Anal.*, 1976, *9*, 417–431.

JENKINS, C. D., ROSENMAN, R. H., AND ZYZANSKI, S. J. Cigarette smoking: Its relationship to coronary heart disease and related risk factors in the Western Collaborative Group Study. *Circulation*, 1968, *38*, 1140–1155.

KANNEL, W. B., CASTELLI, W. P., AND MCNAMARA, P. M. Cigarette smoking and risk of coronary heart disease: Epidemiologic clues to pathogenesis. *Nat. Cancer Inst. Monogr.*, 1968, *28*, 9–20.

KINSEY, A. C., POMEROY, W. B., AND MARTIN, C. E. *Sexual behavior in the male.* Philadelphia: W. B. Saunders, 1948.

KINSEY, A. C., POMEROY, W. B., AND MARTIN, C. E. *Sexual behavior in the female.* Philadelphia: W. B. Saunders, 1953.

KRASNER, L. Behavior modification: Ethical issues and future trends. In H. Leitenberg (Ed.), *Hand-*

book of behavior modification and behavior therapy. Englewood Cliffs, N.J.: Prentice-Hall, 1976.

KRISTEIN, M., ARNOLD, C., AND WYNDER, E. Health economics and preventive care. *Science*, 1977, *195*, 457–462.

LALONDE, M. *A new perspective on the health of Canadians*. Ottawa, Canada: Ministry of Health and Welfare, 1974.

LAPIDES, J., SWEET, R., AND LEWIS, L. Role of striated muscle in urination. *J. Urol.*, 1957, *77*, 247–250.

MACCOBY, N., FARQUHAR, J., WOOD, P., AND ALEXANDER, J. Reducing the risk of of cardiovascular disease: Effects of a community-based campaign on knowledge and behavior. *J. Community Health*, 1977, *3*, 100–114.

MAHONEY, M., AND THORESEN, C. *Self-control: Power to the person*. Monterey, Calif.: Brooks/Cole, 1974.

MASTERS, W., AND JOHNSON, V. *Human sexual response*. Boston: Little, Brown, and Company, 1966.

MATTHEWS, D., AND HINGSON, R. Improving patient compliance. In A. Reading and T. N. Wise (Eds.), *Psychiatry in internal medicine (Medical clinics of North America)*. Philadelphia: W. B. Saunders, 1977, pp. 879–889.

MECHANIC, D. *Research and analytic report, Series Number 14-74*. Madison, Wisc.: Health Economics Research Center, University of Wisconsin, 1974.

MEYER, A. J., AND HENDERSON, J. B. Multiple risk factor reduction in the prevention of cardiovascular disease. *Prev. Med.*, 1974, *3*, 225–236.

METROPOLITAN LIFE. Mortality among overweight men. *Stat. Bull. Metropol. Life Ins. Co.*, 1960, *41*, 6–10.

MILLER, N. E. Learning of visceral and glandular responses. *Science*, 1969, *163*, 434–445.

MINISTRY OF HEALTH AND WELFARE, CANADA, LONG RANGE HEALTH PLANNING PROGRAMS. *Hospital morbidity and total mortality in Canada: Data for priorities and goals*. Ottawa, Canada: Ministry of Health and Welfare, 1974.

MORRIS, J. N. *Uses of epidemiology*. London: E. and S. Livingstone, Ltd., 1957.

MORRIS, J. N., AND CRAWFORD, M. D. Coronary heart disease and physical activity of work: Evidence of a national necropsy survey. *Br. Med. J.*, 1958, *2*, 1485–1496.

NATIONAL CENTER FOR HEALTH STATISTICS. *Leading components of upturn in mortality for men in the United States*, Series 20, Number 11. Washington, D.C.: United States Government Printing Office, 1973.

PAFFENBARGER, R. S. Prevention of heart disease. *Postgrad. Med.*, 1972, *51*, 74–78.

PAVLOV, I. P. *Conditioned reflexes*. New York: Dover Publications, 1927.

PENICK, S. B., FILION, R., FOX, S., AND STUNKARD, A. J. Behavior modification in the treatment of obesity. *Psychosom. Med.*, 1971, *33*, 49–55.

POMERLEAU, O. F. On behaviorism in behavioral medicine (Editorial). *Behav. Med. Newsletter*, 1978, *1*(3), 2.

POMERLEAU, O. F. Why people smoke: Current psychobiological models. In P. Davidson (Ed.), *Behavioral medicine: Changing health life-styles*. New York: Brunner/Mazel, 1979.

POMERLEAU, O. F., ADKINS, D., AND PERTSCHUK, M. Predictors of outcome and recidivism in smoking-cessation treatment. *Addict. Behav.*, 1978, *3*, 65–70.

POMERLEAU, O. F., BASS, F., AND CROWN, V. The role of behavior modification in preventive medicine. *N. Engl. J. Med.*, 1975, *292*, 1277–1282.

POMERLEAU, O. F., BOBROVE, P., AND SMITH, R. Rewarding psychiatric aides for the behavioral improvement of assigned patients. *J. Appl. Behav. Anal.*, 1973, *6*, 383–390.

POMERLEAU, O. F., PERTSCHUK, M., ADKINS, D., AND BRADY, J. P. A comparison of behavioral and traditional treatment for middle-income problem drinkers. *J. Behav. Med.*, 1978, *1*, 187–200.

QUILITCH, H. R. A comparison of three staff-management procedures. *J. Appl. Behav. Anal.*, 1975, *8*, 59–66.

RACHLIN, H. *Introduction to modern behaviorism*. San Francisco: W. H. Freeman and Company, 1970.

RACHLIN, H., AND GREEN, L. Commitment, choice, and self-control. *J. Exp. Anal. Behav.*, 1972, *17*, 87–109.

RISLEY, T., AND BAER, D. Operant behavior modification: The deliberate development of behavior. In B. Caldwell and H. Ricciuti (Eds.), *Review of child development research* Vol. 3. Chicago: University of Chicago Press, 1973.

RODIN, J. Has the internal versus external distinction outlived its usefulness? In G. Bray (Ed.), *Advances in obesity research*, Vol. 2. London: Newman Press, 1978.

ROGERS, C. R., AND SKINNER, B. F. Some issues concerning the control of human behavior. *Science*, 1956, *124*, 1057–1066.

RUBIN, E., AND LIEBER, C. S. Fatty liver, alcoholic hepatitis and cirrhosis produced by alcohol in primates. *N. Engl. J. Med.*, 1974, *290*, 128–135.

SACKET, D. L., HAYNES, R. B., GIBSON, E. S., HACKETT, B. C., TAYLOR, D. W., ROBERTS, R. S., AND JOHNSON, A. L. Randomized clinical trial of strategies for improving medication compliance in primary hypertension. *Lancet*, 1975, *1*, 1205–1207.

SCHMIDT, W., AND DE LINT, J. Mortality experiences of male and female alcoholic patients. *Q. J. Stud. Alc.*, 1969, *30*, 112–118.

SCHNEIDERMAN, N., WEISS, T., AND ENGEL, B. Modification of Psychosomatic behaviors. *In* R. S. Davidson (Ed.), *Experimental analysis of clinical phenomena*. New York: Gardner Press, 1978.

SCHWARTZ, G., AND WEISS, S. What is behavioral medicine? *Psychosom. Med.*, 1977, *36*, 377–381.

SHAPIRO, D. A monologue on biofeedback and psychophysiology. *Psychophysiology*, 1977, *14*, 213–227.

SKINNER, B. F. *The behavior of organisms*. New York: Appleton-Century-Crofts, 1938.

SKINNER, B. F. *Science and human behavior*. New York: Macmillan, 1953.

STIMSON, G. V. Obeying doctor's orders: A view from the other side. *Soc. Sci. Med.*, 1974, *8*, 97–104.

STUART, R. B. Behavioral control of overeating. *Behav. Res. Ther.*, 1967, *5*, 357–365.

STUART, R. B., AND DAVIS, B. *Slim chance in a fat world: Behavioral control of obesity*. Champaign, Ill.: Research Press, 1971.

STUNKARD, A. J. New therapies for eating disorders. *Arch. Gen. Psychiatry*, 1972, *26*, 391–398.

STUNKARD, A. J. From explanation to action in psychosomatic medicine: the case of obesity. *Psychosom. Med.*, 1975, *37*, 195–236.

TAUB, E., AND EMURIAN, C. S. Feedback-aided self-regulation of skin temperature with a single feedback locus: I. Acquisition and reversal training. *Biofeedback Self-Regulation,* 1976, *1,* 146–168.

TERRACE, H. S. Stimulus control. In W. K. Honig (Ed.), *Operant behavior: Areas of research and application.* New York: Appleton-Century-Crofts, 1966, pp. 271–344.

THORNTON, E. W., AND VAN TOLLER, C. Effects of immunosympathectomy on operant heart rate conditioning in the curarized rat. *Physiol. Behav.,* 1973, *10,* 197–201.

TURNER, R., AND BALL, K. Prevention of coronary heart disease: A counter blast to present inactivity. *Lancet,* 1973, *2,* 1137–1140.

ULRICH, R. Behavior control and public concern. *Psychol. Rec.,* 1967, *17,* 229–234.

UNITED STATES DEPARTMENT OF HEALTH, EDUCATION, AND WELFARE. *Vital Statistics Report for 1972,* Volume 21, Number 13 (HSM 73-1121). Washington, D.C.: United States Government Printing Office, 1973.

UNITED STATES PUBLIC HEALTH SERVICE. *The Forward Plan for Health: FY 1978–82.* Washington, D.C.: United States Government Printing Office, 1976.

WALKER, A. R. P. Can expectation of life in western populations be increased by changes in diet and manner of life? *S. Afr. Med. J.,* 1968, *42,* 144–150.

WEINER, H. *Psychobiology and human disease.* New York: Elsevier, 1977.

WEIR, J. M., AND DUNN, J. E. Smoking and mortality: A prospective study. *Cancer,* 1970, *25,* 105–112.

WEISS, T. Biofeedback training for cardiovascular dysfunctions. In A. Reading and T. N. Wise (Eds.), *Psychiatry in internal medicine (Medical clinics of North America).* Philadelphia: W. B. Saunders, 1977, pp. 913–928.

WOLPE, J. *The practice of behavior therapy.* New York: Pergamon Press, 1969.

YATES, A. *Behavior therapy.* New York: Wiley, 1970.

YATES, A. *Theory and practice in behavior therapy.* New York: Wiley, 1975.

Basic Concepts

Behavioral Epidemiology

MARY MCDILL SEXTON, PH.D.

Associate Professor
Department of Epidemiology and Preventive Medicine
University of Maryland School of Medicine
Baltimore, Maryland

1

Behavior and Mortality

Epidemiology is the study of the etiology of disease and death in humans (Macmahon and Pugh, 1970). In this pursuit, studies have included components of clinical medicine, and more recently those of the health care delivery system and of social and personal behaviors. Evidence has accumulated that factors which are not entirely controlled by present and traditional medical technology have a major effect on the health status of the individual (White and Henderson, 1976).

More and more frequently, diseases have come to be linked to the life style of the individual. The way of life determines the way of death. William Farr, a physician in the late 1800's, may have had the seeds of this idea when he reported mortality statistics by characteristics, such as marital status and occupation (Humphreys, 1885). Perhaps these tabulations were meant to suggest that individuals known to vary in their manner of living would die for different reasons. His method of analysis of mortality data is generally regarded as the forerunner of epidemiological research (Lilienfeld, 1976) because his reports emphasized population data.

Figure 1.1 shows that the leading causes of death have changed in the last several decades. In 1900 infectious diseases, such as influenza, pneumonia, and tuberculosis, were the main causes of morbidity and mortality. Today an altogether different challenge faces the medical community—that of preventing and controlling chronic diseases. The nature of these diseases calls for an entirely new approach because their onset and progression are slow and insidious. By the time the individual experiences symptoms, the possibility of control has already diminished considerably. Attendant with the shift to chronic disease has been the increasing involvement of individual behavior in causing death and disease.

A review of present knowledge suggests a behavioral component associated with at least nine of the leading causes of death. Table 1.1 lists selected behaviors and cites some of the studies documenting the relationship between cause of death and particular patterns of behavior. The table is intended merely as an illustration of the extent to which behaviors have been related to causes of morbidity and mortality and should not be taken as an exhaustive list of either references or behaviors. As the table suggests, the interest in and study of the role of behavior in disease and death have increased. Consequently, a growing number of epidemiological studies focus on the relationship of behavior to health. Epidemiological evidence shows that the distribution of the above diseases in the population is not random. The level of risk of morbidity and mortality from these diseases is related to life style. As will be developed later, such evidence strongly suggests that the prevention and control of the major causes of death in the United States will involve

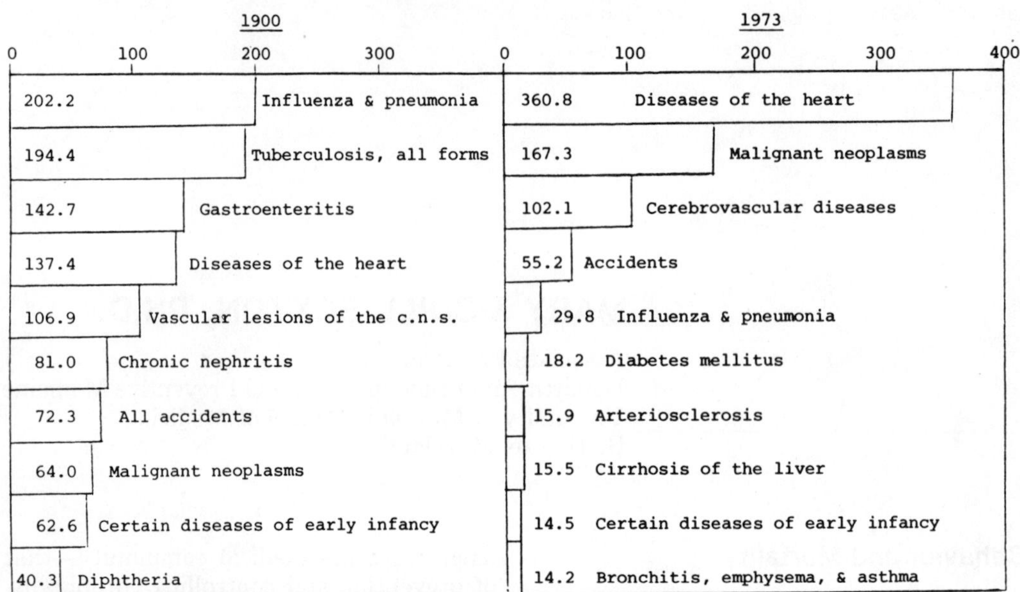

Figure 1.1. Death rates for the 10 leading causes of death per 100,000 population, United States, 1900 and 1973. (Compiled from data in the United States Bureau of the Census. *Statistical Abstract of the United States: 1958,* 79th ed. and *Statistical Abstract of the United States: 1975,* 96th ed. Washington, D.C.: United States Government Printing Office, 1975.)

management of the life style or personal behavior of the individual. Epidemiological studies of the etiology of these diseases have shown, for example, that smokers are at higher risk of coronary heart disease (CHD) as well as most cancers and stroke.

In the Report of Inter-Society Commission for Heart Disease Resources (1972), a large number of studies relevant to heart disease was reviewed: the conclusion was that cigarette smokers in the United States have a 70% increase in the risk of developing coronary heart disease. In the report, data from the National Cooperative Pooling Project were included. These are shown in Figure 1.2. Individuals who smoke a pack or more of cigarettes have a CHD death rate of 60 per 1000, a two-fold increase over lighter smokers (34/1000) and a three-fold increase over those who have never smoked (20/1000). Although the exact physiological mechanism by which cigarette smoking produces increased risk is not yet completely understood, studies are attempting to elucidate this process. Smokers, for example, are found to have an increased prevalence of raised lesions of the aorta based on autopsy findings (Friend, 1967). In the American Cancer Society study (Hammond and Garfinkel, 1969) of over one million men and women, death rates for cerebrovascular diseases were consistently higher for smokers than for nonsmokers. This was found for both men and women. As will be shown later, an association between cigarette smoking and cancer has been reported in a large number of studies (Health Consequences of Smoking—A Report of the Surgeon General, 1972). Thus, smoking has been implicated in each of the three leading causes of death. It is an obvious conclusion that abstinence from smoking would do a great deal to increase health status in this country.

Behavior of the individual is related to deaths from accidents, the fourth leading cause of death. Alcohol has been associated with accidental drownings (Dietz and Baker, 1974) and has been estimated to be related to more than one-third of adult male drownings (Plueckhahn, 1972; Giertsen, 1970). Even more evidence is available relating alcohol to traffic accidents (Hossack and Brown, 1974). At least half of the deaths from motor vehicle accidents involve excessive alcohol intake (Kaye, 1975;

Table 1.1
Behaviors Associated with Leading Causes of Death

Underlying Cause	Behaviors	References
Diseases of the heart	Eating excessive animal fats	Keys, 1970
	Smoking	Report of the Inter-Society Commission for Heart Disease Resources, 1972
	Inadequate physical activity	Paffenbarger, Hale, Brand, et al., 1977
	Excessive calorie consumption	Dawber, 1975
	Type A behavior	Rosenman, Brand, Jenkins, et al., 1975
Malignant neoplasms	Smoking	Armstrong and Doll, 1974
	Insufficient fiber in diet	Burkitt, Walker, and Painter, 1974
	Sexual habits	Gagnon, 1950
Cerebrovascular diseases	Smoking	Kannel, 1971
	Excessive dietary sodium	Freis, 1976
	Excessive calorie consumption	Chiang, Perlman, and Epstein, 1969
Accidents	Excessive alcohol consumption	Kaye, 1975
	Non-use of seat belts	Galasko and Edwards, 1975
Influenza and pneumonia	Smoking	Finklea, Sandifer, and Smith, 1969
Diabetes	Excessive caloric consumption	Bray, 1973
	Excessive dietary sugar	Moss and Mayer, 1977
Arteriosclerosis	Smoking	Auerbach, Hammond, and Garfinkel, 1965
Cirrhosis of the liver	Excessive alcohol intake	Terris, 1967
Bronchitis, emphysema, and asthma	Smoking	Mueller, Keble, Plummer, et al., 1971
	Stress reaction	McLean and Ching, 1973

Bako, MacKenzie, and Smith, 1977). One study showed that in two-thirds of motorcycle fatalities, a measurable amount of alcohol was found in the driver (Baker and Fisher, 1977). Alcohol has also been related to accidents involving cutting tools (Karaharju and Stjernvall, 1974).

A large percentage, approximately 73% (United States Department of Health, Education, and Welfare 1974), of total mortality is accounted for by the four leading causes of death. For each of these at least one behavioral factor has been implicated. Therefore, inroads into the prevention of these particular causes of death should make a major contribution to the protection of health and life.

The primary motivation for determining the etiology of disease is to prevent and control it. If research is limited to those individuals who have already developed the disease and who seek medical care, unanswered questions are left concerning the natural history and the prevention of the disease. Individuals seeking care may not be representative of all those with the disease, which again limits the knowledge about control. The one feature of epidemiological research which, more than any other, distinguishes it from clinical research has been the study of disease and death in *groups* of individuals (Mausner and Bahn, 1974). Usually, epidemiological investigations, concentrating on community-based studies, include individuals with a wider range of characteristics than the more traditional clinical research, which often studies a few individuals intensively. The methodology used allows the findings and their applicability to be described in a rigorous and precise way.

Behavioral science and medical science

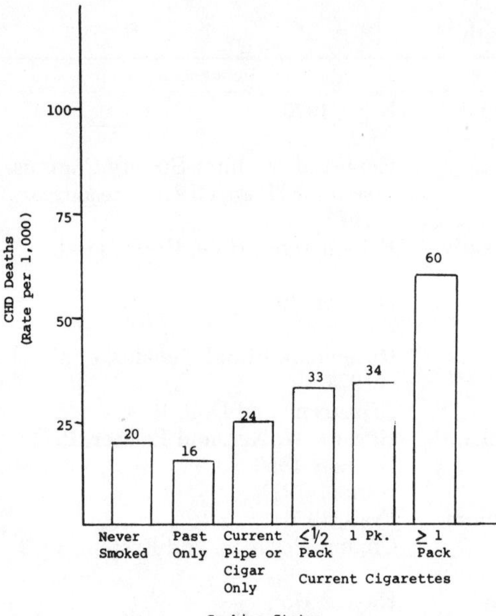

Figure 1.2. CHD death rate by smoking status among United States white males, ages 30–59. (Adapted from Figure 10, Report of Inter-Society Commission for Heart Disease Resources. Primary prevention of the atherosclerotic diseases. *Circulation*, 1972, *42*, 1–4.)

are two facets of biology with the same ultimate scientific aim of understanding human responses for the purpose of developing principles for application. The objective of each is to acquire knowledge necessary to change the natural course of a disease or disorder. To do so requires a clear understanding of the natural history of the disease and the possible points of intervention. This understanding becomes even more crucial when prevention is the goal of intervention. The epidemiological study concerned with the behavioral determinants of health status can be called behavioral epidemiology. The objectives of behavioral epidemiology are to (1) identify potential behavioral factors which influence health status, (2) formulate hypotheses, and (3) test hypotheses. These differ from other studies only in their relative emphasis on behavior; the overall methodology is the same. However, one point is worth noting here which will be discussed later. In order to test hypotheses concerning the relationship of one or more behaviors to health status, it is necessary to be able to change behavior. As the present volume indicates, this is now possible in several areas of behavior.

The Epidemiological Approach

Pickering (1949) pointed out that our understanding of natural phenomena arises from the complementary methods of observation and experimentation, a subdivision of method which is of central importance in the present discussion. In an experiment the investigator intervenes deliberately on the course of nature. It is characteristic of the scientific method that it begins with simple observation and continues through experimentation until a more complete explanation and understanding have been achieved and documented. Science in any field, however, proceeds in a less orderly way than might be supposed if looked at from afar. The discovery of the structure of DNA, for example, was told in a fascinating, personal way by Watson (1968) who recounted the errors in logic, the pursuits of unscientific paths, and the construction of ludicrous models preceding the breakthrough. How does one progress in epidemiological knowledge, from identifying something new in the field of health to using it to improve health status? If one is not unduly encumbered by reality, it is possible to approximate the steps of an orderly sequence through which most scientific studies proceed. Such an orderly sequence disregards foreshortening the procedure because of ingenuity or sheer luck in following one's curiosity; also, the genius is able to see short-cuts and to take advantage of rare, fortuitous events. Similarly, setbacks because of unanticipated difficulties may also occur. In these instances, the sequence may be disrupted or aborted. Epidemiological knowledge is acquired first from observation and second, if possible, from experiment.

OBSERVATIONS

Most epidemiological observations are from studies planned for the purpose of answering a question, but not always. Sometimes a chance, elemental observation is made. We refer to this as an unplanned observation.

UNPLANNED. An unplanned observation can be contrasted with a planned one in which the investigator knows the specific question he or she wishes to pose and plans the observation in such a way as to get the answer. An unplanned or chance observation is the one—if proven right—for which scientific recognition most often is given. The answer is given even before the question is posed. The discovery of penicillin by Fleming was one, among many, such chance observations that have contributed greatly to scientific knowledge. In epidemiology, these elemental observations are apt to be less dramatic but nevertheless should not be dismissed lightly. As Northrop has said "One cannot observe what exists when one is not observing" (1947, p. 41). Schneiderman (1977), for example, suggests four sources of ideas for epidemiological studies in cancer (although they apply as well to other fields): clinical observations, organized data reports, other epidemiological studies, and cross-discipline communications. Some of these sources consist of data reports produced routinely for administrative purposes and not produced by the scientist for his or her own use. The data reports may be the basis of a "chance observation" analogous to an unplanned finding in the laboratory. A clustering of disease among family members, among groups of workers, among residents of a particular location, or among those with some other common characteristics might be noticed and insight into the etiology of disease gained. Since no morality is attached to how discoveries are made, the investigator needs to be concerned only with an appropriate analysis and interpretation of his or her observation.

The first step in acquiring knowledge, regardless of the source, is to notice an existing thing in a new way: the recognition of heterogeneity, for example—that one is observing two diseases, not what was previously thought to be one. The observation could be of non-randomness—the idea that a second factor heretofore unnoticed is related to a particular disease. The practicing physician is pivotal in noting new characteristics and linking factors, for he or she observes disease and death with the least interference and distortion. It remains a mystery as to how one "sees" that two factors, previously thought to be unrelated, are occurring together. Sometimes it is done in a more pedestrian way than other times. However, one dramatic example is the clinical observation of a relationship between cancer of the vagina among young women whose mothers had taken diethylstilbestrol during pregnancy.

Between 1966 and 1969, seven cases of adenocarcinoma of the vagina were seen at the Gynecological Service of the Massachusetts General Hospital. A particularly striking feature was the age of the women; all were younger than 22 years. Adenocarcinoma of the vagina previously had been observed only in women at least 30 and mostly in much older women (Herbst, Ulfelder, and Poskanzer, 1971). As one author related, the possibility of a systematic phenomenon was discussed on an elevator. A study with two purposes was planned: (1) to document at other hospitals the incidence of cancer of the vagina among young women and (2) to identify factors which might account for an increased incidence, if found (Poskanzer and Herbst, 1977). The study showed that mothers of these young women were more likely to have had diethylstilbestrol prescribed for threatened miscarriage during their pregnancy than mothers with similar demographic characteristics who delivered at the same hospital during the same time period. Even though diethylstilbestrol therapy had already been discontinued and the number of potential cases was small, the seriousness of the disease made a follow-up of potential cases essential (Herbst, Cole, Colton, et al., 1977). The initial study illustrates several points. The first and foremost is the astuteness of the clinical observation; with a very small number of cases, an unusual occurrence was recognized. Second, the potential etiological factor of diethylstilbestrol was identified despite a long latent period of 15 to 20 years between exposure during pregnancy and manifestation of disease. The small numbers and the latent period together make it quite remarkable that such a linkage was made. Further, the findings were of particular significance because of the new observation of transplacental carcinogenesis.

PLANNED. Most epidemiological knowledge comes from observational studies which have been planned and systematically conducted. However, the investigator may plan a combination of current, future, or even past data, some of which were not personally recorded. The most common distinction of these types of studies is between retrospective and prospective ones.

Retrospective Studies. Once a disease

and a suspected characteristic are linked hypothetically, the epidemiological investigator seeks to document this relationship, or having observed it in a restricted way, he or she may wish to extend the observation to a broader range. This was precisely what occurred in the example just given of vaginal cancer among young females; the experience of a large number of hospitals and physicians was sought. Frequently, the confirmation of an idea will begin with a retrospective study. A retrospective study is one in which people with a disease—the cases—are compared with those without that particular disease—the controls—to determine whether they differ on some suspected factor which occurred prior to, and therefore may account for, the disease. The data on the suspected factor are obtained from past records or recall by the individual or someone else. The purpose is to show, for one of the groups, a higher rate of exposure to the factor, thereby implicating the factor in the etiology of the disease. Because there are a multitude of ways in which the results from retrospective studies can be misleading (Hill, 1977), the process is usually a slow accumulation of evidence from many studies. Retrospective studies require relatively small numbers of subjects; if the disease is a rare one, as with the previous example of adenocarcinoma of the vagina, this is an important advantage. Furthermore, they are among the least expensive to conduct and yield results within a relatively short period of study since the disease has already occurred. In some instances, they are the only type of study which can be reasonably considered. With an idea that is somewhat tentative, retrospective study is a good way to begin. The main weakness of a retrospective study is that the investigator cannot guarantee that all bias has been removed and hence that the conclusions are valid. Ideally the controls would have all factors in common with the cases except the suspected etiological variable. This can never be achieved in reality and the investigator can never determine how close he or she is to the ideal condition, despite trying to assure that the controls and cases are similar on all important factors known to influence the outcome.

The earliest studies which established smoking as an etiological factor in lung cancer were retrospective ones. Wynder and Graham (1950) were among the first to report such a study. It was a carefully constructed investigation in which the problem of differential reporting was addressed within the study. The authors reasoned that there might be different recall of smoking history among those with and those without lung cancer, or that a history of smoking might be sought with more vigor and care from patients with lung cancer than from others; either possibility could make the reported smoking status different, even if the actual (real) status did not differ. In the study of Wynder and Graham, a nonmedical interviewer without knowledge of the disease interviewed the cases of lung cancer and the controls, as a lack of reliability in the smoking history would make any finding of a relationship between smoking and lung cancer questionable. First, 100 cancer patients and 186 patients with diseases of the chest other than lung cancer were interviewed and the data were used to detect interviewer bias. Second, 83 male patients with cancer of the lungs in other cities were interviewed independently by physicians. Both of these activities should detect a bias which would render the smoking data unreliable; none was found. Smoking habits were then obtained from 780 general hospital patients for comparison with the 684 cases of proven bronchiogenic cancer. The data reported in this comparison are shown in Figure 1.3. As can be seen, there is an excess of very heavy smokers among the lung cancer patients. Because of the care taken to obtain unbiased measurements of smoking and lung cancer, this study illustrates how confidence in the findings from retrospective studies can be increased by an awareness of possible sources of bias.

One of the authors designed a second retrospective study to document the relationship between lung cancer and smoking among physicians, a group easy to follow-up. Using death notices in the *Journal of the American Medical Association,* Wynder and Cornfield (1953) sent letters to the last known address of the physician, requesting information from the next of kin. The response rate was about 60%. Identification of death from lung cancer or some

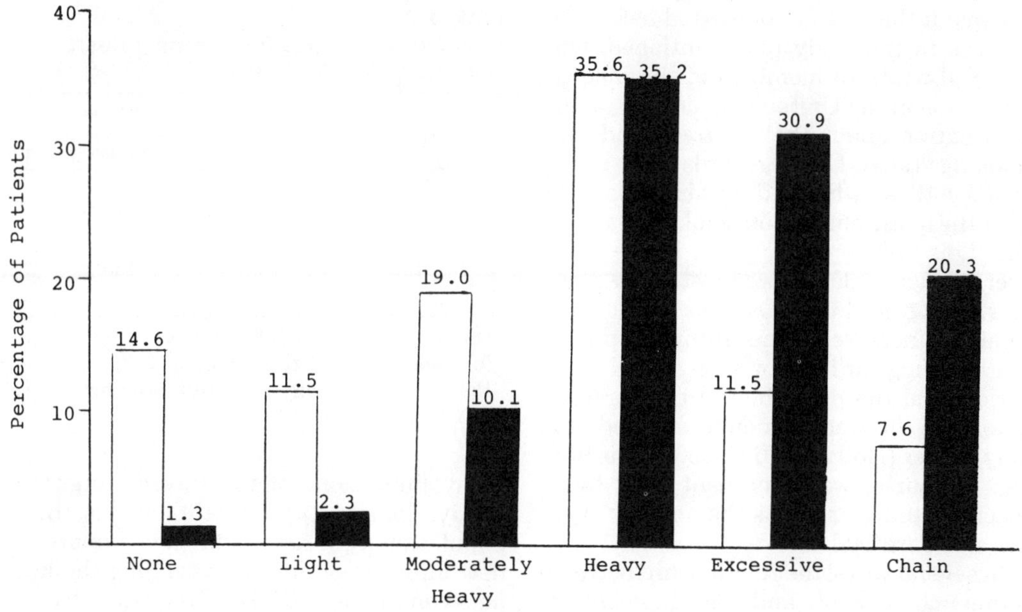

Figure 1.3. Percentages for amount of smoking among 605 male patients with cancer of the lungs (black bars) and 780 men in the general hospital population without cancer (white bars) with the same age and economic distribution. (Reprinted by permission from Wynder, E. L., and Graham, E. A., Tobacco smoking as a possible etiologic factor in bronchiogenic carcinoma. *J.A.M.A.*, 1950, *143*, 329–336. Copyright 1950, American Medical Association.)

other type of cancer was obtained from the death certificate. Even with far from ideal data, a relationship between lung cancer and smoking was found. Without their consistency with a substantial number of retrospective studies, the findings from the physician study could have been easily dismissed. It could have been argued convincingly that the incompleteness of responses made the findings impossible to interpret. There remain a few scientific purists who deny intellectually the proof of a causal link and more than a few smokers who deny emotionally a causal link between smoking and lung cancer, despite a preponderance of evidence from thousands of studies which have consistently shown smoking to be a health risk (National Clearinghouse for Smoking and Health, 1977).

Prospective Studies. The nature and purpose of prospective studies can be well illustrated by pursuing the example of smoking and lung cancer studies. The controversy concerning smoking and disease was a very intense one (Berkson, 1958). Doll and Hill (1954) designed a prospective study to determine the relationship between mortality and smoking among physicians. They summarized the reason for their design, and since it applies to many prospective studies, it is worth quoting:

> Further retrospective studies of that same kind would seem to us unlikely to advance our knowledge materially or to throw any new light upon the nature of the association. If, too, there were any undetected flaw in the evidence that such studies have produced, it would be exposed only to some entirely new approach. That approach we considered should be "prospective." It should determine the frequency with which the disease appeared, in the future, among groups of persons whose smoking habits were already known (p. 1451).

A prospective study is one in which data are obtained on a factor suspected of being related to a disease. The investigator then follows his cohort over time to see how many develop the disease. With these data, a relationship between the factor and the disease is determined. The main advantage of a prospective study compared to a retrospective one is that the investigator can document that the factor existed before the disease. In the study just mentioned, Doll and Hill wrote to members of the medical profession in the United Kingdom to obtain information about their current and past smoking status. Death records were examined for those who died within 29 months after the questionnaire on smoking was sent out. This first report for men in the study over the age of 35, showed a steadily rising mortality from lung cancer as the level of smoking increased. The authors updated these findings in 1956 for a longer follow-up period, and the data showed the same relationship between amount smoked and lung cancer (Doll and Hill, 1956). This finding, of course, was congruent with retrospective studies, such as the ones by Wynder and Cornfield.

In several ways, the relationship between serum cholesterol and development of CHD parallels that of smoking and disease. One prospective study in this area will be cited because it is an international, collaborative one. Investigators from several countries cooperated to provide standard information about coronary heart disease in the Seven Countries Study (Keys, 1970). The effort necessary for a collaborative study is of a completely different magnitude from that for a study with one or two investigators. By the mid-1950's, the prevalence of mortality from CHD in the United States had risen over several decades; some individuals saw it as epidemic, analogous to earlier infectious disease epidemics.

For example, the 1964 incidence rates tabulated in the Report of Inter-Society Commission (1972) are similar to those seen in the past (Table 1.2). It was known that the styles of life were different among countries with varying rates of CHD; this was especially true of the diet because of cultural practices, food preferences, and availability of certain foods. As in all countries, individuals in the United States were relatively homogeneous in their diet. With care in the selection of several countries, a greater range of dietary intake could be obtained than would be possible with the selection and study of any one country. Furthermore, a prospective study would determine whether the risk factor of diet was antecedent to the disease; this could not be done in a retrospective study. Recognizing many limitations of the Seven Countries Study, the investigators still felt that these population cohorts would give important new information in understanding the link between diet and CHD. They explicitly realized, for example, that multiple factors were related to CHD and took many of these into account.

Table 1.2
1964 Mortality Rates for Coronary Heart Disease, Males, Ages 45–54

Country	CHD Rates per 100,000 Population
Finland	442
U.S.A.*	354*
Netherlands	162
Italy	133
Japan	51

(Source: Report of Inter-Society Commission for Heart Disease Resources, 1972, p. 3).
* For white males only, mortality rates are: CHD = 355.

Some preliminary work was necessary to determine the feasibility of a collaborative approach. Participation of countries, and of individual men within them, proved to be quite high. Any differences among those who enrolled and those who did not would be minimized because such a large proportion of the men volunteered for the study. Thus, a long-range study of 5 to 10 years appeared to be quite reasonable and the International Cooperative Study on Cardiovascular Epidemiology was started, with Japan, Greece, Yugoslavia, Italy, Netherlands, United States, and Finland participating (Keys, 1970). Extensive effort was made to standardize study procedures, such as ECG recordings, assessments of diet, medical histories, and physical examinations.

At the end of 5 years, a remarkably high follow-up of over 95% of those alive was obtained. The data from the 5-year follow-up show that dietary intake of saturated fats and of cholesterol is related to the incidence of CHD. These data are shown in Figures 1.4 and 1.5. A positive relationship between serum cholesterol and CHD was found. In this prospective study, elevation of cholesterol before the onset of CHD was documented in a group of heterogeneous countries. One could be confident that the disease itself did not cause the elevation in cholesterol. The study provided further evidence that dietary factors should be pursued for an understanding of CHD incidence.

With neither a retrospective study nor a prospective study can the investigator rule out the possibility that a third factor is the key to the etiology of the disease. It is always possible that a third factor, perhaps known, has led to both the disease and the second factor. This was argued for a long time concerning cigarette smoking and lung cancer. Some people choose to smoke, while others do not. In that sense, cigarette smoking as a causal factor has not been established definitively. Similarly, there could be a genetic factor, for example, accounting for both elevated serum cholesterol and coronary heart disease. As will be discussed below, evidence from an experiment is the most convincing way in ruling out the possibility of unknown, competing etiological factors.

It should be pointed out that prospective studies also allow the natural history of the disease to be observed. Often, studies combine the objectives of identifying risk factors that relate to one or more diseases with those of observing onset, progression, and death from disease. The Framingham Study (Dawber, Meadors, and Moore, 1951) is one in which these objectives were combined. Data on factors suspected of increasing risk of CHD as well as data on the onset and progression of CHD were collected. It was possible to obtain distributions of cholesterol, blood pressure, and smoking for males and females, for example, and to relate these to the occurrence of heart disease and death at subsequent follow-ups. Furthermore, natural changes in risk factors like smoking or weight could be documented. Prospective studies provide data from which hypotheses can be sharpened so that an experiment is feasible.

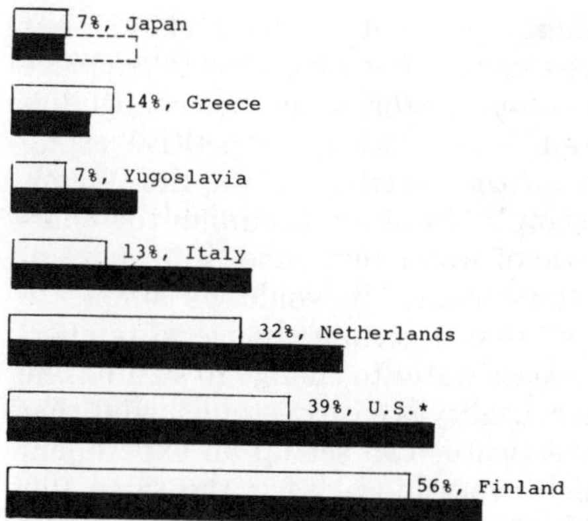

Solid black bars show CHD incidence rate. (Age-standardized average yearly CHD incidence rates per 10,000 of 12,529 men aged 40-59, judged to be free of CHD at the outset, followed for five years. Non-fatal CHD incidence in Japan is not precisely indicated because the relevant 5-year clinical and ECG records were not independently reviewed at the University of Minnesota center. CHD is equal to death, infarct, angina, or specific clinical and ECG criteria.

*Cohort of Railroad men.

Figure 1.4. Percentage of men with serum cholesterol values over 250 mg/dl. (Reprinted from Keys, A. (Ed.). *Coronary heart disease in seven countries,* American Heart Association Monograph Number 29. New York: American Heart Association, 1970, p. 51, by permission of the American Heart Association, Inc.)

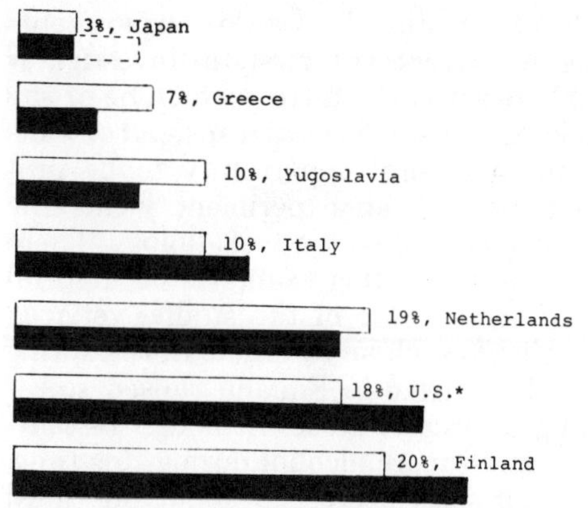

Solid black bars show CHD incidence rate. (Age-standardized average yearly CHD incidence rates per 10,000 of 12,529 men aged 40-59, judged to be free of CHD at the outset, followed for five years. Non-fatal CHD incidence in Japan is not precisely indicated because the relevant 5-year clinical and ECG records were not independently reviewed at the University of Minnesota center. CHD is equal to death, infarct, angina, or specific clinical and ECG criteria.

*Cohort of Railroad men.

Figure 1.5. Average percentage of total dietary calories provided by saturated fatty acids. (Reprinted from Keys, A. (Ed.). *Coronary heart disease in seven countries,* American Heart Association Monograph Number 29. New York: American Heart Association, 1970, p. 51, by permission of the American Heart Association, Inc.)

EXPERIMENTS

The experiment, according to Cochran (1955), is a study in which the investigator plans to *interfere* with nature. Compared with observational studies, experiments have two advantages. First, the investigator is able to select the factors which he or she thinks are most informative instead of waiting for a natural opportunity to be provided. Second, an experiment yields the most convincing evidence of etiology. There are some interesting examples of "natural experiments." One of the studies referred to earlier is such an example. In the spring of 1972, a strike in Finland caused stores selling alcohol to close. Although restaurants served more alcohol during this time, the total sales decreased about one-third during the 6-week strike. Karaharju and Stjernvall (1974) took advantage of this phenomenon to compare accidents requiring hospital admission during the strike period with those during an earlier period. The decrease in accidents during these two periods was quite reasonably assumed to be related to lowered consumption of alcohol.

Most experiments are planned after evidence from observational studies suggests that one mode of treatment may be more beneficial than a second. As Cochran (1955) indicates, the question of experimental research should always be raised. In far too many instances, the possibility of an answer obtained by an experiment is ruled out without full exploration. Some investigations seem to experience discomfort with hypothesis testing with human subjects. Except for those instances in which no differences in efficacy among the competing treatments are found, one treatment will be found more beneficial than others, a fact that is known before the experiment begins. During the course of testing hypotheses then, it is almost inevitable that some individuals in the study will be subjected to a greater risk than others even though it is not evident who they are at the beginning; the study is trying to determine that. This problem is seen most clearly in considering the effectiveness of a drug compared with a placebo: the drug may be beneficial or it may be harmful. If a strong *opinion* regarding the outcome is widespread, then the concern about ethics may preclude the research. If the study is to be done then, the thought that there will almost certainly be an inequity of benefit is not easily put aside. Restricting the study to participants with certain characteristics, such as those whose diastolic blood pressure is below 120 mm Hg, etc., may sometimes make an experiment more acceptable ethically.

Are two factors merely co-existing or are they interrelated? The answer is an all important one in modifying the natural course of a disease. In order to intervene, a risk factor must be modifiable; this is not always the case in health. A host of factors are eliminated from experimentation because they cannot be modified. Such is currently the case with genetic factors, although they may sometimes be offset by therapy. Some demographic factors such as age, sex, and race cannot be changed. As we increase our knowledge, unmodifiable factors may yield to information about modifiable ones.

Experiments establish etiological links between factors. When variation in one factor is related to variation in another, an association exists. As Susser (1973) notes, epidemiologists are interested in distinguishing causal and noncausal relationships. If variation occurs in a factor only when variation occurs in a second factor, then the two are presumed to be causally linked—variation in the first is dependent on variation in the second. The difficulty is in making sure that no other change has occurred except that which has taken place in the second factor; if another change has occurred, it becomes a competitive explanation for the variation in the first factor. For example, variation occurs in the characteristic of water (outcome) if heat is applied (treatment). It would be simple to establish that a certain change in temperature causes water to change to steam. The reason causality is easily established is that the investigator can set up an experiment in which everything else is the same (for example, the hardness of the water, the equipment, the time of day, as well as any other thing which might vary)—all other things are equal—except the application of heat.

Obviously, one way to achieve an answer about causality is to assure that no changes occur during the experiment except those of the treatment itself. This is difficult, but not always impossible, in human experiments. It is difficult because the treatment itself usually introduces differences. Take, for example, the study of a very simple question about drug compliance by number of doses. Specifically, you want to know whether there is greater compliance if one tablet a day is prescribed compared with two tablets a day. Assume that the tablet is made of inert ingredients with no side effects and that you are able to obtain an accurate count of the tablets consumed. If the experiment is set up so that the individual takes one tablet for 6 months and then two tablets for 6 additional months, any difference in compliance could be attributed to a difference in adhering to the regimen (or other learning variable—whether good or bad) which occurred, rather than a difference in the number of tablets taken. While there are several ways an experiment can be devised to answer this particular question (Barlow, Hersen, and Jackson, 1973), the problem illustrates the point: assuring that nothing has changed presents special difficulties in human research. Noncomparability in two phases of an experiment (presence and absence of treatment or two levels of treatments) almost always precludes such an approach with humans. Occasionally, it is possible to have a within-subject control and equalize "all other things" in the two phases. Thus, in short-term drug trials, it is sometimes reasonable to assume that a first drug has no influence on the effect of the second drug. There are times when this is an acceptable assumption. At other times, a more sophisticated experimental cross-over design may solve the problem. Usually, the approach is applicable in short-term trials in which there is little opportunity to introduce other factors.

The person has served as his or her own control in at least one long-term study. In the Diabetic Retinopathy Study (1976), patients were randomly allocated to treatment with either argon or xenon arc laser. Only one eye was treated while the other remained untreated (selected by random) and served as the control eye. The study is an unusual one in that it is seldom possible for a person to be his or her own control in epidemiological studies. In studies in which mortality is the outcome variable, no such possibility exists.

In experiments, such as the above, it is necessary to keep all experimental parameters, except the one under study, constant. In human experiments, accomplishing this is a challenge. Fisher's (1960) method of random allocation in which each individual in the experiment has an equal chance of being in any one of the experimental groups has not been improved upon. Random allocation to groups remains the dictum of experiments designed to demonstrate a relationship between factors such that when one is changed the other changes.

Clinical trials are experiments which usually involve large numbers of randomized individuals observed over a long period of time. These randomized clinical trials are becoming a specialized experimental discipline which usually requires several investigators working in a collaborative effort to answer a question which would be impossible for one investigator alone to answer. The primary reason for a collaborative effort is that the number of study subjects required makes assessment by any one investigator or accumulation in any one geographical location difficult. The approach has the advantage of making the results applicable to individuals over a wider geographical base. Several of the studies already mentioned used this method. A recent article (Byar, 1977) has synthesized a large amount of literature to point out some of the methodological issues in clinical trials. For many scientific questions involving mortality, the collaborative clinical trial is the only type of experiment which has the potential to provide a definitive answer, because of the large sample size needed.

Regardless of the size and outcome of a clinical trial, many unanswered questions will still remain, such as the generalizability of the results—just as in smaller studies. For example, the Veterans Administration Cooperative Studies (1967, 1970) showed that treatment of hypertension in male veterans lowered cerebrovascular morbidity. The question remained as to whether this benefit could be shown for men and women, as well, in a community setting. The Hypertension Detection and Follow-up Program (HDFP) (1976) was designed to answer this question. The study is a randomized clinical trial in which one group is treated by a standardized, stepped-care drug protocol and the other group is referred for treatment in the community. The referred group may receive treatment varying from very poor to excellent. The efficacy of lower morbidity and mortality will be determined for a special, standard protocol of treatment specified in advance versus treatment in the community. In this case, accurate documentation of the community treatment is not feasible. Thus, it has become more common, as in the HDFP, to compare "usual" treatment versus "special" treatment. Such comparisons make many randomized experiments possible which otherwise could not be carried out.

The results from one additional clinical trial will be reviewed here, both because of its relevance to determination of effective lipid-lowering intervention and because it raised a somewhat different question from the studies cited above. In the Coronary Drug Project (1975), it was found that clofibrate, a lipid-lowering drug, gave no additional protection from subsequent myocardial infarctions. Because all individuals had had at least one myocardial infarction before entering the trial, the study did not answer the question of whether cholesterol-lowering by drug is beneficial to individuals who have never had a myocardial infarction, that is, would clofibrate be beneficial for primary prevention of coronary heart disease?

This section would be incomplete without returning to the primary task faced in behavioral epidemiology—accurate interpretation of empirical evidence. Only a small proportion of medical research is experimental epidemiology and an even smaller proportion of research concerned with behavior and health status is experimental. One exception to this is Donovan's clinical trial (1977) in which pregnant smokers were randomized to a smoking cessation-treatment group or a control group and the birthweight of their infants was compared. Some of the details of this study will be discussed later.

Without experimental evidence, inferences drawn from data about causal relationships are much more susceptible to error. The decision as to whether the observed relationship is causal or not is a crucial one because of the conclusions which follow. If the relationship is causal, then intervention can be planned to disrupt the natural course of events. Since interpretation and inferences are central to epidemiological inquiry, many attempts have been made to develop guidelines for deciding whether causation exists when the design of the study permits the establishment of association only. As Hill (1977) states, "This interpretation of statistical data turns, it should be seen, not so much on technical methods of analysis but on the application of common sense to figures and on elementary rules of logic" (p. 294). The seven criteria he proposes are outlined below. For simplicity in the discussion, the relationship assumed is that of a possible causal factor for disease.

Strength of the Association. The suggestion of causality is proportional to the observed difference: that is, the larger the observed difference in the comparative groups, the stronger the suggestion. (The comparison may refer to the proportion of subjects with the potential causal factor among those subjects with and without the disease, or the comparison may be between the proportion with the disease among those subjects with and without the potential causal factor.)

Consistency. The larger the number of studies with diverse populations and with different research designs that have the same result, the more the evidence suggests causality. (This is analogous to replicability in experimental research.)

Specificity. The more one factor is related to one and only one disease, the more confidence one has in the possibility of a causal relationship.

Time Relationship. The probability of a causal relationship is increased if it is known that the factor preceded the disease.

Biological Gradient. The observation that the higher the level of exposure to the factor, the more intense the resulting disease, strengthens the suggestion of causality. This is often referred to as a dose-response phenomenon.

Biological Plausibility. A causal relationship should be considered a more reasonable possibility if it is compatible with current biological knowledge.

Coherence. A causal relationship should be reconcilable with other facts bearing on the factor and on the disease.

Regardless of how carefully the investigator guards against an error in the interpretation of the data, there is no way to provide complete protection. Because of these difficulties, Hill (1971) has been a strong advocate for the use of experiments in medicine. He describes them as "the strongest weapon in the scientist's armoury" (p. 47). The investigator should not be misled into thinking that the weaknesses inherent in a nonexperimental approach can be overcome even by applying the well-developed criteria outlined above. One way to strengthen the possibility of a correct inference from research in behavioral epidemiology, however, is to be aware of some of the fundamental issues in such studies.

Issues in Behavioral Epidemiology

In research on behavior and health, concerns about methodology and interpretation of findings are much the same as those confronted in other types of epidemiological studies. Some of these concerns were discussed in the preceding section. However, the study of behavior complicates some issues and creates additional problems. For example, in comparison with drug treatment, behavioral treatment or intervention is much more elusive and difficult to specify precisely. One of the primary reasons is that most behavioral programs consist of a dynamic, interactional process in which both the participant and the therapist and their relationship influence the effectiveness of the treatment program. The total process is hard to capture with precision. Even more easily described characteristics which may affect treatment results have not always been reported. A current survey of the literature reveals only sketchy descriptions of the exact behavioral technique utilized, the length of the treatment program, the types of treatment personnel, and the demography of the study population—any one of which may be an important factor in determining the efficacy of the intervention itself. Describing treatment or intervention becomes important in research efforts, both because of the scientific need for critical evaluation and interpretation of reported results and because of the practical need for knowledge so that the outcome can be reproduced for clinical purposes.

In behavioral epidemiology, several points are crucial if other investigators are to make an informed assessment of the research findings. This can be illustrated by a hypothetical behavioral study of the relationship between smoking and lung cancer. To present the issues as simply as possible, we will take as our example an experiment with random allocation to two study groups, one of which receives a smoking-cessation treatment and the other of which receives no intervention. Even with such an uncomplicated design, there are several points about which information would be needed to interpret the results. Table 1.3 outlines several dimensions which will help focus the discussion: the interval of time involved in certain phases, the main factors included, and the characterization of these factors in the comparative groups. Regardless of the outcome of such a study, the results might not be the same with different kinds of smokers. Amount of smoking is related both to success in quitting and to incidence of lung cancer. What kind of smokers were included in the study? Did randomization balance the number of heavy smokers with a lengthy history of smoking in the two groups? These are two very reasonable questions. To answer them and others which are equally reasonable, we would need an accurate measurement of smoking at several phases of the study. As we shall show below in a discussion of the

Table 1.3
Hypothetical Example of Study

Time Interval	Study Factors	Comparative Groups: Group A (treatment)	Comparative Groups: Group B (no treatment)
1	Behavioral factor 1	Smoking	Smoking
2	Treatment intervention	Hypnosis	None
3	Behavioral factor 1′	Reduction in smoking	Reduction in smoking
4	Morbidity or mortality outcome	Reduction in lung cancer	Reduction in lung cancer

Donovan study, some measurements might not be reliable enough to answer these questions. Regardless of the proportion of non-smokers found in the two groups when smoking is measured after the treatment phase, the actual number of former smokers classified as not smoking might be due to the type of treatment program or might be simply because of a bias in measuring smoking behavior.

To arrive at a reasonable conclusion about the efficacy of the treatment program, some additional details would also be needed. If the smoking-cessation treatment consisted of hypnosis, as assumed in the example, one might ask about the number of sessions conducted and over what period of time and by whom. When and how was smoking behavior determined after the treatment? Would most of the recidivism among the ex-smokers have occurred by that time, so that the proportion of non-smokers could be expected to remain stable? Finally, how was lung cancer determined and for what period of time in follow-up?

With but a few exceptions, such as use of seat belts, behavioral change must be sustained over a long period of time to influence morbidity and mortality. The column, "time interval" was added in the example to emphasize this point as well as others in which temporal factors play a paramount role in interpretation, such as lag time before health benefits can be expected. In order to demonstrate a link between the change and reduction, behavior has to be measured in such a way that change can be documented, a point to which we will return below. It can be seen from this simple example that some very difficult issues arise in behavioral epidemiology. Some of the general issues that are particularly important will be discussed further.

MEASUREMENT OF BEHAVIOR

As Blalock and Blalock note (1968), for scientific knowledge to be useful, it must say something about the nature and importance of a particular variable in relation to one or more others and must verify these statements by empirical findings. As we have seen, empirical verification may be accomplished by a number of approaches but specification of the nature and a measurement of the factors under study is always called for.

The behavior should be specified so that there is no ambiguity about what is being measured, and the measurement should be valid and replicable. These common sense goals have proven to be difficult in some cases. Many measurements of behavior involve self-reports in one way or another. This has been especially true of behaviors associated with chronic disease. Social and behavioral scientists have long been aware that individuals may give inaccurate information sometimes—even the well-intentioned who merely do so to please the investigator. This phenomenon has plagued researchers attempting to measure behaviors such as smoking or food intake by self-reports.

As reviewed earlier, Wynder and Graham (1950) went to considerable effort to rule out bias in the reporting of cigarettes smoked. Smoking history was taken from the respondent at one point, which was sufficient for the documentation needed in that study. Quite a different situation emerged in a study referred to earlier. Donovan (1977) presented evidence of discrepant reporting by the same respondent, with respect to number of cigarettes smoked and age at which smoking started: when pregnant women in his study were asked the same questions, both at entry into the trial (sometime before the 30th week of gestation) and postnatally, their responses differed. Some 18% had a discrepancy of 2 years or more in their answers as to how old they were when they began to smoke. A similar percentage of those previously stating that they had stopped early in their pregnancy claimed to have stopped before pregnancy when they were asked the same questions postnatally.

A more serious problem in the above study is that the postnatal answer of the treatment group (which received smoking-cessation advice) indicated a higher number of cigarettes in early pregnancy than the first answer; whereas, in the control group, the postnatal answer was a lower number of cigarettes than the first answer. In order to overcome some of the problems experienced in the Donovan study, a more objective measure of behavior should be obtained. It is possible to measure cigarette smoking by biochemical measures of expired carbon monoxide (Vogt, Selvin, Widdowson, et al., 1977), carboxyhemoglobin (Longo, 1977), serum, urinary, or salivary thiocyanate (Barylko-Pikielna and Pangborn, 1968), or cotinine (Zeidenberg, Jaffe, Kanzler, et al., 1977). As a practical matter, however, these measures cannot be used in all situations. As discussed in the preceding references, these are measures of immediate behavior and thus, only under the condition that the consistent behavior is the same as the immediate one, is a valid measure of sustained behavior obtained. If the participant changes his or her behavior around the time of the measurement, then problems similar to those of self-reporting are encountered.

In summary, for research purposes, it is often possible to detect group differences, even though the current methods of behavioral measurement have weaknesses. Special care should be given to assuring that a systematic bias does not exist in self-reporting among the different groups; as we have noted, such problems can occur in intervention studies as well as in observational studies. When possible, self-report should be substantiated by more objective measures, for such a procedure greatly increases the validity of the conclusions.

CHANGE IN BEHAVIOR

In behavioral epidemiology, the ultimate goal is to produce scientifically sound evidence that a change in behavior produces a change in morbidity or mortality. To provide that evidence, a change in behavior large enough to produce a change in health status must be achieved. The magnitude of such a change is related to the magnitude of the change in morbidity. We shall not discuss this intriguing point further except to recognize that the change in morbidity which would be considered clinically significant—and therefore worth achieving—is a matter of judgment, and therefore the magnitude cannot always be determined by completely objective criteria. Our discussion will try to illustrate some of the more practical issues involved in documenting behavioral change.

Donovan (1977) observed no statistically significant differences in the birthweight of infants born to mothers in the smoking-cessation intervention group (3172g) from birthweight in the control group (3184g). One of the problems which he identified in discussing these results was whether the counseling intervention had been received or acted upon sufficiently to affect the infant's weight. Although the general practitioners and local authority physicians were asked to reinforce the advice given to the treatment group, only 31% of the women said they had received such advice; very nearly the same percentage of the control group reported receiving similar admonitions adventitiously. While his results do not support the hypothesis that maternal smoking is an etiological factor in low birthweight, a true test was probably not made in the study. If smoking reduction differences were too modest to affect birthweight, the correct conclusion should be that the hypothesis was not tested, rather than that maternal smoking is not an etiological factor in low birthweight. It should be emphasized that the two conclusions lead to decidedly different courses of action.

Because a behavior can be measured and related to a health outcome does not, in and of itself, guarantee that the behavior can be changed. The same is true for nonbehavioral risk factors related to disease. Accurate measurement of blood pressure, for instance, was possible for a long time before drugs were identified for its control and the efficacy of such blood pressure change on health was demonstrated (Veterans Administration Cooperative Study Group on Antihypertensive Agents, 1967). Another of the risk factors for coronary heart disease provides further illustration. In addition to the more widely documented risk factors of smoking, hypertension, and hyperlipidemia, the evidence relating a coronary-prone pattern of behavior to heart disease has become quite compelling (Jenkins, Rosenman, and Zyzanski, 1974; Rosenman, Friedman, Straus, et al., 1970). The longest prospective study on the subject is the Western Collaborative study in which coronary-prone, Type A behavior was measured by information from a personal interview. The Type A pattern is characterized by enhanced aggressiveness, ambition, competitive drive, and a chronic sense of time urgency. Glass (1977) has conducted studies to verify that these components are indeed what Type A measures. The follow-up results from the Western

Collaborative study, based on 8½ years' experience with middle-aged males, have been reported (Rosenman, Brand, Jenkins, et al., 1975): striking differences were shown in the rate of CHD between Type A and Type B patterns within several risk categories such as smoking, hyperlipidemia, and hypertension. These findings have excited a great deal of interest, but, except for two very recent investigations (Roskies, Spevack, Surkis, et al., 1978; Suinn and Bloom, 1978), there has not been much evidence to suggest that Type A behavior can be changed. Clearly, more studies—especially those with objective validation using standard biochemical risk indicators such as serum cholesterol and triglycerides, blood pressure, and changes in autonomic and endocrine reactivity to stress challenge (Roskies, 1979)—will be needed to settle the issue.

Although a behavior may be modifiable, change may or may not be actually achievable in practice. This concern is illustrated by the problem of determining whether a fat-modified diet would reduce coronary heart disease. Over the past several decades, control of coronary heart disease has been a major challenge in the United States and knowledge has indicated that primary prevention is the most promising way to lower CHD death rates (Report of Inter-Society Commission for Heart Disease Resources, 1972). The Framingham Study (Dawber, Moore, and Mann, 1957) has been one of the main sources of information concerning the identification of risk factors for CHD. Framingham, as well as a large number of other studies, have shown a positive relationship between serum cholesterol and CHD (Doyle, Heslin, Hilleboe, et al., 1957; Epstein, Napier, Block, et al., 1970; Hames, 1971; Keys, Taylor, Blackburn, et al., 1963). Earlier studies had shown a relationship between dietary intake and serum cholesterol (Anderson, Keys, and Grande, 1957; DenHartog, Buzina and Findanza, 1968; DenHartog, Van Schaik, and Dalderup, 1965). However, the question of whether change in diet would *prevent* CHD remained unanswered.

An Executive Committee on Diet and Heart Disease, established in 1960, concluded that a mass field trial of 100,000 men followed for 4 years was needed to determine whether change in diet would reduce the incidence of first heart attacks. There was no good information about the feasibility of such a trial: a free-living population, for example, might not be willing to make the recommended dietary changes. The Diet-Heart feasibilty study was conducted to provide information for a more rational decision on whether such a large research project should be undertaken (National Diet-Heart Study Research Group, 1968). The Diet-Heart study used a double-blind design, providing special, low-fat foods to men from the general population and to residents of mental institutions. In all centers, the serum cholesterol levels (which were about the same as the average for healthy men in the United States), were reduced by the experimental diets. Some change took place within 2 weeks and the lowest serum cholesterol levels were reached in about 6 weeks; the drop-out rate from the study was less than 10%. The study showed very clearly that serum cholesterol reductions could be obtained through dietary changes. The number of subjects required, the expense, and the ethical issues involving control groups, precluded the initiation of a large randomized dietary study. Such a study may never be conducted. An answer to the question of preventing CHD through changes in diet alone may remain unanswered, even though the feasibility of dietary change was established.

As can be seen from the above discussion, there are three points central to demonstrating changes in behavioral patterns: (1) is the behavior susceptible to modification, (2) if so, is it possible to achieve large enough differences in comparable groups to test the hypothesis adequately, and (3) can the change be documented?

DEFINITION OF INTERVENTION

Several points about intervention have already been made in the previous sections. It can be seen that behavioral intervention should be clearly specified so that the results of the magnitude of change, both in the behavior itself and in health status, can be evaluated from knowledge about intervention. If an intervention is demonstrated to be effective, a question which arises in the application of the findings is what exactly is the "treatment" that is needed to reproduce the outcome. This question will probably be faced even more frequently in the future, for the use of a placebo or no-treatment group will often be contra-indicated for ethical reasons, and it is more likely that the experiment will be designed to make comparisons among a number of different treatments. Even so, how much of the effect is a placebo response? Since patients do improve as a result of attention, as well as from drugs or other types of intervention, determining the amount of benefit which might be expected from a minimal intervention is a problem which must be solved. Furthermore, the investigator who knows the group to which a particular patient has been assigned may unintentionally influence the outcome. In other words, it is difficult to conduct a blind behavioral study and even more so to conduct a double-blind one, although it was done in the Diet-Heart Study.

DEMONSTRATION OF BENEFIT

The goal of epidemiology is to provide research results which will lay the foundation for prevention and control of disease. A demonstration of the effect of behavioral change on morbidity and mortality, therefore, is crucial to attaining this goal. There are presently few investigations that make such a demonstration. Some of the reasons have been touched on. The two major reasons—resources and time—are worth restating: In focusing on one behavior, such as dietary intake, the resources needed to show an effect on mortality may be so large as to preclude the research. Also, the time between modification of the behavioral risk factor and the benefit to health is often quite long. Many of the diseases which involve behavioral risk factors are chronic or may involve an extended period of time between the onset of behavior, such as smoking, and the manifestation of disease, such as lung cancer. Additionally, demonstrating a health benefit may require such a long follow-up period that it is sometimes not feasible for a single investigator to conduct the study.

Conclusion

The shift in the leading causes of morbidity and mortality from acute, infectious diseases to chronic diseases and accidents has required a corresponding change in the methods used for prevention and control. As an increasing number of social and behavioral variables have been shown to constitute risk factors for disease, interest in and emphasis on behavioral epidemiology has increased. Given that important conclusions about the causes and management of illness are being drawn from retrospective, prospective, and experimental studies, researchers, clinicians, and all those who might interpret such data should familiarize themselves with the strengths—and weaknesses—of epidemiological and group survey methods as they apply to problems in behavior.

References

Anderson, J. T., Keys, A., and Grande, F. The effects of different food fats on serum cholesterol concentration in men. *J. Nutr.,* 1957, *62,* 421–444.

Armstrong, B., and Doll, R. Bladder cancer mortality in England and Wales in relation to cigarette smoking and saccharin consumption. *Br. J. Prev. Soc. Med.,* 1974, *28,* 233–240.

Auerbach, O., Hammond, E. C., and Garfinkel, L. Smoking in relation to atherosclerosis of the coronary arteries. *N. Eng. J. Med.,* 1965, *273,* 775–779.

Baker, S. P., and Fisher, R. S. Alcohol and motorcycle fatalities. *Am. J. Public Health,* 1977, *67,* 246–249.

Bako, G., MacKenzie, W. C., and Smith, E. S. O. Drivers in Alberta with previous impaired driving records responsible for fatal highway accidents: A survey, 1970–1972. *Can. J. Public Health,* 1977, *68,* 106–110.

Barlow, D. H., Hersen, M., and Jackson, M. Single-case experimental designs: Uses in applied clinical research. *Arch. Gen. Psychiatry,* 1973, *29,* 319–325.

Barylko-Pikielna, N., and Pangborn, R. M. Effect of cigarette smoking on urinary and salivary thiocyanate. *Arch. Environ. Health,* 1968, *17,* 739–745.

Berkson, J. Smoking and lung cancer: Some observations on two recent reports. *J. Am. Stat. Assoc.,* 1958, *53,* 28.

Blalock, H. M. and Blalock, A. B. *Methodology in social research.* New York: McGraw-Hill, 1968.

Bray, G. A. (Ed.). *Obesity in perspective.* Washington, D.C.: United States Government Printing Office, 1973.

Burkitt, D. P., Walker, A. R. P., and Painter, N. S. Dietary fiber and disease. *J.A.M.A.,* 1974, *229,* 1068.

Byar, D. P. Sound advice for conducting clinical trials. *N. Eng. J. Med.,* 1977, *297,* 553–554.

Chiang, B. N., Perlman, L. V., and Epstein, F. H. Overweight and hypertension. A review. *Circulation,* 1969, *39,* 403–421.

Cochran, W. G. Research techniques in the study of human beings. *Milbank Mem. Fund Q.,* 1955, *33,* 121–136.

Coronary Drug Project Research Group. Clofibrate and niacin in coronary heart disease. *J.A.M.A.,* 1975, *231,* 360–381.

Dawber, T. R. *Risk factors for atherosclerotic disease.* Kalamazoo, Mich.: The Upjohn Company, 1975.

Dawber, T. R., Meadors, G. F. and Moore, F. E., Jr. Epidemiological approaches to heart disease; the Framingham Study. *Am. J. Public Health,* 1951, *41,* 270–286.

Dawber, T. R., Moore, F. E., and Mann, G. V. Coronary heart disease in the Framingham study. Am. J. Public Health, 1975, *47,* 4–23.

DenHartog, C., Buzina, R., and Findanza, F. (Eds.). *Dietary studies and epidemiology of heart disease.* The Hague: Sticht. Wetensch. Voorlichting Voedingsgebied, 1968.

DenHartog, C., Van Schaik, Th. F. S. M., and Dalderup, L. M. Diet of volunteers participating in a long term epidemiological field survey on coronary heart disease at Zutphen, Netherlands. *Voeding,* 1965, *26,* 184.

(The) Diabetic Retinopathy Study Research Group. Preliminary report on effects of photocoagulation therapy. *Am. J. Ophthalmol.,* 1976, *81,* 383–395.

Dietz, P. E., and Baker, S. P. Drowning: Epidemiology and prevention. *Am. J. Public Health,* 1974, *64,* 303–312.

Doll, R., and Hill, A. B. The mortality of doctors in relation to their smoking habits: A preliminary report. *Br. Med. J.,* 1954, *1,* 1451–1455.

Doll, R., and Hill, A. B. Lung cancer and other causes of death in relation to smoking: A second report on the mortality of British doctors. *Br. Med. J.,* 1956, *2,* 1071–1081.

Donovan, J. W. Randomised controlled trial of anti-smoking advice in pregnancy. *Br. J. Prev. Soc. Med.,* 1977, *31,* 6–12.

Doyle, J. T., Heslin, A. S., Hilleboe, H. E., Formel, P. F., and Korns, R. F. A prospective study of degenerative cardiovascular disease in Albany: Report of three years' experience. I. Ischemic heart disease. *Am. J. Public Health,* 1957, *47* (Part 2), 25–32.

Epstein, R. H., Napier, J. A., Block, W. D., Hayner, N. S., Higgins, M. P., Johnson, B. C., Keller, J. B., Matzner, H. L., Montaye, H. J., Ostrander, L. D., and Ullman, B. M. The Tecumseh Study. Design, progress and perspectives. *Arch. Environ. Health,* 1970, *21,* 402–407.

Finklea, J. F., Sandifer, S. H., and Smith, D. D. Cigarette smoking and epidemic influenza. *Am. J. Epidemiol.,* 1969, *90,* 390–399.

Fisher, R. A. *The design of experiments,* 7th ed. New York: Hafner, 1960.

Freis, E. D. Salt, volume, and the prevention of hypertension. *Circulation,* 1976, *53,* 589–595.

Friend, B. Nutrients in United States food supply—A review of trends, 1909–1913 to 1965. *Am. J. Clin. Nutr.,* 1967, *20,* 907.

Gagnon, F. Contribution to the study of the etiology and prevention of cancer of the cervix of the uterus. *Am. J. Obstet. Gynecol.,* 1950, *60,* 516–522.

Galasko, D. S. B., and Edwards, D. H. The use of seat belts by motor car occupants involved in road traffic accidents. *Injury,* 1975, *6,* 320–324.

Giertsen, J. C. Drowning while under the influence of alcohol. *Med. Sci. Law,* 1970, *10,* 216.

Glass, D. C. Stress, behavior patterns, and coronary disease. *Am. Sci.,* 1977, *65,* 177–187.

Hames, C. G. Evans Country cardiovascular and cerebrovascular epidemiologic study. Introduction. *Arch. Intern. Med.,* 1971, *128,* 883–886.

Hammond, E. C., and Garfinkel, L. Coronary heart disease, stroke, and aortic aneurysm—Factors in the etiology. *Arch. Environ. Health,* 1969, *19,* 167.

Health consequences of smoking—A report of the surgeon general. Washington, D.C.: United States Government Printing Office, 1972.

Herbst, A. L., Cole, P., Colton, T., Robboy, S. J., and Scully, R. E. Age-incidence and risk of diethylstilbestrol-related clear cell adenocarcinoma of the vagina and cervix. *Am. J. Obstet. Gynecol.,* 1977, *128,* 43–50.

Herbst, A. L., Ulfelder, H. and Poskanzer, D. C. Adenocarcinoma of the vagina: Association of maternal stilbestrol therapy with tumor appearance in young women. *N. Engl. J. Med.,* 1971, *284,* 878–881.

Hill, Sir Austin Bradford. *Principles of medical statistics.* New York: Oxford University Press, 1971.

Hill, Sir Austin Bradford. *A short textbook of medical statistics.* Philadelphia: J. B. Lippincott, 1977.

Hossack, D., and Brown, G. The hard facts of the influence of alcohol on serious road accident casualties. *Med. J. Aust.,* 1974, *2,* 473–479.

Humphreys, N. A. (Ed.). *Vital statistics: A memorial volume of selections from the reports and writings of William Farr, 1807–1883.* London: The Sanitary Institute of Great Britain, 1885.

Hypertension Detection and Follow-up Cooperative Group. The hypertension detection and follow-up program. *Prev. Med.,* 1976, *5,* 207–215.

Jenkins, C. D., Rosenman, R. H., and Zyzanski, S. J. Prediction of clinical coronary heart disease by a test for the coronary-prone behavior pattern. *N. Eng. J. Med.,* 1974, *290,* 1271–1275.

Kannel, W. B. Current status of the epidemiology of brain infarction associated with occlusive arterial disease. *Stroke,* 1971, *2,* 295–318.

Karaharju, E. O., and Stjernvall, L. The alcohol factor in accidents. *Injury,* 1974, *6,* 67–69.

Kaye, S. Alcohol and traffic deaths. *Med. Times,* 1975, *103,* 88–89.

Keys, A. (Ed.). *Coronary heart disease in seven countries,* American Heart Association Monograph Number 29. New York: American Heart Association, 1970.

Keys, A., Taylor, H. L., Blackburn, H., Brozek, J., Anderson, J. T., and Simonson, E. Coronary heart disease among Minnesota business and professional men followed fifteen years. *Circulation,* 1963, *28,* 381–395.

Lilienfeld, A. M. *Foundations of epidemiology.* New York: Oxford University Press, 1976.

Longo, L. D. The biological effects of carbon monoxide on the pregnant woman, fetus, and newborn infant. *Am. J. Obstet. Gynecol.,* 1977, *129,* 69–103.

Macmahon, B., and Pugh, T. F. *Epidemiology: Principles and methods.* Boston: Little, Brown, and Company, 1970.

Mausner, J. S., and Bahn, A. K. *Epidemiology: An introductory text.* Philadelphia: W. B. Saunders, 1974.

McLean, J. A., and Ching, A. Y. T. Follow-up study of relationships between family situation and bronchial asthma in children. *J. Am. Acad. Psychiatry,* 1973, *12,* 142–161.

Moss, N. H. and Mayer, J. (Eds.). *Food and nutrition in health and disease.* New York: The New York Academy of Sciences, 1977.

Mueller, R. E., Keble, D. L., Plummer, J., and Walker,

S. H. The prevalence of chronic bronchitis, chronic airway obstruction, and respiratory symptoms in a Colorado city. *Am. Rev. Respir. Dis.*, 1971, *103*, 209–228.

National Clearinghouse for Smoking and Health. *Bibliography on smoking and health.* Atlanta: Center for Disease Control, 1977.

National Diet-Heart Study Research Group. *The National Diet-Heart Study final report,* American Heart Association Monograph Number 18. New York: American Heart Association, 1968.

Northrop, F. S. C. *The logic of the sciences and the humanities.* New York: Macmillan, 1947.

Paffenberger, R. S., Jr., Hale, W. E., Brand, K. J., and Hyde, R. T. Work-energy level, personal characteristics and fatal heart attack: A birth-cohort effect. *Am. J. Epidemiol.*, 1977, *105,* 200–213.

Pickering, G. W. The place of the experimental method in medicine. *Proc. R. Soc. Med.*, 1949, *42,* 229–234.

Plueckhahn, V. D. The aetiology of 134 deaths due to drowning in Geelong during the years 1957 to 1971. *Med. J. Aust.*, 1972, *2,* 1183.

Poskanzer, D. C., and Herbst, A. L. Epidemiology of vaginal adenosis and adenocarcinoma associated with exposure to stilbestrol in utero. *Cancer,* 1977, *39,* 1892–1895.

Report of Inter-Society Commission for Heart Disease Resources. Primary prevention of the atherosclerotic diseases. *Circulation,* 1972, *42,* 1–44.

Rosenman, R. H., Brand, R. J., Jenkins, C. D., Friedman, M., Straus, R., and Wurm, M. Coronary heart disease in the Western Collaborative Group Study: Final follow-up of 8½ years. *J.A.M.A.*, 1975, *233,* 872–877.

Rosenman, R. H., Friedman, M. F., Straus, R., Jenkins, C. D., Zyzanski, S. J., and Wurm, M. Coronary heart disease in the Western Collaborative Group Study: A follow-up experience of 4½ years. *J. Chronic Dis.*, 1970, *23,* 173–190.

Roskies, E. Considerations in developing a treatment program for the coronary-prone (Type A) behavior pattern. In P. Davidson (Ed.), *Behavioral medicine: changing health life-styles,* New York: Brunner/Mazel, 1979.

Roskies, E., Spevack, M., Surkis, A., Cohen, C., and Gilman, S. Changing the coronary prone (Type A) behavior pattern in a non-clinical population. *J. Behav. Med.*, 1978, *1,* 201–216.

Schneiderman, M. A. The numerate sciences—Epidemiology and biometry. *J. Nat. Cancer Inst.*, 1977, *59,* 633–644.

Suinn, R. M., and Bloom, L. J. Anxiety management training for pattern A behavior. *J. Behav. Med.*, 1978, *1,* 25–36.

Susser, M. *Causal thinking in the health sciences: Concepts and strategies of epidemiology.* New York: Oxford University Press, 1973.

Terris, M. Epidemiology of cirrhosis of the liver: National mortality data. *Am. J. Public Health,* 1967, *57,* 2076–2088.

United States Bureau of the Census. *Statistical Abstract of the United States: 1958,* 79th ed. Washington, D.C.: United States Government Printing Office, 1958.

United States Bureau of the Census. *Statistical Abstract of the United States: 1975,* 96th ed. Washington, D.C.: United States Government Printing Office, 1975.

United States Department of Health, Education, and Welfare, Public Health Service. *Vital Statistics of the United States, 1974. Volume II—Mortality. Part B.* Washington, D.C.: United States Government Printing Office, 1976.

Veterans Administration Cooperative Study Group on Antihypertensive Agents. Effects of treatment on morbidity in hypertension. Results in patients with diastolic blood pressures averaging 115 through 129 mm Hg. *J.A.M.A.*, 1967, *202,* 116–122.

Veterans Administration Cooperative Study Group on Antihypertensive Agents. Effects of treatment on morbidity in hypertension. II. Results in patients with diastolic blood pressure averaging 90 through 114 mm Hg. *J.A.M.A.*, 1970, *213,* 1143–1152.

Vogt, T. M., Selvin, S., Widdowson, G., and Hulley, S. B. Expired air carbon monoxide and serum thiocyanate as objective measures of cigarette exposure. *Am. J. Public Health,* 1977, *67,* 545–549.

Watson, J. D. *The double helix.* New York: New American Library, 1968.

White, K. L., and Henderson, M. M. (Eds.). *Epidemiology as a fundamental science. Its uses in health services planning, administration, and evaluation.* New York: Oxford University Press, 1976.

Wynder, E. L., and Cornfield, J. Cancer of the lung in physicians. *N. Engl. J. Med.*, 1953, *248,* 441–444.

Wynder, E. L., and Graham, E. A. Tobacco smoking as a possible etiologic factor in bronchiogenic carcinoma. *J. A.M.A.*, 1950, *143,* 329–336.

Zeidenberg, P., Jaffe, J. H., Kanzler, M., Levitt, M. D., Langone, J. J., and Van Vunakis, H. Nicotine: Cotinine levels in blood during cessation of smoking. *Compr. Psychiatry,* 1977, *18,* 93–101.

Learning and Conditioning

JOSEPH V. BRADY, PH.D.

Professor and Director
Division of Behavioral Biology
The Johns Hopkins University School of Medicine
Baltimore, Maryland

2

Historical Perspectives

The current resurgence of interest in behavioral research methodologies and their applications to clinical medicine reflects the strong empirical and conceptual influence of the experimental learning and conditioning laboratory. In this regard, it is of somewhat more than coincidental interest that the historical roots of an extensive research literature in the field can be traced to the early studies of Pavlov and Sherrington before the turn of the century, focused upon the central role of learning and conditioning in the physiological adaptations and adjustments of the internal environment (Pavlov, 1927, 1928; Sherrington, 1906). Of at least as great import, however, was the foundation provided by these early investigations, as well as by those of Bechterev (1932) in the Soviet Union and Thorndike (1898) in the United States, for conceptualizing the behavioral interactions between organism and environment within the framework of an orderly and systematic body of scientific knowledge based upon observation and experiment. Several streams of development have, of course, intervened between this emerging "behaviorism" of Russian and American origins early in the century and the current applications of learning and conditioning procedures in clinical medicine.

During the 1920's and 1930's, for example, the writings of Watson and Rayner (1920), Jones (1924), Mowrer and Mowrer (1938), among others in the United States, suggested an early trend toward the application of learning and conditioning principles in clinical settings. At about the same time, Soviet psychophysiologists (Ivanov-Smolensky, 1928; Krasnagorski, 1933), adhering closely to conceptualization derived directly from laboratory research, became increasingly involved in the treatment of clinical disorders, and by the 1940's, the experimental work of Gantt (1944), Liddell (1938), and Masserman (1943), has begun to establish a laboratory conditioning and learning base for the clinical applications of "Pavlovian Psychiatry" (Astrup, 1965) in America.

The clinical and experimental innovations of the 1950's and 1960's within the framework of developments emerging from the learning and conditioning laboratory were focused, for the most part, upon applications involving the treatment of behavioral disorders. The work of Wolpe (1958), for example, based upon laboratory learning research and the neurophysiological conceptualizations of Sherrington focused initially upon an experimental analysis of "emotional conditioning" in cats before introducing "conditioning therapy" in the treatment of neurotic disorders in clinical populations. An equally important influence in this development emerged in London around 1950 under the aegis of Eysenck and Shapiro who emphasized experimental analysis and hypothesis testing in the application of the behavior therapies in an attempt to bridge what they perceived to be a distressingly wide gap between laboratory-based learning and conditioning principles, on the one hand, and clinically oriented treatment practices, on the other (Shapiro, 1951, 1961; Eysenck, 1952).

The dominant and perhaps most enduring influence upon the application of learning and conditioning procedures in clinical treatment settings, however, can be seen to have developed as a direct result of the innovative contributions of Skinner (1938) to the experimental analysis of behavior emphasizing the laboratory study of individual organism-environment interactions and focusing upon the effects or consequences of such interactions as the major determinant of behavior. Unlike more traditional "psychological" approaches occupied with the average behavior of groups, Skinner and his early collaborators in both the laboratory and the clinic (notably Ferster, Lindsley, and Azrin, among others) emphasized the experimental analysis of learning and conditioning in the individual as the basis for the application of behavioral research methodologies in clinical settings (Lindsley and Skinner, 1954; Ferster and DeMeyer, 1961; Ayllon and Azrin, 1965, 1968).

There have, of course, been legitimate concerns expressed about the extent to which the evident temporal ordering of laboratory investigative activity and behavioral treatment development justifies the "ideological excesses" which have at times characterized "learning theory" accounts of clinical practices (London, 1972). Indeed, it is important to recognize that the conceptual contributions of the experimental learning and conditioning laboratory as they bear upon the problems of clinical medicine have been less a matter of applying comprehensively formulated scientific "laws" and "theories" than of providing a paradigmatic and cohesive operational framework for analysis of the complex environmental-behavioral interactions involved. In this regard, it would seem fair to say that methodological influences have been and probably will continue for some time to be the dominant ones, emphasizing detailed and objective descriptions with the focus upon functional analysis of observable and quantifiable behavioral interactions rather than upon inferred unobserved (and in many instances unobservable) processes. The treatment approaches conceptualized within the framework of this experimentally based learning and conditioning analysis can also be seen to emphasize systematic manipulation of environmental and behavioral variables, with assessment of outcomes carried out in the same objective, quantifiable terms that characterized both the initial problem analysis and formulation of the treatment program. Performance changes based upon observed and recorded behavior are the objective criteria which either validate the initial analysis or require re-examination, to include additional data collection, as necessary.

The extent to which these methodological and procedural similarities bear upon the relationship between the learning and conditioning laboratory on the one hand, and currently emerging treatment practices in behavioral medicine on the other, is perhaps most convincingly reflected in the performance histories of those investigators who have made the most innovative contributions to such clinical applications. With few exceptions, their clinical initiatives were preceded by extended and, in many cases, illustrious laboratory investigative careers in "learning and conditioning." This appears to be as true for the "founding fathers" (e.g., Pavlov, Watson, Mowrer, Gantt, Skinner) as it does for the latter-day luminaries (e.g., Azrin, Ferster, Sidman, Wolpe), and suggests that the foundations provided by learning and conditioning studies may well have influenced both the conceptual and methodological advances which are the "raison d'etre" for the present volume.

Basic Concepts and Principles

Within the limits defined by these somewhat immodest attributions regarding the derivations of behavioral treatment applications, a brief over-view of basic concepts and principles may serve to reflect the range of fundamental observations and experiments which have provided the building blocks for the systematic formulations of the learning and conditioning laboratory (Skinner, 1965). The elements of a behavioral interaction between organism and environment, as scrutinized experimentally in the learning and conditioning laboratory, are conventionally represented in terms of stimulus and response events. At the most fundamental level, stimuli are identified with environmental segments, and responses are defined by the activities of individual organisms. The technical referents of both terms, however, are far more complex than their common usage would suggest.

The environment, for example, can be divided into several stimulus classes based upon the functional role of such events in behavioral interactions. One such class of *eliciting stimuli* regularly precedes and elicits reflexive or relatively fixed and stereotyped responses (e.g., patellar tap). A second class of *reinforcing stimuli* (i.e., "reinforcers") consists of environmental events that follow as the consequence of responses and influence the frequency with which those responses will reoccur in future behavioral interactions (e.g., social or financial rewards). The third major class of behaviorally relevant environmental events, *discriminative stimuli,* function as antecedent or concurrent occasioning events or circumstances. In contrast to eliciting stimuli, discriminative stimuli do not elicit responses in the reflexive sense, but rather they influence the frequency of (i.e., set the occasion for) those responses which have previously been followed by reinforcers in their presence (e.g., traffic signals).

In similar fashion, the activities of individual organisms can be generally categorized into two broad classes based principally upon the temporal ordering of relevant stimulus and response events (Rachlin, 1970). The first class of reflexive responses or *respondents* is predominantly under the influence of prior-occurring eliciting stimuli and is basically determined by the "involuntary" constitutional reflex endowment of the organism (e.g., salivation, startle). The second class of instrumental responses or *operants* is comprised of emitted activities influenced for the most part by the occurrence of reinforcing stimuli which follow as a consequence of such "voluntary" responses (e.g., locomotion, manipulation).

Since at least the time of Pavlov, these "stimulus" and "response" concepts have provided a scientifically useful basis for describing and experimentally analyzing increasingly more complex organism-environment interactions of direct relevance to behavioral medicine. Early laboratory studies, for example, provided the first systematic respondent conditioning account of how a conditional stimulus or CS (e.g., the sound of a bell), initially ineffective in changing response activities, can come to elicit a conditional response or CR (e.g., salivation) when paired repeatedly with an unconditional stimulus or UCS (e.g., food). If the sound of a bell as the CS is subsequently presented a number of times without food as the UCS, the magnitude and frequency of the salivation elicited by the CS diminish, and respondent extinction occurs. When a period of time intervenes between such extinction sessions and subsequent presentations of the CS, however, spontaneous recovery is observed in the form of temporary reappearance of the CR elicited by the CS.

The power to elicit a respondent, which is developed in one CS by conditioning, extends to other stimuli with the degree of this *stimulus generalization* determined by the similarities and differences between the other stimuli and the CS. Because the stimuli other than the CS differ with respect to the magnitude and frequency with which they elicit the CR, *stimulus discrimination* also occurs. Indeed, discrimination can be made increasingly more pronounced by repeated pairings of the UCS only with the specific CS (i.e., respondent conditioning) while ensuring that the occurrence of other stimuli is not paired with the UCS.

These basic observations with regard to respondent conditioning have been elaborated in numerous laboratory and clinical-experimental studies since Russian researchers first introduced this systematic approach to behavior analysis. It has been convincingly demonstrated, for example, that second- or higher-order conditioning can occur when a well-established CS is paired with a neutral stimulus. The neutral stimulus acquires the power to elicit the respondent CR. Although it has not been empirically determined just how far this process can be carried, the development of eliciting properties by CSs two or three steps removed from the original UCS is not uncommon. And the intensive investigative effort, principally Russian in origin, to extend the conceptual framework of respondent conditioning to encompass verbal stimuli and semantic responses (Razran, 1961) suggests potentially important directions for development of the theory and the practice of behavioral medicine.

Elicited respondents of the type that have provided the primary focus for such basic and important Pavlovian or classical conditioning analyses must nonetheless be seen to represent only a relatively small proportion of the behavioral interactions of higher organisms. The most prominent aspects of such advanced repertoires are represented by the instrumental or operant category for which there is no environmental eliciting stimulus and which is generally described as "voluntary" or emitted. The frequency of occurrence of an operant is chiefly determined by the environmental consequating events that follow the emitted response. When these environmental consequences involve the appearance of stimuli that increase the probability that the response they followed will recur in the future, the term appetitive or positive reinforcer is applied. When, on the other hand, the disappearance or postponement of an environmental stimulus as a consequence of an operant response results in the increased probability that the response will recur in the future, an aversive or negative reinforcer is defined. That is, reinforcers are always defined by their effects on the subsequent frequency of the immediately preceding response: both positive and negative reinforcers increase the frequency of the preceding response.

Over the past three decades, a broad range of animal laboratory and human experimental studies have provided important insights into the principles that determine the acquisition, maintenance, and modification of such operant behavior (Honig, 1966; Honig and Staddon, 1976). The basic observation is that the rate of emission of an operant response already in the organism's repertoire can be readily increased by following occurrences of the response with a reinforcing stimulus (*operant conditioning*). Beyond this, it has been possible to make explicit the process called *shaping,* whereby a combination of operant conditioning and *extinction* (i.e., withholding reinforcers) can shape existing simple responses into new and more complex performances. Of critical importance for this shaping process is the observation that a reinforcing stimulus not only strengthens the particular response that precedes it, but also results in an increase in the frequency of many other bits of behavior (i.e., *response generalization*) and in effect raises the individual's general activity level.

Thus, the shaping of behavior proceeds, as reinforcers are initially presented following a response similar to or approximating the desired one. Since this tends to increase the strength of various other similar behaviors, a response still closer to the desired can be selected from this new array and followed by reinforcing stimuli. Continued narrowing and refinement of the response criteria required for reinforcement leads progressively to new arrays of available behavior. In this way, by successive and progressive approximation, a new and desired performance can be shaped. The importance of this simple but fundamental and powerful shaping process for the development and modification of behavior cannot be overstated, since the weight of available evidence suggests that a careful and systematic application of such procedures with effective reinforcing stimuli is sufficient to establish or alter any operant performance of which the organism is physically capable. This shaping process is obviously of enormous clinical importance in behavioral medicine since many patient performances can only be changed effectively in this way. Without shaping, one might wait for inordinately long periods before a patient performs some critical health-related behavior for which a reinforcer has been scheduled.

The fact that changes in behavior are not always brought about by deliberate and systematic manipulation of the environment, however, has led to an analysis of *superstitious* behavior. An environmental stimulus may, by chance, follow a response, resulting in the adventitious strengthening of that response. If this sequence of events reoccurs even infrequently (i.e., *intermittent reinforcement* as described below), the individual may learn quite elaborate sequences of superstitious behavior which have absolutely nothing to do with the reinforcing stimuli that are influencing their occurrence (e.g., the exhortations of the gambler do not produce winning dice combinations; they persist because they are occasionally followed by "7" or "11").

The powerful effects of reinforcing stimulus consequences in establishing and maintaining operant behavior suggest that withholding or withdrawing of such reinforcers (i.e., *extinction*) will have comparably powerful effects on the strength of responses previously followed by reinforcing stimuli. Indeed, such extinction procedures do reduce the frequency of response, although the reduction is not usually immediate. Rather, after the onset of extinction, the initial effect is often a brief increase in the frequency as well as the force and variability of the responding previously followed by reinforcement. The extent to which operant responding persists in the absence of reinforcing environmental stimulus consequences (*resistance to extinction*) depends, of course, on the interaction of many complex influences including motivational factors (e.g., level of deprivation). However, both laboratory and clinical experimental evidence now confirms the fact that the single most important variable affecting the course of operant extinction is the *schedule of reinforcement* on which the performance was previously maintained.

Whenever a reinforcing environmental stimulus follows some but not all occurrences of an operant response, a schedule of intermittent reinforcement is operating. Accordingly then, *intermittent reinforcement* is defined when only selected occurrences of an operant are followed by a reinforcer. Every reinforcer occurs according to some schedule or rule, although some schedules are so complicated that detailed analysis is required to formulate them precisely. Simple schedules of intermittent reinforcement can be classified into two broad categories: ratio and interval schedules. *Ratio schedules* prescribe that a certain number of responses be emitted before one response is reinforced, the term "ratio" referring to the relationship between the required response total (e.g., 50) and the one response followed by the reinforcing stimulus (e.g., "piece-work" schedule requiring 49 discrete labor units before the single 50th performance is followed by "payoff"). *Interval schedules,* on the other hand, prescribe that a given interval of time elapse before an emitted response can be followed by a reinforcing stimulus. The relevant interval can be measured from any event, but the occurrence of a previous reinforcer is usually used (e.g., "salaried" pay schedules). The recuperative properties of interval schedules under which the mere passage of even long time periods brings an opportunity for a single response to be followed by a reinforcer, contrasts with the "strain" potential of high ratio schedule requirements under which the performance may extinguish before a sufficient number of responses are emitted for one to be followed by a reinforcer (Rachlin, 1970).

Even simple ratio and interval schedules can in turn be classified into two general categories based upon whether the required number of responses or lapse of time are *fixed* or *variable,* and all known schedules of reinforcement can be reduced to variations of these basic ratio and interval parameters. A single operant performance, in addition, may be followed by a reinforcer in accordance with the requirements of two or more schedules at the same time (*compound schedules*). Two or more responses may be followed by a reinforcer according to the requirements of two or more schedules at the same time (*concurrent schedules*). Perhaps the most ubiquitous case of reinforcement schedule complexity is represented by the *multiple schedule* under the requirements of which two or more independent schedules developed and maintained simultaneously in the same organism are called forth sequentially under discriminably different environmental stimulus conditions. Virtually all operant behavior is followed by reinforcing stimuli according to multiple, compound, and concurrent schedules built out of the same basic elements as the simple ratio and interval schedules. Each schedule, simple or complex, generates and maintains its own characteristic performance, and when reinforcement is discontinued, the course and character of extinction are prominently influenced by the preceding schedule of reinforcement. Significantly, it has also become increasingly clear in the laboratory and the clinic that at least the frequency (or rate) of a given operant performance can usually be more effectively controlled by reinforcement schedule manipulation than by any other means.

The detailed experimental analysis of schedules of reinforcement has also served to emphasize another very important set of relationships between operant performances and environmental events encompassed within the general conceptual framework of *stimulus control.* The occurrence of a reinforcer following an operant not only increases the probability that the response will reoccur, but it also contributes to bringing that performance under the control of other environmental stimuli present when the operant is reinforced. After the responses composing the operant have been reinforced in the presence of a particular stimulus a number of times, that stimulus comes to control the operant (i.e., the frequency of those responses is high in the presence of the stimulus and lower in its absence). A *discriminative stimulus* is thus defined by this process as one in whose presence a particular operant performance is highly probable because the behavior has previously been reinforced in its presence. It is important to recognize, however, that discriminative stimuli do not elicit performances as in the respondent or reflex case, but rather set the *occasion* for operant responses in the sense that they provide the circumstances under which the performance has previously been reinforced. This "controlling" power of a discriminative stimulus develops gradually and at least several occurrences of the reinforcer following the response in the presence of the stimulus are required before the stimulus effectively controls the performance.

Such discriminative stimulus control is not an entirely selective process, however, since reinforcement of a performance in the presence of one stimulus increases the tendency to respond not only in that stimulus but also in the presence of other stimuli with similar properties (i.e., *stimulus generalization*). It is not always clear from simple observation, of course, which stimulus or which property of a stimulus is controlling an operant performance and both laboratory and clinical experiences have documented the hazard of assuming that the similarity casually observed between stimuli provides an adequate explanation of such generalization. There is unfortunately no substitute for experiment in differentiating the many detailed aspects of a stimulus complex which may exercise critical control. Furthermore, related *response generalization* effects have also been observed to occur when following an operant with a reinforcer results not only in an increase in the frequency of the responses composing that operant but also in an increase in the frequency of similar responses.

This very sensitivity to the differential aspects of stimulus and response complexes provides the basis for the other major cornerstone of the stimulus control process identified as *discrimination.* A discrimination between two stimuli is defined when an organism behaves differently in the presence of each. Such *stimulus discrimination* is pronounced under conditions which provide *differential reinforcement,* and this process is seen to operate in the *formation of a discrimination* when there is a high probability that a reinforcer will follow a given response in the presence of one stimulus and a low or zero probability that the reinforcing stimulus will follow the response in the presence of another stimulus. The extent of the generalization between two stimuli will, of course, influence the rapidity and stability with which a discrimination can be formed, and it is important to recognize that the antecedents of a performance that occurs under one set of stimulus conditions may include events which have occurred under quite different stimulus conditions. The careful application of differential reinforcement procedures can, however, bring about remarkably precise control of an operant performance by highly selective aspects of a stimulus complex, and this *attention* to specific properties of a stimulus can be facilitated and enhanced by the use of *instructional stimuli* which, in essence, tell the organism about features of the environment which are currently relevant to the occasioning of reinforcement (e.g., a treasure map). Furthermore, this precise stimulus control (i.e., *attention*) can be transferred from one group of stimuli or stimulus properties to another by simultaneous presentation of the two together followed by the gradual withdrawal (i.e., "*fading*") of the original stimulus.

The intimate and continuing association between discriminative environmental stimulus events and the occurrence of reinforcers endows at least some originally nonreinforcing stimuli with acquired reinforcer properties. These stimuli have come to be designated as *secondary* or *conditioned reinforcers* (e.g., fraternity pins, stock market quotations, etc.) to distinguish them from innate, primary, or unconditioned reinforcers which require no experience to be effective. Such conditioned reinforcers can, of course, be either *appetitive* (*positive*), strengthening a prior-occurring response by their appearance, or *aversive* (*negative*), in which case their disappearance or postponement is reinforcing. Under any circumstances, the development or acquisition of conditioned reinforcing properties by a stimulus is usually a gradual process, as is the case with discriminative stimuli in general, and a common interpretive view of the process suggests that conditioned reinforcers may owe their effectiveness to the fact that they function as discriminative stimuli for later members of a response chain which are maintained by the occurrence of reinforcers in their presence.

Response chaining refers to the observationally and experimentally verified occurrence of a composed series of performances joined together by environmental stimuli that act both as conditioned reinforcers and as discriminative stimuli. A chain (e.g., party-going) usually begins with the occurrence of a discriminative stimulus (e.g., phone invitation) in the presence of which an appropriate response (e.g., acceptance) is followed by a conditioned reinforcer (e.g., "Glad you can make it.") This conditioned reinforcer is also the discriminative stimulus occasion for the next appropriate response (e.g., washing, dressing) which in turn, is followed by another conditioned reinforcer (e.g., leaving the house, catching a cab, etc.) which is also a discriminative stimulus for the next response (e.g., joining the party), and so on. While it is doubtless true that the entirety of such chains is most often maintained by the terminal occurrence of potent environmental consequences (e.g., social interactions, food, etc.), laboratory experiments have clearly demonstrated that the overlapping links in the chain (i.e., discriminative stimulus→ operant response→conditioned reinforcer) are held together primarily by the dual (and demonstrably separable) discriminative and conditioned reinforcing functions of environmental stimuli. The significance of this general chaining principle must, of course, be seen to reside in the fact that virtually all behavioral interactions occur as chains of greater or lesser length and that even performances usually treated as unitary phenomena (e.g., golf, bowling, etc.) can be usefully analyzed at various component levels for purposes of modification or proficiency enhancement.

Perhaps the most important aspect of this complex analysis of environmental stimulus events in relation to behavioral interactions is the clear implication that some degree of independence can be gained from the factors limiting conditioned reinforcer potency by the formation of conditioned reinforcers based upon two or more primary reinforcers. Such conditioned stimulus events (*generalized reinforcers*) gain potency from all the reinforcers on which they are based, and the most prominent operant performances in the human repetoire (e.g., verbal behavior) as well as the most valued stimulus consequences in the social environmental (e.g., money) can be seen to share these broadly based discriminative and generalized conditioned reinforcing properties.

This necessarily abbreviated overview of experimentally derived concepts and principles basic to the theory and practice of behavioral medicine has thus far maintained the generally accepted differentiation between operants and respondents, based principally upon procedural distinctions identified in the laboratory. The independent and distinctive features of these two coextensive processes are seldom apparent, however, in the course of even detailed natural observation. In no investigative aspect of the behavioral universe is the complex interaction between operants and respondents more pronounced than in the experimental analysis of aversive control procedures represented (or *mis*represented!) by the technical terms *escape, avoidance,* and *punishment,* and the corollary concepts of "emotion" and "motivation."

Empirical and theoretical accounts of those aspects of behavioral medicine concerned with disordered performances have frequently assigned a central role to historical and contemporary environmental interactions involving aversive stimuli. Operationally characterized in terms of their behavioral effects, *aversive stimuli* are defined as environmental events which decrease the subsequent frequency of the operant responses they follow, on the one hand, and/or increase the subsequent frequency of operant responses which remove or postpone them. When an aversive stimulus follows and is dependent upon the occurrence of an operant, a *punishment* condition is defined. Punishment may be made contingent upon the occurrence of an operant which has never before been followed by a reinforcer, an operant currently being maintained by appetitive (positive) or aversive (negative) reinforcement, or an operant that is undergoing extinction. Under each condition, the short- and long-term effects of punishment will vary as a function of complex operant-respondent interactions, and both discriminative stimulus control and reinforcement schedule factors may operate to further influence the subsequent form and frequency of the operant performance.

An *escape* condition is defined when a response terminates an aversive stimulus *after* the stimulus has appeared. The interaction between operants and respondents is especially prominent in escape situations since the aversive stimulus usually elicits reflexive responses which eventually result in or accompany an operant performance followed by withdrawal of the aversive stimulus. Strong generalization effects appear during initial exposures to escape situations, but the gradual development of discriminative properties by the aversive stimulus narrows the performance and very low intensities of the aversive stimulus may eventually *maintain* an operant escape performance requiring a much more intense aversive stimulus to *establish.* Reinforcement schedule effects similar in all essential respects to positive reinforcement are observed when withdrawal of an aversive stimulus is the reinforcer, and disappearance of an operant escape response occurs rapidly when presentation of the aversive stimulus is discontinued, or more slowly and erratically if the occurrence of the operant is no longer reinforced by withdrawal of the reoccurring aversive stimulus (extinction).

An *avoidance* condition is defined by the occurrence of an operant response which postpones an aversive stimulus. Avoidance performances may be established and maintained either in the presence or absence of an exteroceptive environmental event (i.e., "warning stimulus") which precedes the aversive stimulus. When an exteroceptive warning stimulus precedes the aversive stimulus, respondent conditioning effects operate to endow the warning stimulus with aversive properties, the termination of which following the operant avoidance response probably combines with the continued absence of the aversive stimulus to act as a reinforcer. The complexity of the avoidance process is suggested by the functionally simultaneous properties acquired by the conditioned aversive "warning" stimulus as (1) an eliciting environmental event for respondents, (2) a conditioned aversive (negative) reinforcer, withdrawal of which strengthens the operant avoidance performance, and (3) a discriminative stimulus which provides the occasion for the operant avoidance response to be followed by a reinforcer. In the absence of an exteroceptive warning stimulus (e.g., Sidman avoidance), a temporal respondent conditioning process provides discriminative cues, and the temporal stimulus correlated with the aversive environmental event acquires the same three simultaneous functions as an exteroceptive stimulus.

Such an analysis of aversive control emphasizes the simultaneous operation of operant and respondent conditioning processes in ongoing behavior segments. Whenever the conditioned stimulus in a respondent conditioning procedure is an appetitive (positive) or aversive (negative) reinforcer, operant conditioning occurs at the same time as respondent conditioning. Similarly, whenever the reinforcer in an operant procedure is an unconditioned stimulus, respondent conditioning proceeds at the same time as operant conditioning. Thus, insofar as the eliciting and reinforcing stimulus classes are composed of the same environmental events, operant and respondent processes are coextensive.

Physiological Relationships and Interactions

The relevance of these basic principles to the methodological developments which have characterized the recent advances in behavioral medicine is perhaps most clearly reflected in the experimental analysis of relationships between such learning and conditioning procedures, on the one hand, and physiological response measures, on the other. For the most part, such investigative activities have emphasized the effects of learning and conditioning procedures upon response measures commonly referred to as "visceral" or autonomic (e.g., heart rate, blood pressure, gastric motility), and can be seen to fall into three broad categories based upon the temporal ordering of behavioral and physiological events. In the first category, respondent or *classical conditioning,* the physiological event that is conditioned appears initially as an unconditional response (e.g., salivation) to an unconditional stimulus (e.g., food) and is subsequently observed to occur (although not necessarily in identical form) during presentation of a conditional stimulus (e.g., bell) which has been paired repeatedly with the unconditional stimulus. The second category, *concurrent learning and conditioning,* is defined by experimental approaches that depend primarily upon operant learning procedures to establish and maintain ongoing performances (e.g., lever pressing) while concurrently measuring physiological changes (e.g., hormone elevations) which show systematic relationships to the instrumental learning behaviors. And in the third category, *instrumental learning,* an essential feature of the procedure emphasizes a contingency relationship between antecedent physiological changes (e.g., heart rate increase) and experimentally programmed environmental consequences (e.g., food delivery and/or shock avoidance). (The procedure has become known, popularly, as biofeedback.)

Over the past decade, animal studies within the framework of these three learning and conditioning paradigms clearly have focused more upon some physiological response systems (e.g., cardiovascular) than others (e.g., gastrointestinal), and this differential emphasis will be necessity be reflected in this summary overview. To a considerable extent, this uneven distribution of physiological measures is a function of the technological and methodological developments which have paced the emergence of a scientifically operational laboratory psychophysiology (Obrist, Black, Brener, et al., 1974). As such advances increase the ease and accessibility of physiological measurement techniques, an ever-broadening range of biological events of direct relevance to behavioral medicine will doubtless be exposed to experimental scrutiny in relationship to learning and conditioning procedures.

CLASSICAL CONDITIONING

The pioneering work of Pavlov and Sherrington has been extended over the past half-century or more and elaborated in numerous volumes which document the effects of classical conditioning procedures upon physiological processes in general (Prokasy, 1965; Razran, 1961; Beecroft, 1966) and autonomic responses, in particular (Ádám, 1967; Dykman, 1967; Harris and Brady, 1974). In the past decade alone, for example, a veritable tidal wave of classical cardiac conditioning studies has all but inundated the literature in this once-pristine area of experimental inquiry. The basic issue posed by the rhetorical question, "Can the heart learn?", has, of course, been addressed extensively, with the answers providing convincing evidence of the wide-ranging variability in the *form* (i.e., acceleration or deceleration) of the classically conditioned cardiac response (Shearn, 1961). Although attempts to examine experimentally the conditions under which such form variations occur have probably contributed more to the complexity of the process than to its clarification, several reports have described a characteristically biphasic cardiac response pattern which emerges after repeated CS-UCS pairings in a range of different laboratory species (Dykman and Gantt, 1958; Schoenfeld, Matos, and Snapper, 1967; Ramsay, 1970). The form in which this pattern has been observed (i.e., an early heart rate acceleration followed by a cardiac deceleration) suggests that separable response components (e.g., "orienting") may participate differentially in the temporal course of such classical cardiovascular conditioning (Kakigi, 1971), and that ongoing behavioral interactions (e.g., "effect of person") may significantly influence the physiological consequences of classical conditioning (Anderson and Gantt, 1966).

Several reports over the past decade have also provided support for the Law of Initial Values (LIV) as a determinant of the physiological effects associated with classical conditioning procedures (Black, Carlson, and Solomon, 1962; Ramsay, 1970; Snapper, Pomerleau, and Schoenfeld, 1969). In all these studies, an inverse relationship was observed between the magnitude of the conditioned heart rate response and the cardiac rate recorded during the time interval immediately preceding the CS presentation. Controlling the pre-CS heart rate with a cardiac pacemaker, however, did not reveal systematic relationships between the classically conditioned heart rate response and the paced pre-CS heart rate level (Snapper et al., 1969), suggesting that the interactions which define the Law of Initial Values effects, so well documented in human cardiovascular conditioning studies (Lacey and Lacey, 1962), probably reflect more the participation of central than peripheral factors.

Of particular etiological significance would appear to be the observation that single-trial classical conditioning can occur as described by Newton and Gantt (1966) in an experiment with dogs in which one CS-UCS (i.e., tone-shock) pairing produced a classically conditioned heart rate response which persisted over extended time intervals during repeated extinction trials involving tone presentations in the absence of shock. Partial reinforcement effects in increasing resistance to extinction of classically conditioned autonomic responses have also been repeatedly confirmed (Fitzgerald, 1966; Wagner, Seigel and Fein, 1967), and discrimination effects have been well documented in experiments which show that the magnitude of the conditioned cardiac response is significantly greater to a CS presentation followed by the UCS than to a CS presentation that has not been followed by the UCS (Paré, 1970; Tighe, Groves, and Riley, 1968).

Other circulatory responses, including blood pressure, blood flow, peripheral vasomotor activity, and catecholamine levels have also been shown to change systematically in relationship to classical conditioning procedures, although the correlations (or lack thereof) between these effects and the differentiation of "orienting" or "startle" components from "true" conditioned autonomic response patterns continue to provide areas of controversy and disagreement (Kakigi, 1971). There are, nonetheless, studies involving determinations made with dogs under both curarized and noncurarized conditions which suggest at least some degree of independence between such classically conditioned cardiovascular responses, on the one hand, and respiratory and skeletal muscle changes, on the other (Newton, 1967).

Clearly, however, the documented role of central regulatory and homeostatic mechanisms for the control of classically conditioned cardiovascular responses would seem to require that a broader biological perspective be maintained with regard to the range of interacting visceral and somatic systems which in concert provide for the adjustments and adaptations of the internal environment. Within this context, for example, the relationship between heart rate and other visceral and motor components of a "total" classically conditioned response has provided the focus for a range of investigative accounts which emphasize both the independent variations of multiple interacting systems (Black, 1965; Yehle, 1968), and the complex interrelationships between such response measures (Hein, 1969; Obrist and Webb, 1967). Probably the most parsimonious view of the complexities involved would recognize that all possible combinations and permutations can and do occur under some circumstances, and that it remains a continuing research challenge to delineate and define the range of independent circumstances under which classical autonomic conditioning effects are established and maintained.

CONCURRENT LEARNING AND CONDITIONING

Although lacking the long-standing and prestigious background enjoyed by classical conditioning, an active and productive research interest in the measurement of performance-related concurrent learning and conditioning effects has emerged over the past several decades. As reviewed initially by Brady (1966) and more recently by Brady and Harris (1976), several groups of laboratory studies in this area have focused upon the experimental production of altered physiological states emphasizing, for the most part, endocrine, cardiovascular, and gastrointestinal changes. Significantly, there has also been an increasing emphasis upon enduringly chronic preparations (Brady, 1965; Findley, Brady, Robinson, et al., 1971; Forsyth, 1969; Herd, Morse, Kelleher, et al., 1969), and aversive control procedures of established effectiveness, including conditioned suppression (Estes and Skinner, 1941) and free-operant avoidance (Sidman, 1953), continue to receive close psychophysiological attention as progressively more refined analysis of observed relationships is reflected in a range of concurrent learning and conditioning studies.

Systematic increases in plasma 17-hydroxycorticosteroid (17-OH-CS) levels have now been described, for example, in relationship to the acquisition of conditioned suppression (i.e., "conditioned emotional response") with monkeys (Mason, Brady, and Tolson, 1966), and the course of cardiovascular changes during the development and maintenance of such conditioned suppression has also been extensively studied in chronically catheterized primates with monitoring of heart rate and both systolic and diastolic blood pressure (Brady, Kelly, and Plumlee, 1969). Dramatic reversals in both the direction and magnitude of such blood pressure and heart rate changes were observed to occur in response to repeated clicker-shock (CS-US) pairings. Initially the development of conditioned behavioral suppression over the first 8 to 10 trials for all five rhesus monkeys in the study was accompanied by a consistent and systematic decrease in both heart rate and blood pressure in response to the 3-minute clicker presentations. Continued daily pairings of clicker and shock superimposed upon the lever-pressing performance, however, produced abrupt and sustained reversals in both the direction and magnitude of the cardiovascular response. Significantly, these changes were observed to persist as large magnitude increases in heart rate and both systolic and diastolic blood pressure in response to the behaviorally suppressing clicker presentations for from 50 to 100 daily conditioning trials. The results were interpreted as reflecting the differential temporal development of the early conditioned emotional response instrumental performance suppression (with the initial cardiovascular "suppression" related to decreases in motor activity during the clicker) followed by the later-appearing "conditioned cardiac respondent" component as sustained cardiovascular activation during clicker presentations. It is also of some interest to contrast the form of these concurrent biphasic cardiovascular changes with the biphasic form of the classically conditioned heart rate response described above. To some extent at least, these several findings provide a basis for explaining the recurrent conflicting reports (DeToledo and Black, 1966; DeVietti and Porter, 1970; Smith and Nathan, 1967; Snapper et al., 1969; Stebbins and Smith, 1964) regarding CER effects upon the cardiovascular system and point conspicuously to the temporal course over which some experimental observations are made as a critical source of contributory variance. More importantly, the results of these studies seem to argue for "causal independence" of the separable but interacting physiological and behavioral responses defining such "emotional" conditioning.

The extended analysis of behaviorally induced endocrine and cardiovascular changes, however, has focused even more extensively upon conditioned avoidance models, predominantly of the free-operant or Sidman variety (Sidman, 1953). In addition to multiple reconfirmations (Brady, 1965, 1967) of the two-fold to four-fold elevations in 17-OH-CS levels associated with even relatively brief, shock-free experimental exposures to this performance requirement, marked differences in the hormone response have been observed (Mason et al., 1966) when the free-operant avoidance procedure includes a discriminable exteroceptive warning signal or when "free" shocks are superimposed upon the performance baseline. Significantly, the corticosteroid response was consistently reduced during "discriminated" avoidance sessions including an exteroceptive auditory stimulus presented 5 seconds before shock whenever 15 seconds had elapsed since a previous response, although removal of the "warning signal" resulted in the immediate reappearance of the steroid elevations. Conversely, superimposing "free" or unavoidable shocks upon a well-established avoidance performance without a "warning signal" has been reported to produce more than a 100% increase over the elevated corticosteroid levels observed during the regular nondiscriminated Sidman avoidance procedure.

Significant advances have also been made in determining the endocrine and cardiovascular consequences of free-operant avoidance performance requirements during long-term studies over months and even years. A report by Brady (1965), for example, describes the effects of repeated exposure to continuous 72-hour avoidance over periods up to, and in some cases exceeding, 1 year upon patterns of thyroid, gonadal, and adrenal hormone secretion in a series of five chair-restrained rhesus monkeys. Two of the five monkeys participated in the 72-hour avoidance experiment on six separate occasions over a 6-month period with an interval of approximately 4 weeks between each exposure. The remaining three animals performed on a schedule which repeatedly programmed 72-hour avoidance cycles followed by a 96-hour nonavoidance or "rest" cycles (3 days "on" and 4 days "off") for periods up to and exceeding 1 year.

The two animals exposed to repeated 72-hour avoidance at monthly intervals for 6 months showed a progressively increasing lever-pressing response rate with each of the six successive 72-hour avoidance sessions. In contrast, shock frequencies over this same period showed a sharp decline within the first two 72-hour avoidance sessions and remained at a stable low level for the remaining four 72-hour avoidance cycles. Hormone changes related to the repeated 72-hour avoidance cycles showed consistent and replicable patterns over the 6-month experimental period for both animals. During the initial experimental sessions both monkeys showed approximately three-fold elevations in 17-OH-CS levels during 72-hour avoidance and returned to near baseline levels about 6 days afterward. The remaining four monthly experiments were characterized by substantial, although diminished, steroid responses (approximately two-fold elevations in 17-OH-CS levels) during avoidance, with essentially the same 6-day period required for recovery to basal levels. Significant changes related to the extended avoidance performance were also observed in catecholamine, gonadal, and thyroid hormone levels, with recovery cycles extending in some instances (thyroid) for 3 weeks following the 72-hour avoidance period. A detailed experimental and interpretive analysis of such multiple hormone changes induced by exposure to the 72-hour Sidman procedure has been provided in an exhaustive multi-authored monograph (Mason, 1968) describing this most systematic laboratory study series yet to appear in the psychoendocrine literature.

The three remaining monkeys described in the Brady (1965) report as performing on the 3 days "on", 4 days "off" avoidance schedule showed an initial increase in lever-pressing response rates for approximately the first 10 avoidance sessions similar to that seen with the two animals described above. By approximately the 20th weekly session with these animals, however, lever-pressing response rates during the 72-hour avoidance period had decreased to a value well below that observed during the initial avoidance sessions, and the performance tended to stabilize at this new low level for the ensuing weeks of the experiment. In contrast, shock frequencies for all animals quickly approximated a stable low level within the first two or three exposures to the avoidance schedule and seldom exceeded a rate of two shocks per hour for the remainder of the experiment. The initial 72-hour avoidance sessions were also characterized by significant elevations in 17-OH-CS levels. In the succeeding weeks, 17-OH-CS levels gradually declined but rose again by the 30th week. The general pattern obtained was replicated with all three animals with only minor variations, although the change in responsivity of the pituitary-adrenal system to the avoidance stress with continued exposure to this procedure over extended time periods was perhaps the most consistent and striking observation. These findings are somewhat at variance with the repeated observations made in many previous acute studies (Brady, 1965, 1966; Mason, et al., 1966) of a close positive relationship between steroid elevations and avoidance performance and indicate that continued exposure to this repeated performance requirement on the time schedule programmed in this experiment produces an apparent dissociation between the avoidance performance and the 17-OH-CS response. Although a definitive analysis of such interactions is not possible on the basis of these data alone, a critical role of the temporal parameters (work-rest cycles) is clearly indicated, and the relationship of these phasic hormone changes to the previously described classical and concurrent cardiovascular conditioning effects would seem to require detailed investigation.

A trend toward more extended periods of experimental observation and measurement has been apparent also in concurrent avoidance studies focusing upon cardiovascular changes, particularly in primates. Both rhesus (Forsyth, 1969) and squirrel monkeys (Herd et al., 1969) have been reported to develop hypertensive blood pressure levels with recurrent exposure to free-operant avoidance requirements for periods up to and exceeding 12 months. Chair-restrained baboons (Findley, Robinson and Gilliam, 1971) performing on a discrete-trial fixed-ratio instrumental escape-avoidance procedure, however, were not found to maintain elevated blood pressure levels over the year or more during which they participated in the study (Findley et al., 1971). Indeed, the baboons in this extended study did show substantial pressure increases during the actual escape-avoidance performance intervals within the daily experimental sessions, and there were some periods during the first several months on the program which were characterized by general elevations in both blood pressure and heart rate. However, the chronically high cardiac output levels (i.e., heart rate) maintained apparently by the extended exposure to work-activity requirements of the ratio escape-avoidance schedule in this study suggest a potentially important "physical exercise" factor which may account, at least in part, for the long-term return to normotensive pressure levels not recovered in previous studies (Forsyth, 1969; Herd et al., 1969) with exposures of comparable duration to less demanding free-operant avoidance requirements.

A recent series of studies on cardiovascular changes associated with operant avoidance procedures (Anderson and Brady, 1971; Anderson and Tosheff, 1973) provides further evidence which is at least consistent with the hypothesized relationship between muscle activity and the dynamic interplay between cardiac output and peripheral resistance in the behavioral pathogenesis of hypertensive conditions. The focus of these studies with dogs has been upon continuous monitoring of blood pressure and heart rate during free-operant (panel press) shock avoidance and, significantly, during a fixed-interval pre-avoidance period systematically programmed to precede the required avoidance performance. Under these conditions, a unique divergence between heart rate and blood pressure changes was observed during pre-avoidance intervals up to 15 hours in length, with virtually all animals showing a characteristic systolic and diastolic increase accompanied by either a decrease or no change in heart rate. Comparisons involving similar performance requirements on a variable-interval *food* reinforcement schedule revealed a markedly different pre-performance cardiovascular pattern characterized by systematic increases in both heart rate and blood pressure. This differential "preparatory" pattern was confirmed both between individual animals maintained separately on each of the procedures and "within" the same animal alternately performing on the avoidance and food reinforcement schedule. Moreover, direct measurements of cardiac output in dogs prepared with aortic flow probes during exposure to the avoidance program confirmed that the pre-avoidance pressure changes were attributable to increased peripheral resistance, while the pressure increases during the avoidance performance per se occurred as the peripheral resistance was actually observed to decrease and the cardiac output increased markedly. Additional studies involving β-adrenergic blockade with the drug propranolol during the same experimental procedure, however, clearly showed that peripheral resistance levels do increase to maintain elevated pressure levels during avoidance when drug-induced heart rate reductions produce decreases in cardiac output (Anderson and Brady, 1973).

The results of these experiments establish firm relationships between a broad range of endocrine and cardiovascular response processes and free-operant behavioral performances. Both general and specific support for these findings have now been provided by numerous published reports with rodents, carnivores, and primates (Banks, Miller, and Ogawa, 1966; Black, 1959; Brady, 1967; Forsyth, 1968; Kelleher, Morse, and Herd, 1972; Mason, Brady, and Rose, 1969; Miller, Banks, and Caul, 1967; Morse, Herd, Kelleher, et al., 1971; Stern and Word, 1962; Swadlow, Hosking, and Schneiderman, 1971). In many respects, the changes in the absolute levels of selected hormones and autonomic activity can be viewed as reflecting relatively undifferential consequences of arousal states associated with behavioral responses under aversive conditions. The definite temporal course of visceral and steroid changes under such conditions and the quantitative nature of the relationship between degree of behavioral involvement and level of physiological response have been well documented. In addition, the critical role of an organism's behavioral history in determining the nature and extent of autonomic-endocrine response to performance situations has been convincingly demonstrated. Clearly, however, the most meaningful dimension for hormone and visceral analysis in relationship to more chronic behavioral interactions would appear to be the broader patterning or balance of secretory and visceral changes in many interdependent autonomic and endocrine systems which in concert regulate metabolic events. The extensive and prolonged participation of these fundamental systems in behavioral interactions suggests a relationship between such physiological activity and the more durable consequences of performances under aversive control. Indeed, the differentiation of such autonomic-endocrine response patterns in relationship to the historical and situational aspects of behavioral events may well provide a first approximate step in the direction of identifying distinguishable intra-organismic consequences associated with both episodic and persistent behavioral interactions.

The concurrent learning and conditioning research literature concerned with physiological relationships and interactions also reflects an abiding interest in the effects of such behavioral processes upon the gastrointestinal system (Ader, 1971). Of particular interest would seem to be the rather prominent controversy over the factors that influence the incidence of peptic ulcers in rodents and primates under aversive behavioral control. Some further support for the efficacy of "conflict" and related conditioning procedures in the production of gastric lesions in laboratory rats has been provided by studies focusing upon a variety of social-psychological and physiological parameters (Sawrey and Sawrey, 1966), but replication and confirmation of the reported relationships continue to present problems (Ader, Beels, and Tatum, 1960). Similarly, recurrent descriptions of avoidance conditioning effects upon the gastrointesinal system have characteristically presented something less than a consistent picture with regard specifically to the conditions under which erosions of the gastric mucosa are most likely to occur. The reported incidence of peptic ulcers in rhesus monkeys intermittently exposed to a free-operant shock-avoidance procedure (Brady, Porter, Conrad, et al., 1958) has proved difficult to repeat under some laboratory conditions (Folz and Miller, 1964), including those under which the study originated (Brady, 1964). Additionally, several investigations with laboratory rats on escape-avoidance procedures have failed to find an incidence of gastric lesions in experimental animals which exceeded that of controls, and in some instances yoked control animals receiving unavoidable shocks alone showed a greater degree of ulceration than their avoiding partners (Moot, Cebulla, and Crabtree, 1970; Weiss, 1971a).

To some extent, a clarification and at least partial reconciliation of these apparently conflicting developments in the delineation of concurrent learning and conditioning effects upon the gastrointestinal system has been suggested by Weiss (1970, 1971b). Starting with the observation that laboratory rats receiving intermittent tail shock following presentation of a 10-second beeping tone developed significantly less gastric ulceration than animals receiving the same shock without the "predictability" provided by the pre-aversive "warning" stimulus, Weiss examined the effects of adding an operant escape-avoidance ("coping") panel-press to the procedure. Under these conditions markedly fewer gastric lesions were found in the experimental animals when compared with "helpless" controls similarly exposed to warning signals and shocks (one per minute for 21 hours) but without escape-avoidance responses. When the interactions between warning signals and the escape-avoidance responses were tested in a subsequent experiment involving groups differentiating between two types of pre-aversive stimuli ("beeping" tone and an "added clock"), presence or absence of escape-avoidance wheel-turning, and appropriate "yoked" controls, the results provided a basis for reconciling the apparent contradictions between the rat and monkey studies. While the outcome of this rather mammoth 180-rat experiment confirmed the prepotence of the operant escape-avoidance conditioning in reducing the incidence of ulcers, the addition of a warning signal to the procedure was found to attenuate the development of gastric pathology even further. It is of some interest to note that a similar warning stimulus procedure has been found to reduce the steroid response to operant avoidance performance requirements in the monkey (Mason et al., 1966).

In Weiss' view, these findings indicate that the incidence of peptic ulcers may be a function of the interaction between strength of the escape-avoidance performance (i.e., the frequency of "coping" responses) and the probability of discriminable response-contingent signals associated with the absence of aversive stimuli (i.e., "feedback" about shock-free conditions). Within the framework of this interpretive analysis, the incidence of peptic ulcers in free-operant avoidance monkeys would be accounted for in terms of a high response frequency in the absence of warning stimuli and the relatively low "feedback" discriminability of "safe" signals produced by those responses. The yoked-control monkeys, in contrast, characteristically emitted "avoidance" responses only infrequently, received only a few shocks well distributed in time (due to the high performance rates of the experimental animals), and were found to be free of gastrointestinal pathology. Some further confirmation of this formulation has been provided by Weiss in a subsequent series of experimental manipulations which increased the frequency of ulcers in avoidance rats punished with shock for responding, and decreased the incidence of ulcers in animals producing a brief tone with each shock-postponing panel-press (Weiss, 1971b,c).

INSTRUMENTAL LEARNING

Laboratory studies concerned with the experimental analysis of instrumental physiological learning effects represent a relatively recent development in the basic science foundations of behavioral medicine (Harris and Brady, 1974). The systematic series of investigations undertaken at Yale in the mid-1960's by Miller and his colleagues (Miller and Carmona, 1967; Miller and DiCara, 1967), for example, can be seen to have activated a productive decade of "operant" learning research involving visceral and autonomic processes. There were, of course, notable precedents established in the earlier human experimental literature (Kimmel, 1967), and many reports had previously appeared on the "voluntary" control of physiological responses by yoga and related meditative techniques (Wenger and Bagchi, 1961). However, the significant recent advances of laboratory animal research in this area would seem to be attributable, at least in part, to the prominent experimental focus upon explicit contingency relationships between specific antecedent physiological events, on the one hand, and programmed environmental consequences, on the other.

The initial animal instrumental physiological learning experiments by Miller and Carmona (1967) showed that marked increases in salivation could be produced in fluid-deprived dogs given access to water contingent upon such salivatory responses. The magnitude of this effect was emphasized by the 14-fold difference in salivation rate between these animals and similarly deprived dogs given water only when no salivation occurred. This dramatic instrumental physiological learning effect has been confirmed more recently in an experiment using food to operantly reinforce *decreases* in salivation (Shapiro and Herendeen, 1975), the results contrasting sharply with well-documented classical conditioning effects in the opposite direction. Equally convincing demonstrations of instrumental heart rate learning have emphasized the bidirectional control over both increases and decreases in cardiac rate which can be established in laboratory rats (DiCara and Miller, 1969) and rhesus monkeys (Engel and Gottlieb, 1970), while large magnitude, enduring heart-rate elevations have been operantly conditioned in dog-faced baboons (Harris, Gilliam, and Brady, 1976).

The specificity of physiological response effects suggested by such instrumental learning studies has, in fact, been documented in operant conditioning experiments showing independent control of heart rate and intestinal contractions (Miller and Banuazizi, 1968). Instrumentally learned increases or decreases in the P-R interval of the EKG has also been shown to be independent of changes in the P-P interval (Fields, 1970). Perhaps the most dramatic demonstration of such specificity, however, is the reported selective instrumental learning of vasomotor tone increases in one ear of the laboratory rat and vasomotor tone decreases in the other ear of the same animal (DiCara and Miller, 1968). Significantly, these instrumentally learned blood flow changes were not correlated with heart rate, rectal temperature, or vasomotor tone in the tail, suggesting a remarkable and previously unrecognized localization of sympathetic action. Subsequent replications and confirmations of these findings with respect to the specificity of instrumentally learned physiological responses have included the observation that operantly conditioned blood pressure effects can occur independently of changes in heart rate and skeletal muscle activity (Pappas, DiCara, and Miller, 1970).

Instrumental learning experiments have also focused upon the analysis of bidirectional changes in blood pressure with both rats (Pappas et al., 1970) and monkeys (Benson, Herd, Morse, et al., 1969), and impressive operantly conditioned blood pressure elevations of large magnitude have been reported with the dog-faced baboon (Harris, Findley, and Brady, 1971). Significantly, these latter studies involved the application of operant "shaping" techniques with both the amplitude and duration of blood pressure elevations required to avoid shock and obtain food systematically increased in small progressive steps to diastolic pressure levels 50 to 60 mm Hg above resting levels. More chronic studies of instrumentally learned blood pressure changes with the baboon have emphasized the analysis of such procedures under conditions which provide for enduring elevations of 25 to 30 mm Hg above baseline during daily 12-hour "conditioning" sessions alternating with 12-hour "rest" periods (Harris, Gilliam, Findley, et al., 1973). Figure 2.1, for example, shows the stable response pattern (right-hand panel) developed after exposure to such daily instrumental blood pressure learning sessions for 2 to 3 months. Characteristically, sustained elevations of 30 mm Hg or more in both systolic and diastolic blood pressure were maintained throughout the 12-hour "conditioning on" periods accompanied by elevated but progressively decreasing heart rate over the course of the 12-hour interval. During the ensuing 12-hour "conditioning off" recovery period, heart rate continued to fall somewhat precipitiously, and blood pressure returned to approximately basal levels (or slightly above) within 6 to 8 hours. That these large magnitude sustained elevations in blood pressure were related directly and specifically to the programmed contingency requirements of the instrumental learning procedure was further confirmed by the results obtained with an additional group of baboons in the same experiment exposed to virtually identical conditions except that food reward and shock avoidance were made contingent upon *decreases* in blood pressure. Extended exposure (i.e., 6 months or more) to this instrumental blood pressure lowering procedure (including exposure to all of the same surgery and chronic catheterization, confinement and chair restraint, food deprivation and reward, and, of course, electric shocks) was observed to produce only small (i.e., nonsignificant) *decreases* in blood pressure under the same general laboratory conditions prevailing for the animals which showed instrumentally learned blood pressure elevations.

The role of autonomic mediation in these operantly conditioned circulatory changes has also been evaluated by assessing the effects of specific pharmacological α- and β-adrenergic blockers on the instrumentally learned blood pressure increases in

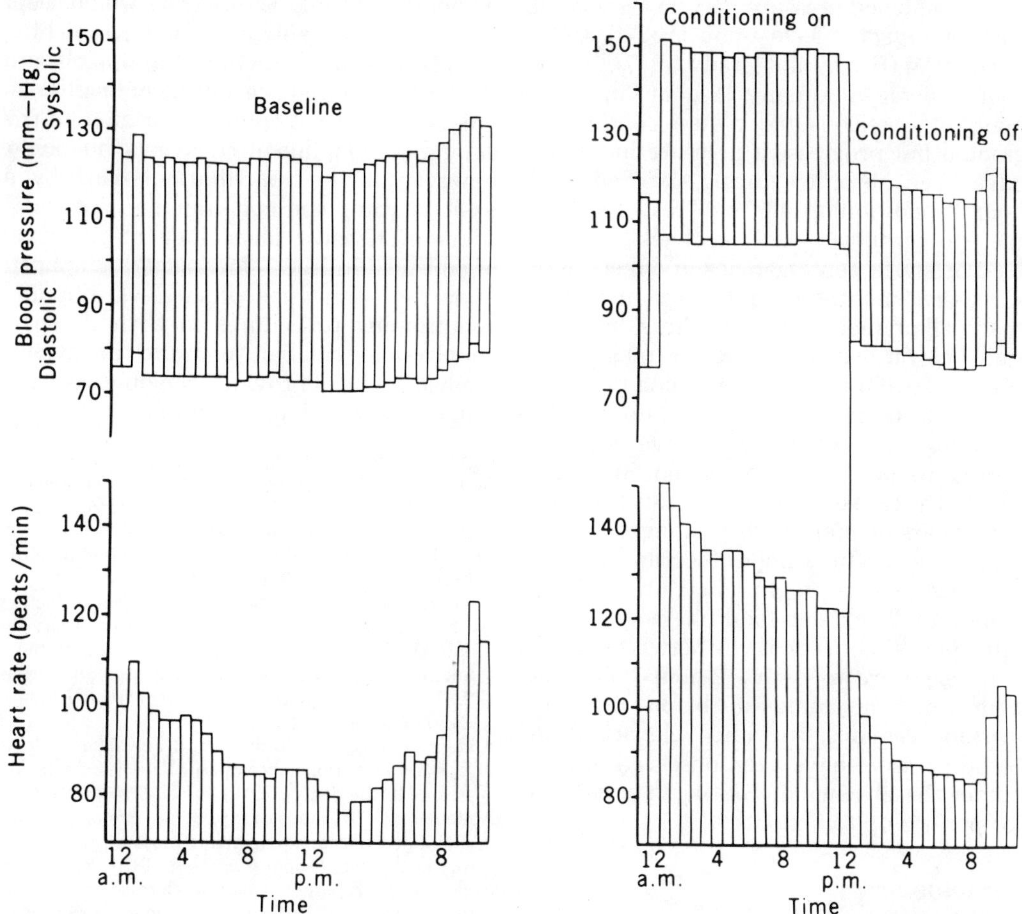

Figure 2.1. Average blood pressure and heart rate values for four baboons over consecutive 40-minute intervals during sixteen pre-experimental baseline determinations (left panel) compared with sixteen 12-hour conditioning on, 12-hour conditioning off sessions (right panel) (Harris et al., 1973).

baboons (Goldstein, Harris, and Brady, 1977a). β-Adrenergic blockade, for example completely eliminated the heart rate increases accompanying instrumentally learned blood pressure elevations without attenuating the pressure increase. Similarly, α-blockade of adrenergically mediated peripheral vasoconstriction did not significantly alter the instrumentally learned blood pressure elevation response. Although combined α-and β-adrenergic blockade did substantially reduce the magnitude of the operant blood pressure increase, the continued appearance of a significant instrumentally learned elevation in both systolic and diastolic blood pressure despite combined blockade suggests nonadrenergic participation in such instrumental autonomic learning effects. In addition, the sensitivity of the arterial baroreflex changes systematically in relation to the instrumental blood pressure learning procedure with marked *decreases* during the 12-hour conditioning sessions occurring in the context of significant *increases* during the rest periods as compared to initial pre-experimental baseline baroreceptor sensitivity levels (Goldstein, Harris, and Brady, 1977b).

Of particular importance would seem to be the observations made over the past several years with the baboons in these instrumental blood pressure learning studies which suggest that continued exposure to such recurrent experimental procedures involving sustained large-magnitude increases in blood pressure may be associated with emergent effects upon the "resting" circulation (Harris and Brady, 1977). In the course of repeated daily 12-hour "on", 12-hour "off" sessions under these conditions, gradual but progressive pressure increases have been observed during the daily 12-hour "conditioning off" or "rest" periods (i.e., no cardiovascular "feedback" and no food or shock contingencies in effect) over successive months of the program in virtually all animals. Although these "rest period" elevations are of lesser magnitude (i.e., 15–20 mm Hg) than the blood pressure increases observed during the 12-hour "conditioning on" sessions, they have been reported to persist for extended intervals. And in the case of selected animals followed for 2 years or more with prolonged "vacations" (i.e., no instrumental cardiovascular learning sessions programmed, no feedback stimuli or shock, and food freely available) interspersed between the otherwise continuous exposure to daily 12-hour "on", 12-hour "off" instrumental blood pressure learning sessions, sustained elevations in blood pressure have been observed to persist in the absence of contingency control for periods up to 5 months.

Conclusion

There are, of course, many unresolved procedural, interpretive, and theoretical problems in the analysis of learning and conditioning processes which bear importantly upon the basic and applied aspects of behavioral medicine. The prominent focus upon "mediational" issues, for example, has not only generated physiological controversies about interrelationship between autonomic-visceral and somato-motor mechanisms (e.g., DiCara, 1970; Black, 1968), but has as well emphasized the need to reexamine some of the conventional distinctions between types of learning and conditioning (e.g., Schoenfeld, 1972). Disagreements regarding mechanism and methodology notwithstanding, the evidence that learning and conditioning procedures, however mediated, can exert orderly and systematic effects upon the functional characteristics of biochemical, anatomical, and physiological systems seems incontrovertible. Clearly, the experimental analysis of such interactions involving behavioral and somatic processes would seem to hold considerable promise for enriching both laboratory and clinical approaches to the treatment and preventing of health disorders. Of at least equal importance to the emerging discipline of behavioral medicine, however, is the contribution made by a basic learning and conditioning analysis to a comprehensive physiology of the total organism. Indeed, increasing emphasis upon the application of such learning and conditioning procedures in both the psychophysiology laboratory and behavioral medicine clinic provides tangible recognition of this developing frontier.

References

Ádám, G. *Interoception and Behavior.* Budapest, Hungary: Akademiai Kiado Publishing House of the Hungarian Academy of Sciences, 1967.

Ader, R. Experimentally induced gastric lesions. *Adv. Psychosom. Med.,* 1971, *6,* 1–39.

Ader, R., Beels, C. C., and Tatum, R. Social factors affecting emotionality and resistance to disease in animals. I. Susceptibility to gastric ulceration as a function of interruptions in social interactions and the time at which they occur. *J. Comp. Physiol. Psychol.,* 1960, *53,* 455–458.

Anderson, D. E., and Brady, J. V. Pre-avoidance blood pressure elevations accompanied by heart rate decreases in the dog. *Science,* 1971, *172,* 595–597.

Anderson, D. E., and Brady, J. V. Prolonged pre-avoidance effects upon blood pressure and heart rate in the dog. *Psychosom. Med.,* 1973, *35,* 4–12.

Anderson, D. E., and Tosheff, J. Cardiac output and total peripheral resistance changes during pre-avoidance periods in the dog. *J. Appl. Psychol.,* 1973, *34,* 650–654.

Anderson, S., and Gantt, W. H. The effect of person on cardiac and motor responsivity to shock in dogs. *Conditional Reflex,* 1966, *1,* 181–189.

Astrup, C. *Pavlovian Psychiatry.* Springfield, Ill.: Charles C Thomas, 1965.

Ayllon, T., and Azrin, N. H. The measurement and reinforcement of behavior of psychotics. *J. Exp. Anal. Behav.,* 1965, *8,* 357–383.

Ayllon, T., and Azrin, N. H. *The Token Economy.* New York: Appleton-Century-Crofts, 1968.

Banks, J. H., Miller, R. E., and Ogawa, N. The development of discriminated autonomic and instrumental responses during avoidance conditioning in the rhesus monkey. *J. Genet. Psychol.,* 1966, *108,* 199–211.

Bechterev, V. *General principles of reflexology,* Translation: E. Murphy and W. Murphy. London: Hutchinson, 1932.

Beecroft, R. S. *Classical conditioning.* Goleta, Calif.: Psychonomic Press, 1966.

Benson, H., Herd, J. A., Morse, W. H., and Kelleher, R. T. Behavioral inductions of arterial hypertension and its reversal. *Am. J. Physiol.,* 1969, *217,* 30–34.

Black, A. H. Heart rate changes during avoidance learning in dogs. *Can. J. Psychol.,* 1959, *13,* 229–242.

Black, A. H. Cardiac conditioning in curarized dogs: The relationship between heart rate and skeletal behavior. In W. F. Prokasy (Ed.), *Classical conditioning: A symposium.* New York: Appleton-Century-Crofts, 1965.

Black, A. H. Operant conditioning of autonomic responses. *Conditional Reflex,* 1968, *3,* 130.

Black, A. H., Carlson, N. J., and Solomon, R. L. Exploratory studies of the conditioning of autonomic responses in curarized dogs. *Psychol. Monogr.,* 1962, *76* (29, Whole No. 548), 1-31.

Brady, J. V. Behavioral stress and physiological change: A comparative approach to the experimental analysis of some psychosomatic problems. *Trans. N.Y. Acad. Sci.,* 1964, *26,* 483-496.

Brady, J. V. Experimental studies of psychophysiological responses to stressful situations. In *Symposium on Medical Aspects of Stress in the Military Climate,* Walter Reed Army Institute of Research. Washington, D.C.: United States Government Printing Office, 1965.

Brady, J. V. Operant methodology and the production of altered physiological states. In W. Honig (Ed.), *Operant behavior: Areas of research and application.* New York: Appleton-Century Crofts, 1966.

Brady, J. V. Emotion and the sensitivity of the psychoendocrine systems. In D. Glass (Ed.), *Neurophysiology and emotion.* New York: The Rockefeller University Press, 1967.

Brady, J. V., and Harris, A. H. The experimental production of altered physiological states. In W. K. Honig and J. E. R. Staddon (Eds.), *Handbook of Operant Behavior.* Englewood Cliffs, N.J.: Prentice-Hall, 1976.

Brady, J. V., Kelly, D., and Plumlee, L. Autonomic and behavioral responses of the rhesus monkey to emotional conditioning. *Ann. N.Y. Acad. Sci.,* 1969, *159,* 959-975.

Brady, J. V., Porter, R., Conrad, D., and Mason, J. Avoidance behavior and the development of gastroduodenal ulcers. *J. Exp. Anal. Behav.,* 1958, *1,* 69-72.

DeToledo, L., and Black, A. H. Heart rate: Changes during conditioned suppression in rats. *Science,* 1966, *152,* 1404-1406.

DeVietti, T. L., and Porter, P. B. Heart rate response during aversive conditioning. *Psychol. Rep.,* 1970, *27,* 651-658.

DiCara, L. V. Learning in the autonomic nervous system. *Sci. Am.,* 1970, *222* (1), 30-39.

DiCara, L. V., and Miller, N. E. Instrumental learning of vasomotor responses by rats: Learning to respond differentially in the two ears. *Science,* 1968, *159,* 1485-1486.

DiCara, L. V., and Miller, N. E. Transfer of instrumentally learned heart rate changes from curarized to noncurarized state: Implications for a mediational hypothesis. *J. Comp. Physiol. Psychol.,* 1969, *62* (2, Part 1), 159-162.

Dykman, R. A. On the nature of classical conditioning. In C. C. Brown (Ed.), *Methods in psychophysiology.* Baltimore, Williams & Wilkins, 1967.

Dykman, R. A., and Gantt, W. H. Cardiovascular conditioning in dogs and in humans. In W. H. Gantt (Ed.), *Physiological Bases of Psychiatry.* Springfield, Ill.: Charles C Thomas, 1958.

Engel, B. T., and Gottlieb, S. H. Differential operant conditioning of heart rate in the restrained monkey. *J. Comp. Physiol. Psychol.,* 1970, *73,* 217-225.

Estes, W. K., and Skinner, B. F. Some quantitative properties of anxiety. *J. Exp. Psychol.,* 1941, *29,* 390-400.

Eysenck, H. J. Discussion on the role of the psychologist in psychoanalytic practice: The psychologist as technician. *Proc. R. Soc. Med.,* 1952, *45,* 447-449.

Ferster, C. B., and DeMeyer, M. K. The development of performances in autistic children in an automatically-controlled environment. *J. Chronic Dis.,* 1961, *13,* 312-345.

Fields, C. Instrumental conditioning of the rat cardiac control systems. *Proc. Nat. Acad. Sci.,* 1970, *65,* 293-299.

Findley, J. D., Brady, J. V., Robinson, W. W., and Gilliam, W. Continuous cardiovascular monitoring in the baboon during long-term behavioral performances. *Commun. Behav. Biol.,* 1971, *6,* 49-58.

Findley, J. D., Robinson, W. W., and Gilliam, W. A restraint system for chronic study of the baboon. *J. Exp. Anal. Behav.,* 1971, *15,* 69-71.

Fitzgerald, R. D. Some effects of partial reinforcement with shock on classically conditioned heart rate in dogs. *Am. J. Psychol.,* 1966, *79,* 242-249.

Folz, E. L., and Miller, F. E. Experimental psychosomatic disease states in monkeys. I. Peptic ulcer "executive monkeys." *J. Surg. Res.,* 1964, *4,* 445-453.

Forsyth, R. P. Blood pressure and avoidance conditioning. *Psychosom. Med.,* 1968, *30,* 125-135.

Forsyth, R. P. Blood pressure responses to long-term avoidance schedules in the restrained rhesus monkey. *Psychosom. Med.,* 1969, *31,* 300-309.

Gantt, W. H. *Experimental basis of neurotic behavior.* New York: Hoeber-Harper, 1944.

Goldstein, D. S., Harris, A. H., and Brady, J. V. Sympathetic adrenergic blockade effects upon operantly conditioned blood pressure elevations in baboons. *Biofeedback Self Regulation,* 1977a, *2,* 93-105.

Goldstein, D. S., Harris, A. H., and Brady, J. V. Baroreflex sensitivity during operant blood pressure conditioning. *Biofeedback Self Regulation,* 1977b, *2,* 127-138.

Harris, A. H., and Brady, J. V. Animal learning: Visceral and autonomic conditioning. *Annu. Rev. Psychol.,* 1974, *25,* 107-133.

Harris, A. H., and Brady, J. V. Long-term studies of cardiovascular control in primates. In G. E. Schwartz and J. Beatty (Eds.), *Biofeedback: Theory and research,* New York: Academic Press, 1977.

Harris, A. H., Findley, J. D., and Brady, J. V. Instrumental conditioning of blood pressure elevations in the baboon. *Conditional Reflex,* 1971, *6,* 215-226.

Harris, A. H., Gilliam, W. J., and Brady, J. V. Operant conditioning of large magnitude 12-hour heart rate elevations in the baboon. *Pavlovian J. Biol. Sci.,* 1976, *11,* 86-92.

Harris, A. H., Gilliam, W. J., Findley, J. D., and Brady, J. V. Instrumental conditioning of large magnitude daily 12-hour blood pressure elevations in the baboon. *Science,* 1973, *183,* 175.

Hein, P. L. Heart rate conditioning in the cat and its relationship to other physiological responses. *Psychophysiology,* 1969, *5,* 455-464.

Herd, J. A., Morse, W. H., Kelleher, R. T., and Jones, L. G. Arterial hypertension in the squirrel monkey during behavioral experiments. *Am. J Physiol.,* 1969, *217,* 24-29.

Honig, W. K. (Ed.). *Operant behavior: Areas of research and application.* New York: Appleton-Century-Crofts, 1966.

Honig, W. K., and Staddon, J. E. R. (Eds). *Handbook of operant behavior.* Englewood Cliffs, N.J.: Prentice Hall, 1976.

Ivanov-Smolensky, A. G. The pathology of conditioned reflexes and the so-called psychogenic depression. *J. Nerv. Ment. Dis.,* 1928, *67,* 346–350.

Jones, M. C. The elimination of children's fears. *J. Exp. Psychol.,* 1924, *7,* 382–390.

Kakigi, S. Cardiovascular generalization and differentiation—The relationship between heart rate and blood pressure. *Conditional Reflex,* 1971, *6,* 191–204.

Kelleher, R., Morse, W., and Herd, J. A. Effects of propanolol, phentolamine, and methylatropine on cardiovascular function in the squirrel monkey during behavioral experiments. *J. Pharmacol. Exp. Ther.,* 1972, *182,* 204.

Kimmel, H. D. Instrumental conditioning of autonomically mediated behavior. *Psychol. Bull.,* 1967, *67,* 337–345.

Krasnagorski, N. I. Physiology of cerebral activity in children as a new subject of pediatric investigation. *Am. J. Dis. Child.,* 1933, *46,* 473–494.

Lacey, J. L., and Lacey, B. C. The law of initial values in the longitudinal study of autonomic constitution: Reproducibility of autonomic responses and response patterns over a four-year interval. *Ann. N.Y. Acad. Sci.,* 1962, *98,* 1257–1289.

Liddell, H. S. The experimental neuroses and the problem of mental anguish. *Am. J. Psychiatry,* 1938, *94,* 1035–1043.

Lindsley, O. R., and Skinner, B. F. A method for the experimental analysis of behavior of psychotic patients. *Am. Psychol.,* 1954, *9,* 419–420.

London, P. The end of ideology in behavior modification. *Am. Psychol.,* October 1972, 913–920.

Mason, J. W. Organization of psychoendocrine mechanisms. *Psychosom. Med.,* 1968, *30,* 565–808.

Mason, J. W., Brady, J. V., and Rose, R. M. Adrenal responses to maternal separation and chair adaptation in experimentally-raised rhesus monkeys (*Macaca mulatta*). *Proc. Second Int. Congress Primatol.,* 1969, *1,* 211–218.

Mason, J. W., Brady, J. V., and Tolson, W. W. Behavioral adaptations and endocrine activity. In R. Levine (Ed.), *Proceedings of the association for research in nervous and mental diseases.* Baltimore, Williams & Wilkins, 1966.

Masserman, J. H. *Behavior and neurosis.* Chicago: University of Chicago Press, 1943.

Miller, N. E., Banks, J. H., and Caul, W. F. Cardiac conditioned responses in avoidance and yoked-control rats. *Psychosom. Sci.,* 1967, *9,* 581–582.

Miller, N. E., and Banuazizi, A. Instrumental learning by curarized rats of a specific visceral response, intestinal or cardiac. *J. Comp. Physiol. Psychol.,* 1968, *65,* 1–7.

Miller, N. E., and Carmona, A. Modification of a visceral response, salivation in thirsty dogs, by instrumental training with water reward. *J. Comp. Physiol. Psychol.,* 1967, *63,* 1–6.

Miller, N. E., and DiCara, L. Instrumental learning of heart rate changes in curarized rats: Shaping, and specificity to a discriminative stimulus. *J. Comp. Physiol Psychol.,* 1967, *63,* 12–19.

Moot, S. A., Cebulla, R. P., and Crabtree, J. M. Instrumental control and ulceration in rats. *J. Comp. Physiol. Psychol.,* 1970, *71,* 405–410.

Morse, W. H., Herd, J. A., Kelleher, R. T., and Gross, S. A. Schedule-controlled modulation of arterial blood pressure in the squirrel monkey. In H. Kimmel (Ed.), *Experimental psychopathology: Recent research and theory.* New York: Academic Press, 1971.

Mowrer, O. H., and Mowrer, W. M. Enuresis—A method for its study and treatment. *Am. J. Orthopsychiatry,* 1938, *8,* 436–459.

Newton, J. E. Blood pressure and heart rate changes during conditioning in curarized dogs. *Conditional Reflex,* 1967, *2,* 158.

Newton, J. E., and Gantt, W. H. One trial cardiac conditioning in dogs. *Conditional Reflex,* 1966, *1,* 251–265.

Obrist, P. A., Black. A. H., Brener, J., and DiCara, L. V. (Eds.). *Cardiovascular psychophysiology.* Chicago: Aldine Publishing Co., 1974.

Obrist, P. A., and Webb, R. A. Heart rate during conditioning in dogs: Relationship to somatic-motor activity. *Psychophysiology,* 1967, *4,* 7–34.

Pappas, B. A., DiCara, L. V., and Miller, N. E. Learning of blood pressure responses in the noncurarized rat: Transfer to the curarized state. *Physiol. Behav.,* 1970, *5,* 1029–1032.

Paré, W. P. The development of a three-stimulus cardiac discrimination problem in three mammalian species. *Psychophysiology,* 1970, *6,* 629–630.

Pavlov, I. P. *Conditioned reflexes,* Translation: G. V. Anrep. London: Oxford University Press, 1927.

Pavlov, I. P. Lectures on conditioned reflexes, Translation: W. H. Gantt. New York: International Press, 1928.

Prokasy, W. F. (Ed.). *Classical conditioning: A symposium.* New York: Appleton-Century-Crofts, 1965.

Rachlin, H. *Introduction to modern behaviorism.* San Francisco, W. H. Freeman and Company, 1970.

Ramsay, D. A. Form and characteristics of the cardiovascular conditional response in rhesus monkeys. *Conditional Reflex,* 1970, *5,* 36–51.

Razran, G. The observable unconscious and the inferable conscious in current Soviet psychophysiology: Interoception conditioning, semantic conditioning, and the orienting reflex. *Psychol. Rev.,* 1961, *68,* 81–147.

Sawrey, J. M. and Sawrey, W. L. Age, weight, and social effects on ulceration rate in rats. *J. Comp. Physiol. Psychol.,* 1966, *61,* 464–466.

Schoenfeld, W. N. Problems of modern behavior theory. *Conditional Reflex,* 1972, *7,* 33–65.

Schoenfeld, W. N., Matos, M. A., and Snapper, A. C. Cardiac conditioning in the white rat with food presentation as unconditional stimulus. *Conditional Reflex,* 1967, *2,* 56–67.

Shapiro, M. B. An experimental approach to diagnostic psychological testing. *J. Ment. Sci.,* 1951, *97,* 748–764.

Shapiro, M. B. The single case in fundamental clinical psychological research. *Br. J. Med. Psychol.,* 1961, *34,* 255–262.

Shapiro, M. M., and Herendeen, D. L. Food-reinforced inhibition of conditioned salivation in dogs. *J. Comp. Physiol. Psychol.,* 1975, *88,* 628–632.

Shearn, D. W. Does the heart learn? *Psychol. Bull.,* 1961, *58,* 452–458.

Sherrington, C. S. *The integrative action of the nervous system,* 1947 ed. Cambridge: Cambridge University Press, 1906.

Sidman, M. Avoidance conditioning with brief shock

and no exteroceptive warning signal. *Science*, 1953, *118*, 157–158.

Skinner, B. F. *The behavior of organisms*. New York: Appleton-Century-Crofts, 1938.

Skinner, B. F. *Science and human behavior*. New York: The Free Press, 1965.

Smith, O. A., and Nathan, M. A. The development of cardiac and blood flow conditional responses during the acquisition of a differentiated "conditioned emotional response" in monkeys. *Conditional Reflex*, 1967, *2*, 155–156.

Snapper, A. G., Pomerleau, O. F., and Schoenfeld, W. N. Similarity of cardiac CR forms in the rhesus monkey during several experimental procedures. *Conditional Reflex*, 1969, *4*, 212–220.

Stebbins, W. C., and Smith, O. A. Cardiovascular concomitants of the conditioned emotional response in the monkey. *Science*, 1964, *144*, 881–883.

Stern, J. A., and Word, T. J. Heart rate changes during avoidance conditoning in the male albino rat. *J. Psychonomic Res.*, 1962, *6*, 167–175.

Swadlow, H. A., Hosking, K. E., and Schneiderman, N. Differential heart rate conditioning and level lift suppression in restrained rabbits. *Physiol. Behav.*, 1971, *7*, 257–260.

Thorndike, E. L. Animal intelligence—an experimental study of the associative processes in animals. *Psychol. Monogr.*, 1898, *2*, 1–106 (Mongr. Suppl. Whole No. 8).

Tighe, T. J., Groves, D. M., and Riley, C. A. Successive reversals of a classically conditioned heart-rate discrimination. *J. Exp. Analy. Behav.*, 1968, *11*, 199–206.

Wagner, A. R., Seigel, L. S., and Fein, G. G. Extinction of conditioned fear as a function of percentage of reinforcement. *J. Comp. Physiol. Psychol.*, 1967, *63*, 160–164.

Watson, J. B., and Rayner, R. Conditioned emotional reactions. *J. Exp. Psychol.*, 1920, *3*, 1–14.

Weiss, J. M. Somatic effects of predictable and unpredictable shock. *Psychosom. Med.*, 1970, *32*, 297–408.

Weiss, J. M. Effects of coping behavior in different warning signal conditions on stress pathology in rats. *J. Comp. Physiol. Psychol.*, 1971a, *77*, 1–13.

Weiss, J. M. Effects of punishing the coping response (conflict) on stress pathology in rats. *J. Comp. Physiol. Psychol.*, 1971b, *77*, 14–21.

Weiss, J. M. Effects of coping behavior with and without a feedback signal on stress pathology in rats. *J. Comp. Physiol. Psychol.*, 1971c, *77*, 22–30.

Wenger, M. A., and Bagchi, K. Studies of autonomic functions in practitioners of yoga in India. *Behav. Sci.*, 1961, *6*, 312–323.

Wolpe, J. *Psychotherapy by reciprocal inhibition*. Stanford, Calif.: Stanford University Press, 1958.

Yehle, A. L. Divergences among rabbit response systems during three-tone classical discrimination conditioning. *J. Exp. Psychol.*, 1968, *77* (3, Part 1), 468–473.

Biofeedback*

DAVID SHAPIRO, PH.D.

Professor
Department of Psychiatry
University of California, Los Angeles
Los Angeles, California

RICHARD S. SURWIT, PH.D.

Associate Professor of Medical Psychology
Department of Psychiatry
Duke University Medical Center
Durham, North Carolina

3

Biofeedback methodology and experimentation represent a major recent advance in the investigation of the role of behavior and the environment in the regulation of physiological processes. It is probably the single most significant development to occur in psychophysiological research since the methods of Pavlov were first developed and elaborated early in the twentieth century, as evidenced by the many books and collections of reprints that have been published on basic and clinical research in the area (Barber, DiCara, Kamiya, et al., 1976; Beatty and Legewie, 1977; DiCara, Barber, Kamiya, et al., 1975; Kamiya, Barber, Miller, et al., 1977; Schwartz and Beatty, 1977; Shapiro and Surwit, 1976; Stoyva, Barber, Kamiya, et al., 1978).

Biofeedback is significant not only because it widened the scope and increased the capability of behavioral models of experimentation and analysis in research on physiological functioning, but also because it provoked a renewed interest in behavioral models of etiology and treatment of psychophysiological disorders. In addition, it suggested new approaches to the modification of emotional states and the study of consciousness. This chapter will define and discuss the basic concepts and methods of biofeedback, outline some of the theoretical frameworks for the phenomena of biofeedback, review some basic empirical biofeedback research on selected physiological responses, give some examples of the use of biofeedback in clinical practice, and consider clinical issues in biofeedback relevant to behavioral medicine. The chapter will conclude with a general appraisal of the current status of clinical biofeedback research and the potential of biofeedback in behavioral medicine.

To begin with, we can define biofeedback in terms of the application of operant conditioning methods to the control of visceral, somatomotor, and central nervous system activities. The objectivity of observation and recording, precise definition and quantitative analysis of behavioral change, and systematic investigation of the effects of environmental stimuli contingent on be-

* Preparation of this chapter was supported in part by National Institutes of Health Grant RO1-HL-22547, National Institute of Mental Health Research Grant MH-26923, and Office of Naval Research Contract N00014-75-C-0150, NR201-152.

havioral change which are inherent in the methods of operant conditioning contributed significantly to the rise of empirical biofeedback research. The basic experimental procedure can be outlined as follows. The individual is placed in a controlled environment in which various physiological responses are identified, recorded, measured, and counted. Whenever a response of interest occurs, e.g., increase in heart rate, decrease in systolic blood pressure, reduction in integrated muscle activity, or increase in electroencephalographic activity in a given frequency range, a reinforcer is presented to the individual. The reinforcer may be a rewarding (or punishing) event, or information that is provided to the subject about the physiological activity, or whether a particular physiological change has occurred or not. The effects of such contingent stimuli are evaluated by examining changes in response rate over time (e.g., criterion skin conductance responses or blood pressure changes), tonic level of physiological activity over given time periods (e.g., average heart rate in beats per minute, average blood volume), or variability in such dependent measures.

In the informational sense of biofeedback, the appropriate change in physiological activity may be signaled to the subject by a discrete stimulus, such as a flash of light or a tone. Continuous feedback, such as a varying light, tone, or meter reading, which changes in direct correspondence with fluctuations in the physiological response, is also commonly used. Simple digital numerical information, e.g., skin temperature in degrees centigrade, blood pressure in millimeters of mercury, or heart rate in beats per minute, is an alternative to tones, lights, or meter fluctuations.

In recent research, computer techniques are being employed to produce continuously changing graphic displays (Lang, 1974). Computer-generated displays may help correct for individual differences in range and variability of the physiological response being studied, for differences in difficulty of control of the particular response, or for variations in ongoing success and failure in the task (Reeves, Shapiro, and Cobb, in press). Computer techniques allow potentially more effective shaping of the desired behavior in terms of actual changes in performance and more flexible selection of response characteristics or patterns of response for feedback. They also enlarge the scope and enhance the credibility of experimental control and random feedback techniques, e.g., feedback contingent on other responses, inconsistent feedback, or intermittent feedback. Finally, through mass storage of experimental data, capabilities for the analysis of results are greatly enhanced by computer methods.

Reinforcers commonly used in biofeedback research vary greatly depending on the subject population. In human research, a tone or light may signal a monetary bonus, simply points, or success in a task. Interesting stimuli (e.g., music, slides of paintings, puzzle completions) are also used. In animal research, food, water, escape and avoidance of noxious stimuli, and rewarding brain stimulation have been commonly utilized as reinforcers.

Informational and reinforcing properties are both involved in the biofeedback stimuli and procedure. Thus, aside from its reinforcing properties, the reinforcer itself may also be informational, indicating to the subject that the desired response has occurred. Aside from its informational characteristics, the biofeedback stimulus may be reinforcing, indicating to the subject that he or she has done the right thing, has achieved the desired result, or has been successful in the task. Typically in clinical applications, informational and reinforcing properties of the biofeedback stimuli (lights, tones, meter readings) are merged together, thereby capitalizing on both influences so as to maximize effects. One can think of the biofeedback method in the human situation as a self-regulation procedure in which the nature of the biological information and the contingencies of reinforcement are completely defined and understood by the individual. In clinical situations, the elements of reinforcement and information as well as other aspects of the setting and relationship between doctor and patient that have a bearing on the patient's perception of and approach to the biofeedback task have to be thoroughly considered and appreciated. In research, whether with humans or animals, the various elements involved in the process can be examined in isolation or in various combinations.

Aside from reinforcement and informational properties, interpretation of results obtained by means of the biofeedback procedure requires a consideration of numerous other factors, which may or may not be taken into account in the experimental design, choice of independent variables and controls, or selection of dependent measures. For example, the biofeedback stimuli may reflexively elicit the responses of interest. Response frequency may be a function of the instructions employed or of the perceptions of the subject regarding the task, over and above the specific effects of the stimuli as feedback or as reinforcers. Or, the subject may be able to produce the desired result through the voluntary control of certain previously learned behaviors which elicit the responses of interest. The issues of mechanism and causal mediation, which will be discussed below, have been debated widely. They provide explanations for the phenomena of biofeedback over and beyond the relatively atheoretical operant conditioning and simple informational frameworks (Katkin and Murray, 1968). In this regard, the biofeedback paradigm has served to stimulate further research from a large variety of perspectives on a whole variety of means of achieving voluntary control or self-regulation of physiological processes.

Historical Background and Fundamentals

The first important discussion of the concept of biofeedback in research on autonomic functions was in Razran's monograph (1961) on research in the Soviet Union and Eastern Europe concerned with interoceptive conditioning, semantic conditioning, and the orienting reflex. Razran described an experiment by Lisina indicating that subjects could learn to control their vasomotor activity to avoid noxious stimulation, but only under the condition of observing their own polygraph record of the continuous physiological changes. At the same time, electrodermal activity, or the galvanic skin response, was a prime target for many early studies of learned autonomic nervous system control by means of operant conditioning (Fowler and Kimmel, 1962; Shapiro, Crider, and Tursky, 1964).

Research on the modification of apparently "involuntary" somatomotor activities such as minute muscle twitches or isolated muscular contractions associated with individual motor units represented a major early application of operant conditioning and biofeedback to the control of "covert" somatomotor activities. In this case, electromyographic recordings of muscle activities were used to produce visual or auditory displays or behavioral consequences (Basmajian, 1963; Hefferline, Keenan, and Harford, 1959). In research on central nervous system responses, the early investigations of Kamiya (summarized in Kamiya, 1969) on the control of brain wave activity (alpha EEG activity of 8–12 Hz) stimulated much research to follow. Kamiya was initially concerned with the ability of subjects to discriminate changes in their own alpha rhythm activity, and then went on to study the ability of subjects to increase or decrease this activity and to evaluate associated changes in subjective reports of "mental" activity. Although this early research in human subjects involved complications of subject cooperation and motivation, individual differences, and the like, it is of historical interest that much of it preceded the more highly controlled animal work to follow. We shall begin with a more complete description of specific research on the control of electrodermal activity in human subjects as a means of laying out some of the basic research issues in historical perspective.

Early in 1960's, several laboratories reported that the human electrodermal response, either measured as a skin resistance or skin potential change, could be relatively increased or decreased in frequency by contingent reinforcement (Fowler and Kimmel, 1962; Johnson, 1963; Shapiro et al., 1964). The electrodermal response is usually considered a reflexive or "involuntary" response, but it also occurs spontaneously, without being correlated with external stimuli, and it can thus be considered as an unelicited or emitted response. Moreover, the spontaneous electrodermal response is relatively discrete in nature, and it occurs intermittently. Unlike continuously varying biological functions such as heart rate, blood pressure, or skin temperature, the fact that the electrodermal response is discrete and unelicited by external stimuli lends it still further to operant analysis and experimentation. It thus can be treated like a simple response of the skeletal muscles and analyzed by the traditional methods of operant conditioning.

One study in this series (Shapiro et al., 1964) is emphasized because it was one of the first to deal with certain critical issues that have concerned basic researchers in this field. In this study, a spontaneous fluctuation of palmar skin potential of a given amplitude was selected as the response to be brought under control by means of operant conditioning. All subjects were given the same instructions, that the purpose of the experiment was to study the effectiveness of various devices for measuring thought processes and that the task was to think actively about emotional experiences. Subjects were instructed that each time the apparatus detected an "emotional thought" they would hear a tone and earn a small monetary reward. One group of subjects was given a reward each time a skin potential response occurred, and a second group was given the same number of rewards but at times when the response was absent. The first group showed increases in response rate relative to the second group which showed a decrement in response rate over time. The fact that the same reward, particularly with instructions held constant, could be used either to enhance *or* to diminish the autonomic behavior eliminated the explanation that the eliciting effect of the reinforcer itself on the electrodermal response could account for the observed differences.

An even more significant result emerged from this study. Learned variations in electrodermal response rate were found not to be associated with such physiologically related functions as skin potential level and heart rate. Nor were the variations obviously associated with changes in rate of breathing or in breathing irregularities. Cognitive factors, to the extent they could be assessed by blind ratings of recorded post-session interviews, were not associated with the observed effects. Response contingent and non-response contingent subjects reported the same moderate relationship between the reinforcer (tone indicating bonus) and their thoughts or ideation; level of involvement in the task was also about the same for the two groups.

The basic implication of the study was that the reinforcement contingency was critical in selecting out a given response and shaping its frequency while at the same time presumably related responses did not covary. If an operant procedure could have a selective effect on an autonomically mediated behavior such as the skin potential response, it made a convincing argument for the value of exploring autonomic regulation of specific functions or patterns of functions with operant conditioning methods. Such methods could also provide a means of investigating the extent to which a given autonomic response could be differentiated from other autonomic and somatic behaviors. That is, by providing feedback for reinforcing a given response, the degree to which other presumably related responses change in the same direction would to some degree indicate their actual functional relationship. Research on the biofeedback control of various components of cardiovascular functions (see below) provided additional critical data on the issues of specificity of conditioning and the usefulness of biofeedback methods in dissociating one physiological response from other associated responses.

The association between learned electrodermal responding and somatomotor responses was explored in several studies (Birk, Crider, Shapiro, et al., 1966; Crider, Shapiro, and Tursky, 1966). From these and other research (Rice, 1966; Van Twyver and Kimmel, 1966) it could be seen that the role of somatomotor and other mediating activities was not entirely consistent. As Birk et al. concluded, "Whether these variables [somatomotor] are to be classified as "mediating" phenomena cannot be decided until such questions are phrased in terms of known physiological mechanisms or testable hypotheses (p. 166)." The curare research discussed below also tackled similar questions.

Although the foundations for biofeedback research were laid down in these early human investigations, the animal research of Miller, DiCara, and associates on the topic of visceral learning (as reviewed in Miller, 1969) was a major influence in the subsequent growth of research. Their goal was to establish that operant conditioning of heart rate and other visceral functions was not necessarily dependent on peripheral somatomotor activity. They used curare to paralyze animals and examined the degree to which such animals could learn to control visceral activities in an operant conditioning procedure. They employed brain stimulation or shock escape and avoidance as reinforcers. Their initial results were positive in many experiments in rats and cats on various physiological systems. Rather substantial increases and decreases in physiological response rate were obtained in the curarized animals (Miller, 1969). However, recent difficulties in replicating these experiments resulted in a slowing down of animal research (Miller and Dworkin, 1974; see also Brener, Eissenberg, and Middaugh, 1974; Dworkin and Miller, 1977; Howard, Galosy, Gaebelein, et al., 1974; Roberts, 1978). The use of muscular paralysis does not rule out the influence of central nervous system motor innervation. Such central somatomotor influences could affect peripheral cardiovascular changes (Black, 1972; Obrist, 1976; Obrist, Howard, Lawler, et al., 1974). Current research has played down the critical necessity or desirability of demonstrating learned visceral control in animals paralyzed by curare. Rather, the conclusion of many researchers seems to be that there can be some independence of somatic and autonomic activities and that peripheral muscular activity can probably be ruled out as a *necessary* requirement for learned visceral control. On the other hand, somatomotor and autonomic functions often vary together according to different behavioral settings and demands (Cohen and Obrist, 1975; Obrist, 1976). They are coupled together in various ways at all levels of the nervous system. Moreover, the curare preparation involves many difficult methodological problems (e.g., control of respiratory parameters, possible direct autonomic effects of curare itself, and possible central nervous effects of curare). Alternative approaches in animal research are to assess physiological mechanisms in other ways, e.g., use of lesions and ablations, biochemical and drug influences, etc. Studies of humans with neurological and neuromuscular diseases are also pertinent (Miller, 1975; Pickering, Brucker, Frankel, et al., 1977). Another strategy is to assess patterns of somatomotor and visceral changes in biofeedback studies or to modify patterns of such activity as a means of elucidating processes of learned change (Black, 1972; Engel, 1972; Fetz and Finocchio, 1971; Schwartz, 1972, 1977). From a purely clinical standpoint, moreover, the fact that self-regulation is mediated by somatomotor or cognitive processes is of no great consequence so long as the desired goal of physiological change can be achieved and maintained and there are no unwanted "side effects" of such mediating processes. In fact, as already stated, in searching for alternative explanations of biofeedback studies, investigators uncover alternative pathways to physiological control.

Further definitive research is needed to examine the size of the effects and the comparability of changes achieved by specific biofeedback methods and those achieved by alternative methods of behavioral regulation, e.g., simple instructional effects, suggestions, thoughts, imagery, and physical strategies (breathing changes, muscular relaxation and tension). These comparisons have both theoretical and practical clinical interest. For example, to the extent that alternative methods to biofeedback produce as large and as persistent changes, the need for the rather elaborate instrumentation is diminished or eliminated.

In our view, the single most remarkable feature of biofeedback is the potential for selective control of specific responses or patterns of response, and this feature may be of particular significance in the management of certain specific symptoms of psychophysiological disorders. Whether or not alternative methods of behavioral control can be used to achieve comparable specificity remains to be seen. In applications in which control of specific patterns of response is not critical, this feature of biofeedback methodology is of no particular value, and behavioral approaches which emphasize more global effects may be more suitable.

Theoretical Frameworks

Research on the regulation and voluntary control of visceral and neural processes by means of biofeedback and operant conditioning has grown considerably in the past

15 years. General reviews of both animal and human research have been published by Kimmel (1967), Katkin and Murray (1968), Miller (1969), DiCara (1970), Shapiro and Schwartz (1972), Engel (1972), Schwartz (1973), Blanchard and Young (1973, 1974), and Shapiro and Surwit (1976). Various theoretical positions have been advanced by Katkin and Murray (1968), Crider, Schwartz, and Shnidman (1969), Black (1971, 1972), Lang (1974), Brener (1974, 1977), Lazarus (1977), Black, Cott, and Pavloski (1977), Mulholland (1977), Schwartz (1977), and Shapiro (1977). The major theoretical positions or models may be grouped under the following rubrics, each identified with particular experimental strategies and points of view: operant conditioning (Black et al., 1977), complex skills learning (Lang, 1974, 1977), discrimination and awareness of internal bodily responses and processes (Brener, 1977), "mediation" of physiological responses and control through somatomotor and cognitive change (Katkin and Murray, 1968), cybernetic formulations derived from electrical engineering and control systems theory (Anliker, 1977; Mulholland, 1977), and psychobiological patterning models (Schwartz, 1977). Each theoretical position can be supported by empirical data, and there are a number of studies that attempt to isolate and differentiate the effects of the different hypothesized variables. At this stage of our knowledge, there is no exceptionally strong empirical evidence to support one viewpoint over another. The viewpoints seem to be stressing processes and mechanisms that are not exclusive of one another. Three of the major frameworks will be discussed in further detail: operant conditioning, informational process, and skills learning.

The operant conditioning framework is basically atheoretical. It emphasizes the use of reinforcements (rewards and punishments) that are made contingent on selected ongoing physiological responses and a learning process that follows. This kind of research has proceeded using a variety of conditioning procedures, physiological responses, and subjects, including man, rats, monkeys, and cats. In some instances, investigators have attempted to examine in detail similarities and differences between the conditioning of skeletal motor and visceral or neural processes. By and large, systematic exploration of operant techniques per se in the study of human physiological regulation has not occurred, e.g., study of different schedules, intermittent reinforcement, or avoidance and punishment techniques (see, for example, Shapiro and Crider, 1967; Crider, Schwartz, and Shapiro, 1970; Shapiro and Watanabe, 1971; Johnson and Schwartz, 1967). As mentioned previously, the application of operant procedures to human visceral learning has been productive, and the notation of operant conditioning has been useful in designing experiments and in yielding interpretable results. However, it is obvious that the study of human learning is more complex than the study of animal learning. Methodological issues arise in human research in regard to the appropriateness and selection of reinforcers, prior learning history of the subjects, set, expectancy and other cognitive factors, and so on. Moreover, the principles of operant learning derived from animal research do not necessarily hold in the same fashion for humans. The pattern of acquisition may be different, and typical learning effects shown in animals (such as schedule effects) may not be found in humans. The value of analogies between human biofeedback findings and supposed principles and patterns derived from animal studies may be questionable. Even within the framework of operant conditioning, the adequacy of reinforcing stimuli typically employed in biofeedback studies has been questioned by Garcia and Rusiniak (1977). To quote them, " . . . it is clear that behavioral models derived from animals actively coping with external problems, informative distal signals and discrete distal goals are inappropriate for biofeedback training. The hedonic changes sensed by peripheral receptors are more intimately related to the control of the diffuse sluggish vegetative processes, as sought in biofeedback training." They question the value of immediate reinforcement for small changes in response as compared with delayed signals for larger and more appropriate changes in state, and they also question the use of "telereceptive" biofeedback signals as compared with heat, cold, or other reinforcing stimuli having "hedonic" value.

A second major line of inquiry has stemmed from the concepts and techniques of biofeedback as an informational model. In biofeedback training, the individual is fed back information about his own biological responses. The information is a sensory analog (usually auditory or visual) of the actual simultaneously occurring responses. The information is provided to the subject at the same instant that the physiological activity is occurring, or after a very brief delay. Hence the term biofeedback—"bio" meaning that the information is biological, and "feedback" meaning that the information is precisely coupled in time with the ongoing biological events. From a purely cybernetic standpoint, the feedback concept means that some part of the output of a process is introduced into the input of a process so as to alter the process. Cybernetic and control systems formulations of biofeedback have been advanced by Mulholland (1977) and Anliker (1977), but such a model has not been applied extensively. In the informational model, the biofeedback stimuli may be conceived of as essentially symbolic representations of the physiological events, and the individual engages in some behavior either to augment or diminish the feedback stimuli and therefore the activity. In this sense, the biofeedback is seen as neutral with respect to its direct effect on the physiological activity, and it may be thought of as a physiological monitor (see Schwartz, 1973). Research stemming from this orientation has attempted to compare various characteristics of the feedback stimuli themselves (e.g., amount or frequency of feedback—Gatchel, 1974; Lang and Twentyman, 1974; Shapiro, Tursky, and Schwartz, 1970b; type of sensory modality—Blanchard and Young, 1972).

In a third framework not unrelated to the informational model, emphasis has been given to learned physiological control as a form of complex human learning, such as the learning of motor skills (Brener, 1974; Lang, 1974). The biofeedback functions to guide individuals in the learning process, and it may serve to implement awareness of sensations accompanying the physiological responses or to sensitize the individual to other responses more directly under his control as a means of mediating voluntary control over the physiological changes. In this line of reasoning, a theory of voluntary control has been developed by Brener (1974, 1977). He has proposed that the externalized sensory feedback is used by the individual as a means of *calibrating* the afferent feedback of his own visceral responses against the external sensory referent, thereby facilitating greater awareness of the visceral activities and greater control. Brener gives the analogy of a deaf person being trained to talk by calibrating the responses of his own muscular vocal apparatus against vibratory sensations in the fingers produced by talking. These sensations substitute for the usual auditory sensations (feedback) occurring in normal people. After practice and learning, such a feedback crutch can be dispensed with. Brener regards visceral learning and self-regulation as an analogous process. This general framework has generated research on the role of instructions in learned physiological control (Beatty, 1972; Bergman and Johnson, 1972; Blanchard, Scott, Young, et al., 1974a; Johnston, 1976, Shapiro, 1973) and the role of actual discrimination and awareness of the internal changes (Blanchard, Young, and McLeod, 1972; Brener and Jones, 1974; Epstein and Stein, 1974). With no feedback provided, instructions are clearly effective in the control of certain functions, such as heart rate, and relatively ineffective in the control of other functions, such as electrodermal activity (Roberts, 1977) or blood pressure (Shapiro, 1973). The degree to which the particular function itself or other bodily activities closely associated with the function can be discriminated by the individual appears to be significant in explaining such differences. Research on the ability of subjects to detect visceral activity or to improve in such detection through training has produced some positive evidence (Brener and Jones, 1974; Hamano, 1977), but there is little in the way of published literature indicating the extent to which training in such detection has an influence on subsequent control during biofeedback training.

In one of the most suggestive studies employing a skills learning framework, Schwartz, Young, and Vogler (1976) examined "the value of conceptualizing complex visceral skills as reflecting learned patterns of underlying neurophysiological abilities."

They compared the ability of subjects to develop "strength and endurance control" versus "reaction time control," the former requiring subjects to increase or decrease heart rate maximally and sustain the change for 1 minute and the latter requiring subjects to produce a small, 3 second burst of increased or decreased heart rate as quickly as possible at the onset of a trial. Subjects trained in one skill showed improvements in that skill and not in the other. There was no evidence of transfer of one heart rate skill to the other.

The field of biofeedback is sorely in need of further theoretical developments with associated critical experiments on the nature of the behavioral control and processes of learning involved. Such basic investigation on mechanisms will permit a more rational and effective exploitation of the procedures in the clinical sphere.

Review of Empirical Research on Selected Responses and Clinical Examples

This section reviews empirical research on particular responses for which there has been substantial basic biofeedback investigation and related clinical applications. The review is not intended to be exhaustive, and the emphasis on cardiovascular functions, particularly blood pressure, is in line with our own research interests and previous writings on the topic of essential hypertension (Shapiro, Mainardi, and Surwit, 1977; Surwit, Shapiro, and Good, 1978).

BLOOD PRESSURE

Basic Research. Basic research on biofeedback in the regulation of blood pressure includes data from both animal and human experiments. In the curarized rat, instrumental conditioning of systolic blood pressure was demonstrated using shock escape and avoidance (DiCara and Miller, 1968b). Learned changes in pressure were about 20% of baseline in both increase and decrease directions, and they were not associated with changes in heart rate or rectal temperature. In a subsequent study in noncurarized rats, changes obtained were about 5% of baseline (Pappas, DiCara, and Miller, 1970). Diastolic pressure elevations of large magnitude (50–60 mm Hg) were obtained in the rhesus monkey using a shock avoidance procedure in which the elevations functioned as an avoidance response (Plumlee, 1969). In the dog-faced baboon, substantial elevations in blood pressure were established by an operant procedure in which food delivery and shock avoidance were made contingent upon increases in diastolic pressure (Harris, Findley, and Brady, 1971; Harris, Gilliam, Findley, et al., 1973). In their recent work, these investigators reported sustained increases of about 30 to 40 mm Hg in both systolic and diastolic blood pressure. The changes in blood pressure were associated with elevated but progressively decreasing heart rates (Harris and Brady, 1974). Long-term studies of such cardiovascular control in primates and associated physiological mechanisms are discussed further in Harris and Brady (1977). Benson, Herd, Morse, et al. (1969) put squirrel monkeys on a work schedule in which they were required to press a key in order to avoid electric shock. Prolonged and persistent elevations in blood pressure resulted. Then, the schedule was reversed, and a decrease in pressure became the criterion for shock avoidance. Pressures were shown to decline 10 to 20 mm Hg. It is not known whether similar reversals can occur in animals with chronic high levels of pressure.

Most of the human studies on blood pressure control with biofeedback methods follow the procedures first described in Shapiro, Tursky, Gershon, et al. (1969). The "constant cuff" technique was devised to obtain a relative measure of blood pressure on each beat of the heart so as to be able to provide continuous feedback to subjects. In the constant cuff method, a blood pressure cuff is wrapped around the upper arm, and a crystal microphone is placed over the brachial artery under the distal end of the cuff. The cuff is inflated to about average systolic pressure and held constant at that level. Whenever the systolic pressure rises and exceeds the occluding cuff pressure, a Korotkoff sound is detected from the microphone. When the systolic level is less than the occluding pressure, no Korotkoff sound is detected. Using a regulated low-pressure source and programming apparatus, it is possible to find a constant cuff pressure at which 50% of the heart beats yield Korotkoff sounds. This pressure is by definition median systolic pressure. Inasmuch as the time between the R-wave in the electrocardiogram and the occurrence of the Korotkoff sound is approximately 300 msec, it is possible to detect either the presence of the Korotkoff sound (high systolic pressure relative to the median) or its absence (low systolic pressure relative to the median) on each heart beat. In this way, the system provides information about directional changes in pressure relative to the median on each successive heart beat, and this information can be used in a biofeedback procedure. Subjects are provided with binary (yes-no) feedback of either relatively high, or low, pressure on each heart beat. After a prescribed number of feedback stimuli or a change in median pressure, rewarding slides or other incentives are presented.

Initial studies with the constant cuff method attempted to determine whether normal volunteer subjects could learn to modify their systolic or diastolic blood pressure. Complete details of the experiments may be found in Shapiro et al., (1969), Shapiro, Tursky, and Schwartz (1970a), Shapiro et al. (1970b), Schwartz, Shapiro, and Tursky (1971), Schwartz (1972), and Shapiro, Schwartz, and Tursky (1972b). In these studies, subjects were told that the feedback represented information about "a physiological response usually considered involuntary." Subjects were told to make the feedback stimulus occur as much as possible and thereby to earn as many rewards as possible. They were not told that the feedback was being given for changes in blood pressure, nor were they told whether to increase it or decrease it. This procedure controlled for any results that are due to the natural ability of subjects to control their pressure "voluntarily," and tested the specific effects of feedback and reward contingency. Voluntary control of blood pressure and other circulatory changes has been reported in some individuals (Ogden and Shock, 1939). Such voluntary control of blood pressure unassisted by external feedback could not be demonstrated in a sample of normal subjects (Brener, 1974; Shapiro, 1973).

To summarize the normal blood pressure biofeedback studies, normal subjects were able to modify their blood pressure with feedback and reward. Average differences in systolic pressure between increase and decrease conditions for groups of subjects at the end of a single session of training varied from 3 to 10% of baseline. The best results were obtained for diastolic pressure (Shapiro et al., 1972b) with individuals showing increases up to 25% and decreases up to 15% of baseline values. Heart rate was not associated with learned changes in systolic pressure, and systolic pressure was not associated with learned changes in heart rate (Shapiro et al., 1970b). However, Fey and Lindholm (1975), using the constant cuff method, reported that heart rate increased or decreased in groups receiving contingent feedback for increasing and for decreasing systolic blood pressure, respectively. Brener (1974), citing data in which continuous recordings of heart rate, chin electromyogram, and respiratory activity were obtained while subjects were given both increase and decrease feedback training for diastolic blood pressure, reported that the training effects were specific to blood pressure. However, Shapiro et al. (1972b) reported that heart rate was not independent of learned changes in diastolic pressure. Further evidence is needed on the specificity of control of blood pressure and other associated cardiovascular functions.

To explain the conditions under which specificity of conditioning occurs, Schwartz (1972) hypothesized that when feedback is given for one response, simultaneous learning of other responses will depend on the degree to which these other responses are directly associated with the response for which feedback is given. He developed an on-line procedure for tracking both phasic and tonic patterns of blood pressure and heart rate in real time and showed that subjects could learn to control patterns of simultaneous changes in both functions. Subjects learned to integrate systolic blood pressure and heart rate (i.e., make both increase or both decrease simultaneously) and to some extent to differentiate both functions (i.e., make one increase and the other decrease simultaneously). Further analysis of the patterning of both functions over time, of natural tonic reactivity in this situation, and of homeostatic mechanisms made it possible to predict the extent and time course of pattern learning in the different conditions (Schwartz, 1974). It is of interest that subjective reports of a "relaxed" state were associated with learned reductions in both systolic pressure and heart rate.

Although the average curves suggest that it is easier to obtain reductions rather than increases in pressure in a single session (Shapiro et al., 1969), further data under conditions of random reinforcement indicated a tendency for baseline pressure values to habituate over time (Shapiro et al., 1970a). Therefore, increases in pressure over baseline values may be more likely in normal subjects. Unpublished data (Shapiro, Note 1) indicated that the same pattern of pressure reduction occurs whether subjects try to reduce their pressure with or without feedback or simply rest in the laboratory and do nothing. On the other hand, Fey and Lindholm (1975), using the constant cuff method and unrestricted subjects, reported reliable decreases in systolic blood pressure over three 1-hour sessions of feedback training for reduced pressure as compared with no changes in no-feedback, random, or increase training groups. Surwit, Hager, and Feldman (1977) conducted a study in which normal subjects were instructed to increase and decrease their blood pressure. Subjects were given either contingent beat-to-beat feedback, noncontingent beat-to-beat feedback, noncontingent feedback randomly associated with the heart beat, or no feedback at all. No clear differences between training conditions were observed in this one session study. This calls into question the utility of feedback when instructions are given. Also, as previously noted, blood pressure increases were easier to obtain than blood pressure decreases. As in the case of heart rate, the processes involved in increasing blood pressure may be different from those involved in decreasing pressure (Engel, 1972; Lang and Twentyman, 1974). In normal subjects, typical resting pressures are close to minimal waking values, but there is a potential for large increases above baseline. For individuals having significantly elevated pressure levels, significant decreases may be more likely.

Recently, Steptoe and Johnston (1976) and Steptoe (1977) demonstrated that pulse transit time from the R-wave of the electrocardiogram to the foot of the radial pulse upstroke can be used as a source of blood pressure feedback in the voluntary training of blood pressure in normal subjects. Steptoe (1977) demonstrated that this type of feedback training led to greater modifications than instructions alone.

All told, blood pressure biofeedback research suggests that blood pressure can be self-regulated by normal subjects with a fair degree of consistency and specificity. The degree of change achieved, especially in a decrease direction, is relatively small. Most of the human research consists of one-session experiments in subjects already low in pressure to begin with. More work is needed to determine whether larger and persistent changes can be brought about with long-term training. Other techniques for recording and measuring blood pressure need to be explored. Pattern feedback techniques need to be exploited, particularly with the aid of computer techniques. The effects on blood pressure of biofeedback for other cardiovascular parameters also needs to be explored more systematically. The direction of such future basic research will derive from a variety of perspectives and from clinical research described below which is rapidly accumulating observations and critical questions, answers to which will permit a more rational and comprehensive approach to clinical application.

Clinical Applications. The basic laboratory data discussed above provided a foundation for the clinical application of biofeedback to hypertension. Benson, Shapiro, Tursky, et al. (1971) used feedback techniques in the lowering of systolic blood pressure in seven patients, five of whom had been diagnosed as having essential hypertension. Medication dosage, diet, and other factors were kept constant during the course of the study. Of the other two patients, one did not have elevated systolic pressure and the other had renal artery stenosis. No reductions were observed in as many as 15 pretreatment control sessions. The five patients responding positively showed decreases of 34, 29, 16, 16, and 17 mm Hg with 33, 22, 34, 31, and 12 sessions of training, respectively.

Using the constant cuff procedure, Goldman, Kleinman, Snow, et al. (1975) reported average decreases of 4 and 13% in systolic and diastolic pressure, respectively, in seven patients with average baseline values of 167/109 mm Hg who were diagnosed as having essential hypertension and who were willing to participate in the study prior to having medication. Although feedback was given for systolic pressure, the significant reductions occurred only in diastolic pressure over the course of the nine training sessions. Those patients who showed the greatest decreases in both systolic and diastolic pressure during biofeedback training also showed the greatest improvement on the Category Test of the Halstead-Reitan Neuropsychological Test Battery for Adults (Reitan, 1966). As this test is related to cognitive dysfunctioning, the results imply that biofeedback may be useful in lowering pressure *and* in overcoming a cognitive impairment associated with hypertension. This kind of impairment has been suggested in previous research (Reitan, 1954; Richter-Heinrich and Läuter, 1969). Moreover, the improvement in cognitive functioning suggests that the effects of biofeedback training may not be entirely laboratory-specific.

Miller (1975) attempted to train 28 patients with essential hypertension to reduce their diastolic blood pressure. A few patients appeared to reduce their blood pressure, but, after reaching a plateau, the pressure drifted up again. One patient showing good results was trained to alternate in increasing and decreasing her pressure. Over a period of 3 months, this patient acquired the ability to change pressure over a range of 30 mm Hg. Her baseline pressure decreased from 97 to 76 mm Hg, and similar decreases were observed on the ward; medication was discontinued. Later on, she lost voluntary control as a result of life stresses and was put back on drugs. When the patient came back to training 2½ years later, she rapidly regained a large measure of control. Such multiple courses of treatment need to be attempted more often.

Kristt and Engel (1975) reported evidence that patients with essential hypertension having a variety of cardiovascular and other complications can learn to control and reduce their pressure over and above the effects produced by drugs. In phase 1, the patients took their pressure at home daily over a 7-week period and mailed in their reports to the laboratory. In phase 2, patients were trained to raise, to lower, and to alternately raise and lower systolic blood pressure. The constant cuff method (Shapiro et al., 1969) was used to record pressure and provide feedback. In phase 3, the patients again took their pressure at home and mailed in daily reports. Learned control of pressure was observed in all patients during the training sessions, and reductions in pressure of about 10 to 15% were observed from pretraining baselines to values recorded at a 3-month follow-up. Although feedback training was provided for systolic pressure, diastolic pressure was also reduced.

Since systolic blood pressure has been found to be more closely associated with morbidity and mortality than diastolic pressure in males over 45 years of age, reductions in systolic pressure could be a treatment of choice for this particular age-sex population. Also, morbidity and mortality in females seem to be more dependent upon systolic than diastolic pressure at almost all ages (Kannel, Gordon, and Schwartz, 1971). In younger men, diastolic pressure is more closely associated with morbidity and mortality (Kannel et al., 1971), in agreement with traditional concepts of hypertension (Merrill, 1966). Diastolic pressure is thought to be more critical in later or final stages of hypertension because of its closer relation to peripheral resistance (Merrill, 1966). Preliminary research (Benson, Shapiro, and Schwartz, Note 2) suggests that it is difficult to reduce abnormally high diastolic levels in patients with hypertension (Schwartz and Shapiro, 1973). Part of the problem may be related to unreliability in obtaining consistent diastolic values over repeated sessions. Learned control of diastolic pressure was observed in a single-session study of normal subjects, with consistent changes occurring in almost all subjects (Shapiro et al., 1972b). However, positive results of biofeedback training for decreases in diastolic pressure have been reported in other laboratories. Using feedback and verbal praise, 20 to 30% reductions in diastolic pressure were obtained in patients diagnosed as essential hypertensives (Elder, Ruiz, Deabler, et al., 1973). None of the 18 patients studied were under antihypertensive medication, although many were on central nervous system depressants. As discussed previously, other clinical studies have reported significant reductions in diastolic pressure, even though the feedback training was related to control of systolic pressure.

Surwit et al. (1978) reported findings of a clinical study in which two types of biofeedback training were compared to a form of meditation in the treatment of borderline hypertension. Twenty-four borderline hypertensives served as subjects and were evenly divided into three treatment conditions. All subjects received two 1-hour baseline sessions and eight 1-hour biweekly treatment sessions. The first treatment group received binary feedback for simultaneous reductions of blood pressure and heart rate (Schwartz, Shapiro, and Tursky, 1972). The second group received analog feedback for combined forearm and frontalis electromyographic activity. The third group received a meditation-relaxation procedure (Benson, 1975). Six weeks following the last treatment session, all subjects received a 1-hour treatment follow-up session. Data analysis indicated that the three treatment groups all showed significant reductions in pressure over trials during each session, implying that each of the behavioral methods tested was equally effective as a clinical intervention. Carryover effects from session to session or in a 1 year follow-up were not significant. Borderline or labile patients may reveal normal pressure levels in a quiet laboratory, suggesting that the conditions of training may not be appropriate for retraining purposes. Related to this issue, high levels of pressure may be under the control of particular situational events, and patients would therefore need to learn to reduce their reactivity in relation to such triggering stimuli. Biofeedback training under quiet, non-stimulating conditions may not be appropriate.

The above clinical studies provide supportive evidence concerning the potential of biofeedback techniques in the direct reduction of blood pressure in patients with essential hypertension. Similar biofeedback procedures have been used in independent laboratories with relatively consistent positive results. However, wide differences exist in characteristics of patients studied, duration of treatments, availability of follow-up data, and amount of systematic documentation of physiological effects and changes in drug regimes. The total number of patients studied is still small, and only large scale clinical trials accompanied by comprehensive medical, physiological, and psychological evaluations can provide the information required before biofeedback can be routinely applied in essential hypertension.

We have not presented in this chapter a detailed consideration of alternative behavioral methods as they have been applied in the management of hypertension. Relaxation approaches, have been utilized widely: for example, certain meditative disciplines, progressive relaxation, autogenic training, metronome-conditioned relaxation, and the like. In concluding a recent review of hypertension treatments, Reeves and Shapiro (1978) state,

> Since biofeedback and relaxation techniques have by and large resulted in equivalent BP reductions, it would seem that the less costly and simpler relaxation procedures would be the treatment of choice. However, the combination of biofeedback and relaxation has produced the most substantial pressure reductions. Unfortunately, studies combining biofeedback and relaxation have employed designs which make it impossible to assess the relative contributions of biofeedback and relaxation to such reductions. At any rate, research addressing whether biofeedback itself adds anything unique, over and above simpler relaxation techniques, is needed.

Finally, comparative studies of biofeedback and other behavioral methods with traditional medical approaches to hypertension (e.g., antihypertensive medication) are also needed. Single-case experimental designs (Barlow and Herson, 1973) may be a valuable alternative to the time-consuming and often awkward group-outcome designs typically employed in clinical research on hypertension and on other disorders as well.

HEART RATE

Basic Research. There is an extremely large literature on the use of biofeedback in the voluntary regulation of heart rate.

Heart rate changes have been repeatedly demonstrated in animals (DiCara and Miller, 1968a; Miller and DiCara, 1967; Trowill, 1967) and in humans (Brener and Hothersall, 1966; Engel and Hansen, 1966; Hnatiow and Lang, 1965; Shapiro et al., 1970b). Although procedures for blood pressure feedback are extremely complicated, heart rate is an easy function to monitor. With the use of surface electrodes, heart rate can be monitored continuously and presented either as an analog function of rate or heart period (i.e., the time between R-waves in the electrocardiogram) or as a dichotomous binary signal indicating whether or not the subject is above or below criterion on each beat of the heart. Perhaps because of the great ease with which this function can be monitored, the literature on heart rate control contains more citations than any other area of human biofeedback.

As with blood pressure, it is easier to train an increase in heart rate than a decrease. Studies have reported average heart rate increases in excess of 10 bpm (Blanchard, Young, Scott, et al., 1974b; Colgan, 1977; Obrist, Galosy, Lawler, et al., 1975). Wells (1973) reported that six out of nine subjects produced heart rate increases of greater than 15 bpm. The remainder of this sample failed to produce heart rate increases above 7 bpm. This dichotomy of ability is characteristic of the great individual differences reported by most investigators exploring heart rate control (Bell and Schwartz, 1975; Colgan, 1977; Stephens, Harris, Brady, et al., 1975).

Although individual differences appear to play a role in voluntary heart rate slowing there seems to be less of an ability for subjects to decrease their heart rate from a stable baseline than to increase their heart rate. Only a few studies (Colgan, 1977; Sirota, Schwartz, and Shapiro, 1974, 1976) have reported mean heart rate decreases of greater than 5 bpm. However, the data from the Sirota *et al.* studies are complicated by the fact that only short 5-minute adaptation periods are used, and subjects are exposed to the threat of a noxious stimulus during the course of training. The discrepancy between the ability of subjects to increase and decrease their heart rate voluntarily when provided with heart rate feedback has led to speculations that heart rate increases and decreases might be mediated by different physiological mechanisms (Bell and Schwartz, 1975; Lang, Troyer, Twentyman, et al., 1975). Thus, it appears that heart rate, like blood pressure, is more easily increased than decreased. In addition, it appears that large individual differences exist in the ability to control this variable.

As with blood pressure, investigators have asked the question as to whether or not heart rate can be manipulated with equal facility both with and without feedback in instructed subjects. Bergman and Johnson (1971) demonstrated that heart rate could be voluntarily controlled to some degree without feedback. Furthermore, Bergman and Johnson (1972) reported that the addition of heart rate feedback did not significantly improve the performance of subjects simply instructed to control their heart rate. More recently, studies have reported that increases in heart rate are significantly larger in subjects given feedback as well as instructional control (Bell and Schwartz, 1975; Davidson and Schwartz, 1976; Lang and Twentyman, 1974, 1976). In the control of heart rate decreases the facilitatory effect of feedback is not as clear (Davidson and Schwartz, 1976; Young and Blanchard, 1974). This may be in part due to the fact that these studies are only able to produce minimal heart rate decreases.

As mentioned earlier, heart rate feedback is presented either as an analog or binary signal. Analog signals usually consist of some type of visual display in which the change of the signal is proportional to the heart rate change. Binary signals provide the subject with yes/no information on a beat-by-beat or time-period basis. This type of feedback is computed by setting a criterion of rate or interbeat interval and then comparing the ongoing heart rate to this criterion during discrete time periods. The subject then sees a signal informing him as to whether or not he is higher or lower than this target at any given point in time. Three of five studies comparing analog to binary feedback have demonstrated a clear superiority for analog feedback in increasing heart rate (Blanchard et al., 1974b; Colgan, 1977; Lang and Twentyman, 1974). Most investigators have found no differences between types of feedback when subjects are trained to decrease heart rate (Blanchard et al., 1974b; Lang and Twentyman, 1974; Manuck, Levenson, Hinrichsen, et al., 1975; Young and Blanchard, 1974).

CLINICAL APPLICATIONS. Despite the enormous number of studies on the manipulation of heart rate through biofeedback in normals, there is relatively little published on the successful application of heart rate training to clinical problems. A number of applications do exist, however, and they are worthy of note. Several groups of investigators have reported heart rate feedback to be useful in the treatment of cardiac arrhythmias. Engel and Bleecker (1974) demonstrated that paroxysmal atrial tachycardia could be brought under control with heart rate feedback. Of significant clinical interest is the finding that patients with ventricular arrhythmias, secondary to coronary artery disease, can learn to decrease the frequency of these arrhythmias through heart rate training. Weiss and Engel (1971), Engel and Bleecker (1974), and Miller (1975) showed that such patients with premature ventricular contractions could demonstrate a significant and often sustained change in the frequency of arrhythmias. Finally, Bleecker and Engel (1973) and Weiss and Engel (1975) have reported that heart rate feedback might be beneficial in the control of certain coronary conduction defects.

The finding that heart rate feedback is useful in the treatment of pathologically high heart rates as in sinus tachycardia suggests some interesting possibilities. Although biofeedback may not aid in producing heart rate decreases below those observed in a resting baseline in normal subjects, it may prove useful in the reduction of excessively high heart rates produced by stress and/or cardiac pathology. Sirota et al. (1974, 1976) have demonstrated that subjects can learn to slow their heart rates in response to the threat of an electric shock and in doing so reduce the aversiveness of the shock. Victor, Mainardi, and Shapiro (1978) have also demonstrated a similar effect to a cold pressor situation. Sirota et al. (1974) point out that the validity and utility of biofeedback in stress reduction may only show itself in such a coping situation.

PERIPHERAL VASOMOTOR ACTIVITY

BASIC RESEARCH. Control of digital skin temperature through biofeedback and instrumental learning has been cited as a clinical tool for the control of migraine headaches (Sargent, Green, and Walters, 1973) and Raynaud's disease (Surwit, 1973). Since the peripheral vasculature is innervated exclusively by the sympathetic nervous system (Patton, 1965), control of digital temperature provides one of the clearest examples of voluntary control of the sympathetic nervous system available in human experimentation. Indeed, the earliest demonstration that an autonomic response may be learned with the aid of feedback occurred in the vasomotor system (Lisina, 1958). This investigator trained subjects to vasodilate in the forearm in order to escape an electric shock. Such escape training was not possible until the subjects were able to watch their responses on the polygraph. Snyder and Noble (1968), using a plethysmograph, demonstrated that subjects could learn to voluntarily vasoconstrict in the digits when skeletal-muscular mediation was controlled for. Roberts, Kewman, and Macdonald (1973) and Roberts, Schuler, Bacon, et al. (1975) demonstrated that subjects could learn to raise differentially the temperature in digits of the two hands with and without hypnosis when feedback of these temperature changes was provided to them. Surwit, Shapiro, and Feld (1976) demonstrated that following 2 days of baseline training voluntary decreases in digital temperature and pulse amplitude were much easier to obtain than voluntary increases. Whereas subjects could readily produce temperature decreases in excess of 2°C, temperature increases were much more modest (0.25°C). These investigators pointed out that earlier demonstrations of voluntary vasodilatation had failed to control adequately for baseline effects. Thus, the literature on voluntary digital vasodilatation, like that of blood pressure and heart rate, suggests that increases in arousal are easier to obtain than decreases in arousal.

CLINICAL APPLICATIONS. Although thermal feedback is an extremely popular form of clinical biofeedback, until recently there have been no controlled studies to demonstrate its utility. Surwit, Pilon, and Fenton (1978) recently demonstrated that patients suffering from idiopathic Raynaud's disease could be taught to maintain their temperature voluntarily with the aid of autogenic training. Trained subjects were shown to have 50% fewer vasospasms than untrained subjects and were able to show a 4°C improvement in digital temperature during the 1-hour exposure to a cold challenge. Half of the subjects in this study were given temperature feedback and half were not. While temperature feedback and autogenic instructions were shown to produce temperature control superior to autogenic instructions alone during training, feedback did not provide any clinical benefit in terms of reduction of vasospastic attacks or resistance to cold challenge.

Blanchard and Silver (Note 3) recently compared digital vasomotor training to progressive relaxation in patients suffering from migraine headaches. Both treatment procedures proved equally effective in producing a reduction in frequency and intensity of migraine headaches. Bradner, Surwit, and Birk (Note 4) found that autogenic training and temperature feedback were less effective than a simple relaxation technique (Benson, 1975) in producing relief of migraine. Thus, it appears that at present there is little data to indicate that digital vasomotor feedback offers a unique contribution to clinical problems.

ELECTROMYOGRAPHIC (EMG) ACTIVITY

Muscular activity can be measured either on the surface of the skin or intramuscularly by recording small voltage changes produced as motor units fire. Because the skeletal muscular system is already under voluntary control, it is no surprise that subjects can learn to control EMG with feedback. What is surprising is that with feedback, subjects can learn control otherwise not possible. The earliest report of EMG feedback facilitating voluntary muscular control comes from the physical rehabilitation literature. Basmajian (1977) reports that since 1943 physicians had been employing EMG feedback from needle electrodes inserted into the affected limb and allowing patients to attend to the unprocessed EMG signal. Hefferline and Perera (1963) used EMG feedback to teach subjects to discriminate a small muscle twitch not perceptible otherwise. In 1963, Basmajian demonstrated that single motor units could be trained discretely when needle electrodes were inserted into a muscle. The feedback signal was the actual recorded sound of the EMG. EMG feedback has been utilized in numerous studies to treat paralysis secondary to polio (Marinacci, 1968) and paralysis secondary to cerebral vascular accidents (Andrews, 1957; Basmajian, Kulkulka, Narayan, et al., 1975; Brudny, Korein, Grynbaum, et al., 1976; Brudny, Korein, Levidow, et al., 1974; Johnson and Garton, 1973; Marinacci and Horande, 1960; Takebe, Kulkulka, Narayan et al., 1976). EMG feedback has also been used in the treatment of torticollis (Brudny, Grynbaum, and Korein, 1974; Cleeland, 1973), nerve injuries (Booker, Rubow, and Coleman, 1969; Jacobs and Felton, 1969), temporomandibular joint pain (Carlsson, Gale, and Ohman, 1975), and bruxism (Solberg and Rugh, 1972). The literature on the applications of EMG feedback in muscular rehabilitation has recently been reviewed by Keefe and Surwit (1978). They conclude that, although EMG feedback is perhaps the oldest form of clinical biofeedback, adequate research is lacking to support the notion that it offers the unique approach to the treatment of any disorder.

EMG feedback has also been used as a method of relaxation training. Typically, electrodes are attached to the frontalis muscle, and subjects are taught to relax the facial musculature using an auditory analog of the frontalis EMG (Budzynski and Stoyva, 1969). This type of feedback has been used, often in combination with progressive relaxation, for the treatment of muscle contraction headaches (Budzynski, Stoyva, and Adler, 1970; Budzynski, Stoyva, Adler, et al., 1973), asthma (Davis, Saunders, Creer, et al., 1973; Sheer, Crawford, Sergent, et al., 1975), essential hypertension (Moeller, 1973; Surwit et al., 1978; Weston, 1974), insomnia (Freedman and Papsdorf, 1976), chronic anxiety (Townsend, House, and Addario, 1975), phobias (Reeves and Mealiea, 1975), and cerebral palsy (Finley, Niman, Standler, et al., 1976). Surwit and Keefe (in press) recently reviewed the literature on the application of frontalis EMG feedback to these disorders. These authors concluded that while EMG feedback seems useful in treating many of these problems, it is far from clear whether or not EMG frontalis feedback training has any distinct advantage over more conventional procedures such as progressive relaxation.

CENTRAL NERVOUS SYSTEM ACTIVITY

Although, as we have seen, much of the early work on biofeedback dealt with the regulation of sympathetic nervous system activity in humans and animals, it was the early work on biofeedback and the control of the EEG (discussed in Kamiya, 1969) that stimulated most popular interest in biofeedback. Studies on the use of biofeedback to control brain activity can be subdivided according to the area and frequency of the activity recorded and controlled. The first reports on the control of EEG were concerned with alpha rhythms. These 8 to 13 Hz wave forms are of high amplitude and are easily observed in the waking EEG. In 1967, Carmona reported an ability to train cats to increase and decrease the EEG amplitude when electrical brain stimulation was used as a reinforcement. Two years later, Kamiya (1969) reported that human subjects could show voluntary control of alpha frequency with the aid of discrimination training consisting of a feedback signal indicating the presence or absence of alpha activity. Paskewitz and Orne (1973) conducted an experiment which elucidated the mechanisms of alpha control and downplayed the importance of feedback in the regulation of alpha. Using binary auditory feedback of alpha activity in the occipital area, Paskewitz and Orne attempted to train two groups of volunteers to increase alpha activity over a no task resting baseline. Although subjects trained in an illuminated room with eyes opened showed some ability to increase alpha when provided with feedback of its occurrence, subjects were not able to increase alpha activity above that observed in an eyes-closed baseline measure. When subjects were trained to increase alpha in a dark room, the presence of feedback did not produce any significant difference in the amount of alpha activity observed. Thus, it appears that successful regulation with biofeedback of alpha activity is accomplished by reducing visual system activity. This is supported by data from Hord, Naitoh, and Johnson (1973).

Attention has also been given to the control of theta rhythms (3.5–7.5 Hz). This activity is of low amplitude and relatively poorly organized in comparison to alpha. Beatty (1977) reports that reinforcement of theta can lead to statistically reliable discriminatory control of the posterior theta activity.

Still a third EEG frequency reported to be controllable via feedback and reinforcement is the sensory motor rhythm or SMR. This rhythm consists of a 12 to 14 Hz signal appearing over the sensory motor cortex. It is usually associated with the suppression of movement. The rhythm has been operantly trained in cats (Sterman, LoPresti, and Fairchild, 1969) and in humans (Sterman, 1973). Of all the EEG biofeedback techniques, learning control of the SMR promises to be the most useful. Epileptic patients trained to increase the predominance of SMR characteristically show a decrease in seizure activity (Lubar and Bahler, 1976; Sterman, 1977; Sterman, Macdonald, and Stone, 1974). Attempts at achieving similar results by training of alpha frequencies have proven ineffective (Kaplan, 1975). Although there is still a controversy over whether or not the effects of this type of training are specifically due to direct changes in the EEG as opposed to nonspecific behavioral control (Mostofsky and Balaschak, 1977), this technique does appear to be promising.

Finally, Beatty (1977) has reported that subjects trained in suppression of theta activity show an increase in vigilance as compared to subjects trained to increase theta activity. Ironically, regulation of the alpha rhythm has not proved to be a clinically useful technique. Although increase in alpha output by the use of EEG biofeedback has become a popular technique for relaxation training, there is almost no evidence indicating that it can be reliably used for this purpose (Beatty, 1977; Orne and Wilson, 1977).

OTHER RESPONSES

Various other physiological responses have also been brought under voluntary control through the use of feedback and reinforcement.

Rosen (1973) demonstrated that direct feedback for penile tumescence was more effective than instructions alone in suppressing erections elicited by tape recorded erotic stimuli. Quinn, Harbison, and McAllister (1970) used iced lime to reinforce heterosexually stimulated penile tumescence in a homosexual patient who had been water deprived for 18 hours. In addition, Rosen, Shapiro, and Schwartz (1975) demonstrated that normal subjects could develop erections without external stimulation simply by utilizing analog feedback of penile tumescence. Csillag (1976) utilized a penile feedback method to facilitate erection in six patients with psychogenic impotence. He reported that all patients showed improvement during 16 training sessions.

Gastric acidity has also been voluntarily regulated utilizing feedback and reward. Whitehead, Renault, and Goldiamond (1975) demonstrated that subjects rewarded for increases or decreases in gastric pH could voluntarily produce these decreases if given feedback for appropriate changes. Gastric pH was measured by having subjects swallow a pH meter. One of the more outstanding clinical applications of biofeedback methods to gastrointestinal control is found in the work of Engel, Nikoomanesh, and Schuster (1974). Using biofeedback for sphincteric responses, six patients with severe fecal incontinence and evidence of external sphincter impairment were taught to produce external sphincter contraction in synchrony with internal sphincter relaxation. These responses were induced by rectal distention.

Vachon and Rich (1976) demonstrated that asthmatic adult subjects given feedback of respiratory resistance could learn to decrease the total respiratory resistance. Similar procedures appeared to be promising in a pilot study of asthmatic children (Feldman, 1976).

SUMMARY AND OVERVIEW

From this overall review of the biofeedback literature several points become clear. In experimental studies, through the use of biofeedback methodology, animals and humans have demonstrated various degrees of voluntary control of both autonomic and central nervous system processes heretofore thought to be involuntary. Biofeedback seems to allow discrete control of the response system fed back to the subject. For example, one component of sympathetic activity can be modified without other sympathetic systems being called in to play. Specific EEG patterns can be modified and discrete muscle groups as small as single motor units can be trained independently with the use of feedback. However, in the autonomic nervous system, it appears that increases in arousal-like activity are easier to obtain than decreases in arousal-like activity. Thus, researchers have more consistently demonstrated voluntary blood pressure increases, heart rate increases, and skin temperature decreases than the opposite of these processes. There is some indication (Sirota et al., 1974, 1976; Victor et al., 1978) that feedback may be more useful in lowering high levels of arousal such as those associated with clinical stress conditions or pathological states. Thus, that decreases in arousal-like activity are difficult to produce with feedback may be more a result of the nature of the experimental training situation in which nonstressful baselines are employed than of the lack of ability of subjects to learn to develop a coping response to stress.

Although the extent of voluntary control of physiological processes through the use of biofeedback has been extensively explored, the question as to the clinical utility of this type of training is as of yet largely unanswered. There are very few large scale controlled clinical outcome studies on the efficacy of biofeedback as compared to other behavioral techniques in the management of many physiological disorders. Those that do exist (Surwit et al., 1978, in press) do not find that biofeedback provides a distinct advantage over other behavioral procedures. The selectivity of physiological control often achieved by biofeedback methods would suggest that the methods would have a unique advantage in disorders in which the symptom is quite specific, for example, cardiac arrhythmias, seizure disorders, various neuromuscular disorders, certain varieties of asthma, etc. Clearly, more research is needed to demonstrate whether or not this advantage is a practical reality. Such questions concerning the relative clinical utility of different behavioral methods in medicine are discussed elsewhere in this volume.

Technical Issues

No effort will be made in this chapter to consider in detail certain basic and technical questions about biofeedback methods and their application. Examples of questions typically raised by those interested in clinical application of biofeedback methods are: 1) Does it make any difference whether the feedback is presented in an auditory, visual, or tactile form? Which is more effective? 2) Is it advantageous to give continuous moment-to-moment biofeedback information as compared with discrete, relatively intermittent information? 3) How important is it that the feedback be immediate rather than delayed? 4) How many sessions of biofeedback treatment are needed to test whether it is really useful for a patient? 5) In repeated treatment sessions, how should they be spaced? Daily? Twice weekly? Weekly? 6) Is it advisable to coach the patient to try to utilize certain specific aids in training (e.g., visualizations, self-suggestions, certain thoughts) or is it better to emphasize more of a trial-and-error exploration of strategies of self-control? 7) How important is it to have the individual focus on internal sensations correlated with the response of interest? 8) What transformations, if any, should be made of the physiological information? Linear? Logarithmic? Reciprocal? 9) Is it desirable, and appropriate, to give training in both increase and decrease directions as a means of facilitating control of the physiological response? How does such bidirectional training compare with unidirectional training in terms of amount and persistence of change? 10) What kinds of individuals are likely to respond positively to biofeedback training?

These questions cannot readily be addressed or discussed in this chapter. Related hypotheses have been posed, and some relevant experimental data exist and have been reported in the publications cited in this chapter. By and large, however, the mass of such data is not substantial, and it would be premature to make recommendations as if they were based on well-established facts.

The specific form and structure of the biofeedback training must depend largely on the individual characteristics of the patient, the physiological symptoms in question, the particular physiological system for which feedback is to be given, the nature of the disorder itself, and so on. Through an accumulation of knowledge gained through basic and clinical research, including systematic case studies, certain generalizations may be possible. At this time, they are not. The clinician has to choose a specific procedure on the basis of all the facts in the case and his or her own understanding of the current technology and state of research knowledge. Through trial-and-error and close observation of clinical outcomes as they happen in a given patient, the clinician can proceed in a step-by-step fashion. The field is too young to expect much standardization of methods. There have been few, if any, large scale clinical trials of the methods in given disorders. As such trials are completed, and as more experimental data are gathered, we may be in a better position to make more specific generalizations about the various technical questions posed above.

What about the instrumentation itself, particularly the various portable devices that are widely advertised in certain professional journals? By and large, scientific research in this field is conducted in specialized laboratories devoted to research in psychophysiology. In such research, multichannel physiological recorders and highly sophisticated experimental control apparatus are employed. On the basis of this work, certain specialized devices have been developed and packaged in a convenient form for nontechnically oriented practitioners. The devices that are currently widespread include instruments for the measurement and feedback of electromyographic activity, skin temperature, electrodermal activity (skin conductance, skin resistance, skin potential), and EEG rhythms. Pulse wave velocity and heart rate devices are beginning to appear on the market. By and large, the various devices are oriented to a few cardiovascular, electrodermal, and electromyographic functions that are relatively easily measured noninvasively.

The entire range of functions that are of medical significance and that may be pertinent for biofeedback experimentation and clinical application is, of course, much greater. With a knowledge of the basic principles involved, it should be possible to adapt almost any instrument that obtains measurements of physiological function, particularly continuous measurements, for purposes of biofeedback. In medical settings, especially where engineering expertise is available, such new ventures may readily be undertaken. In any case, whatever the device, care must be taken to be clear about its specifications, how it works, and what it purports to measure. Information about the technical features of the equipment, and its safety, has to be evaluated by competent people before such equipment is used routinely, and some effort has been made to evaluate and compare the characteristics of various devices (Paskewitz, 1975; Schwitzgebel and Rugh, 1975). Given the rapid advances in electronics and miniature apparatus, we may expect in the future that portable instruments that are flexible in operation and easy to use will become more and more available.

We should also emphasize the importance of "hard copy," that is, of some permanent record, such as on paper or on magnetic tape, of the actual changes achieved by the patient, whether the training be carried out in a clinic, hospital, or by the patient himself at home. Such a record is necessary to document the critical changes occurring within a session and from session to session. Unfortunately, such record-keeping is not yet routine in much clinical biofeedback practice—a situation to be deplored.

An outstanding example of a portable instrument embodying many excellent features is an electroencephalographic device developed by M. B. Sterman and his associates for clinical biofeedback research with epileptic patients. This machine permits the clinician, after making a small adjustment, to set one of several EEG frequency band passes as the feedback criterion. Other circuts inhibit the feedback signal if certain other frequencies occur, or if spike discharges or seizures reflected in the EEG occur. The feedback signals are clear and straightforward, and, finally, the machine contains within it a paper record indicating that the patient used the machine and including a count of the critical events.

Clinical Issues

As we have seen, there is evidence that biofeedback methods can help in the remediation of physical problems usually thought to be treatable only by somatic therapies. However, further research is needed before biofeedback can be advocated as a standard treatment for any disorder. In addition to the numerous questions of efficacy and comparative effects of biofeedback and other behavioral methods, there are a host of practical issues which need to be dealt with in considering the possible role of biofeedback in the treatment of disease.

The first and perhaps most obvious question of practical concern in the evaluation of biofeedback as a clinical tool is the question of economy. How much time and effort on the part of both the patient and the practitioner are needed to obtain a clinically useful result? Even if biofeedback techniques can be shown to be therapeutically effective, what patient would opt for a costly time-consuming training course if equal therapeutic benefit could be obtained from a pill? It is true that there are no medications which are completely effective for Raynaud's disease, tension headache, and cardiac arrhythmias. However, in many cases medication can be a simple, effective and painless way to remedy hypertension, epilepsy, and migraine headaches. Unless the side effects of the medication are serious or the efficacy of biofeedback shown to be superior to that of medication, it seems unlikely that biofeedback will be considered a treatment of choice. On the other hand, the long-term consequences of a continuing course of medication, for example, in the treatment of essential hypertension, have not been thoroughly evaluated. Compliance with medication itself, perhaps because of unpleasant or undesired side effects, may not be optimal, and biofeedback used in conjunction with medication may foster general compliance with treatment.

A related issue has to do with patient motivation. Several articles (Schwartz,

1973; Schwartz and Shapiro, 1973; Shapiro and Schwartz, 1972; Shapiro and Surwit, 1976; Surwit, 1973) have commented on the importance of patient motivation in any biofeedback treatment program. It is not sufficient to assume that feedback indicating therapeutic improvement will, in and of itself, act as a reinforcer and maintain the persistent practice required to gain therapeutic benefit. Indeed, those who have used biofeedback clinically have noted this problem. In one case, Surwit (1973) reported that a patient who had made a long trip to receive biofeedback training complained of being bored during the training sessions and made no progress.

One of the reasons for this problem has been elaborated on by Shapiro and Schwartz (1972). Many of the disorders to which biofeedback might be applied have no short-term aversive consequences. Hypertension works its insidious destruction within the cardiovascular system without usually causing any serious discomfort to the patient, except as the disorder becomes more severe. By the time a painful heart attack occurs, it is too late to correct the damage. It is only the knowledge that the patient has hypertension in conjunction with the knowledge that this disorder is not good for him that provides motivation to undergo treatment. However, in light of the fact that most hypertensive patients will not even take their medication regularly, it is doubtful whether biofeedback training which requires a long period of practice will prove useful for most patients. Similar problems can be seen for any disorder in which the practice of biofeedback is not immediately reinforcing. Conversely, one might expect biofeedback treatments as most appropriate for disorders such as tension headaches and Raynaud's disease where training can lead to immediate relief from pain. Unfortunately, no data exist on the comparative effectiveness of biofeedback in treating disorders such as hypertension as opposed to tension headache. Other behavioral techniques of reinforcing compliance with biofeedback should be considered as an essential ingredient of a behavioral treatment program.

A second motivational problem encountered in the clinical application of biofeedback is that the symptom itself may be reinforcing for the patient. In other words, the disorder may have secondary gain. A striking example of this was reported by Surwit (1973). A patient who was involved in intensive biofeedback treatment for Raynaud's disease spontaneously expressed her ambivalence of "giving up" her illness because she did not know how to relate to people without it. She was aware of using her Raynaud's disease as an excuse for a poor social life and dependent relationship with her mother. In this case, social training was carried out to attempt to remedy the problem. Patients suffering from psychosomatic illnesses often use their well-known sensitivity to emotional situations to manipulate others (Lachman, 1972). A therapy based on "voluntary control" would tend to undermine their manipulations and consequently might not be seen as desirable by the patient. Although early models of behavior therapy tended to ignore the more subtle contingencies implicit in some behavioral problems, more recent writers are taking them into account (Kraft, 1972; Lazarus, 1971). In that some of these contingencies might not be known to the patient explicitly, they may be considered as unconscious. A behavioral therapy designed to treat a disorder supported by secondary gain would therefore have to include techniques aimed at making up any social deficit left by the removal of the symptom. These might include setting up family contingencies and/or working on alternative means of social interaction. When the patient himself does not see the need for such additional procedures, an insight-oriented approach may be called for as a first step.

A third possible area of motivational difficulty may arise from other behaviors strongly entrenched in the patient's repertoire which are in conflict with the aim of therapy. This is best illustrated in a case discussed by Schwartz (1973). A patient was treated for essential hypertension and over a week of treatment lowered his blood pressure by as much as 20 mm Hg. Over the weekend his pressure would become elevated again. The difficulty turned out to be that the patient liked to gamble at the race track on weekends and persisted in doing so despite the fact that such activities were countertherapeutic. This last point is extremely important. There is good evidence that certain schedules of reinforcement can induce ulcers and hypertension in normal animals (Benson et al., 1969, 1970; Brady, 1958; Harris et al., 1973). It would seem futile to attempt to treat a disorder by biofeedback unless work were also done on analyzing and correcting contingencies that may be aggravating the problem.

An issue closely related to motivation and equally important in the successful application of biofeedback techniques is transfer of training. It is often all too easy to forget, even for psychologists, that learning techniques cannot be administered as are most medical treatments. There is no reason to believe that biofeedback, like radiation therapy and diathermy, can be expected to produce sustained effects outside the treatment session. It is completely logical that a patient may show perfect control over his problem during a feedback session and no control at home. In basic research in normal subjects, some investigators have explored the use of intermittent reinforcement schedules as an aid to generalization (Greene, 1966; Shapiro and Crider, 1967; Shapiro and Watanabe, 1971), but the evidence is too scanty to conclude that partial reinforcement increases resistance to extinction in the case of visceral responses. Weiss and Engel (1971) in their study of the control of premature ventricular contractions phased the feedback out gradually, making it available all the time at first, then 1 minute on and 1 minute off, then 1 on and 3 off, and finally 1 on and 7 off. The purpose of the procedure was to wean the patient from feedback and also enable the patient to become more aware of his arrhythmia through his own sensations and less dependent upon feedback. Surwit et al. (in press) asked patients suffering from Raynaud's disease to practice warming their hands 30 times a day, 30 seconds at a time. Patients were given little gold stars which they were told to paste around the home, office, and car to remind them to practice. They recorded the total number of practice periods each day on a small counter. This systematic programmed practice was felt by many patients to be responsible for their reported improvement. There is also evidence for the short-term maintenance of learned control of diastolic pressure (Shapiro et al., 1972b), but the need is great for comprehensive research on extinction processes and on self-control without feedback in autonomic learning.

A related but more complex issue c cerns the need of patients to control th reactivity to stressful stimuli or situations In most cases, biofeedback procedures are applied in resting, nonstimulating laboratory settings. Will the patient be able to transfer this training to the relevant situations in everyday life? Sirota et al. (1974, 1976) attempted to explore the effects of feedback-assisted voluntary control of heart rate to facilitate adaption to noxious events. An earlier study (Shapiro, Schwartz, Nelson, et al., 1972a), combined skin resistance feedback and reinforcement with a variant of a desensitization procedure in attempting to facilitate adaptation of phobic subjects to the feared stimuli (snakes). The methodology of this research follows from several studies indicating that discrete electrodermal responses to stimuli in human subjects can be relatively increased or decreased by means of reinforcement for the appropriate response, and that these changes may have consequences for performance related to these stimuli (Kimmel et al., 1967; Shnidman, 1969, 1970; Shnidman and Shapiro, 1971).

In the Sirota et al. (1974) study, in anticipation of receiving noxious electrical stimulation, subjects learned to control their heart rate when provided with external heart rate feedback and reward for appropriate changes. In this study, subjects were also informed about the actual physiological response required for reward. The results showed that voluntary slowing of heart rate led to a relative reduction in the perceived aversiveness of the noxious stimuli, particularly for those subjects who reported experiencing cardiac reactions to fear situations in their daily life. Sirota et al. concluded, "Taken together, the results support the general conclusion that direct feedback control of autonomic functions which are appropriate for given subjects in terms of their normal fear responding and/or whose relevance for fear has been instructionally induced may possibly be used in systematic desensitization to inhibit anxiety from occurring in response to phobic stimuli and as an adjunct to other therapeutic techniques for the prevention and reduction of anxiety and fear reactions" (p. 266). In a related study (Victor et al., 1978), similar methods were used to show that subjects could learn to vary their heart rate, by means of biofeedback training, in response to the cold pressor test, immersion of the hand in ice water for 30 seconds. The variations in heart rate were associated with different perceptions of the intensity of the painful cold water stimulus. Procedures such as these should be studied to increase the potential of transfer of learned control of relevant situations for the individual. In the case of different psychosomatic disorders, to the extent that they involve behavioral and physiological reaction patterns specific to certain types of eliciting stimuli or situations, a physiological desensitization procedure can be designed accordingly. Biofeedback may turn out to have practical application to the management of anxiety and phobic reactions, in addition to the control of symptoms triggered by specific stimuli (Blanchard and Abel, 1976; Gatchel and Proctor, 1976).

In addition to motivation, Shapiro and Schwartz (1972) have pointed out that patient characteristics must also be considered in determining the feasibility of biofeedback as a treatment. Because most clinical and experimental work on biofeedback has been done with highly educated, motivated individuals, it is presently unclear how the variables of intelligence, socioeconomic status, and overall adjustment are related to treatment outcome. Surwit, Bradner, Fenton, et al. (Note 5) have shown that personality variables can predict success in the behavioral treatment of Raynaud's disease. Specifically, low scorers on the Alienation scale of the Psychological Screening Inventory (Lanyon, 1970, 1973) show significantly more vasomotor control after training than high scorers. Older subjects were found to do better than younger subjects. Until more data shed light on these questions, therapists should be cognizant of the particular characteristics of the population from which successful behavior therapy patients have been drawn.

Because biofeedback involves the treatment of disease, it is one area of psychological practice where the medical model of illness cannot be dismissed. While many physical disorders can be exacerbated by emotional and environmental variables, most of them have a distinct physical etiology and may represent the "symptom" of a more profound physiological dysfunction. Also, certain disorders which have resulted in permanent destruction and/or alteration of tissue may not be amenable to a behavioral treatment. In many cases, it is conceivable that medication should be used as a valuable concomitant to biofeedback. Engel (Note 6) has noted that propranolol seems to facilitate heart rate control in subjects suffering from angina pectoris. It is probably wise to employ an eclectic strategy in determining the treatment of any physiological disorder. As Pinkerton (1973) aptly remarked, "no single factor is of overriding importance in symptom production [in psychosomatic illness]. The clinical outcome is always determined by a composite etiological sequence, so that the key to successful management lies in correctly evaluating each factor's importance in any given case" (p. 462).

In any event it is clearly not up to the psychologist alone to decide how biofeedback will contribute to the treatment of a physical problem. Consequently, biofeedback should be used clinically only after a competent medical diagnosis has been made and the examining physician has decided that biofeedback may be valuable. Patients coming directly to psychologists for biofeedback or other behavioral treatments of a physical disorder should be referred first to a medical specialist for a thorough examination and work up. The need for medical participation in any biofeedback case is both an ethical and legal responsibility of the psychological practitioner. Conversely, it is also the ethical responsibility of a physician who wishes to employ biofeedback in treatment to consult with a psychologist for the behavioral aspects of the proposed therapy. Medical training does not provide the in-depth knowledge of behavioral variables of which the practitioner must be cognizant in order for training to be successful. Therefore, the use of biofeedback in therapy for various physiological disorders should be a collaborative endeavor involving both medical and behavioral specialists.

Conclusions

This chapter has presented a review of methodology, theory, basic research, and clinical applications of biofeedback as a means of regulating visceral, somatomotor, and neural processes. Less than 20 years old, biofeedback has spawned hundreds of basic and clinical papers, dozens of books, scores of workshops, many portable biofeedback devices, and quite a few specialized biofeedback clinics and training programs. Although the field may have overextended itself, and the popular fascination with the methods and their potential may in part account for that, biofeedback represents a highly significant development in basic research and clinical practice. It provides a valuable *behavioral* strategy of dealing with physiological processes, of examining behavioral and environmental influences on physiological functioning, and of modifying symptoms of psychophysiological and other disorders. Biofeedback research has developed techniques which have enabled therapists to place physiological activities of the body under the control of environmental contingencies, in much the same way as has been done with other types of behavior. It provides another means, in addition to the other methods discussed in this book, of extending the full scope of behavior modification into the domain of medicine.

However one regards the theoretical foundations and empirical evidence in this field, the essential concept of providing the individual a means of monitoring his own bodily activities as they are occurring in real time as a means of regulating such activities is intuitively appealing. The very simplicity of the concept, however, can also be misleading, inasmuch as the processes of physiological self-regulation are as complicated as the processes of behavioral self-regulation. The kind of learning or physiological change involved in biofeedback depends upon numerous social and biological constraints and influences. Like any method or technique, biofeedback does not operate in a vacuum.

With these words of caution and the field seen in proper perspective, biofeedback should become one of the mainstays of research concerned with the role of behavior in the etiology, development, treatment, rehabilitation, and prevention of disease. In many respects, the biofeedback approach to disease probably comes closer than any other psychological method to the approach of conventional medicine in which a treatment is rationally devised to deal directly with the symptom or with the cause of the disease. That is, biofeedback is akin to the use of specific drugs or surgery to correct a deficiency or eliminate a symptom. This potential has its origins in basic research, reviewed in this chapter, which shows that specific physiological responses or patterns of responses can be modified by biofeedback methods. Thus, a rationale for the clinical use of biofeedback is especially clear in cases in which the symptom is quite specific, such as high blood pressure in essential hypertension, degree of muscular activity in various neuromuscular disorders, or heart rate dependent cardiac arrhythmias. Biofeedback can also be used as an indirect means of influencing the course of particular disorders, such as by facilitating relaxation, calming the individual, or reducing overall physiological arousal levels.

From a purely practical standpoint, much more research will be needed to demonstrate the utility of biofeedback. How effective is it in comparison with relaxation and other behavioral methods, for which disorders, for which kinds of people? Are the effects long lasting? What methods can be used to sustain them? How can laboratory training be generalized to everyday situations? Does biofeedback provide a viable alternative for individuals for whom drug treatment is ineffective or causes unacceptable side effects?

At this point in time, a great deal of attention is being paid to comparative studies of the different behavioral methods with one another, including biofeedback, and with standard medical treatments, and time will tell. There is no question, however, that the methods will grow in importance in behavioral medicine, particularly as they continue to grow out of the collaborative efforts of behavioral scientists, physiologists, psychologists, and physicians.

Reference Notes

1. Shapiro, D. Unpublished data, 1972.
2. Benson, H., Shapiro, D., and Schwartz, G. E. Unpublished data, 1972.
3. Blanchard, E. B., and Silver, B. V. Personal communication, December, 1977.

4. Bradner, M. N., Surwit, R. S., and Birk, L. A comparison of biofeedback with the relaxation response in the treatment of migraine headache. In preparation.
5. Surwit, R. S., Bradner, M. N., Fenton, C. H., and Pilon, R. N. Individual differences in response to the behavioral treatment of Raynaud's disease. In preparation.
6. Engel, B. T. Personal communication, October, 1977.

References

Andrews, J. M. Electromyography. *J. Am. Osteopathol. Assoc.*, 1957, *56*, 354–355.

Anliker, J. Biofeedback from the perspectives of cybernetics and systems science. In J. Beatty and H. Legewie (Eds.), *Biofeedback and behavior.* New York: Plenum, 1977.

Barber, T. X., DiCara, L. V., Kamiya, J., Miller, N. E., Shapiro, D., and Stoyva, J. (Eds.). *Biofeedback and self-control 1975/76: An Aldine Annual on the regulation of bodily processes and consciousness.* Chicago: Aldine, 1976.

Barlow, D. H., and Hersen, M. Single case experimental designs: Uses in applied clinical research. *Arch. Gen. Psychiatry*, 1973, *29*, 319–325.

Basmajian, J. V. Control and training of individual motor units. *Science*, 1963, *141*, 440–441.

Basmajian, J. V. Learned control of single motor units. In G. E. Schwartz and J. Beatty (Eds.), *Biofeedback: Theory and research.* New York: Academic Press, 1977.

Basmajian, J. V., Kulkulka, C. G., Narayan, M. G., and Takebe, K. Biofeedback treatment of a foot-drop after stroke compared with standard rehabilitation technique: Effects on voluntary control and strength. *Arch. Phys. Med. Rehabil.*, 1975, *56*, 231–236.

Beatty, J. Similar effects of feedback signals and instructional information on EEG activity. *Physiol. Behav.*, 1972, *9*, 151–154.

Beatty, J. Learned regulation of alpha and theta frequency activity in the human electroencephalogram. In G. E. Schwartz and J. Beatty (Eds.), *Biofeedback: Theory and research.* New York: Academic Press, 1977.

Beatty, J., and Legewie, H. (Eds.). *Biofeedback and behavior.* New York: Plenum, 1977.

Bell, I. R., and Schwartz, G. E. Voluntary control and reactivity of human heart rate. *Psychophysiology*, 1975, *12*, 339–348.

Benson, H. *The relaxation response.* New York: William Morrow & Co., 1975.

Benson, H., Herd, J. A., Morse, W. H., and Kelleher, R. T. Behavioral induction of arterial hypertension and its reversal. *Am. J. Physiol.*, 1969, *217*, 30–34.

Benson, H., Herd, J. A., Morse, W. H., and Kelleher, R. T. Behaviorally induced hypertension in the squirrel monkey. *Circ. Res.* (Suppl. 1), 1970, *26-27*, 21-26.

Benson, H., Shapiro, D., Tursky, B., and Schwartz, G. E. Decreased systolic blood pressure through operant conditioning techniques in patients with essential hypertension. *Science*, 1971, *173*, 740–742.

Bergman, J. S., and Johnson, H. J. The effects of instructional set and autonomic perception on cardiac control. *Psychophysiology*, 1971, *8*, 180–190.

Bergman, J. S., and Johnson, H. J. Sources of information which affect training and raising of heart rate. *Psychophysiology*, 1972, *9*, 30–39.

Birk, L., Crider, A., Shapiro, D., and Tursky, B. Operant electrodermal conditioning under partial curarization. *J. Comp. Physiol. Psychol.*, 1966, *62*, 165–166.

Black, A. H. The direct control of neural processes by reward and punishment. *Am. Sci.*, 1971, *59*, 236–245.

Black, A. H. The operant conditioning of central nervous system electrical activity. In G. H. Bower (Ed.), *The psychology of learning and motivation: Advances in research and theory.* New York: Academic Press, 1972.

Black, A. H., Cott, A., and Pavloski, R. The operant learning theory approach to biofeedback training. In G. E. Schwartz and J. Beatty (Eds.), *Biofeedback: Theory and research.* New York: Academic Press, 1977.

Blanchard, E. B., and Abel, G. G. An experimental case study of the biofeedback treatment of a rape-induced psychophysiological disorder. *Behav. Ther.*, 1976, *7*, 113–119.

Blanchard, E. B., Scott, R. W., Young, L. D., and Edmundson, E. D. Effect of knowledge of response on the self-control of heart rate. *Psychophysiology*, 1974a, *11*, 251–264.

Blanchard, E. B., and Young, L. D. Relative efficacy of visual and auditory feedback for self-control of heart rate. *J. Gen. Psychol.*, 1972, *87*, 195–202.

Blanchard, E. B., and Young, L. D. Self-control of cardiac functioning: A promise as yet unfulfilled. *Psychol. Bull.*, 1973, *79*, 145–163.

Blanchard, E. B., and Young, L. D. Clinical applications of biofeedback training: A review of evidence. *Arch. Gen. Psychiatry*, 1974, *30*, 573–589.

Blanchard, E. B., Young, L. D., and McLeod, P. G. Awareness of heart activity and self-control of heart rate. *Psychophysiology*, 1972, *9*, 63–68.

Blanchard, E. B., Young, L. D., Scott, R. W., and Haynes, M. R. Differential effects of feedback and reinforcement in voluntary acceleration of human heart rate. *Percep. Mot. Skills*, 1974b, *38*, 683–691.

Bleecker, E. R., and Engel, B. T. Learned control of cardiac rate and cardiac conduction in the Wolff-Parkinson-White syndrome. *N. Engl. J. Med.*, 1973, *288*, 560–562.

Booker, H. E., Rubow, R. T., and Coleman, P. J. Simplified feedback in neuromuscular retraining: An automated approach using EMG signals. *Arch. Phys. Med. Rehabil.*, 1969, *50*, 621–625.

Brady, J. V. Ulcers in "executive" monkeys. *Sci. Am.*, 1958, *199*, 95–103.

Brener, J. A general model of voluntary control applied to the phenomena of learned cardiovascular change. In P. A. Obrist, A. H. Black, J. Brener, and L. V. DiCara (Eds.), *Cardiovascular psychophysiology.* Chicago: Aldine, 1974.

Brener, J. Visceral perception. In J. Beatty and H. Legewie (Eds.), *Biofeedback and behavior.* New York: Plenum, 1977.

Brener, J., Eissenberg, E., and Middaugh, S. Respiratory and somatomotor factors associated with operant conditioning of cardiovascular responses in curarized rats. In P. A. Obrist, A. H. Black, J. Brener, and L. V. DiCara (Eds.), *Cardiovascular psychophysiology*. Chicago: Aldine, 1974.

Brener, J., and Hothersall, D. Heart rate control under conditions of augmented sensory feedback. *Psychophysiology*, 1966, *3*, 23–28.

Brener, J., and Jones, J. M. Interoceptive discrimination in intact humans: Detection of cardiac activity. *Physiol. Behav.*, 1974, *13*, 763–767.

Brudny, J., Grynbaum, B. B., and Korein, J. Spasmodic torticollis: Treatment by feedback display of the EMG. *Arch. Phys. Med. Rehabil.*, 1974, *55*, 403–408.

Brudny, J., Korein, J., Grynbaum, B. B., Friedmann, L. W., Weinstein, S., Sachs-Frankel, G., and Belandres, P. V. EMG feedback therapy: Review of treatment of 114 patients. *Arch. Phys. Med. Rehabil.*, 1976, *57*, 55–61.

Brudny, J., Korein, J., Levidow, L., Grynbaum, B. B., Lieberman, A., and Friedmann, L. W. Sensory feedback therapy as a modality of treatment in central nervous system disorders of voluntary movement. *Neurology*, 1974, *24*, 925–932.

Budzynski, T. H., and Stoyva, J. M. An instrument for producing deep muscle relaxation by means of analog information feedback. *J. Appl. Behav. Anal.*, 1969, *2*, 231–237.

Budzynski, T., Stoyva, J., and Adler, C. Feedback-induced muscle relaxation: Application to tension headache. *J. Behav. Ther. Exp. Psychiatry*, 1970, *1*, 205–211.

Budzynski, T. H., Stoyva, J. M., Adler, C. S., and Mullaney, D. J. EMG biofeedback and tension headache: A controlled outcome study. *Psychosom. Med.*, 1973, *35*, 484–496.

Carlsson, S. G., Gale, E. N., and Ohman, A. Treatment of temporomandibular joint syndrome with biofeedback training. *J. Am. Dent. Assoc.*, 1975, *91*, 602–605.

Carmona, A. Trial and error of the cortical EEG activity. Unpublished doctoral dissertation, Yale University, New Haven, Conn., 1967.

Cleeland, C. S. Behavior techniques in the modification of spasmodic torticollis. *Neurology*, 1973, *23*, 1241–1247.

Cohen, D. H., and Obrist, P. A. Interactions between behavior and the cardiovascular system. *Circ. Res.*, 1975, *37*, 693–706.

Colgan, M. Effects of binary and proportional feedback on bidirectional control of heart rate. *Psychophysiology*, 1977, *14*, 187–191.

Crider, A., Schwartz, G. E., and Shapiro, D. Operant suppression of electrodermal response rate as a function of punishment schedule. *J. Exp. Psychol.*, 1970, *83*, 333–334.

Crider, A., Schwartz, G. E., and Shnidman, S. On the criteria for instrumental autonomic conditioning: A reply to Katkin and Murray. *Psychol. Bull.*, 1969, *71*, 455–461.

Crider, A., Shapiro, D., and Tursky, B. Reinforcement of spontaneous electrodermal activity. *J. Comp. Physiol. Psychol.*, 1966, *61*, 20–27.

Csillag, E. R. Modification of penile erectile response. *J. Behav. Ther. Exp. Psychiatry*, 1976, *7*, 27–29.

Davidson, R. J., and Schwartz, G. E. The psychobiology of relaxation and related states: A multi-process theory. In D. I. Mostofsky (Ed.), *Behavior control and modification of physiological activity*. Englewood Cliffs, N.J.: Prentice-Hall, 1976.

Davis, M. H., Saunders, D. B., Creer, T. L., and Chai, H. Relaxation training facilitated by biofeedback apparatus as a supplemental treatment in bronchial asthma. *J. Psychosom. Res.*, 1973, *17*, 121–128.

DiCara, L. V. Learning in the autonomic nervous system. *Sci. Am.*, 1970, *222*, 30–39.

DiCara, L. V., Barber, T. X., Kamiya, J., Miller, N. E., Shapiro, D., and Stoyva, J. (Eds.). *Biofeedback and self-control 1974: An Aldine Annual on the regulation of bodily processes and consciousness*. Chicago: Aldine, 1975.

DiCara, L. V., and Miller, N. E. Changes in heart rate instrumentally learned by curarized rats as avoidance responses. *J. Comp. Physiol. Psychol.*, 1968a, *65*, 8–12.

DiCara, L. V., and Miller, N. E. Instrumental learning of systolic blood pressure responses by curarized rats: Dissociation of cardiac and vascular changes. *Psychosom. Med.*, 1968b, *30*, 489–494.

Dworkin, B. R., and Miller, N. E. Visceral learning in the curarized rat. In G. E. Schwartz and J. Beatty (Eds.), *Biofeedback: Theory and research*. New York: Academic Press, 1977.

Elder, S. T., Ruiz, Z. R., Deabler, H. L., and Dillenkoffer, R. L. Instrumental conditioning of diastolic blood pressure in essential hypertensive patients. *J. Appl. Behav. Anal.*, 1973, *6*, 377–382.

Engel, B. T. Operant conditioning of cardiac function: A status report. *Psychophysiology*, 1972, *9*, 161–177.

Engel, B. T., and Bleecker, E. R. Application of operant conditioning techniques to the control of the cardiac arrhythmias. In P. A. Obrist, A. H. Black, J. Brener, and L. V. DiCara (Eds.), *Cardiovascular psychophysiology*. Chicago: Aldine, 1974.

Engel, B. T., and Hansen, S. P. Operant conditioning of heart rate slowing. *Psychophysiology*, 1966, *3*, 176–187.

Engel, B. T., Nikoomanesh, P., and Schuster, M. M. Operant conditioning of rectosphincteric responses in the treatment of fecal incontinence. *N. Engl. J. Med.*, 1974, *290*, 646–649.

Epstein, L. H., and Stein, D. B. Feedback-influenced heart rate discrimination. *J. Abnorm. Psychol.*, 1974, *83*, 585–588.

Feldman, G. M. The effect of biofeedback training on respiratory resistance of asthmatic children. *Psychosom. Med.*, 1976, *38*, 27–34.

Fetz, E. E., and Finocchio, D. V. Operant conditioning of specific patterns of neural and muscular activity. *Science*, 1971, *174*, 431–435.

Fey, S. G., and Lindholm, E. Systolic blood pressure and heart rate changes during three sessions involving biofeedback or no feedback. *Psychophysiology*, 1975, *12*, 513–519.

Finley, W. W., Niman, C., Standler, J., and Ender, P. Frontal EMG biofeedback training of athetoid cerebral palsy patients: A report of six cases. *Biofeedback Self-Regulation*, 1976, *1*, 169–182.

Fowler, R. L., and Kimmel, H. D. Operant conditioning of the GSR. *J. Exp. Psychol.*, 1962, *63*, 563–567.

Freedman, R., and Papsdorf, J. D. Biofeedback and progressive relaxation treatment of sleep onset insomnia. *Biofeedback Self-Regulation*, 1976, *1*, 253–271.

Garcia, J., and Rusiniak, K. W. Visceral feedback and the taste signal. In J. Beatty and H. Legewie (Eds.), *Biofeedback and behavior*. New York: Plenum, 1977.

Gatchel, R. J. Frequency of feedback and learned heart rate control. *J. Exp. Psychol.*, 1974, *103*, 274-283.

Gatchel, R. J., and Proctor, J. D. Effectiveness of voluntary heart rate control in reducing speech anxiety. *J. Consult. Clin. Psychol.*, 1976, *44*, 381–389.

Goldman, H., Kleinman, K. M., Snow, M. Y., Bidus, D. R., and Korol, B. Relationship between essential hypertension and cognitive functioning: Effects of biofeedback. *Psychophysiology*, 1975, *12*, 569–573.

Greene, W. A. Operant conditioning of the GSR using partial reinforcement. *Psychol. Rep.*, 1966, *19*, 571–578.

Hamano, K. Studies on self regulation of internal activity: Preliminary report on transaction with interoceptive feedback in the discrimination of cardiac activity. *Jpn. Psychol. Res.*, 1977, *19*, 143–148.

Harris, A. H., and Brady, J. V. Animal learning—Visceral and autonomic conditioning. In M. R. Rosenzweig and L. W. Porter (Eds.), *Annual review of psychology*, Vol. 25. Palo Alto: Annual Reviews, Inc., 1974.

Harris, A. H., and Brady, J. V. Long-term studies of cardiovascular control in primates. In G. E. Schwartz and J. Beatty (Eds.), *Biofeedback: Theory and research*. New York: Academic Press, 1977.

Harris, A. H., Findley, J. D., and Brady, J. V. Instrumental conditioning of blood pressure elevations in the baboon. *Conditional Reflex*, 1971, *6*, 215–226.

Harris, A. H., Gilliam, W. J., Findley, J. D., and Brady, J. V. Instrumental conditioning of large magnitude, daily, 12-hour blood pressure elevations in the baboon. *Science*, 1973, *182*, 175–177.

Hefferline, R. F., Keenan, B., and Harford, R. A. Escape and avoidance conditioning in human subjects without their observation of the response. *Science*, 1959, *130*, 1338–1339.

Hefferline, R. F., and Perera, T. B. Proprioceptive discrimination of a covert operant without its observation by the subject. *Science*, 1963, *139*, 834–835.

Hnatiow, M., and Lang, P. J. Learned stabilization of cardiac rate. *Psychophysiology*, 1965, *1*, 330–336.

Hord, D., Naitoh, P., and Johnson, L. C. EEG spectral features of self-regulated high alpha states. In D. Shapiro, T. X. Barber, L. V. DiCara, J. Kamiya, N. E. Miller, and J. Stoyva (Eds.), *Biofeedback and self-control 1972: An Aldine Annual on the regulation of bodily processes and consciousness*. Chicago: Aldine, 1973, (Abstract).

Howard, J. L., Galosy, R. A., Gaebelein, C. J., and Obrist, P. A. Some problems in the use of neuromuscular blockade. In P. A. Obrist, A. H. Black, J. Brener, and L. V. DiCara (Eds.), *Cardivascular psychophysiology*. Chicago: Aldine, 1974.

Jacobs, A., and Felton, G. S. Visual feedback of myoelectric output to facilitate muscle relaxation in normal persons and patients with neck injuries. *Arch. Phys. Med. Rehabil.*, 1969, *50*, 34–39.

Johnson, H. E., and Garton, W. H. Muscle re-education in hemiplegia by use of electromyographic device. *Arch. Phys. Med. Rehabil.*, 1973, *54*, 320–323.

Johnson, H. J., and Schwartz, G. E. Suppression of GSR activity through operant reinforcement. *J. Exp. Psychol.*, 1967, *75*, 307-312.

Johnson, R. J. Operant reinforcement of an autonomic response. *Diss. Abstr.*, 1963, *24*, 1255–1256.

Johnston, D. Criterion level and instructional effects in the voluntary control of heart rate. *Biol. Psychol.*, 1976, *4*, 1–17.

Kamiya, J. Operant control of the EEG alpha rhythm and some of its reported effects on consciousness. In C. Tart (Ed.), *Altered states of consciousness*. New York: Wiley, 1969.

Kamiya, J., Barber, T. X., Miller, N. E., Shapiro, D., and Stoyva, J. (Eds.). *Biofeedback and self-control 1976/77: An Aldine Annual on the regulation of bodily processes and consciousness*. Chicago: Aldine, 1977.

Kannel, W. B., Gordon, T., and Schwartz, M. J. Systolic versus diastolic blood pressure and risk of coronary heart disease. *Am. J. Cardiol.*, 1971, *27*, 335–343.

Kaplan, B. J. Biofeedback in epileptics: Equivocal relationship of reinforced EEG frequency to seizure reduction. *Epilepsia*, 1975, *16*, 477–485.

Katkin, E. S., and Murray, E. N. Instrumental conditioning of autonomically mediated behavior: Theoretical and methodological issues. *Psychol. Bull.*, 1968, *70*, 52–68.

Keefe, F. J., and Surwit, R. S. Electromyographic biofeedback—Behavioral treatment of neuromuscular disorders. *J. Behav. Med.*, 1978, *1*, 13–24.

Kimmel, H. D. Instrumental conditioning of autonomically mediated behavior. *Psychol. Bull.*, 1967, *67*, 337–345.

Kimmel, H. D., Pendergrass, V. E., and Kimmel, E. B. Modifying children's orienting reactions instrumentally. *Conditional Reflex*, 1967, *2*, 227–235.

Kraft, T. The use of behavior therapy in a psychotherapeutic context. In A. A. Lazarus (Ed.), *Clinical behavior therapy*. New York: Brunner/Mazel, 1972.

Kristt, D. A., and Engel, B. T. Learned control of blood pressure in patients with high blood pressure. *Circulation*, 1975, *51*, 370–378.

Lachman, S. J. *Psychosomatic disorders: A behavioristic interpretation*. New York: Wiley, 1972.

Lang, P. J. Learned control of human heart rate in a computer directed environment. In P. A. Obrist, A. H. Black, J. Brener, and L. V. DiCara (Eds.), *Cardiovascular psychophysiology*. Chicago: Aldine, 1974.

Lang, P. J. Research on the specificity of feedback training: Implications for the use of biofeedback in the treatment of anxiety and fear. In J. Beatty and H. Legewie (Eds.), *Biofeedback and behavior*. New York: Plenum, 1977.

Lang, P. J., Troyer, W. G., Jr., Twentyman, C. T., and Gatchel, R. J. Differential effects of heart rate modification training on college students, older males, and patients with ischemic heart disease. *Psychosom. Med.*, 1975, *37*, 429–446.

Lang, P. J., and Twentyman, C. T. Learning to control heart rate: Binary versus analogue feedback. *Psychophysiology*, 1974, *11*, 616–629.

Lang, P. J., and Twentyman, C. T. Learning to control heart rate: Effects of varying incentive and criterion of success on task performance. *Psychophysiology*, 1976, *13*, 378–385.

Lanyon, R. I. Development and validation of a psychological screening inventory. *J. Consult. Clin. Psychol. Monogr.*, 1970, *35* (1, Part 2).

Lanyon, R. I. *The Psychological Screening Inventory: Manual.* Goshen, N.Y.: Research Psychologists Press, 1973.

Lazarus, A. *Behavior therapy and beyond.* New York: McGraw-Hill, 1971.

Lazarus, R. S. A cognitive analysis of biofeedback control. In G. E. Schwartz and J. Beatty (Eds.), *Biofeedback: Theory and research.* New York: Academic Press, 1977.

Lisina, M. I. The role of orientation in the transformation of involuntary into voluntary reactions. In L. G. Voronin, A. N. Leontiev, A. R. Luria, E. N. Sokolov, and O. S. Vinogradova (Eds.), *Orienting reflex and exploratory behavior.* Moscow: Akad. Pedag. Nauk RSFSR, 1958 (in Russian); Washington, D.C.: American Psychological Association, 1965 (in English).

Lubar, J. F., and Bahler, W. W. Behavioral management of epileptic seizures following EEG biofeedback training of the sensorimotor rhythm. *Biofeedback Self-Regulation*, 1976, *1*, 77–104.

Manuck, S. B., Levenson, R. W., Hinrichsen, J. J., and Gryll, S. L. Role of feedback in voluntary control of heart rate. *Percept. Mot. Skills*, 1975, *40*, 747–752.

Marinacci, A. A. *Applied electromyography*. Philadelphia: Lea & Febiger, 1968.

Marinacci, A. A., and Horande, M. Electromyogram in neuromuscular re-education. *Bull. Los Angeles Neurol. Soc.*, 1960, *25*, 57–71.

Merrill, J. P. Hypertensive vascular disease. In J. V. Harrison, R. D. Adams, I. L. Bennett, W. H. Resnik, G. W. Thorn, and M. M. Wintrobe (Eds.), *Principles of internal medicine.* New York: McGraw-Hill, 1966.

Miller, N. E. Learning of visceral and glandular responses. *Science*, 1969, *163*, 434–445.

Miller, N. E. Applications of learning and biofeedback to psychiatry and medicine. In A. M. Freedman, H. I. Kaplan, and B. J. Sadock (Eds.), *Comprehensive textbook of psychiatry-II.* Baltimore: Williams & Wilkins, 1975.

Miller, N. E., and DiCara, L. Instrumental learning of heart rate changes in curarized rats: Shaping, and specificity to discriminative stimulus. *J. Comp. Physiol. Psychol.*, 1967, *63*, 12–19.

Miller, N. E., and Dworkin, B. R. Visceral learning: Recent difficulties with curarized rats and significant problems for human research. In P. A. Obrist, A. H. Black, J. Brener, and L. V. DiCara (Eds.), *Cardiovascular psychophysiology*. Chicago: Aldine, 1974.

Moeller, T. A. Reduction of arterial blood pressure through relaxation training and correlates of personality in hypertensives. Unpublished doctoral dissertation, Nova University, Fort Lauderdale, Fla., 1973.

Mostofsky, D. I., and Balaschak, B. A. Psychobiological control of seizures. *Psychol. Bull.*, 1977, *84*, 723–750.

Mulholland, T. B. Biofeedback method for locating the most controlled responses of EEG alpha to visual stimulation. In J. Beatty & H. Legewie (Eds.), *Biofeedback and behavior.* New York: Plenum, 1977.

Obrist, P. A. The cardiovascular-behavioral interaction—As it appears today. *Psychophysiology*, 1976, *13*, 95–107.

Obrist, P. A., Galosy, R. A., Lawler, J. E., Gaebelein, C. J., Howard, J. L., and Shanks, E. M. Operant conditioning of heart rate: Somatic correlates. *Psychophysiology*, 1975, *12*, 445–455.

Obrist, P. A., Howard, J. L., Lawler, J. E., Galosy, R. A., Meyers, K. A., and Gaebelein, C. J. The cardiac-somatic interaction. In P. A. Obrist, A. H. Black, J. Brener, and L. V. DiCara (Eds.), *Cardiovascular psychophysiology*. Chicago: Aldine, 1974.

Ogden, E., and Shock, N. W. Voluntary hypercirculation. *Am. J. Med. Sci.*, 1939, *198*, 329–342.

Orne, M., and Wilson, S. Alpha, biofeedback and arousal/activation. In J. Beatty and H. Legewie (Eds.), *Biofeedback and behavior.* New York: Plenum, 1977.

Pappas, B. A., DiCara, L. V., and Miller, N. E. Learning of blood pressure responses in the noncurarized rat: Transfer to the curarized state. *Physiol. Behav.*, 1970, *5*, 1029–1032.

Paskewitz, D. A. Biofeedback instrumentation: Soldering closed the loop. *Am. Psychol.*, 1975, *30*, 371–378.

Paskewitz, D. A., and Orne, M. T. Visual effects on alpha feedback training. *Science*, 1973, *181*, 360–363.

Patton, H. D. The autonomic nervous system. In T. C. Rugh, H. D. Patton, J. W. Woodbury, and A. L. Towe (Eds.), *Neurophysiology.* Philadelphia: W. B. Saunders, 1965.

Pickering, T. G., Brucker, B., Frankel, H. L., Mathias, C. J., Dworkin, B. R., and Miller, N. E. Mechanisms of learned voluntary control of blood pressure in patients with generalised bodily paralysis. In J. Beatty and H. Legewie (Eds.), *Biofeedback and behavior.* New York: Plenum, 1977.

Pinkerton, P. The enigma of asthma. *Psychosom. Med.*, 1973, *35*, 461–462.

Plumlee, L. A. Operant conditioning of increases in blood pressure. *Psychophysiology*, 1969, *6*, 283–290.

Quinn, J. T., Harbison, J. J. M., and McAllister, H. An attempt to shape human penile responses. *Behav. Res. Ther.*, 1970, *8*, 213–216.

Razran, G. The observable unconscious and the inferable conscious in current Soviet psychophysiology: Interoceptive conditioning, semantic conditioning and the orienting reflex. *Psychol. Rev.*, 1961, *68*, 81–147.

Reeves, J. L., and Mealiea, W. Biofeedback assisted cue-controlled relaxation for the treatment of flight phobias. *J. Behav. Ther. Exp. Psychiatry*, 1975, *6*, 105–109.

Reeves, J. L., and Shapiro, D. Biofeedback and relaxation in essential hypertension. *Int. Rev. Appl. Psychol.*, 1978.

Reeves, J. L., Shapiro, D., and Cobb, L. F. Relative influences of heart rate biofeedback and instructional set in the perception of cold pressor pain. In N. Birbaumer and H. D. Kimmel (Eds.), *Biofeedback and self-regulation.* Hillsdale, N.J.: Lawrence Erlbaum Associates, in press.

Reitan, R. Intellectual and affective changes in essential hypertension. *Am. J. Psychiatry*, 1954, *110*, 817–828.

Reitan, R. A. A research program on the psychological effects of brain lesions in human beings. In N. R. Ellis (Ed.), *International review of research in men-*

tal retardation, Vol. 1. New York: Academic Press, 1966.

Rice, D. G. Operant GSR conditioning and associated electromyogram responses. *J. Exp. Psychol.*, 1966, *71,* 908–912.

Richter-Heinrich, E., and Läuter, J. A psychophysiological test as diagnostic tool with essential hypertensives. *Psychother. Psychosom.*, 1969, *17,* 153–168.

Roberts, A., Kewman, D. G., and Macdonald, H. Voluntary control of skin temperature: Unilateral changes using hypnosis and feedback. *J. Abnorm. Psychol.*, 1973, *82,* 163–168.

Roberts, A. H., Schuler, J., Bacon, J. R., Zimmerman, R. L., and Patterson, R. Individual differences and autonomic control: Absorption, hypnotic susceptibility, and the unilateral control of skin temperature. *J. Abnorm. Psychol.*, 1975, *84,* 272–279.

Roberts, L. E. The role of exteroceptive feedback in learned electrodermal and cardiac control: Some attractions of and problems with discrimination theory. In J. Beatty and H. Legewie (Eds.), *Biofeedback and behavior.* New York: Plenum Press, 1977.

Roberts, L. E. Operant conditioning of autonomic responses: One perspective on the curare experiments. In G. E. Schwartz and D. Shapiro (Eds.), *Consciousness and self-regulation: Advances in research,* Vol. 2. New York: Plenum, 1978.

Rosen, R. C. Suppression of penile tumescence by instrumental conditioning. *Psychosom. Med.*, 1973, *35,* 509–514.

Rosen, R. C., Shapiro, D., and Schwartz, G. E. Voluntary control of penile tumescence. *Psychosom. Med.*, 1975, *37,* 479–483.

Sargent, J. D., Green, E. E., and Walters, E. D. Preliminary report on the use of autogenic feedback training in the treatment of migraine and tension headaches. *Psychosom. Med.*, 1973, *35,* 129–135.

Schwartz, G. E. Voluntary control of human cardiovascular integration and differentiation through feedback and reward. *Science*, 1972, *175,* 90–93.

Schwartz, G. E. Biofeedback as therapy: Some theoretical and practical issues. *Am. Psychol.*, 1973, *28,* 666–673.

Schwartz, G. E. Toward a theory of voluntary control of response patterns in the cardiovascular system. In P. A. Obrist, A. H. Black, J. Brener, and L. V. DiCara (Eds.), *Cardiovascular psychophysiology.* Chicago: Aldine, 1974.

Schwartz, G. E. Biofeedback and patterning of autonomic and central processes: CNS-cardiovascular interactions. In G. E. Schwartz and J. Beatty (Eds.), *Biofeedback: Theory and research.* New York: Academic Press, 1977.

Schwartz, G. E., and Beatty, J. (Eds.). *Biofeedback: Theory and research.* New York: Academic Press, 1977.

Schwartz, G. E., and Shapiro, D. Biofeedback and essential hypertension: Current findings and theoretical concerns. *Semin. Psychiatry,* 1973, *5,* 493–503.

Schwartz, G. E., Shapiro, D., and Tursky, B. Learned control of cardiovascular integration in man through operant conditioning. *Psychosom. Med.*, 1971, *33,* 57–62.

Schwartz, G. E., Shapiro, D., and Tursky, B. Self control of patterns of human diastolic blood pressure and heart rate through feedback and reward. *Psychophysiology*, 1972, *9,* 270 (Abstract).

Schwartz, G. E., Young, L. D., and Vogler, J. Heart rate regulation as skill learning: Strength-endurance versus cardiac reaction time. *Psychophysiology,* 1976, *13,* 472–478.

Schwitzgebel, R. L., and Rugh, J. D. Of bread, circuses, and alpha machines. *Am. Psychol.*, 1975, *30,* 363–378.

Shapiro, D. Role of feedback and instructions in the voluntary control of human blood pressure. *Jpn. J. Biofeedback Res.*, 1973, *1,* 2–9 (in Japanese).

Shapiro, D. A monologue on biofeedback and psychophysiology. *Psychophysiology,* 1977, *14,* 213–227.

Shapiro, D., and Crider, A. Operant electrodermal conditioning under multiple schedules of reinforcement. *Psychophysiology,* 1967, *4,* 168–175.

Shapiro, D., Crider, A. B., and Tursky, B. Differentiation of an autonomic response through operant reinforcement. *Psychonom. Science*, 1964, *1,* 147–148.

Shapiro, D., Mainardi, J. A., and Surwit, R. S. Biofeedback and self-regulation in essential hypertension. In G. E. Schwartz and J. Beatty (Eds.), *Biofeedback: Theory and research.* New York: Academic Press, 1977.

Shapiro, D., and Schwartz, G. E. Biofeedback and visceral learning: Clinical applications. *Semin. Psychiatry*, 1972, *4,* 171–184.

Shapiro, D., Schwartz, G. E., Nelson, S., Shnidman, S., and Silverman, S. Operant control of fear-related electrodermal responses in snake-phobic subjects. *Psychophysiology,* 1972a, *9,* 271 (Abstract).

Shapiro, D., Schwartz, G. E., and Tursky, B. Control of diastolic blood pressure in man by feedback and reinforcement. *Psychophysiology,* 1972b, *9,* 296–304.

Shapiro, D., and Surwit, R. S. Learned control of physiological function and disease. In H. Leitenberg (Ed.), *Handbook of behavior modification and behavior therapy.* Englewood Cliffs, N.J.: Prentice-Hall, 1976.

Shapiro, D., Tursky, B., Gershon, E., and Stern, M. Effects of feedback and reinforcement on the control of human systolic blood pressure. *Science*, 1969, *163,* 588–590.

Shapiro, D., Tursky, B., and Schwartz, G. E. Control of blood pressure in man by operant conditioning. *Circ. Res.* (Suppl. 1), 1970a, *26–27,* 27–32.

Shapiro, D., Tursky, B., and Schwartz, G. E. Differentiation of heart rate and systolic blood pressure in man by operant conditioning. *Psychosom. Med.*, 1970b, *32,* 417–423.

Shapiro, D., and Watanabe, T. Timing characteristics of operant electrodermal modification: Fixed interval effects. *Jpn. Psychol. Res.*, 1971, *13,* 123–130.

Sheer, M. S., Crawford, P. L., Sergent, C. B., and Sheer, C. A. Effect of biofeedback techniques on chronic asthma in a summer camp environment. *Ann. Allergy*, 1975, *35,* 289–295.

Shnidman, S. R. Avoidance conditioning of skin potential responses. *Psychophysiology*, 1969, *6,* 38–44.

Shnidman, S. R. Instrumental conditioning of orienting responses using positive reinforcement. *J. Exp. Psychol.*, 1970, *83,* 491–494.

Shnidman, S., and Shapiro, D. Instrumental modification of elicited autonomic responses. *Psychophysiology*, 1971, *7,* 395–401.

Sirota, A. D., Schwartz, G. E., and Shapiro, D. Voluntary control of human heart rate: Effect on reaction to aversive stimulation. *J. Abnorm. Psychol.*, 1974, *83,* 261–267.

Sirota, A. D., Schwartz, G. E., and Shapiro, D. Voluntary control of human heart rate: Effect on reaction to aversive stimulation: A replication and extension. *J. Abnorm. Psychol.*, 1976, *85,* 473–477.

Snyder, C., and Noble, M. E. Operant conditioning of vasoconstriction. *J. Exp. Psychol.*, 1968, *77,* 263–268.

Solberg, W. K., and Rugh, J. D. The use of biofeedback devices in the treatment of bruxism. *J. S. Calif. Dent. Assoc.*, 1972, *40,* 852–853.

Stephens, J. H., Harris, A. H., Brady, J. V., and Shaffer, J. W. Psychological and physiological variables associated with large magnitude voluntary heart rate changes. *Psychophysiology*, 1975, *12,* 381–387.

Steptoe, A. Blood pressure control with pulse wave velocity feedback: Methods of analysis and training. In J. Beatty and H. Legewie (Eds.), *Biofeedback and behavior*, New York: Plenum, 1977.

Steptoe, A., and Johnston, D. The control of blood pressure using pulse-wave velocity feedback. *J. Psychosom. Res.*, 1976, *20,* 417–424.

Sterman, M. B. Neurophysiologic and clinical studies of sensorimotor EEG biofeedback training: Some effects on epilepsy. *Semin. Psychiatry*, 1973, *5,* 507–525.

Sterman, M. B. Effects of sensorimotor EEG feedback training on sleep and clinical manifestations of epilepsy. In J. Beatty and H. Legewie (Eds.), *Biofeedback and behavior.* New York: Plenum, 1977.

Sterman, M. B., LoPresti, R. W., and Fairchild, M. D. *Electroencephalographic and behavioral studies of monomethylhydrazine toxicity in the cat*, Technical Report AMRL-TR-69-3, Wright-Patterson Air Force Base, Ohio, Air Systems Command, 1969.

Sterman, M. B., Macdonald, L. R., and Stone, R. K. Biofeedback training of the sensorimotor electroencephalogram rhythm in man: Effects on epilepsy. *Epilepsia*, 1974, *15,* 395–416.

Stoyva, J., Barber, T. X., Kamiya, J., Miller, N. E., and Shapiro, D. (Eds.), *Biofeedback and self-control 1977/78: An Aldine Annual on the regulation of bodily processes and consciousness.* Chicago: Aldine, 1978.

Surwit, R. S. Biofeedback: A possible treatment for Raynaud's disease. *Semin. Psychiatry*, 1973, *5,* 483–490.

Surwit, R. S., Hager, J. L., and Feldman, J. The role of feedback in voluntary control of blood pressure in instructed subjects. *Psychophysiology*, 1977, *14,* 97 (Abstract).

Surwit, R. S., and Keefe, F. J. Frontalis EMG feedback training: An electronic panacea? *Behav. Ther.*, in press.

Surwit, R. S., Pilon, R. N., and Fenton, C. H. Behavioral treatment of Raynaud's disease. *J. Behav. Med.*, 1978, *1,* 323–335.

Surwit, R. S., Shapiro, D., and Feld, J. L. Digital temperature autoregulation and associated cardiovascular changes. *Psychophysiology*, 1976, *13,* 242–248.

Surwit, R. S., Shapiro, D., and Good, M. I. A comparison of cardiovascular biofeedback, neuromuscular biofeedback, and meditation in the treatment of borderline essential hypertension. *J. Consult. Clin. Psychol.*, 1978, *46,* 252–263.

Takebe, K., Kulkulka, C. G., Narayan, M. G., and Basmajian, J. V. Biofeedback treatment of a footdrop after stroke compared with standard rehabilitation technique. Part II: Effects on nerve conduction velocity and spasticity. *Arch. Phys. Med. Rehabil.*, 1976, *57,* 9–11.

Townsend, R. E., House, J. F., and Addario, D. A comparison of biofeedback mediated relaxation and group therapy in the treatment of chronic anxiety. *Am. J. Psychiatry*, 1975, *32,* 598–601.

Trowill, J. A. Instrumental conditioning of the heart rate in the curarized rat. *J. Comp. Physiol. Psychol.*, 1967, *63,* 7–11.

Vachon, L., and Rich, E. S., Jr. Visceral learning in asthma. *Psychosom. Med.*, 1976, *38,* 122–130.

Van Twyver, H. B., and Kimmel, H. D. Operant conditioning of the GSR with concomitant measurement of two somatic variables. *J. Exp. Psychol.*, 1966, *72,* 841– 846.

Victor, R., Mainardi, J. A., and Shapiro, D. Effect of biofeedback and voluntary control procedures on heart rate and perception of pain during the cold pressor test. *Psychosom. Med.*, 1978, *40,* 216–225.

Weiss, T., and Engel, B. T. Operant conditioning of heart rate in patients with premature ventricular contractions. *Psychosom. Med.*, 1971, *33,* 301–321.

Weiss, T., and Engel, B. T. Evaluation of an intracardiac limit of learned heart rate control. *Psychophysiology*, 1975, *12,* 310–312.

Wells, D. T. Large magnitude voluntary heart rate changes. *Psychophysiology*, 1973, *10,* 260–269.

Weston, A. Perception of autonomic processes, social acquiescence, and cognitive development of a sense of self-control in essential hypertensives trained to lower blood pressure using biofeedback procedures. Unpublished doctoral dissertation, Nova University, Fort Lauderdale, Fla., 1974.

Whitehead, W. E., Renault, P. F., and Goldiamond, I. Modification of human acid secretion with operant-conditioning procedures. *J. Appl. Behav. Anal.*, 1975, *8,* 147–156.

Young, L. D., and Blanchard, E. B. Effects of auditory feedback of varying information content on the self control of heart rate. *Psychophysiology*, 1974, *11,* 527–534.

Self-management

MICHAEL J. MAHONEY, PH.D.
Professor
Department of Psychology
The Pennsylvania State University
University Park, Pennsylvania

DIANE B. ARNKOFF
Department of Psychology
The Pennsylvania State University
University Park, Pennsylvania

4

There is a strong and growing conviction in the health professions that the management and prevention of medical disorders are largely under the control of the individual. Behavior patterns such as diet, exercise, and stress reactions are thought to relate directly to health. In this view, disease is less a matter of random misfortune than the result of a failure to develop health-enhancing behavior. There is now increasing consensus on several components of a health-promoting life-style: sound nutrition, regular exercise, and adequate coping skills for stress management. Individuals are held responsible for maintaining their health through developing health patterns.

This trend toward personal responsibility may be recent, but a belief in the virtues of self-development is not at all new. Humans have long valued a person's ability to direct and maintain their own behavior. Indeed, almost all of our efforts as parents, educators, and health professionals are directed at teaching independence and self-sufficiency. Our ideas of maturity and psychological adjustment are filled with vague notions of self-definition and individuality. Among other things, the mature and adapting person is supposed to be capable of coping with stress, making responsible decisions, and executing life changes which will promote greater happiness or personal growth. Our rather high standards for personal development are poignantly specified in Rudyard Kipling's famous poem:

IF

If you can keep your head when all about you
  Are losing theirs and blaming it on you;
If you can trust yourself when all men doubt you,
  But make allowance for their doubting too;
If you can dream—and not make dreams your master;
  If you can think—and not make thoughts your aim;
If you can meet triumph and disaster
  And treat those two impostors just the same;
If you can force your heart and nerve and sinew
  To serve your turn long after they are gone,
And so hold on when there is nothing in you
  Except the Will which says to them: "Hold on";
If you can fill the unforgiving minute
  With sixty seconds' worth of distance run—
Yours is the Earth and everything that's in it,
  And—which is more—you'll be a Man, my son!*

Aside from its rather sexist ending and the fact that it overlooks smoking and obesity, this poem conveys many of the explicit and implicit demands which are placed on individuals in today's society. Two of the most salient themes in Kipling's poem might be called *balance* and *perseverance.*

* "If," copyright 1910 by Rudyard Kipling from *Rewards and Fairies* by Rudyard Kipling. Used by permission of Doubleday & Company, Inc.

The mature, well-rounded person is supposed to avoid the extremes in life (e.g., conceit versus overwhelming self-doubt) and to also "force their heart and nerve and sinew" well beyond their capacity.

Now what does Kipling have to do with the topic of self-control? Basically this: he is but one of many eloquent writers over the last twenty centuries who have been specifying the ideal forms of human conduct. In company with Plato, Shakespeare, Goethe, and even Ben Franklin, he has set down a formidable list of human "virtues." All of these literary figures have agreed that one important ideal is that of "self-development." Although they have referred to it with different words, they have agreed on the critical importance of self-control in the ideal human. One of the most frustrating things in their writing, however, is that—while they seem eager to reflect on the goals of human conduct—few have offered any constructive suggestions for the means of achieving those goals. We are told where to go, but not how to get there.

One of the most likely culprits in this historical crime is the concept of *willpower*. Like his predecessors, Kipling was quick to invoke the idea that a strong will is the key to success. Even today it is not unusual to hear people talking about the importance of willpower in self-control efforts. Mary's loss of 30 pounds is attributed to her fortunate possession of sufficient willpower, while John's failure to quit smoking is credited to his deficiency in this category. How do we know Mary has willpower? Well, she did lose 30 pounds, didn't she? Likewise, it is obvious that John couldn't have enough "gumption"—otherwise he would be an ex-smoker. The problem here, of course, is that willpower as it is used here is a tautology. Our only evidence of Mary's inferred willpower is her weight loss. Citing "willpower" brings us no farther logically. In fact, we may have taken a step backwards—we have taken a behavior, attributed it to an inferred state, and then returned to the behavior as our only defense of the inference. We have gone around in a logical circle and—what may be worse—we have deluded ourselves into thinking that we have explained something when we have only re-described it.

The problem with the concept of willpower is not that it is inferential, but that it is tautologous. As we will see a bit later, there are other forms of anchored inference which may dramatically enhance our understanding of self-control patterns. Historically, however, people have been content to equate self-regulation with willpower and to close the issue. The inference made by many persons was that willpower is some mysterious inborn strength with which the fortunate in our race are blessed. Even today our smoking clinics, weight control programs, and waiting rooms are filled with people who believe they lack the "intestinal fortitude" which accounts for the happiness of their peers. Human patterns ranging from alcoholism to sexual dysfunction are perceived as stemming from a deep-seated and unchangeable trait of personal inadequacy.

One of the most valuable contributions of behavioral approaches to life intervention was their early and vigorous challenge of fatalistic traits and their emphasis on the malleability of the adapting human. Behaviorists were quick to recognize the logical as well as empirical problems with trait psychology, and so they suggested functional analyses as an alternative to trait diagnoses (Mischel, 1968, 1973; Skinner, 1953). This was no less the case in the area of self-control, where behavioral researchers were quick to reject the notion of a static internal strength called willpower. With an open invitation to functional analyses, Skinner (1953) was the first to outline clearly how self-control might be more adequately explained by principles of learning rather than inherited strengths. In *Science and Human Behavior,* he wrote:

> When a man controls himself, chooses a course of action, thinks out the solution to a problem, or strives toward an increase in self-knowledge, he is *behaving*. He controls himself precisely as he would control the behavior of anyone else—through the manipulation of variables of which behavior is a function (p. 228).

It was not until more than a decade later, however, that another behaviorist took up the banner of self-regulation. In an article titled "Self-Control Procedures in Personal Behavior Problems," Goldiamond (1965) reiterated Skinner's assertion that self-control is basically a self-application of principles which govern all human behavior:

> Behavior is not an emergent property of an organism nor a property solely of its environment, but is described by a functional relation between the two. More technically, given a specified behavior B and a specified environmental variable, x, a lawful relationship can be found, such that B = f(x), under certain empirical constraining conditions c. . . . When the subject himself sets x at that value, *he* will get his own B, as stipulated. This defines self-control (p. 852).

The essence of Goldiamond's argument, of course, is that it should make no practical difference whether it is a therapist or the client who establishes the conditions which lead to the desired behavior.

At about this same time, Ferster and his colleagues were translating these analyses into actual procedures which could be implemented by a client (Ferster, Nurnberger, and Levitt, 1962). Their creative suggestions for a behavioral approach to weight control laid the foundations for Stuart's (1967) still classic study and have remained a core ingredient in many subsequent obesity programs (Stunkard and Mahoney, 1976). By 1970, self-control had been identified as a rapidly developing area of interest among behavioral researchers (Bandura, 1969, 1971; Cautela, 1969; Kanfer, 1970a, 1971; Stuart, 1972). In fact, by 1972, there was enough research to warrant a review (Mahoney, 1972) and books on the topic were soon to follow (Goldfried and Merbaum, 1973; Mahoney and Thoresen, 1974; Thoresen and Mahoney, 1974).

Although interest in self-regulatory processes was pioneered by persons who were primarily operant conditioners in orientation, this situation began to change in the mid and late 1960's. In their two separate laboratories, Bandura (1969, 1971) and Kanfer (1970a, 1971) were conducting studies which laid the foundations for much later work. Their investigations were also influential in suggesting strategies for clinical application. As we move up to the present day, it is clear that self-regulation constitutes an enduring theme in both basic and applied research (Bandura, 1977; Mahoney and Arnkoff, 1978; Masters and Mokros, 1974).

In the applied field of behavioral medicine, self-management strategies have already been extensively utilized in treating problems such as obesity and smoking. Three related functions for self-control techniques in behavioral medicine can be identified:

1. The emerging technology of self-control provides psychological methods for dealing with behaviors which frequently have been defined as medical problems. The challenge now is to extend the use of these methods to problems such as hypertension which until recently have been treated almost exclusively with traditional medical techniques. If self-control techniques continue to show promise, their advantages make them an attractive alternative or adjunct to established medical practices. For example, self-management procedures appear to be less problematic in terms of side effects than drug treatments. Further, training individuals in self-control techniques may provide them with skills which they can transfer to other situations. For example, the obese individual who learns to use self-control methods to lose weight may also use them to quit smoking. A therapeutic bonus of this type is unlikely with more traditional medical approaches since the intervention is both externally imposed and non-transferable from one illness to another.

2. In addition to their use as a primary treatment, self-control techniques may be used as an adjunct in more traditional treatments. Most importantly, the techniques of self-control may be useful in gaining adherence to a medical treatment (Dunbar and Stunkard, 1977). Medication for hypertension, for example, can only be effective if the individual takes it regularly. However, nonadherence to such a medical procedure is common. This is particularly likely when, as in the case of hypertension, the person does not experience current discomfort. The use of self-control techniques for ensuring compliance would appear to be promising. The function of the self-control procedures would be both to remind the person of the treatment at the necessary time and to provide immediate motivation for adhering to it.

3. The final application of self-control techniques in behavioral medicine involves

a behavior change for prevention of disorders. The methods used to modify a current problem may be utilized in the primary or secondary prevention of those same problems. For example, the long-term regulation of diet and exercise are commonly thought to contribute to the prevention of heart disease. Such regulation generally involves the exchange of short-term negative consequences like self-denial of sweets for the long-term positive gains of health. Rather than relying on a mystical force called willpower for aid in self-denial, self-control methods provide a realistic means for the individual to effect long-term goals.

The promise of self-control has spawned an impressive volume of investigations into techniques and effective ingredients. One might expect that this vigorous inquiry has harvested an equally impressive body of knowledge. It is safe to say that our understanding of self-control processes has dramatically improved over the last decade. Unfortunately, it is equally clear that our understanding is sorely inadequate. In the sections which follow we shall explore our occasional glimpses of enlightenment amid the continuing shadows of our ignorance. By way of preview, however, it might be worth noting that our progress has been satisfying and that continuing efforts in this area would seem to be amply warranted.

Conceptual Issues

Although it has increased in popularity, the topic of self-control has also stimulated considerable debate among behavior researchers. Much of this discussion has focused on the definition of self-control and the processes which account for it. Let us take a moment here to examine these topics briefly.

DEFINITIONS OF SELF-CONTROL

What exactly is "self-control"? According to Skinner (1953) and Goldiamond (1965), self-control is a behavioral sequence in which an organism manipulates environmental influences in accordance with learning principles in order to alter a specific behavior. Aside from being somewhat general and non-operational, this definition flirts with teleological problems. That is, the *intent* or purpose of the self-initiated change appears to be a crucial element. This is also the case with Cautela's (1969) assertion that "self-control is conceptualized as the response of an organism made to control the probability of another response (p. 324)." In 1974, Thoresen and Mahoney attempted to spell out more operational criteria:

> A person displays self-control when, in the relative absence of immediate external constraints, he engages in behavior whose previous probability has been less than that of alternatively available behaviors (involving lesser or delayed reward, greater exertion or aversive properties, and so on). This response pattern is often influenced by delayed environmental consequences. . . . The designation of a behavior pattern as self-regulatory is a socially relative labeling process (p. 12).

This definition may have been an improvement in some respects, but its inadequacies are also apparent. How does one assess the momentary probability of a response, for example, or the "availability" of alternative behaviors?

An enduring source of confusion in this search for an adequate definition has been the implicit assumption that there is a certain quality which is present in self-regulatory patterns and absent in others. This assumption seems to have led many writers on a frantic search for the key characteristic which would distinguish self-control from other patterns of behavior. At this point, however, there is a growing consensus that self-control patterns are not distinguishable from any other human behaviors on the basis of their topography. Does this mean that there is no such thing as "self-control"? Not necessarily.

The viewpoint endorsed here is that self-control is not a quality inherent in some behaviors and absent in others. Rather, *self-control is a social label which is differentially applied to some behavior patterns*. In other words, an adequate definition must take into account the criteria of a labeler. These criteria may vary from one person to the next and are clearly different in various cultures. In contemporary western societies, however, there are several contextual features which increase the likelihood that a behavior pattern will be labeled self-control.

HUMAN PERFORMANCE. For the most part, psychologists and the lay public restrict the term "self-control" to human beings. The sources of this bias are probably multiple and include the reluctance of experimental psychologists to *anthropomorphize*—i.e., to attribute human qualities to infrahumans. Also responsible here may have been the fear that an ascription of self-control implied an ascription of a "self," and most humans are reluctant to grant such a precious fiction to an animal.

The reluctance of researchers to use the term "self-control" in reference to animals came to light when it was first demonstrated that pigeons could be trained to exhibit an apparently puritanical pattern of behavior (Mahoney and Bandura, 1972). In 1953, Skinner had noted that:

> Self-reinforcement . . . presupposes that the individual has it in his power to obtain reinforcement but does not do so until a particular response has been emitted (pp. 237–238).

This pattern was demonstrated in two pigeons which, after training, pecked a disc despite the presence of freely available grain and the absence of external constraints on their behavior. That is, they had the opportunity to obtain reinforcement but did not do so until after they had emitted a disc-pecking response. Subsequent experiments replicated and extended these findings and suggested that the pattern was easily produced and not attributable to ethological variables or the phenomenon of "negative automaintenance" (Bandura, Mahoney, and Dirks, 1976; Mahoney, Bandura, Dirks, et al., 1974). The same pattern was demonstrated in monkeys, and it was shown that a dog could be trained not only to respond in the presence of free food, but also to repeatedly interrupt his reinforcement, return to "work," resume consumption of his reinforcers, and so on (Bandura and Mahoney, 1974). This last exhibition was closest to that observed in humans who are ostensibly rewarding themselves for ongoing performance.

Were these animal experiments demonstrations of "self-control"? Not in the eyes of many beholders. Critics were quick to invoke a variety of arguments which either restricted that label to humans or questioned its meaningfulness in any context (Catania, 1975; Goldiamond, 1976; Rachlin, 1974). The original design and interpretation of these experiments did not invoke willpower, intent, or even a "self" in the pigeon. In fact, their results were congruent with Skinner's early assertions that patterns labeled as "self-control" can be developed by simple extrapolation of learning principles. Moreover, it was shown that—in animals as well as humans—the maintenance of a self-regulatory pattern is dependent upon such factors as the schedule of consequences during earlier training. Aside from this, professional reactions to the animal studies make it clear that the label "self-control" is reserved for featherless bipeds.

CONSPICUOUS IMMEDIATE INFLUENCE. A second feature which seems to affect the likelihood of self-control labeling is the conspicuousness of immediate external influences. Generally speaking, a behavior pattern is not considered self-regulatory if it is apparent to the labeler that said behavior is receiving prompt reward or punishment. If we stare out of our kitchen window and spot a lonely jogger pushing himself toward exhaustion, we may be inclined to respond with an attribution of self-control. That same jogger—and the same behavior—would earn less of our respect if he were surrounded by 30 military recruits in khaki uniforms. The person who loses weight on a diet may spark our admiration, but the same behavior would be viewed differently if it followed intestinal bypass surgery.

HISTORY AND EFFORT. In general, we do not give people self-control credit for something they seem to have been doing effortlessly for most of their lives. The nonsmoker, for example, is not likely to be credited with self-control when he or she declines the offer of a cigarette. A chain smoker who is in his second day of attempted abstinence, however, may elicit our respect and admiration. The more effortful his behavior, the more likely are we to label it as self-control. This pattern is influenced by temporal variables, however. We tend to attribute more self-control to the person who is just beginning a personal change project. As he or she maintains this change, we often withdraw or reduce our self-regulatory attribution. After 10 years of abstinence, for example, an ex-smoker is not given as much credit when he or she turns down a cigarette.

RESPONSE DESIRABILITY. The label of "self-control" is not equally applied to all responses. We tend to reserve this term for performances which are considered socially appropriate or desirable. The person who overcomes formidable barriers in carrying out an antisocial act is seldom credited with self-control. In fact, we tend to stereotype delinquents and criminals as persons who are lacking in self-control abilities.

PERCEIVED MOTIVATION. No matter how effortful or desirable the response, we seldom consider it self-regulatory unless it is thought to be motivated by noble ideals (e.g., self-improvement, loyalty, etc.). Perceived motives are often an evaluative matter which may be affected by context. When a soldier falls on a grenade to save his comrades, his act of clear and intentional suicide is lauded. Much the same response is considered a reprehensible crime, however, when its motives are thought to be less noble. A person who subjects himself to punishment in an attempt to quit smoking is more positively treated than one who self-inflicts punishment for no apparent reason. The former is viewed as a paragon, the latter as a paradox; and yet the "masochist" is often behaving in a fashion very parallel to that of a self-regulating person.

PERCEIVED SACRIFICE. A sixth factor which seems to influence our ascription of self-control is whether or not the person is demonstrating an obvious sacrifice in terms of immediate consequences. This factor obviously overlaps with the criterion of effort, but it is a bit more complex. In virtually every instance where the term "self-control" is applied, one finds a *reversing-consequence gradient*. As shown in Figure 4.1, the immediate effects of the behavior are opposite to its long-term effects. In *decelerative* self-control—where the target is to reduce or eliminate a response—its immediate effects are usually positive, but its delayed effects are negative. This is obviously the case in smoking, overeating, drug addiction, and alcohol abuse. In *accelerative* self-control the intent is to increase a target behavior and here the immediate effects of the response may be negative but its eventual consequences are more positive. Examples of this are physical exercise, studying, pain tolerance, and saving money.

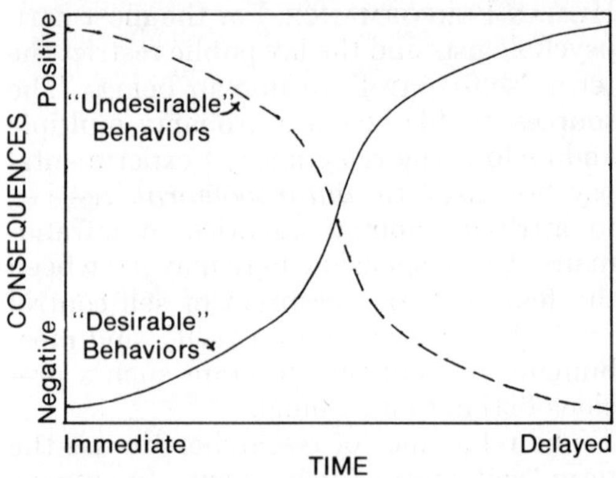

Figure 4.1. Hypothetical reversing-consequences gradient.

In terms of our current understanding, it would therefore appear that "self-control" lies, if anywhere, in the eyes of the beholder. It is not a quality inherent in certain behaviors, but rather a label applied under circumstances which may vary across time, culture, and labelers. In western society, self-control tends to be ascribed more often in reference to (1) a human performance in which (2) external constraints are inconspicuous and (3) the person does not have a recent history of effortless execution of the behavior. More often than not, the self-regulatory response is (4) socially desirable and involves (5) noble motivation and (6) some degree of self-sacrifice.

PRIME MOVER ISSUES

The definition of self-control is not the only conceptual issue which has stimulated professional debate. There have been a number of recent articles which have addressed the topic of primary causation in self-control. This argument basically focuses on the question of "where" self-control resides—inside the person or in his or her external environment. The environmentalists have often taken an explicitly external stance on this matter (Catania, 1975; Gewirtz, 1971; Goldiamond, 1976; Jones, Nelson, and Kazdin, 1977; Rachlin, 1974; Stuart, 1972). Their arguments are essentially those voiced by Skinner in 1953:

> When a man controls himself . . . his behavior in so doing is a proper object of analysis, and eventually it must be accounted for with variables lying outside the individual himself (pp. 228–229).
> . . . little ultimate control remains with the individual. A man may spend a great deal of time designing his own life—he may choose the circumstances in which he is to live with great ease, and he may manipulate his daily environment on an extensive scale. Such activity appears to exemplify a high order of self-determination. But it is also behavior, and we account for it in terms of other variables in the environment and history of the individual. It is these variables which provide the ultimate control (p. 240).

One must be careful here to recognize that the assertions of environmentalists have seemed to reflect two very different arguments. On the one hand, some have espoused the cosmological hypothesis that most human behavior is shaped by environmental influence. This assertion is obviously a controversial one, and it often overshadows a second element in the environmental argument—namely, that we are methodologically restricted to environmental (observable) variables in all scientific analyses.

A debate, of course, requires disagreement, and this has been amply provided by critics of the environmentalist position (Bandura, 1976, 1977; Thoresen and Mahoney, 1974). On the cosmological hypothesis, it has been argued that one-way determinism is logically untenable:

> Are people partial determiners of their own behavior, or are they ruled exclusively by forces beyond their control? The long-standing debate over this issue has been enlivened by Skinner's (1971) contention that, apart from genetic contributions, human behavior is controlled solely by environmental contingencies, for example, "A person does not act upon the world, the world acts upon him" (p. 211). A major problem with this type of analysis is that it depicts the environment as an autonomous force that automatically shapes and controls behavior. Environments have causes as do behaviors. . . . It is true that behavior is regulated by its contingencies, but the contingencies are partly of a person's own making. By their actions, people play an active role in producing the reinforcing contingencies that impinge upon them. Thus, behavior partly creates the environment, and the environment influences the behavior in a reciprocal fashion (Bandura, 1974, p. 886).

In place of one-way determinism, it has been argued that *reciprocal determinism* is a more viable concept. Where Skinner (1953) and Goldiamond (1965) had argued that behavior is a function of environment ($B = f(x)$), the new contention was that the environment is also influenced by behavior ($E = f(b)$). This suggests that the question may be a chicken-egg issue and points up the futility of arguing that either internal or external factors are the "primary" ones in human behavior. It is arbitrary to stop at any one point in an infinite regress and call it "the beginning." Just as mental way stations may masquerade as explanations, it is also possible to invoke environmental variables as explanatory fictions.

This is, of course, a cosmological issue and should not be confused with a separate argument—namely, that our analyses of all human behavior patterns must eventually rest in publicly observable events (i.e., the external environment). These two arguments are sometimes so intertwined that it is difficult to separate them (Rachlin, 1977; Skinner, 1974). An adequate response to the methodological argument would consume more space than is here available and is perhaps superfluous given its availability elsewhere (Mahoney, 1974a, 1977; Paivio, 1975; Reese, 1971; Weimer, 1977). By way of summary, however, it can be said that the focal issue here is not the scientific legitimacy of inferred variables. Inference is not only legitimate but essential to all scientific research. The question is not *whether* to infer, but rather how best to refine those inferences in a manner which will optimize their contribution to our knowledge. Observable anchors are indispensable in this refinement and this has never been disputed by mediational researchers.

Self-control Techniques

To catalog self-control techniques is to impose some organizational structure on a relatively diverse set of procedures. The structure imposed here is therefore arbitrary and the list presented below may not be exhaustive. It does incorporate the five most common strategies now employed by self-control therapists. By way of preview, these are (1) self-monitoring, (2) goal specification, (3) cueing strategies, (4) modification of incentives, and (5) rehearsal. More extensive reviews of these strategies are already available (Goldfried and Merbaum, 1973; Mahoney and Arnkoff, 1978; Mahoney and Thoresen, 1974; Thoresen and Mahoney, 1974).

SELF-MONITORING

The importance of self-awareness is stressed in many psychological treatment models, from psychoanalysis to gestalt therapy. In behavioral self-control, this self-awareness takes the form of self-observation of explicit behaviors. As an assessment device, self-monitoring is a prerequisite to other self-control techniques, by providing accurate information. It can also be an agent of change in its own right.

In early behavioral research many investigators asked subjects to record their performance in structured diaries or on special forms. A variety of self-monitoring devices were soon developed and, by the early 1970's, one could identify self-control enthusiasts at professional conventions by their accoutrements—golf counters, parking meter timers, and bead necklaces and bracelets which served both ornamental and metric functions. The theoretical and practical ramifications of self-monitoring were soon receiving the attention of specialists in the area (Kanfer, 1970b; Kazdin, 1974; Nelson, 1977).

Self-monitoring is a skill which, like other skills from tennis to playing the piano, must be learned. Whenever self-monitoring is to be undertaken, the desired behavior must be carefully explained and demonstrated. Practice of the behavior is also essential; the client should practice several instances of self-monitoring as they are presented by the therapist. Since adherence to a treatment is often a function of whether the procedures have been comprehended (Dunbar and Stunkard, 1977), these steps are an essential part of treatment.

Some clients may require shaping of self-monitoring skills. Initially these clients should be asked to practice with simple self-monitoring tasks (such as the number of cigarettes remaining in a package at the end of a day) before moving gradually to more demanding self-monitoring tasks (social interactions preceding the urge to smoke). Finally, it may be necessary to provide reinforcements for consistent and accurate self-monitoring. Such reinforcements can be as simple as therapist praise or as complex as a contract that the client will purchase a desired item after a certain number of weeks of record-keeping.

Client adherence to a program of self-monitoring depends not only on adequate teaching of skills, but also on a careful consideration of what and how to self-monitor. Clearly the choice of targets depends on the information to be obtained. For example, an assessment of the most likely time of day for overeating would require self-monitoring of caloric intake throughout the day. In contrast, identification of thoughts which cue binge eating would be assessed through a recording of the internal dialogue prior to eating. As treatment proceeds, the choice of behaviors to self-monitor may change as hypotheses about the conditions leading to and following the problematic behavior are revised.

As in the case of what behaviors to self-monitor, the choice of recording instruments is limited only by the imagination of the therapist and client. Mechanisms such as the golf counter and diary are widely used, but the choice of a particular method should be governed by its suitability to the purpose. Golf counters, wrist counters, and the like are suited to monitoring the frequency of behaviors. These methods would be used for observing the number of cigarettes smoked, frequency of Type A behaviors, and so on. Such methods give information on rate and change in rate of responding, but nothing else. Timers provide information on duration of an event such as exercise, or time between events, such as smoking. Other devices are as diverse as their purposes and vary considerably in elaborateness, from the bathroom scale to the portable plethysmograph for measuring pulse rate.

Paper and pencil methods of self-monitoring can provide a richer source of information than the procedures just mentioned. Several variables can be measured at once by this means, and qualitative information can be included (type of food eaten, antecedent events, and so on). Such measures vary from checklists to less systematic formats such as a diary. The diary may be particularly useful at the outset of treatment because of its capacity to include a broad range of variables. After a period of self-monitoring with the diary, those variables which are thought to have particular relevance for the client's problem can then be further investigated.

An example of such a diary is shown in Figure 4.2. For each instance of the behavior being assessed, the client records particulars about the event such as time, place, and what occurred, as well as antecedent and consequent thoughts and actions. Examination of the diary can lead to identification of the patterns surrounding the undesired behavior—time of day most likely for eating, persons associated with smoking, consequences of drinking, etc.

The behavioral diary is an example of a self-monitoring device which provides a broad range of information. More specialized goals may suggest a less elaborate form of self-recording. In addition to considering the goal of the self-monitoring, the choice of techniques should be governed by the likelihood that the client will carry out the self-monitoring consistently. Simplicity of the system, portability, and relative unobtrusiveness are criteria to be considered. For example, keeping a behavioral diary such as that in Figure 4.2 for each instance of eating may be tedious and too obtrusive for a particular client and may lead to haphazard or incomplete self-monitoring. Alternatives such as time or behavior sampling may be preferable with such clients.

To this point self-monitoring has been discussed primarily as an assessment strategy—i.e., a means of collecting relevant information about behavior. This information is then to be used in the ongoing refinement of therapy. An obvious concern here, of course, is the *accuracy* of these self-reports. How much confidence can a therapist place in a client's self-monitoring records? This is an issue which has stimulated considerable research in recent years. At the present time it seems clear that self-monitoring accuracy can vary widely across persons, target behaviors, and self-recording strategies. It is important to note, however, that the therapist can often enhance self-report reliability by following certain guidelines in

Date ______________________________ Target ______________________

Time	Place	Persons Present	Preceding Thoughts	Preceding Actions or Events	Subsequent Thoughts	Subsequent Actions or Events	Comments

Figure 4.2. Generalized self-monitoring diary.

the use of self-monitoring with clients. There is tentative agreement that each of the following may facilitate accuracy and honesty in self-monitoring:

1. a clearly specified target behavior;
2. a simple self-monitoring device;
3. emphasis on the importance of accuracy and honesty in self-reports;
4. demonstration of the self-monitoring strategy;
5. supervised practice in the self-monitoring assignment;
6. therapist-client agreement to allow occasional and unannounced checks on self-monitoring accuracy; and
7. the use of additional outcome measures which may reflect on self-report accuracy.

While these factors may not guarantee accuracy, there is now substantial evidence that they may increase its likelihood.

Self-report accuracy is clearly an important consideration in that a therapist's recommendations and assignments are often influenced by the client's recent progress and current level of functioning. Inaccurate personal data may lead to less than optimal intervention. The diabetic who misreports his or her compliance with a diet or medication regimen may elicit contratherapeutic suggestions. This is why it is so important to emphasize the critical role of honesty in self-recording and to employ additional outcome measures. Laboratory tests have now been developed, for example, to corroborate self-reports of abstinence from nicotine and other drugs. Use of such corroborative tests appears to increase the accuracy of clients' self-report data (Nelson, 1977).

Since it was being employed primarily as an aid in assessment, early self-control researchers tended to view self-monitoring as an important adjunct to treatment. This assumption was vigorously challenged when it became clear that the act of observing and recording one's behavior can be *reactive*—i.e., it can lead to behavior change. In preparation for treatment, many people had been asked to record their baseline (pretreatment) performance of a target behavior (e.g., smoking, eating, studying, etc.). They would often return to their therapist with glowing reports of improvement and these reports were often met with surprise by the therapist (who was waiting to outline the "real" treatment strategy).

It soon became apparent that self-monitoring was more than just an assessment strategy; it was also a potential influence in behavior change. A number of research studies were soon underway—trying to identify the power of self-monitoring and to isolate some of the parameters of its reactivity (Kazdin, 1974; Nelson, 1977). The therapeutic effects of self-monitoring alone can be seen in a representative study by Romancyzk (1974). Subjects in this study were obese individuals averaging more than 50 lb over ideal weight as calculated from actuarial tables. They were assigned to one of five groups: (1) no treatment control; (2) self-monitoring of daily weight; (3) self-monitoring of daily weight plus daily caloric intake; (4) training in behavioral techniques of weight control; and (5) training in behavioral techniques plus daily recording of both weight and caloric intake. At the end of the 4-week treatment program, the group which self-monitored weight and calories was found to be equally as effective as both groups which had therapist contact and behavioral training. All three of these groups had lost significantly more weight than had the no treatment control group. However, the effects of self-monitoring depended on what behavior was recorded; at the end of the treatment phase, the group recording daily weight only had lost no more weight than the no treatment control. Apparently it was not self-monitoring per se, but the act of monitoring particular behaviors which was effective.

The reactive effects of self-monitoring have been widely studied. At the present time it looks as if the reactive effects of self-monitoring are inconsistent and dramatically influenced by a wide range of factors. Reports of early reactivity—i.e., during the first few weeks of self-observation—are not uncommon, but many of these changes seem to be temporary. Unless supplemented by other self-regulatory strategies, it would appear that self-monitoring is often insufficient as a behavior change technique. Its effects are much too variable and short-lived for it to warrant substantial use as the sole method of intervention. These limitations in its power as a treatment strategy should not, however, overshadow its important assessment functions.

GOAL SPECIFICATION

When submitted to a means-ends analysis, self-control can be viewed as an enterprise in which the person is attempting to change in specified ways. The difference between self-regulated change and that normally taking place in our lives is perhaps (a) the presence of specific goals, and (b) the use of techniques which are employed to realize those goals. One could spend considerable time in the elaboration and evaluation of this view, but it is perhaps more useful to simply note that our culture often attaches negative connotations to the pursuit of a life by any philosophy other than means-ends. Individuals who can specify personal goals but are at a loss for means are often viewed as frustrated or unmotivated. They constitute a sizeable percentage of our clientele in the mental health professions. Persons with means—but who lack personal goals—are a somewhat rarer breed. They are, nonetheless, stigmatized as directionless. "Existential dilemmas" may involve some of this pattern. It is very rare, indeed, to find someone who lacks both coping strategies and personal goals, and much more common to encounter a person who exhibits both of these. Needless to say, this four-fold matrix is misrepresentative in its portrayal of means and ends as dichotomous variables. On the other hand, this brief digression may serve to illustrate the implicit cultural assumption that a well adjusted person is one in whom there is little discrepancy between means and ends.

Coming back down to a more practical plane, there have been two basic issues in the experimental analysis of goal-setting as a self-regulatory strategy—(a) whether it facilitates self-change, and (b) whether it is sufficient as a treatment technique. The literature in this regard is somewhat inconclusive and any generalizations offered must therefore be viewed as tentative. At the present time, it would appear that goal-setting is often a facilitative component in self-regulation (Kolb, Winter, and Berlew, 1968; Locke, Cartledge, and Koeppel, 1968). Its facilitative effects are not, however, uniform and they may be influenced by parameters of the goal-setting itself. If the goals are vague or unreasonable, for example, or if they are presented without suggestions as to how they might be achieved, one would not expect much improvement. Three parameters which have received preliminary research attention have corroborated this assertion:

1. In general, a publicly stated goal (e.g., in the form of a witnessed contract) may facilitate change.
2. Goals which focus on *behavior* change rather than other factors (e.g., eating habits rather than bodyweight) may be more effective.
3. Short-range (immediate) goals may be superior to long-range (distant) goals.

The importance of behavioral focus was demonstrated in a study by Mahoney (1974b). Obese subjects were assigned to one of four groups: (1) delayed treatment; (2) self-monitoring of daily weight and eating habits; (3) self-monitoring and self-reinforcement for reaching a weight change goal; and (4) self-monitoring and self-reinforcement for reaching a habit change goal. Figure 4.3 illustrates the finding that the group which self-reinforced for attaining a performance goal showed greater weight change than the other groups, both at the end of treatment (week 8) and at a 4-month follow-up. The superiority of the group that focused on behavior change was maintained at 1 year. Goals which specify performance rather than outcome criteria appear to be superior, perhaps because the behaviors required of the individual are more salient.

The salience issue may also be reflected in the finding that short-range (immediate) goals may be superior to long-range (distant) goals. This is the conclusion of a report by Bandura and Simon (1977). In this study on obesity, control and self-monitoring groups were compared with two groups which were given goals regarding reduction of food intake. One group was given the distal goal of reducing food intake across 1-week periods. The other goal-setting group was given the more proximal goal of reducing intake during four daily time periods. For purposes of analysis, the distal group was divided into those who had reported on

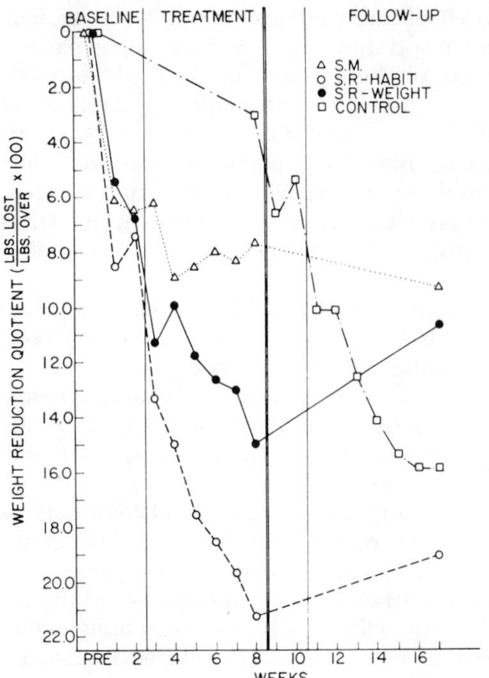

Figure 4.3. Weight loss over time for different groups: self-monitoring of daily weight and eating habits (SM), self-monitoring and self-reinforcement for reaching a habit-change goal (SR-habit), self-monitoring and self-reinforcement for reaching a weight-change goal (SR-weight), and delayed treatment (control). (Reprinted by permission from Mahoney, M. J. Self-reward and self-monitoring techniques for weight control. *Behav. Ther.*, 1974, *5*, 48–57.)

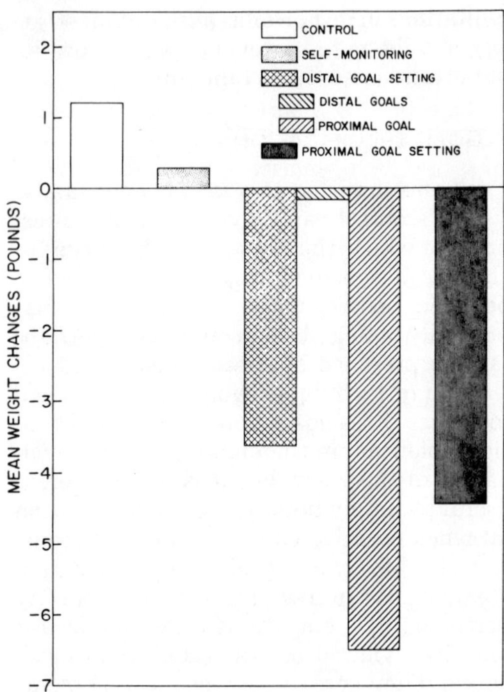

Figure 4.4. Weight change in treatment, comparing proximal and distal goal procedures; subjects were subdivided into groups that followed experimenter-designated goals (Distal and Proximal Goal Groups) and those that set proximal goals for themselves (Distal and Proximal Goal Setting Groups). (Reprinted by permission from Bandura, A. and Simon, K. M. The role of proximal intentions in self-regulation of refractory behavior. *Cognitive Ther. Res.*, 1977, *1*, 177–194.)

a questionnaire that they had retained the distal goal, and those who had created more proximal goals—for example, limits on intake at each meal. Figure 4.4 shows the weight change in each group, with the distal group displayed both as a whole and as subdivided. Although there was no statistical difference between the distal group as a whole and the proximal group, subjects in the distal group who created more proximal goals for themselves lost significantly more weight than did subjects who retained the distal goals set by the experimenter.

The finding regarding immediate and long-range goals is, of course, consistent with the common behavior strategy of *graduated performance demands.* In desensitization and shaping, for example, clients are asked to make very small and gradual improvements. The gradation of these goals may be an important component in the success of these popular techniques.

It is worth noting that the unreasonableness of a person's goals may often contribute to their psychological distress (Beck, 1976; Mahoney, 1974a; Meichenbaum, 1977). A very frequent pattern in clinical situations is that of a person who wants to achieve dramatic personal change in a very brief period and without excessive effort or discomfort. In obesity, for example, it is not unusual to encounter clients who want to lose 50 pounds in 60 days. Besides their unreasonable goals, many clients also harbor naive and sometimes self-defeating notions about their means. They often suggest drastic strategies which are doomed to failure (e.g., a starvation diet). Perhaps the most pernicious assumption in self-regulation is that which demands perfectionistic performance. The *saint or sinner syndrome* (SOS) is a common one in everyday life, and it is probably a significant contributor to the failure of many self-control efforts. This syndrome—if it can be called that—is characterized primarily by (a) dichotomous thinking, and (b) moralistic self-evaluations.

In weight control, for example, the SOS syndrome is apparent in persons who believe that they must either be "on" or "off" a diet. The diet in these cases is usually very structured and prohibitive. Once the individual consumes a forbidden food, their episode of sainthood is ended—they are no longer a perfect dieter and are automatically a failure. Going off the diet is often accompanied by moralistic self-criticism and guilt, and it is not unusual for the fallen dieter to binge. This pattern may be repeated in an endless sequence of restrictive diets and uncontrolled binging—leading to what one expert has called "the rhythm method of girth control." Dichotomization is also apparent in smokers and drinkers who believe that one must either be abstinent or addicted. It is a personal philosophy which is very conducive to feelings of guilt, depression, and overall failure.

There are actually two levels of perfectionism within the SOS syndrome. The adoption of dichotomous and ambitious goals is only one. Another is the assumption that one will achieve those goals without too much difficulty. Recent research on the distinction between "coping" and "mastery" models has begun to unravel some of the consequences of this assumption (Mahoney and Arnkoff, 1978). Where saintly goals might be considered *outcome perfectionism,* saintly means might be called *process perfectionism.* The mastery model is basically one who achieves personal goals with minimal effort, bountiful self-confidence, and no signs of either distress or difficulty. A coping model, on the other hand, exhibits more realistic fallibility and strives toward personal goals with obvious difficulty, occasional self-doubts, and moderate distress. A handful of studies have now examined this process dimension by exposing clients to models who achieved identical outcomes but varied in their ease with this accomplishment. At present, it would appear that the coping model is a much more therapeutic one. The implications of these findings for our own behavior as therapists are worth serious consideration.

CUEING STRATEGIES

Behavior modifiers often talk about the ABC's of human behavior—i.e., the fact that a behavior (B) is sandwiched between antecedents (A) and consequences (C). The alteration of those antecedents and consequences can bring about changes in behavior. In early analyses, these two categories of influence were often restricted to the physical environment. More recently, it has been emphasized that the factors which surround and influence a behavior can be conceptualized as ranging across three overlapping environments—the physical, social, and private. A person's physical environment is comprised of inanimate objects. His or her social environment consists of other persons, and the private environment is comprised of those biological and psychological processes which dictate ongoing behavior. Among the latter processes are the ones confined to the central nervous system which may help to organize and direct behavior.

The distinction between antecedents and consequences and among the three environments is a convenient one for some purposes, but it is hardly an adequate one in other respects. The same stimulus, for example, can serve as both the antecedent and the consequence for a behavior and one can be hard pressed to distinguish clearly between the various environments. With this limitation in mind, however, we can talk about the functions of various events in the regulation of ongoing behavior. The present section will be devoted to cueing functions and we will later turn our attention to incentive influences.

Psychologists have long recognized that "attention" is a critically important feature in learning. Despite problems in defining this concept, attention has continued to dominate a large body of research and to expand into areas other than the learning laboratory. Clinical psychologists, for example, have begun to examine the relevance of this concept for patterns of distress and techniques of adjustment (Mahoney, 1974a). Self-control researchers have been particularly interested in the programming of stimuli in an adaptive fashion.

The earliest attempts to program more adaptive stimulation intentionally were borrowed directly from the animal laboratory. In discrimination training with pigeons, for example, one can produce a pattern called *stimulus control*. This is characterized by rates of responding which are very different depending on the stimuli present. Through differential reinforcement, an organism may come to associate specific stimuli with various contingencies. The possibility that this pattern may also apply to humans was suggested by observations and reports that many "habits" seem to be influenced by prevailing stimulation. The smoker, for example, may report that the likelihood of lighting a cigarette is dramatically increased after a meal or when someone else has started a cigarette. Likewise, the problem eater sometimes reports almost reflexive eating at certain times of the day (particularly evenings) and when food stimuli are conspicuous (e.g., at a party or during television commercials which advertise food).

Stimulus control analyses of dysfunctional behavior led to a variety of early strategies for self-control. All of these techniques were designed to gradually restrict and eliminate stimuli which had come to elicit maladaptive behavior and, simultaneously, to increase the individual's exposure to more desirable stimuli. Thus, the overeater was told to restrict eating to specified times and places, and the smoker was encouraged to break habitual associations between certain events and cigarettes. The potential power of such strategies was suggested by Stuart's (1967) classic report on the treatment of obesity with stimulus control methods. At 1-year contact, Stuart's clients had lost from 26 to 47 pounds. However, weight losses of this magnitude and consistency have, unfortunately, not been typical.

Another application of stimulus control techniques has been in the treatment of insomnia (Bootzin, 1972). Bootzin reasoned that lying in bed may be a cue for being awake rather than asleep for some individuals. This would be the case for individuals who use the bed for activities such as reading or watching TV, or for those who use the time before sleep for rehashing the day's events and worrying. He instructed subjects to use stimulus control techniques such as restricting the bed to sleep and sexual activity and leaving the bedroom if they did not fall asleep within 10 minutes of lying down. In an experimental comparison, the stimulus control treatment was found to be superior to progressive muscular relaxation in reducing time to sleep onset.

Bootzin's study suggests that stimulus control techniques can be powerful, but studies in which stimulus control has been evaluated on its own have been rare in the behavioral literature. It has been far more common for stimulus control to be combined with other techniques such as contingency management. At the present it can only be said that stimulus control procedures are frequent components in successful self-control. Their singular contribution, however, has yet to be adequately assessed (Mahoney and Arnkoff, 1978; Stunkard and Mahoney, 1976).

With the advent of more recent conceptualizations of self-control, the role of private cues has become a popular research theme. There are now dozens of studies suggesting that a person's internal stimulation—i.e., his or her thoughts, images, and fantasies—may exert a powerful influence on both feelings and behavior (Bandura, 1977; Beck, 1976; Mahoney, 1974a; Mahoney and Arnkoff, 1978; Meichenbaum, 1977). At the risk of oversimplification, this research has focused on four basic themes—thoughts about (1) the stimulus, (2) the response, (3) the consequence, and (4) the relationship (i.e., contingency) among these. Investigators have found that a person's response to a stimulus may be affected by their perception of it. If a beverage is *perceived* as containing alcohol, for example, it will produce different results than when this perception is absent (Wilson and Abrams, 1977). Likewise, both obese and nonobese persons respond differently to the same food when they perceive it as either high or low in calories (Wooley, 1972).

A person's perception of the response is another factor which may influence performance. Of particular significance here is the person's perception of his or her ability to perform the response. Bandura (1977) has termed this perception *self-efficacy*. He hypothesizes that psychological treatments may operate through modifying the individual's expectations of effective performance. In two studies investigating self-efficacy in the treatment of snake phobics (Bandura and Adams, 1977), subjects' self-reports of efficacy expectations were an accurate predictor of post-treatment performance. Since the measures are correlational, these studies do not by themselves establish the fact that self-efficacy change was the cause of the performance improvement. Nor is there evidence as of yet to suggest whether self-efficacy expectations are central to problems other than avoidance behaviors. Nevertheless, the hypothesis is intriguing and certainly deserving of further scrutiny.

In addition to perceptions of efficacy, perceptions of reinforcement may predict behavior. It is now becoming more and more apparent than human beings respond in accordance with their perception of contingencies—and these perceptions may sometimes be quite variant from the actual or intended contingency. Finally, a person's attention to and perception of the consequence may dramatically alter his or her behavior. In studies of pain tolerance and delay of gratification, for example, individuals are usually less successful when they focus on the consequences of their behavior. Other experiments have suggested that a person's reactions to a consequence may depend on his or her interpretation of it (Bandura, 1977; Mahoney, 1974a).

This digression into the realms of private stimulation must be necessarily brief, but it should point out that much of a person's behavior may be cued by intrapersonal (cognitive) processes. In addition, it resurrects the oversimplication which is inherent in a linear ABC analysis of human action. Many of the private events are operative before, during, and after a particular response. With the recognition of the complex interdependence among private and external stimulation, it is perhaps not surprising that recent theorists have begun to advocate systems analyses and reciprocal determinism.

MODIFICATION OF INCENTIVES

More research has been devoted to incentive modification than to almost any other self-control strategy. This may be due to the fact that self-reward and self-punishment were direct extrapolations from the mainstay of behavior modification—viz., consequence programming. There are now dozens of studies suggesting that self-presented rewards may be very effective in the development and maintenance of desired behavior patterns (Thoresen and Mahoney, 1974; Mahoney and Arnkoff, 1978).

Self-reinforcement can refer to two different processes (Bandura, 1976), but the differences between these processes have not been extensively investigated. In some studies, self-reinforcement indicates only the self-presentation of consequences, while the criteria for reinforcement have been established by the therapist. For example, the therapist may instruct the client to set aside a specified amount of money toward the purchase of a desired item each time a pre-determined reduction in smoking is achieved. In this case the only difference from external reinforcement is that the client puts the money aside. In other instances, self-reinforcement refers to both self-presentation of the reinforcement and self-selection of the contingencies. The client would determine both the cigarette reduction goals and the nature of the reinforcer to be self-presented. In regard to this second type of self-reinforcement, there is evidence that when individuals determine reinforcement criteria for themselves, they may impose very stringent standards (Bandura and Perloff, 1967). Some clinical populations may be particularly likely to impose strict contingencies on themselves—for example, depressives, and perhaps those displaying the Type A behavior pattern which is implicated in heart disease (Friedman and Rosenman, 1974). For self-reinforcement to be a successful procedure with these individuals, they may first need to learn to set realistic criteria for reinforcing themselves. Learning to be realistic may, in fact, be an integral part of treatment.

Although there seems to be general consensus regarding the promise of self-reinforcement techniques, there has been recent debate about the actual processes underlying their apparent effectiveness (Bandura, 1976; Catania, 1975; Goldiamond, 1976; Jones, Nelson, and Kazdin, 1977; Rachlin, 1974). Some of these discussions have focused on the technical definition of reinforcement and on the role of environmental factors in the maintenance and efficacy of self-reinforcement patterns. It is noteworthy, however, that there has been little disagreement about the potential usefulness of these procedures with certain populations and problems.

An example of the large number of studies which have been performed on self-reinforcement is an obesity study carried out by Bellack (1976). In this instance, self-reinforcement refers to the self-presentation of a reward; the contingencies were determined by the experimenter. The study compared a self-monitoring group with a self-reward group. The reward in this case consisted of self-rating of adherence to the behavioral program at each meal. Assigning a high "grade" to oneself was assumed to be reinforcing. After a 7-week treatment and 7-week follow-up, the self-reward subjects had lost approximately twice as much weight as the subjects who only self-monitored. Such results are typical of the research on self-reward when it is compared with self-monitoring.

Somewhat less enthusiasm has been generated by the strategy of self-punishment. Some promising results with this technique have been noted. An example is the pair of case studies reported by Axelrod, Hall, Weis, et al. (1974). In both cases the contingency of losing money for failure to reduce smoking was associated with a dramatic decrease in number of cigarettes smoked. Such results, however, have not been the norm. More typical is the study on treatment of obesity by Mahoney, Moura, and Wade (1973). Self-reward was compared with self-punishment in this study, with money used for rewards or fines. Subjects were given suggestions on contingencies but were free to self-reward or self-punish as they chose. As Figure 4.5 illustrates, subjects in the self-reward groups lost more weight than subjects in the self-punishment only group. The latter lost no more weight than subjects in the control group. A partial explanation for the lack of efficacy of self-punishment may be the paradoxial finding

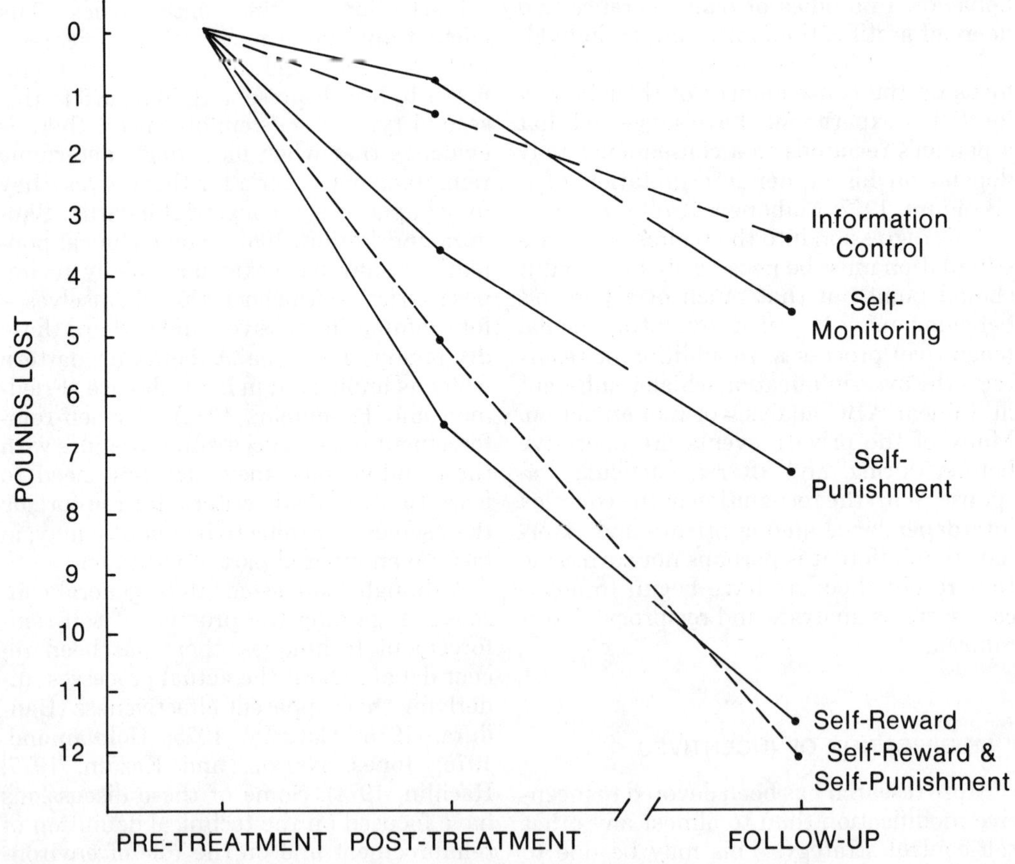

Figure 4.5. Weight loss with different self-management procedures.

that when a self-presented stimulus is aversive enough to be suppressive, there is often a decline in the consistency of its self-application. In contrast to the questionable utility of self-punishment, self-reward strategies emerge as one of the more powerful and promising techniques of self-regulated change.

Individuals can reinforce themselves in a number of ways. Tangible rewards—such as money and gift certificates—have been shown to be effective in many applications. More recently, persons have been trained to self-reward privately (i.e., via a thought) as a means of strengthening or maintaining behavior (Meichenbaum, 1977). Likewise, they may enlist social support for their actions such that their self-reward strategies are supplemented by the compliments and encouragement of family and friends. Recent research in obesity has suggested that this latter strategy—social support engineering—may be a critically important component in successful self-control (Brownell, Heckerman, Westlake, et al., 1977). Persons with cooperative and supportive social environments tend to exhibit greater self-improvement and more enduring achievements. This may sound like a return to environmental control until one realizes that the reaction patterns of family and friends are often influenced and shaped by the behaviors of the client. Training in social skills may help the person to develop a mutual reinforcement loop in which family and friends are praised for their praise of the client.

The promise of the self-reinforcement strategy suggests that it may be a useful adjunct in obtaining adherence to a medical regimen. For example, the self-monitoring of ingestion of medication for essential hypertension could be combined with self-reward for adhering to the treatment regimen. An adherence program for nonadhering hyperlipidemia patients has been carried out (Dunbar and Agras, 1977). In this case, self-monitoring was combined with external supervision in the form of a telephone call. There was some evidence of lowered cholesterol levels in experimental subjects, particularly among those who had higher but erratic rates of adherence before intervention (35–50% adherence as opposed to 5–34% adherence). The next step would seem to be to combine the self-monitoring with self-reward, since the reactive effects of self-monitoring alone are generally short-lived.

REHEARSAL

The fifth-control technique is rehearsal—the systematic practice of a performance. This can be done via analog tasks which are graduated in difficulty. The unassertive person, for example, may be asked to practice assertion skills with a friend before applying them to a target performance. More recently, investigators have begun to explore the promise of *covert rehearsal*—i.e., practicing a performance via imagery. This technique is not unfamiliar to the lay public and has received the attention of sport psychologists. In several dozen studies of "mental practice" in athletes, there is evidence to suggest that this strategy can be helpful (Corbin, 1972). Recent applications to such problems as test anxiety, unassertiveness, and animal phobias have also rendered results which are encouraging.

An example of the covert modeling strategy can be seen in Kazdin's (1973) study on mastery and coping models in the treatment of snake phobics. The coping-mastery distinction has been described above. A previous study (Meichenbaum, 1971) had shown that a coping model was more effective in inducing reduction in phobic avoidance than a mastery model. In the Kazdin study, the subjects were told to imagine the models performing the task. A coping covert model group, in which subjects imagined an initially fearful model who coped, was compared with a mastery covert modeling group and two control groups. The results presented in Figure 4.6 demonstrate that both modeling groups produced more behavior change than the control groups. Moreover, the covert coping model strategy was significantly more effective than the covert mastery model in reducing snake avoidance behavior. This study, among others, suggests the potential of the covert rehearsal strategy. In behavioral medicine, applications of the covert modeling approach would seem to be a promising direction. For example, covert rehearsal could be used as part of a treatment package to modify Type A behavior patterns.

The role of rehearsal in self-control has yet to be fully explored. It is worth noting,

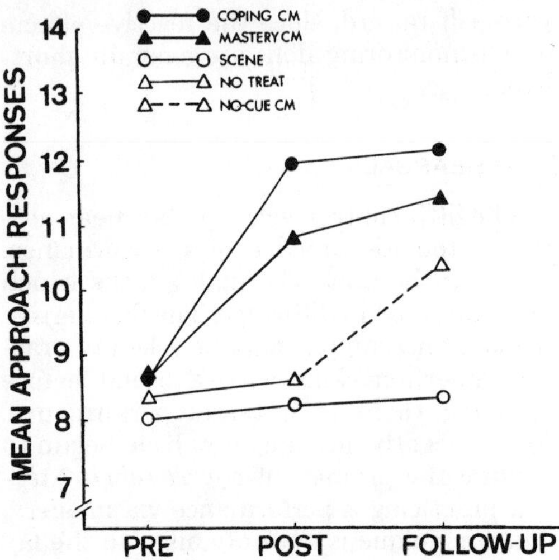

Figure 4.6. Approach responses with different covert modeling (CM) procedures in snake phobics. (From Kazdin, A. E. Covert modeling and the reduction of avoidance behavior. *J. Abnorm. Psychol.*, 1973, *81*, 87–95. Copyright 1973 by the American Psychological Association. Reprinted by permission.)

however, that such rehearsal may serve a variety of functions. In practicing a self-regulatory skill, a person may learn to refine his or her performance and to increase feelings of self-efficacy. Likewise, the rehearsal—whether overt or covert—may serve to prepare the individual for unanticipated problems in the later execution of a response. For example, the pre-assertive person might be asked to role play and rehearse an interview during which he asks his employer for a raise. During this rehearsal, he may realize that the employer's reaction could be defensive or even aggressive. Anticipation of these reactions may be an important element in the strategy of rehearsal. While they are most often used in the preparatory pre-performance phase of self-control training, rehearsal techniques can also be employed as a means of ongoing skill refinement.

Methods for Training Self-control Skills

We have now discussed the five most common self-control techniques—self-monitoring, goal specification, cueing, incentive modification, and rehearsal. All of these are strategies which are frequently used in more traditional behavior therapy. In self-control applications, however, the client takes more responsibility for implementing these techniques. How does one go about teaching a client to use self-control strategies? In much the same way one teaches almost any other skill—through (1) direct supervision, (2) modeling, (3) bibliographic methods, or (4) a combination of these. In direct supervision, the therapist may instruct the client to self-reinforce, for example, and may intermittently praise the client's self-reward efforts. This direct training can often be enhanced by modeling—offering live or filmed demonstrations of the self-control skill. Bibliographic materials such as a treatment manual may also contribute to skill development.

In many cases of self-control training, these three basic methods are combined. At the present time there are no conclusive comparisons among the three and their integration may be the most pragmatic strategy until more data are available. It is worth noting that other parameters of self-control training are now beginning to receive examination. The gradual fading of therapist involvement may, for example, contribute to development and maintenance of self-control skills. Contrary to some longheld assumptions, relatively dense therapist supervision and support may be countertherapeutic unless gradually withdrawn (Richards, Perri, and Gortney, 1976). Thus, many self-control therapists are now advocating a system in which the counselor assumes considerable responsibility at the beginning of therapy but, as the client develops and refines his or her self-regulatory skills, external supervision is slowly removed. Progress in self-regulation and the gradual assumption of personal responsibility are, of course, reinforced—but the therapist realizes that maintenance may depend on the supportiveness of the client's future environments. Thus, although progressively less frequent *booster contacts* are used to assess and encourage maintenance, more emphasis is placed on developing the client's skills in shaping environmental support.

Interestingly, this concern over maintenance was anticipated by Skinner (1953) in his pioneering analysis of self-control. He pointed out the distinction between the "controlled response" (e.g., smoking, exercise, dietary habits) and the "controlling response" (e.g., cueing, self-reward, etc.). Assuming that it is not a violation of general learning principles, one would not expect the controlling response to be functionally autonomous. To be maintained, it, too, must be cued, reinforced, and so on. This is why the development of skills in environmental influence may be crucially important in successful self-control. Factors which affect maintenance have only recently begun to attract substantial research attention. It is no longer sufficient in the behavioral literature to demonstrate the power of the techniques to change behavior at one point in time. Treatments are now being judged and endorsed on the basis of their power in producing changes which endure. In this regard, self-reinforcement and goal-setting as behavior change techniques appear to merit cautious optimism. As noted earlier in the Mahoney (1974b) obesity study, subjects in the self-reward habit change group were unsurpassed in maintaining their weight loss at the 1-year follow-up.

Another intriguing hypothesis regarding maintenance of behavior change is that it may not be sufficient to focus only on the specific behavior to be altered. Other important aspects of the individual's life, such as internal belief systems and external social processes, may exert a powerful influence toward relapse into old behavior unless these aspects themselves are modified. For example, the use of self-monitoring and self-reinforcement may result in a decrease in cigarette smoking. However, the incidence of smoking may return to its pretreatment level the next time the individual is under stress unless alternative reactions to stress have been taught. Techniques such as Beck's cognitive therapy (1976) may be important in altering the belief systems which contribute to maladaptive behavior. Aspects of the social environment which sustain the problematic behavior may also be made a target of the treatment package. For example, in the recent obesity study of Brownell et al. (1977), the subjects who showed the most change at follow-up were those whose spouse was both cooperative and included in the treatment by the experimenters. Results such as these indicate the necessity to be broad in our treatment focus if we aim for endurance of change.

Levels of Self-control

It should now be apparent that the term "self-control" may be just as misleading as its counterpart—"environmental control"—if either of these is meant to imply total and independent regulation. Self-control patterns often require skills in environmental engineering and, likewise, many instances of environmental control have been potentiated by the person's behavior. In early applications of self-control techniques, the therapist was often an overwhelming part of the client's external environment. Although the client was asked to participate in data collection and implementation of a behavior change strategy, all other aspects of intervention fell primarily to the therapist. Definition of the client's problem and selection of an appropriate self-regulatory strategy, for example, were usually left to the therapist. This arrangement might be called *first-order* self-control since it limits client responsibilities to those of a technician.

Recently, several researchers have begun to explore the feasibility of *second-order* self-control which might be more generally termed "personal problem solving." The goal of personal problem solving therapy is to train the client in a broad range of functional coping skills. Thus, he or she is not simply asked to carry out the assignments of a therapist but is, instead, trained in basic skills of problem definition, functional analysis, generation of possible solutions, and so on. In a sense, the client is trained to be a "personal scientist" who learns to apply scientific problem solving strategies to personal adjustment. One such system (Mahoney and Mahoney, 1976) uses the mnemonic "SCIENCE" to enumerate seven basic stages in personal problem solving:

S Specify general problem
C Collect information
I Identify causes or patterns
E Examine options
N Narrow options and experiment
C Compare data
E Extend, revise, or replace

For example, the client in the first stage (Specify general problem) may decide that her problem is excessive smoking. In the second stage (Collect information), she would self-monitor her smoking behavior, perhaps by means of a diary as in Figure 4. 2. The goal here would be to set the stage for the third phase (Identify causes), in which she would examine the information collected. She may discover that she smokes almost exclusively in situations involving social discomfort—at the office when dealing with co-workers, and at social functions such as parties. In the fourth stage (Examine options), she would generate alternatives, in a "brainstorming," or non-evaluative fashion. The options may range from practicing muscular relaxation whenever she wants a cigarette, to avoiding social situations which are most troublesome. In the fifth phase (Narrow options and experiment), she would examine her alternatives and choose one with which to experiment. If she chose relaxation, she would practice it so that she could use it as an active coping skill whenever she desired to smoke (Goldfried and Trier, 1974). During this time she would still be collecting data, so that in the sixth phase (Compare data), she could assess the success of her experiment. In the last phase (Extend, revise, or replace), she would decide if the experiment required revision—perhaps even starting again at the problem specification phase—or if the experiment succeeded, she would now need to instigate maintenance procedures.

The personal science model is clearly an elaboration and specification of the problem-solving process carried out in some fashion by many people in everyday life. However, serious deficiencies in the particular skills which constitute each stage are common. Many individuals, for example, are poor observers of their own behavior, and many are deficient in their capacity to generate more than one or two alternatives to a problem (Spivack, Platt, and Shure, 1976). The goal of teaching problem solving in the clinic or in the school is to help refine some of the skills which are a part of everyday problem solving. A problem-solving model similar to the personal science model presented here has been offered by Sobell and Sobell (1977) as relevant for the treatment of alcoholism. The goal with every such model is training the skills for managing one's own actions.

Training in such generally applicable skills would appear to set the stage for maintenance of desirable behavior change. If individuals are knowledgeable in problem analysis and change techniques, they may be more able to generate maintenance strategies for themselves. Further, they should be better armed to face future demands. Research on this approach is still preliminary but clearly promising (Mahoney and Arnkoff, 1978; Spivack et al., 1976; Spivack and Shure, 1974). Personal problem solving does, of course, place more responsibility on the client for various aspects of problem analysis and intervention, but the skills developed in the process may be well worth these additional demands.

Conclusion

We have now surveyed a large and expanding set of strategies which have been applied to self-regulation. While some of these strategies have yet to receive adequate experimental scrutiny, their overall promise is clearly indicated by the available literature. Research activity on self-control processes and procedures is extensive, and there are many signs of theoretical and conceptual refinement. Given the recency of scientific exploration and the rapidity with which our knowledge is changing, it would be premature to conclude that we now understand human self-regulation or that we have identified the most powerful techniques in this area. On the other hand, it seems safe to assert that we have made substantial progress after only one decade of concentrated research. Some of our present techniques appear to be consistent and powerful, and more recent innovations have already begun to show therapeutic promise. Self-control theory and technology has not "arrived" at some static state of complacency, but this is hardly unusual in science. Let us not allow the elusiveness of "arrival" rob us of the satisfaction which can be derived from a feeling of movement.

References

Axelrod, S., Hall, R. V., Weis, L., and Rohrer, S. Use of self-imposed contingencies to reduce the frequency of smoking behavior. In M. J. Mahoney and C. E. Thoresen (Eds.), *Self-control: Power to the person.* Monterey, Calif.: Brooks/Cole, 1974, pp. 77–85.

Bandura, A. *Principles of behavior modification.* New York: Holt, Rinehart & Winston, 1969.

Bandura, A. Vicarious and self-reinforcement processes. In R. Glaser (Ed.), *The nature of reinforcement.* New York: Academic Press, 1971, pp. 228–278.

Bandura, A. Behavior theory and the models of man. *Am. Psychol.,* 1974, *29,* 859–869.

Bandura, A. Self-reinforcement: Theoretical and methodological considerations. *Behaviorism,* 1976, *4,* 135–155.

Bandura, A. Self-efficacy: Towards a unifying theory of behavioral change. *Psychol. Rev.,* 1977, *84,* 191–215.

Bandura, A., and Adams, N. E. Analysis of self-efficacy theory of behavioral change. *Cognitive Ther. Res.,* 1977, *1,* 287–310.

Bandura, A., and Mahoney, M. J. Maintenance and transfer of self-reinforcement functions. *Behav. Res. Ther.,* 1974, *12,* 89–98.

Bandura, A., Mahoney, M. J., and Dirks, S. J. Discriminative activation and maintenance of contingent self-reinforcement. *Behav. Res. Ther.,* 1976, *14,* 1–6.

Bandura, A., and Perloff, B. Relative efficacy of self-monitored and externally imposed reinforcement systems. *J. Pers. Soc. Psychol.,* 1967, *7,* 111–116.

Bandura, A., and Simon, K. M. The role of proximal intentions in self-regulation of refractory behavior. *Cognitive Ther. Res.,* 1977, *1,* 177–194.

Beck, A. T. *Cognitive therapy and the emotional disorders.* New York: International Universities Press, 1976.

Bellack, A. S. A comparison of self-reinforcement and self-monitoring in a weight reduction program. *Behav. Ther.,* 1976, *7,* 68–75.

Bootzin, R. R. A stimulus control treatment for insomnia. *Proc. Am. Psychol. Assoc.,* 1972, 395–396.

Brownell, K. D., Heckerman, C. L., Westlake, R. J., Hayes, S. C., and Monti, P. The effect of spouse cooperativeness and couples training in the treatment of obesity. Paper presented at the annual meeting of the Association for the Advancement of Behavior Therapy, Atlanta, December, 1977.

Catania, A. C. The myth of self-reinforcement. *Behaviorism,* 1975, *3,* 192–199.

Cautela, J. R. Behavior therapy and self-control: Techniques and implications. In C. M. Franks (Ed.), *Behavior therapy: Appraisal and status.* New York: McGraw-Hill, 1969, pp. 323–340.

Corbin, C. B. Mental practice. In W. P. Morgan (Ed.), *Ergogenic aids and muscular performance.* New York: Academic Press, 1972, pp. 93–118.

Dunbar, J., and Agras, W. S. A behavioral strategy for improving adherence to medication. Paper presented at the annual meeting of the Association for the Advancement of Behavior Therapy, Atlanta, December, 1977.

Dunbar, J. M., and Stunkard, A. J. Adherence to diet and drug regimens. In R. Levy, B. Rifkind, B. Dennis, and N. Ernst (Eds.), *Nutrition, lipids, and coronary heart disease.* New York: Raven Press, 1977

Ferster, C. B., Nurnberger, J. I., and Levitt, E. B. The control of eating. *J. Mathetics,* 1962, *1,* 87–109.

Friedman, M., and Rosenman, R. H. *Type A behavior and your heart.* New York: Alfred A. Knopf, 1974.

Gewirtz, J. L. The roles of overt responding and extrinsic reinforcement in "self-" and "vicarious-reinforcement" phenomena and in "observational learning" and imitation. In R. Glaser (Ed.), *The nature of reinforcement.* New York: Academic Press, 1971, pp. 279–309.

Goldfried, M. R., and Merbaum, M. (Eds.). *Behavior change through self-control.* New York: Holt, Rinehart & Winston, 1973.

Goldfried, M. R., and Trier, C. S. Effectiveness of relaxation as an active coping skill. *J. Abnorm. Psychol.,* 1974, *83,* 348–355.

Goldiamond, I. Self-control procedures in personal behavior problems. *Psychol. Rep.,* 1965, *17,* 851–868.

Goldiamond, I. Self-reinforcement. *J. Appl. Behav. Anal.,* 1976, *9,* 509–514.

Jones, R. T., Nelson, R. E., and Kazdin, A. E. The role of external variables in self-reinforcement: A review. *Behav. Mod.,* 1977, *1,* 147–178.

Kanfer, F. H. Self-regulation: Research, issues and speculations. In C. Neuringer and J. L. Michael (Eds.), *Behavior modification in clinical psychology.* New York: Appleton-Century-Crofts, 1970a, pp. 178–220.

Kanfer, F. H. Self-monitoring: Methodological limitations and clinical applications. *J. Consult. Clin. Psychol.,* 1970b, *35,* 148–152.

Kanfer, F. H. The maintenance of behavior by self-generated stimuli and reinforcement. In A. Jacobs and L. B. Sachs (Eds.), *The psychology of private events: Perspectives on covert response systems.* New York: Academic Press, 1971, pp. 39–59.

Kazdin, A. E. Covert modeling and the reduction of avoidance behavior. *J. Abnorm. Psychol.,* 1973, *81,* 87–95.

Kazdin, A. E. Self-monitoring and behavior change. In M. J. Mahoney and C. E. Thoresen (Eds.), *Self-control: Power to the person.* Monterey, Calif.: Brooks/Cole, 1974, pp. 218–246.

Kolb, D. A., Winter, S. K., and Berlew, D. E. Self-directed change: Two studies. *J. Appl. Behav. Sci.,* 1968, *4,* 453–471.

Locke, E. A., Cartledge, N., and Koeppel, J. Motivational effects of knowledge of results: A goal-setting phenomenon? *Psychol. Bull.,* 1968, *70,* 474–485.

Mahoney, M. J. Research issues in self-management. *Behav. Ther.,* 1972, *3,* 45–63.

Mahoney, M. J. *Cognition and behavior modification.* Cambridge, Mass.: Ballinger, 1974a.

Mahoney, M. J. Self-reward and self-monitoring techniques for weight control. *Behav. Ther.,* 1974b, *5,* 48–57.

Mahoney, M. J. Reflections on the cognitive learning trend in psychotherapy. *Am. Psychol.,* 1977, *32,* 5–13.

Mahoney, M. J., and Arnkoff, D. B. Cognitive and self-control therapies. In S. L. Garfield and A. E. Bergin (Eds.), *Handbook of psychotherapy and behavior change,* 2nd ed. New York: Wiley, 1978.

Mahoney, M. J., and Bandura, A. Self-reinforcement in pigeons. *Learning Mot.,* 1972, *3,* 293–303.

Mahoney, M. J., Bandura, A., Dirks, S. J., and Wright, C. L. Relative preference for external and self-controlled reinforcement in monkeys. *Behav. Res. Ther.,* 1974, *12,* 157–164.

Mahoney, M. J., and Mahoney, K. *Permanent weight control.* New York: W. W. Norton, 1976.

Mahoney, M. J., Moura, N. G. M., and Wade, T. C. The relative efficacy of self-reward, self-punishment, and self-monitoring techniques for weight loss. *J. Consult. Clin. Psychol.,* 1973, *40,* 404–407.

Mahoney, M. J., and Thoresen, C. E. (Eds.). *Self-control: Power to the person.* Monterey, Calif.: Brooks/Cole, 1974.

Masters, J. C., and Mokros, J. R. Self-reinforcement processes in children. In H. Reese (Ed.), *Advances in child development and behavior,* Vol. 9. New York: Academic Press, 1974.

Meichenbaum, D. H. Examination of model characteristics in reducing avoidance behavior. *J. Pers. Soc. Psychol.,* 1971, *17,* 298–307.

Meichenbaum, D. *Cognitive behavior modification.* New York: Plenum, 1977.

Mischel, W. *Personality and assessment.* New York: Wiley, 1968.

Mischel, W. Toward a cognitive social learning reconceptualization of personality. *Psychol. Rev.,* 1973, *80,* 252–283.

Nelson, R. O. Self-monitoring: Procedures and methodological issues. In J. D. Cone and R. P. Hawkins (Eds.), *Behavioral assessment: New directions in clinical psychology.* New York: Brunner/Mazel, 1977.

Paivio, A. Neomentalism. *Can. J. Psychol.,* 1975, *29,* 263–291.

Rachlin, H. Self control. *Behaviorism,* 1974, *2,* 94–107.

Rachlin, H. Reinforcing and punishing thoughts. *Behav. Ther.,* 1977, *8,* 659–665.

Reese, H. W. The study of covert verbal and nonverbal mediation. In A. Jacobs and L. B. Sachs (Eds.), *The psychology of private events: Perspectives on covert response systems.* New York: Academic Press, 1971, pp. 17–38.

Richards, C. S., Perri, M. G., and Gortney, C. Increasing the maintenance of self-control treatments through faded counselor contact and high information feedback. *J. Counsel. Psychol.,* 1976, *23,* 405–406.

Romanczyk, R. G. Self-monitoring in the treatment of obesity: Parameters of reactivity. *Behav. Ther.,* 1974, *5,* 531–540.

Skinner, B. F. *Science and human behavior.* New York: Macmillan, 1953.

Skinner, B. F. *About behaviorism.* New York: Alfred A. Knopf, 1974.

Sobell, L. C., and Sobell, M. B. Alcohol problems. In R. B. Williams and W. D. Gentry (Eds.), *Behavioral approaches to medical treatment.* Cambridge, Mass.: Ballinger, 1977.

Spivack, G., Platt, J. J., and Shure, M. D. *The problem-solving approach to adjustment.* San Francisco: Jossey-Bass, 1976.

Spivack, G., and Shure, M. B. *Social adjustment of young children: A cognitive approach to solving real-life problems.* San Francisco: Jossey-Bass, 1974.

Stuart, R. B. Behavioral control of overeating. *Behav. Res. Ther.,* 1967, *5,* 357–365.

Stuart, R. B. Situational versus self-control. In R. D. Rubin, H. Fensterheim, J. D. Henderson, and L. P. Ullmann (Eds.), *Advances in behavior therapy.* New York: Academic Press, 1972, pp. 129–146.

Stunkard, A. J., and Mahoney, M. J. Behavioral treatment of the eating disorders. In H. Leitenberg (Ed.), *Handbook of behavior modification and behavior therapy.* New York: Appleton-Century-Crofts, 1976.

Thoresen, C. E., and Mahoney, M. J. *Behavioral self-control.* New York: Holt, Rinehart & Winston, 1974.

Weimer, W. B. *Notes on the methodology of scientific research.* Hillsdale, N.J.: Lawrence Erlbaum Associates, 1977.

Wilson, G. T., and Abrams, D. Effects of alcohol on social anxiety and physiological arousal: Cognitive versus pharmacological processes. *Cogn. Ther. Res.,* 1977, *1,* 195–210.

Wooley, S. C. Physiologic versus cognitive factors in short term food regulation in the obese and nonobese. *Psychosom. Med.,* 1972, *34,* 62–68.

Clinical Applications

Behavioral Pediatrics*

EDWARD R. CHRISTOPHERSEN, PH.D.

Associate Professor
Department of Pediatrics
University of Kansas Medical Center
Kansas City, Kansas, and
Senior Scientist
Bureau of Child Research
University of Kansas
Lawrence, Kansas

MICHAEL A. RAPOFF, M.S. ED.

Graduate Research Assistant
Bureau of Child Research
University of Kansas
Lawrence, Kansas

5

Beginning almost 40 years ago with Anderson's (1930) address to the American Medical Association in which he discussed the increasing emphasis on methods of child training and problems of adjustment in children, the foundation was set for what is now termed "behavioral pediatrics." Major contributors to the later development of this area of medicine include Kagan (1965) and Wright (1967), both of whom discussed and advocated a marriage of sorts between pediatricians and child psychologists. The American Board of Pediatrics in 1951 began stressing the importance of having pediatric training centers assume the responsibility for the day-to-day teaching of growth and development in clinical settings. However, the lack of substantial advancement in education in this area is reflected by the recommendation of the 1978 Task Force on Pediatric Education that one of its top priorities should be in the area of behavioral pediatrics. There has been little advancement until recently as shown by the fact that, in a review of the literature, Christophersen and Rapoff (in press) cited over 100 studies dealing with a wide variety of minor pediatric behavior problems, and approximately 85% of the references were works published in the last decade. This may explain the slow assimilation of behavioral pediatrics into pediatric training programs; that is, until relatively recently, there simply has not been much relevant work carried out in pediatric primary health care systems.

The present chapter is a review of the literature in behavioral pediatrics, beginning with a brief discussion of the prevention and early detection of pediatric behavior problems during well-child visits. The chapter then discusses advances in several major areas either in pediatrics or directly related to it. Where possible, this review will refer to actual experimental studies, avoiding case studies or collections of case studies as much as possible. The review is intended to provide the reader with a working knowledge of the current state of development of behavioral pediatrics.

* Preparation of this manuscript was partially supported by Grant 03144 from the National Institute of Child Health and Human Development to the Bureau of Child Research, University of Kansas.

Prevention and Early Detection of Pediatric Behavior Problems

Brazelton (1975), Christophersen (in press), and Kenny and Clemmens (1975) all stress the importance of scheduling expectant parents for at least one prenatal visit with the pediatrician. Although these authors differ on the specifics of what should be included during this visit, they do agree on the main ingredient, that is, the focus on the parent-child relationship, and on the profound effect that this relationship can have on the child. Each of these authors provides some preliminary guidelines for the pediatrician on what to cover and how to cover it during the prenatal visit. Each is directly in keeping with Friedman's (1975) statement that:

> Behavioral pediatrics maintains the pediatric tradition of emphasizing prevention, with curative and rehabilitative orientation always "second best" to preventing the disease or defect in the first place. Those identified with behavioral pediatrics do not claim expertise in the major psychiatric problems of childhood, but emphasize early prevention and treatment of the less severe problems. There is a special interest in the psychological aspects of physical illness in children and adolescents, and in integrating this concern into the total health care system (p. 515).

Much work has yet to be done to document the effectiveness of prevention of behavioral problems. To date, only anecdotal reports and case studies have been reported. All of these have been well intentioned but have not been scientific. Christophersen (in press) and Christophersen and Rapoff (in press) have also clearly directed the pediatrician on how to conduct a well-child visit in such a way so as to detect problems long before the parent would have specifically scheduled an appointment to talk to the pediatrician about the specific problem. In giving such direction to the pediatrician, one assumes, or makes the value judgment, that a positive and affectionate relationship between the parent and child is of utmost importance. Assuming this, it is necessary to educate the pediatrician in the subtle nuances that serve as indicators that the relationship is beginning to deteriorate. Again, there are no hard data on the effectiveness of the prevention of behavioral problems and the suggestions for prevention are only anecdotal.

What follows is a summary of the data and of case studies (where no data are available) of the kinds of behavioral problems that the practicing pediatrician is likely to encounter on a nearly daily basis. This summary is organized according to major presenting symptoms. The reader, like the authors, will probably be struck by how much work really is necessary for the remediation of some behavioral problems. Hopefully, this awareness will strengthen interest in research on the prevention and early detection of behavioral problems.

Noncompliance

Failure to comply with parental requests is a frequent problem brought to the attention of clinicians. Although most parents encounter this problem and deal with it successfully on their own, others may need varying degrees of professional assistance. Fortunately, there are effective procedures available.

Based on observations of one mother-child pair, Budd, Green, and Baer (1976) identified several parental behaviors which seemed to be related to the child's rate of noncompliance. These included the following: (1) the mother repeated commands excessively; (2) she decreased instructions contingent on the child's inappropriate behavior; (3) she physically intervened to procure compliance and then praised the child; (4) she gave additional attention while an instruction was still pending; and (5) she failed to use any form of time-out for noncompliance. The experimenters then trained the mother to alter these behaviors while taking measures on the child's rate of compliance. Using a multiple baseline design, they demonstrated that the time-out procedure was a necessary component of the training program. Changes in the first four parental behaviors resulted in some desirable changes in the child's behavior, but complete remediation of the child's inappropriate behaviors did not occur until the time-out contingency was established.

In a group study design Roberts, McMahon, Forehand, et al. (in press) compared two treatment strategies designed to alter children's noncompliant behavior with a control group. One group of parents were trained to issue specific commands and wait until the child complied or until 5 seconds elapsed. A second group received "command training" and were also taught to use a time-out procedure contingent on the child's noncompliance (failure to comply within 5 seconds of a parental command). A third group served as a control. Pre- and post-test measures of child compliance indicated that the command only and command plus time-out groups significantly increased child compliance over the control group. Parents in the command plus time-out group obtained significantly higher compliance rates than those in the command only group. These results suggest that teaching parents to alter antecedent events (issuing of commands) can have beneficial results, but the best strategy is to alter both antecedent and consequent events.

Forehand and King (1977) found that teaching parents to alter their children's noncompliant behavior can also produce positive changes in the parents' attitude toward their child. They trained 11 mothers in a clinic playroom setting to alter their children's behavior by issuing specific commands, reinforcing compliance, and consequating noncompliance with time-out. In addition to measures on the child's and mother's behaviors, they took baseline, treatment, and follow-up attitude measures using the Parent Attitude Test. This test purports to reflect the parent's perception of the child's adjustment at home and school. On the behavioral observation measure, predictable results were found: the children were significantly more compliant after treatment and at a 3-month follow-up. In terms of the attitude measures, the mothers rated their children as better adjusted after treatment and at follow-up. The resulting adjustment after treatment was comparable to that of a nonclinic sample using the same behavioral and attitudinal measures.

Using a group design with random assignment, Christophersen, Barnard, Ford, et al. (1976), demonstrated that a home-based intervention program was more effective than a conventional outpatient treatment program in effecting changes in children referred for behavior problems (of which the most frequent was noncompliance). The home-based treatment, although more effective, required more time to implement. Treatment procedures generally involved the use of token systems and time-out. During home visits the therapists modeled and had the parents and children practice behaviors which the therapists and families agreed were important to improve interactions. Frequent home visits were made during the first few weeks of treatment, at times convenient to the families. Visits were also made at those times when problems were known to occur (e.g., at night for bedtime problems).

The few studies which have been reviewed are representative of the literature and suggest that parents can be supplied with effective procedures for managing noncompliant behavior in their children. The study by Christophersen et al. (1976) suggests further that home-based treatment, although more expensive in terms of professional contact, may be a more efficacious approach to treating children with behavior problems. Of course, additional research is needed to replicate these findings. The use of time-out appears to be a necessary component of any effective treatment package—Drabman and Jarvie (1977) offer an excellent discussion of some "pitfalls" that can be encountered by parents attempting to use time-out; they also offer specific remedies for these problems.

In the experience of the authors in a pediatric outpatient clinic, parents can be shown how to manage noncompliant behavior effectively through the combined use of social reinforcement and time-out: during home or clinic visits, they are taught to look specifically for compliant behavior and to praise, hug, etc., their children at these times; in addition, parents are to use a simple time-out procedure for noncompliance. The procedures are modeled for the parents and children and are practiced with feedback from the therapist. (A written handout which details the procedures is available from the authors on request.) Frequent phone contact is maintained with the families during the first few weeks to assist them in handling problems which may occur. The authors have found that if these problems are identified and treated early (when the child is pre-school age), treatment is much easier and the prognosis for the child much more favorable.

Aggression

About one-third of all mental health referrals from parents and teachers are estimated to involve children with out-of-control behavior or problems with aggression (Patterson, Reid, Jones, et al., 1975). The aggressive child presents a substantial challenge to mental health practitioners and educators as well as parents. Although the treatment literature concerning aggressive children in both home and school settings is quite extensive, the present summary will not provide a thorough review of this entire literature. Instead, an attempt will be made to summarize studies representative of behavioral treatment approaches to treating aggressive children which utilize parents as primary change agents. In addition, the work of Wahler and Patterson, two clinical researchers who have made substantial contributions to this literature, will be reviewed in more detail. In sampling the literature and providing specific details of exemplary treatment programs, it is hoped that the reader will gain sufficient understanding of the present technology available for treating aggressive children.

Since 1965 numerous studies, generally involving fewer than five subjects, have appeared in the literature which have demonstrated that parents can be taught to manage the noxious behaviors of their children more effectively (O'Dell, 1974). Hawkins, Peterson, Schweid, et al. (1966) reported on a case involving a 4-year-old child who exhibited aggressive behaviors such as kicking others, calling names, and hitting himself. Treatment procedures were carried out in the home with the experimenters cueing the mother's responses by using "gestural signals." When the child exhibited objectionable behaviors, the mother was signaled to tell him to stop. If he did not stop, the mother was signaled to place the child in his room and lock the door (time-out). The child was to remain in his room 5 minutes and was to be quiet for a short period before he could come out. When the child was behaving appropriately, the mother was signaled to give him special attention, praise, and affectionate physical contact. Through a reversal design it was demonstrated that the child's objectionable behaviors were decreased by the treatment conditions. These changes were maintained at 1-month follow-up. The authors indicated that home treatment may be more effective than treatment in clinic settings, particularly if the undesirable behavior has a low probability of occurrence in the clinic setting. O'Leary, O'Leary, and Becker (1967) successfully modified aggressive interactions in siblings by training the mother to use a token reinforcement system and time-out procedure. The subjects were two male children, 6 and 3 years of age, who frequently kicked, pushed, hit, called names, and threw objects at each other. The procedures were introduced to the children by the experimenters at the same time as they were taught to the mother. The token system involved check marks given for cooperative behavior which could be exchanged for comic books, gum, small toys, and other inexpensive items. The time-out procedure involved isolating the child in the bathroom (with easily removed items absent) for a period of at least 5 minutes, with the requirement that he was to be quiet for at least 3 minutes before being allowed to come out. This procedure was introduced after it was found that the token system alone did not substantially reduce aggressive interactions. Utilizing a reversal design the treatment procedures were shown to be effective in increasing cooperative behavior and decreasing aggressive responses. No follow-up data were reported. The changes did not generalize to the school setting for the 6-year-old child, and he continued sporadically to exhibit aggressive behavior in that setting.

Bernal (1969) described a training format for parents designed to modify the behavior of children who engage in highly aggressive and defiant behaviors. She used the colloquial term "brat" to describe these difficult-to-manage children. The training format involved videotaping parent-child interactions in the home and clinic setting and analyzing the tapes to determine what parental responses elicited and maintained "brat" behaviors. Based on this analysis, "step-by-step instructions" were tailored for each parent indicating more appropriate responses to their child's behavior. During treatment, videotapes were used by the clinician to provide feedback to the parents as they gradually learned to manage their children's behavior. Bernal presented two case studies involving two male children age 5 and 8 years who exhibited high rates of aggressive and destructive behaviors. The mothers were taught to use contingent praise for appropriate behavior, to ignore minor abusive behavior, and to punish physically abusive behavior. Written instructions, videotape feedback, and verbal "coaching" were all used to shape appropriate parental responses. Over a period of 25 weeks both children showed marked improvement in their behavior. Bernal suggested that videotape feedback alone may be sufficient to modify some parental responses but more complex parent-child behavioral chains may require direct instruction plus feedback.

Studies by Hawkins et al., O'Leary et al., and Bernal represent a more extensive, although poorly integrated, body of literature which suggest that parents can be effective mediators of treatments designed to alter aggressive responses of children. The work of Robert Wahler at the University of Tennessee Child Behavior Institute and of Gerald Patterson at the Oregon Social Learning Center (formerly the Oregon Research Institute) and their colleagues will now be reviewed in more detail. Their work represents a more integrated body of literature specifically focused on treatment of the aggressive child. In addition, they offer theoretical formulations regarding the development and maintenance of aggressive behavior in children, stimulating both previous and current research efforts in this area.

Based on numerous hours of observations of aggressive boys in their natural homes, Patterson and his colleagues have suggested that the aggressive child is both "architect" and "victim" of a coercive family system (Patterson, 1976). The child is the architect of his coercive system in the sense that he exhibits coercive behaviors (whining, screaming, hitting, etc.) to shape and control the behavior of other family members. He is a victim of his system in the sense that other family members maintain these responses by providing positive consequences for coercive behaviors at times and by retaliating in like manner at other times. The result is a spiraling increase in coercive interchanges among family members that is reciprocal in nature. Patterson has also found several consistent characteristics of the aggressive child and his parents. The parents are likely to give threats which are seldom backed up and are more likely to provide positive consequences for their children's coercive behaviors. The aggressive child displays higher rates of coercive behaviors which tend to come in spurts, increases his coercive behavior when presented with "garden variety" punishments (spanking and yelling), and is less responsive to adult approval. The general picture is one of a disrupted family system with family members avoiding interactions even of a recreational nature. Given the reciprocal nature of coercive interactions among family members, Patterson reasoned that " . . . changing the aggressive behavior of the child might have been of only limited clinical utility unless accompanied by concomitant changes in other family members" (1976, p. 268).

The treatment package utilized by the Patterson group (1976) involved both a home and school component. In the home component, parents were involved in treatment for a minimum of 1 month; the parents were required to read a programmed text (Patterson and Gullion, 1968) which is based on social learning and child management techniques. They were taught specifically to define, track, and record deviant and prosocial child behaviors. They were then assigned to parent training groups where modeling and role-playing procedures were used to illustrate appropriate techniques. In the group, they were also taught to design contracts specifying contingencies for various problem behaviors which occurred in the home and at school. These contracts specifically involved point losses and gains backed up by a list of privileges. Frequent phone contact was maintained with the families during treatment. When necessary (and this was not specified), training was done in the home. Treatment in the school involved direct intervention by the teaching staff using token systems which earned privileges for the child and his peers and contracts with consequences dispensed at home via a daily report card. For some families, it was necessary to provide additional procedures for the management of marital conflicts (Patterson, Reid, Jones, et al., 1975).

Outcome measures of home treatment were based on direct observational data and parental reports. Direct observations in the home were made at dinner time, with the observer making two 5-minute observations of each family member in a prearranged random order. This sampling procedure produced a sequential account of the target child's behavior and the reactions of family members. Both noxious and prosocial behaviors of family members were sampled, using a code system which contained 29 behavioral categories (Patterson, Ray, Shaw, et al., 1969). The behaviors sampled were expressed as rate per minute with an upper limit of 10 responses per minute for any subject during an observation period. The parental report consisted of a list of problems which the parent had identified as being of greatest concern during an intake interview. The parent simply checked if these behaviors occurred or did not occur on a particular day. Observational data were also collected in the classroom for those children who needed school intervention. In the school, data were collected for a minimum of five sessions prior to treatment, during treatment, at termination, and at 6 and 12 months following termination. Outcome measures for the home treatment were taken 6 to 10 days prior to treatment, following the reading of the text, at the 4th and 8th weeks of treatment, and at termination. The clinician and the family determined the time to terminate treatment. Following termination, outcome data were collected at months 1 to 6 and at months 8, 10, and 12. At any point during the 12-month follow-up period, the parents or the clinician could initiate "booster shot" training in which components of the treatment package were reimplemented.

The treatment outcome data, summarized by Patterson (1976), encompasses work with 27 families treated from January 1968 to June 1972. Details have been presented in two major reports (Patterson, Cobb, and Ray, 1973; Patterson and Reid, 1973). Significant improvements were found on all outcome measures on the target children in both the home and school settings. The average cost of treatment in terms of professional time per family was 31.5 hours for the home intervention and 28.6 hours for the school intervention. During the 12-month follow-up period, an average of 1.9 hours of professional time was spent in "booster shot" training. Although the rates of coercive behaviors significantly decreased for each target child, this was not the case for all family members. Commenting on this finding, Patterson suggested that there is only partial support for the notion that the system changed as a function of treatment: "These findings set further constraints upon our confidence in the likelihood of long-term adjustment for many of these cases" (Patterson, 1976, p. 305). Follow-up data on 14 of the 27 families treated indicated that significant improvements were maintained in both the home and school settings (Patterson, 1974). Patterson's follow-up analyses have not been without criticisms. Kent (1976) has re-analyzed the data and has suggested that Patterson's conclusions regarding maintenance of treatment effects are "unwarranted." Reid and Patterson (1976) have replied to these criticisms. The resolution of the controversy involves questions of experimental design and dependent measures and is beyond the scope of this discussion. The reader should be aware, however, that the controversy over the follow-up data does exist.

Given extensive research and contact with aggressive children and their families, it is Patterson's impression that one-third of these families can be helped by teaching the parents specific techniques for changing their children's behavior. About one-third of families require more extensive intervention (e.g., marital counseling), and about one-third of the families fail to make any significant changes in spite of the clinician's "best efforts" (Patterson, 1976). Patterson and his colleagues emphasize that their work represents a developing technology which is under constant revision based on continued experience and empirical investigations. They have written a manual for professionals which describes in detail their clinical and research procedures (Patterson et al., 1975), although they emphasize that the manual represents the current state of development of their treatment process and is in no way a finished product. The assessment and treatment procedures developed by Patterson and his colleagues represent the most highly refined treatment package available. This technology, although adequately described, should not be applied in a careless manner. Particularly with the problem of aggression, clinicians attempting to use these procedures should have extensive training and experience with behavioral approaches to child management.

The work of Wahler and his associates at the University of Tennessee Child Behavior Institute parallels and, in many respects, complements that of the Patterson group. The clinical populations are quite similar and both groups have published frequently quoted articles since the mid 1960's. In speculating on the development of deviant behavior in children, Wahler (1976) emphasizes the influence of other family members in maintaining the child's behavior. His impression is that the child's deviance is "locked into" a disrupted family system. He describes two types of "trap" situations that develop within a family to promote deviant behaviors. In one situation, "the positive reinforcer trap," the child's behavior (e.g., clinging/dependent behavior) is at first reinforced by the family, but as the child ages these behaviors become aversive to the family. The other situation, which Wahler believes is the most relevant to the development of aggressive/oppositional behaviors, is one that he describes as "the negative reinforcer trap." In this case, the child exhibits aversive behaviors and family members discover that a very efficient way to terminate these behaviors is to provide positive consequences. This terminates the aversive behaviors only temporarily. The example used was of a child screaming and kicking in the supermarket and being given a popsicle by his or her mother in order to stop the offensive behavior. The process continues to develop and extends to other situations, and the child becomes increasingly demanding. Oppositional children, who can be aggressive and defiant or passively noncompliant, do not outgrow these problems, according to Wahler. His description of these children and their parents is similar to Patterson's description of families with aggressive children. The child's coercive behaviors are at times reinforced and at other times punished. In this system positive feedback is often contingent on the very behaviors which the family finds aversive. Wahler has also found that these children are relatively unresponsive to parental approval. Since it is extremely difficult for most of these parents to ignore their children's coercive behaviors, Wahler contends that punishment procedures (time-out) are a necessary component of any intervention strategy for this population.

An early case study involving three children who exhibited high rates of aggressive and defiant behaviors (Wahler, Winkel, Peterson, et al., 1965) exemplifies the approach. For two of the three children, extinction and differential reinforcement applied by their mothers were sufficient to produce appropriate changes in their behavior. For the third child a 5-minute time-out contingency was necessary to bring the child's behavior under control. Using a reversal design, Wahler (1969a) experimentally demonstrated that differential attention and time-out were effective in altering the oppositional behaviors of two children 5 and 6 years of age. In addition, the effectiveness of parental reinforcement increased as a function of the program and the parents described themselves as enjoying their children more after treatment. Wahler suggested that changes in the children's behavior apparently led to changes in the parents' behavior that were more reinforcing to the children. Although significant changes can be made in the home setting, Wahler (1969b) also demonstrated that these changes should *not* be expected to generalize to the school setting. Although the finding would not be considered remarkable at present, it was one of the first empirical demonstrations that the problem of generalization of treatment effects has important implications for clinical practice. It has become obvious since the publication of this study that separate intervention components are necessary for home and school settings.

Recently Wahler and his associates have suggested that the parent-training strategy may not benefit some families, particularly "high risk" families (Wahler, Leske, and Rogers, 1977). These are typically low socio-ecomonic families living in overcrowded, high-crime rate areas who are poorly educated and often have only one parent present in the home. Wahler proposed that these families become "insulated" from their "surrounding social context" as many of their extra-familial interactions are with agencies in which harrassment occurs (e.g., police and social welfare). The families lack a "positive reinforcement network" which can support changes made within the family. According to Wahler, Leske, and Rogers, "friendship may be the missing ingredient in effective therapeutic intervention for high risk families." The implication of this "insularity hypothesis" is that changes need to be made beyond, as well as within, the family. What these specific changes are and how they are to be made is not clear at this time. The possibility that relationships external to the family affect interactions within the family needs to be empirically tested. Once demonstrated, the implications for treating high-risk families may become clearer.

It appears from the theoretical formulations suggested by Patterson and Wahler that treatment of the aggressive child necessitates effecting changes in the family system. The formulations also suggest the need for preventive treatment efforts or anticipatory guidance with parents of young children. For example, parents can be cautioned to avoid "negative reinforcement traps" by not "giving in" to coercive behaviors in their children. Primary health care providers in pediatrics are in an excellent position to offer this type of guidance as they have frequent contact with parents of young children. Training parents in behavioral management procedures can result in a favorable outcome for some families with aggressive children. For others, services such as marital counseling, adult psychological or psychiatric treatment, or extensive school-based treatment may be necessary adjuncts to parental training. In some cases, the resolution of other problems (e.g., marital discord) may be a prerequisite to any attempt to change parent-child interactions. Finally, with some families, the prognosis is unfavorable, regardless of the intensity of therpeutic efforts. The maintenance and generalization of treatment effects, with few exceptions, has *not* been routinely investigated in this literature. The area should be thoroughly explored, as strategies for promoting generalization and maintenance of changes in families need to be developed; ultimately, transfer of training should be the criterion for successful treatment (O'Dell, 1974).

Enuresis

Enuresis, or bed wetting in the absence of any organic etiology, is reported to occur in approximately 10% of children as old as 6 years (Blomfield, 1956). Although there are numerous recommendations about the best time to treat enuresis, the present authors prefer Cohen's (1975) suggestion that treatment should be initiated when enuresis begins to interrupt the normal sequence of social, emotional, or cognitive development. A variety of treatment procedures have been proposed for enuresis, including dry-bed training, self-hypnosis, urine alarm, drugs, urine retention training, and dietary restrictions, each of which will be briefly described and discussed.

The first of these procedures, dry-bed training, has been very well described by Azrin, Sneed, and Foxx (1974). It consists of a multifaceted treatment technique which, in addition to a urine alarm, includes training inhibiting urination, positive reinforcement for correct use of the toilet, training rapid awakening, increased fluid intake, increased social motivation to be non-enuretic, self-correction of accidents, and practicing nighttime use of the toilet. This requires one night of intensive training after which telephone follow-up is usually sufficient to maintain the program. The authors report a mean of one accident during the 1st week, one during the 2nd week, and zero during the 3rd week. During a 6-month follow-up, none of the children relapsed to pretraining levels of enuresis. Doleys and Ciminero (1976) reported a higher relapse rate using the dry-bed procedure. Bollard and Woodroffe (1977) reported an adaptation which eliminates the intensive one-night training by a professional therapist. Although this adaptation has yet to be replicated, eliminating the need for the therapist to make an all-night home visit would surely increase the practicality of the dry-bed training procedures.

Another method for treating enuresis is discussed by Olness (1975): she reported using weekly sessions, over a period ranging from 6 to 28 months, to treat children using a self-hypnosis procedure. She indicated that 77% of the children treated were cured, but presented no data on controls and follow-up. The method probably has considerable appeal for clinicians with a background in clinical hypnosis and those who do not find the dry-bed procedures of Azrin, Sneed, and Foxx (1974) acceptable.

Werry and Cohrssen (1965) compared no treatment, psychotherapy, and urine alarm training. Their results indicated that in addition to being more effective, urine alarm training was more economical in terms of the need for professional supervision. Since urine alarms are readily available commercially, it is possible for parents to carry out treatment without any professional supervision. Taylor and Turner (1975) report a relapse rate of 45.7% and an overall failure rate of 42.6% with the urine alarm training. The original description by Mowrer and Mowrer (1938) of the use of the urine alarm apparatus is a refreshingly detailed and complete description, even by today's standards. They present initial outcome data and follow-up data going up to 2½ years after training, and even devote a significant amount of discussion to the problem of symptom substitution. (There probably has not been a more thorough report in the 40 years since.) When the clinician has neither the time nor the option of introducing the dry-bed training of Azrin, Sneed, and Foxx, the urine alarm training of Mowrer and Mowrer is probably the treatment of choice.

Drugs are also used in the treatment of enuresis, the most common being imipramine (Tofranil). Using imipramine, Perlmutter (1976) reported immediate cessation of enuresis with 40 to 50 percent of patients; however, almost two-thirds of these patients relapsed after discontinuation of the drug. The present authors concur with Gaultieri (1977), who stated that, although imipramine is a useful drug, it is not without risks and, therefore, ought to be reserved only for those cases in which non-prescription therapies have been ineffective.

Another procedure employed to reduce enuresis is urine retention training. Starfield and Mellits (1968) reported 6-month follow-up data on 83 enuretic children who had participated in a bladder training regimen which involved three components: unrestricted amounts of fluid, encouraging the child to retain urine at least once a day to the point of minimum discomfort, and recording the amount of urine passed each day. The children were also instructed to practice starting and stopping their urine stream during daytime micturition. The data demonstrated a relationship between increased bladder capacity and reduced enuresis. However, in a well-controlled study, Harris and Purohit (1977) failed to demonstrate a relationship between increased bladder capacity and decreased frequency of enuresis. A 35-day bladder-training program resulted in a significant mean increase in bladder capacity for experimental subjects over controls, but there was no significant difference in frequency of enuresis. These results were maintained at a 3-month follow-up. The authors stated that their results cast serious doubt on the efficacy of bladder training as the sole means of treating enuresis.

Dietary restrictions have also been studied for their effects on enuresis. In a study comparing restrictions on milk and other dairy products, eggs, citrus fruits, tomatoes, cocoa, carbonated beverages containing coloring agents, and kool-aid, with imipramine and urine alarm training, McKendry, Stewart, Khana, et al. (1975) found that cure rates for dietary restrictions were not significantly greater than spontaneous cure rates; as a result, they did not recommend changes in diet. McKendry and Stewart (1974) suggested dietary changes principally for children with histories of allergies or in cases of resistant diurnal incontinence.

Table 5.1 presents the procedures described above. The table, from Christophersen and Rapoff (1978), provides a comparison of treatment procedures based on the available literature in terms of effectiveness, relapse rate, cost, etc. The dry-bed training procedure of Azrin, Sneed, and Foxx (1974) appears to be the treatment of choice. The Olness (1975) self-hypnosis procedure, if verified by a well-controlled experimental study, has the potential for matching the results achieved with the dry-bed procedure. The urine alarm approach probably represents the most thoroughly investigated procedure ever published in the behavioral literature. Due to the commercial availability of the urine alarms and the large number of investigators who have researched the procedure, this will probably remain the "old standby" of treatment procedures for some time to come. In the absence of very convincing experimental evidence, the other treatment procedures currently available do not warrant much consideration. Drugs may be the principal exception for, in some cases, they are the only procedure that the parents will tolerate; in such situations, the equivocal outcome data and potentially hazardous side effects have to be overlooked.

Table 5.1
Comparison of Treatment Procedures*

Treatment	Effectiveness (% of cases)	Relapse Rate (% of cases)	Cost and Length of Treatment	Immediacy of Treatment Effects	Long-Term Treatment Effects	Results Replicated
Dry-bed training	+	+	+	+	+	+
Self-hypnosis†	+	+	−	+	0	−
Urine alarm	0	−	+	−	+	+
Drugs (imipramine)	0	−	+	+	−	+
Urine retention	−	−	+	−	−	0
Diet restrictions	−	−	+	−	−	−
Psychotherapy	−	−	−	−	−	0

* Key: + = better than average; 0 = average; − = less than average.

Reprinted by permission from Christophersen, E. R., and Rapoff, M. A. Enuresis treatment. *Issues in Comprehensive Pediatric Nursing*, 1978, *2*, 34–52.

† Based on one uncontrolled, unreplicated study; offered as a novel procedure in need of experimental verification.

Encopresis

The term encopresis is used to describe any voluntary or involuntary passage of feces that results in soiling of clothes (Wright, 1973b). Levine (1975) reported that 3% of the pediatric clinic population present with encopresis. Although Levine divided encopresis into either organic or psychogenic, the present review will deal with only the psychogenic type.

Davidson (1958) was one of the first authors to break with the long-standing tradition of attributing all encopresis to underlying psychopathology. He stated that encopresis almost never results from a single cause, but is the result of several factors. These factors include a constitutional predisposition, dietary factors, difficulty with passage of hard stools because of failure to provide leverage, the influence of pain and voluntary resistance causing stool retention, and development of incontinence associated with fecal impaction. Both Wright (1975) and Levine (1975) report that 80% of their patients had fecal impaction accompanying their fecal incontinence at the time of their first visit to the clinic. Levine has revised this estimate to an even higher figure. He now states that, given a thorough review of a simple, non-prepped KUB (an x-ray of the lower abdomen including the kidneys, ureters, and bladder), almost all of the encopretic patients that he sees have some degree of fecal impaction. He has also developed a protocol for a stool retention rating record for plain films of the abdomen (Levine and Barr, 1978), the results of which led him to conclude that stool retention was higher than the previously reported 80%.

Despite the number of authors in both the behavioral and medical literature who either do not address the issue of stool retention or who state that it was not a consideration in their studies, it is probably important to initiate any treatment plan with a careful physical examination (including an examination of the lower abdomen and a rectal examination) and a plain film of the abdomen (since, as Levine reports, the plain film can frequently pick up stool retention that was not discernible on physical examination). There is general agreement that the child should then be thoroughly "cleaned out" with enemas and laxatives before any treatment plan is instituted. Although several authors have reported treatment regimens that did not begin with bowel evacuation, these studies were usually case studies with relatively few subjects, usually no more than three (Doleys and Arnold, 1975; Ayllon, Simon, and Wildman, 1975; Plachetta, 1976).

A recent study in the medical literature appears to lend support to the notion that encopretics frequently have either a congenital or acquired megacolon with decreased sensitivity to rectal pressure. Meunier, Mollard, and Marechal (1976) compared 15 control subjects with 61 children who had radiological megarectum. The experimental procedure involved the insertion of three catheters into the child's rectum. Meunier et al. then artificially produced varying amounts of internal pressure at three different points within the rectum. The data revealed three distinctly different groups of responders. The first, composed of 70% control subjects, responded subjectively to a range of only 10 to 50 ml of pressure in the catheter. The second group, composed of 18% control subjects, responded to 60 to 100 ml of pressure. The third group, composed entirely of children with histories of encopresis, did not respond subjectively until experiencing between 120 and 380 ml of pressure. The study does not prove that fecal impaction or megarectum *causes* decreased rectal sensitivity, but it does adequately demonstrate that children with positive histories of encopresis require considerably more rectal pressure before they sense the urge to defecate. This finding is certainly consistent with the histories that are frequently given by encopretics, namely that they often cannot tell when they have to defecate until after they have already soiled themselves.

Several authors have indicated the necessity for using medication, usually stool softeners, laxatives or suppositories, until the colon can regain its normal muscle tone (Wright and Walker, 1977; Christophersen and Rainey, 1976). The fact that many encopretics, after a period of no soiling but with daily bowel evacuation, will proudly boast that they "had to go to the bathroom," sharply contrasts with the frequent reports prior to treatment that the child "did not feel the stools coming."

At present, two major medical approaches to the management of encopresis are strikingly similar. Davidson (1958) and Levine and Barr (1978) both recommend cleaning out the child with enemas or laxatives initially. Then, they recommend the daily use of mineral oil in order to help stimulate daily bowel movements and to avoid fecal impaction or constipation. Levine and Barr (1978) include a nice touch at this point when they attempt to "de-mystify" the problem of encopresis in an effort to alleviate associated blame and guilt from moral "turpitude." Both studies call for a daily regimen of having the child sit on the toilet for one or two brief periods each day. This is to help the child adjust to daily use of the toilet. The investigations also suggest that the clinician deal with the parent-child relationship; however, both are vague about how this is to be done. Finally, the parents are encouraged to monitor the child's bowel habits to make sure that the child is using the toilet regularly.

Wright (1973b) and Wright and Walker (1977) described a set of procedures similar to Levine's and to Davidson's with several apparently important additions. Wright suggests the use of glycerin suppositories in the morning before breakfast, which when combined with the normal gastro-colic reflex, should result in a bowel movement shortly after breakfast. The advantage of the use of suppositories is that the child's bowel movements can be "timed" much more accurately and the parent and the child know that elimination will usually occur shortly after breakfast. (With the use of mineral oil the timing of bowel movements is much less precise.) With the parents, Wright also discusses in detail how to reinforce the child for correct elimination. In his 1973 article, he suggests that "parental time" be used as a reinforcer for bowel movements in the toilet. The parents are encouraged to spend time with the child, engaging in activity of the child's choice for 15 minutes for each bowel movement in the toilet. Wright also suggests that the parents arrange for a punisher to be used for accidents. He suggests such things as loss of TV privileges, being kept indoors, or having to sit in a chair. Wright also suggests that the clinician point out emphatically the importance of maintaining complete adherence to the treatment regimen by both parents and child.

Christophersen and Rainey (1976) use procedures very similar to Wright's (1973b), with some notable exceptions. They present a copy of a one-page list of instructions that is given to the parents to aid them in their compliance with the treatment regimen. They have the parents keep daily records on their child's bowel movements (number, size, consistency, etc., of each bowel movement). Moreover, they also recommend frequent, almost daily, telephone contact with the parents in order to maintain treatment compliance. During these brief phone contacts the parents are asked to describe exactly what happened since the last phone contact. Christophersen and Rainey discourage the use of any punishment whatsoever. This is consistent with Levine's and with Davidson's suggestions, but not with Wright's.

A major sequel to the Christophersen and Rainey paper is a thesis (Barnard, 1978) which describes a rather simple, but very important set of procedures for doing reliability checks on parental reports of soiling and/or cleanliness. Obviously these reliability checks are not necessary in a clinical setting, but corroboration of some kind is absolutely essential in studies on the effectiveness of treatment. Another important contribution from Barnard's thesis is the use of an experimental design involving a multiple baseline across four subjects. The particular choice is unimportant as long as some experimental design is employed. The studies by Levine (1975), Levine and Barr (1978), Davidson (1958), Davidson, Kugler, and Bauer (1963), Wright (1973b), and Wright and Walker (1977) were, unfortunately, all case studies. The principal redeeming feature of these papers was the large number of subjects—each of the investigators reported on the use of his particular procedure with over 100 children.

Collectively, Levine, Davidson, and Wright have reported treating over 300 encopretic children with similar procedures. They actually treated the encopresis rather than the underlying psychopathology. The next question that might be raised is whether the clinician need be concerned over the possible development of another, equally inappropriate, symptom (i.e., symptom substitution). Levine, Mazonson, and Bakow (1978) directly addressed the problem, using an appropriate comparison group, and demonstrated clearly that symptom substitution was not an issue for concern. The study is described in detail later in this chapter under the separate heading of "Symptom Substitution."

Taken together, these studies demonstrate that even when the physician develops and describes an apparently effective and practical set of procedures for treating a particular clinical problem, the psychologist working in the medical setting (as is the case for both Wright and Christophersen) has expertise in the areas of enhancing patient compliance and developing appropriate reward systems to encourage cooperation with the treatment procedures. The psychologist in this setting can also offer help in research methodology by obtaining reliable recording and devising practical research designs. These contributions are of immense importance in an area of investigation which has been dominated by case studies. Here is yet another example of the physician and psychologist working together to the mutual benefit of the patient.

Anorexia Nervosa

Most of the literature on anorexia nervosa consists of case studies with few subjects (usually only one). This, in itself, is unfortunate, considering that anorexia is a serious illness that occurs with sufficient frequency to demand that pediatricians be trained to diagnose it and, in some locations, to treat it as well. The few collections of case studies (Lucas, Duncan, and Piens, 1976; Bruch, 1974), while presented as "proof" of the correctness of the approaches used, do not really offer the interested clinician sufficient data on the actual effectiveness of the various components.

Case studies with anorectics suggest that operant conditioning (Bachrach, Ervin, and Mohr, 1965), desensitization (Lang, 1965; Schnurer, Rubin, and Ray, 1973), and reinforcement (Bianco, 1972; Neumann and Gaoni, 1975) were each effective in treating a few patients. None of these studies even suggested how the practicing clinician was to decide which treatment approach was likely to be successful for a given patient. Two studies have criticized the use of behavioral treatment alone—that is, behavior modification which does not deal with psychodynamic variables (Lucas et al., 1976; Geller, 1975). A study by Bruch (1974) even questions the use of behavioral management techniques in anything but "mild" cases. Yet, only one of the critics of the behavioral methods reported follow-up data (a 12-month follow-up on one subject by Geller). Bruch, in a scathing attack on the "perils of behavior modification in treatment of anorexia nervosa" (p.1419), criticizes the lack of follow-up data on behavior modification. In the same article, she then proceeds to report the immediate effects of her intervention without giving any follow-up data. In fact, she only presents information on the effects of intervention for two of the three patients discussed in the article. The third patient apparently maintained most of the weight gains from the behavior modification program.

Clearly, the answer to a serious clinical problem like anorexia lies not in vitriolic attacks on opposing methodologies, but in painstaking scientific analysis on the effectiveness of each component of a given intervention technique. This need for scientific analysis, using genuine experimental designs (rather than case studies), is, of course, independent of the treatment method a particular researcher/clinician uses.

Agras, Barlow, Chapin, et al. (1974) reported one of the few controlled investigations of treatment efficacy. Using a within-subject reversal design, the authors demonstrated (rather than speculated) that positive reinforcement in the absence of informational feedback *did not* produce gains in caloric intake or in weight: "The addition of feedback led to gains in caloric intake and weight, and removal of feedback to a drop in both caloric intake and weight" (pp. 284–285).

The authors further demonstrated that the amount of food offered to an anorectic patient affected eating patterns. "The larger the amount of food served, the more is eaten" (p. 285). Based on the data presented, they then suggested a treatment regimen to "encourage weight gain in patients with anorexia nervosa" (p. 286). The fact that Agras et al. did not collect any follow-up data does not detract from their basic single-subject experimental design. The question of the long-term effects of the procedures used by Agras et al., or by anyone else, for management of anorexia is a difficult question that can only be adequately answered with experimental data. Bruch's statement that "it is generally known that true benefit is derived from weight gain *only* if it is part of an integrated treatment program with correction of the underlying individual and family problems" (p. 1421) may well be true. But this has yet to be demonstrated experimentally.

Table 5.2 presents a brief summary of a representative sample of recently published articles on anorexia nervosa (collectively these 10 articles have over 100 different references to earlier papers on anorexia). Several points are obvious from this table:

Table 5.2
Representative Studies: Anorexia Nervosa

Name and Date	N	Mode of Treatment		Research Design	Immediate Effect	Follow-up	Cautions
Bachrach, Erwin, and Mohr, 1965	1	Operant Conditioning	IP*	Case study	Wt gain	18 mo	Yes
Lang, 1965	1	Desensitization	OP*	Case study	?	None	No
Lucas, Duncan, and Piens, 1976	32	Psychotherapy, separation, diet, family therapy	IP	Case study	Wt gain	None	No
Scrignar, 1971	1	Diet, family counseling	OP	Case study	Wt gain	None	No
Bianco, 1972	2	Reinforcement	IP	Case study	Wt gain	None	Yes
Schnurer, Rubin, and Roy, 1973	1	Desensitization	IP	Case study	Wt gain	6 mo	Yes
Neumann and Gaoni, 1975	1	Reinforcement	IP	Case study	Wt gain	30 mo	Yes
Bruch, 1974	3	Psychotherapy	?	Case study	Wt gain	None	No
Agras, Barlow, Chapin, et al., 1974	7	Reinforcement, feedback, meal size	IP IP	Within-subject reversal	Wt gain	None	No
Geller, 1975	1	Reinforcement, feedback, meal size, psychotherapy	IP	Case study	Wt gain	12 mo	No

* IP, inpatient; OP, outpatient.

(1) little experimental work (as opposed to case studies) has been done; (2) most of the studies have few subjects; (3) most of the studies have little or no follow-up data; and (4) a variety of different procedures will lead to immediate benefits, in terms of weight gain. Half of the studies also indicate that their own results should be viewed with caution until more is known about anorexia and more follow-up studies are done.

Future efforts in the area of management of anorexia nervosa need to be directed at the collection of data on treatment effectiveness, both immediate and long-term. Without these data, arguments regarding the superiority of one method over another will remain just that—arguments. Studies patterned after the experimental analysis employed by Agras et al. offer the only hope of solving the perplexing and potentially disastrous problems of anorexia nervosa.

Asthma

Asthma has been defined as "... a diffuse obstructive disease of the airways characterized by a high degree of reversibility with appropriate therapy" (Ellis, 1975, p. 504). The incidence of asthma has been estimated at 5% of the population, and, for those under 17 years of age, asthma is the leading cause of activity limitation (Hindi-Alexander, 1974). There are several etiological factors which vary in their importance across individuals. These include biochemical abnormalities, infections, and immunological and endocrine factors. Although psychological factors are rarely assigned a primary etiological role, they may precipitate asthmatic symptoms (Ellis, 1975; Kagan and Weiss, 1976). Turnbill (1962) has gone as far as to speculate that asthmatic-like behavior may be learned through a combined process of classical and operant conditioning. It is more likely that under certain conditions, with specific individuals, and at specific points in time, asthmatic attacks may be triggered and/or maintained by emotional and behavioral factors. For example, using a structured interview method, White (1975) found that asthmatic children in a high "emotional-precipitant" group received more inappropriate reinforcement for asthmatic symptoms than did children in a low "emotional-precipitant" group. Although the significance of psychological factors is not well understood, there is a developing literature which has examined therapeutic strategies designed to provide symptomatic relief and improve medical treatment of asthmatics. An attempt will be made to review some of this literature.

The role of parental enforcement in maintaining asthmatic symptoms was suggested in a study by Neisworth and Moore (1972). They reported on the treatment of a 7-year-old male asthmatic who exhibited prolonged wheezing and coughing at bedtime. The mother frequently cautioned the child not to overexert himself, to take medications, and to avoid restricted foods. Proceeding from the analysis that the mother was reinforcing "sick" behavior, an extinction procedure was employed which involved having the mother discontinue special attention and medications at bedtime. In addition, if the child coughed less than usual during the night, he was allowed to have lunch money instead of having to take his lunch. Utilizing a reversal design (ABAB), the authors demonstrated a reduction of asthmatic symptoms (duration in minutes of coughing, wheezing, etc.) which was maintained at a follow-up 11 months later. Neisworth and Moore suggested that environmental contingencies may amplify or attenuate symptoms, although they were quick to add that their study "... does not purport to obviate 'organic' factors in the etiology or maintenance of asthmatic responses" (p. 98). It should be noted that the clarity of the treatment effect is lessened somewhat by the absence of reliability assessments on data presented, in this study.

In an uncontrolled case study, Creer, Weinberg, and Molk (1974) reported using "time-out" to modify a behavioral pattern which was labeled "malingering." Malingering was defined as "... the art of attempting to exaggerate symptoms in order to be hospitalized or, if already admitted, to prolong the stay by making complaints that vaguely indicate asthma or other physical ailments" (p. 259). The subject was a 10-year-old asthmatic who, because of difficulties with school and peers, was spending an inordinate amount of time in the hospital.

The setting was a residential treatment facility for asthmatic children. The time-out procedure involved the following requirements: during a hospital stay, the child could not have visitors, could not visit other patients, had only schoolbooks available, could not watch TV, was in a private room, and had to eat meals alone in his room. The procedure was applied for one 2-day stay, and during the 6 months following this single application, the mean days per month spent in the hospital dropped from 11.1 days to 6.8 days, with the duration of each admission dropping from 3.3 days to 2.1 days. A second application produced similar, significant reductions. In addition to the time-out procedure, staff were instructed to reinforce the child for school attendance. The child's parents were given a behavioral management text, were tested on their understanding of the text, and were provided with a written program to help manage the child's behavior at home following discharge. Anecdotal reports from the parents and school indicated gains in school performance, and reductions in "malingering" were maintained. Of course, in the absence of an experimental design, it is difficult to state with certainty that treatment gains were the result of the procedures.

Renne, Nau, Dretiker, et al. (1976) presented details of a "shaping" program designed to teach asthmatic children to monitor their symptoms closely and thus enter treatment in the early stages of an asthma attack. The authors noted that many acute asthmatics unnecessarily delay beginning treatment which is readily available. They reasoned that this may be because asthmatics do not monitor symptoms closely enough to be able to discriminate pulmonary function changes indicative of the need for treatment. The hypothesis was tested with seven children presenting with chronic bronchial asthma in a residential treatment center. The dependent measure was peak expiratory flow rates (PEFR) obtained twice daily using a Wright peak flow meter. The objective of the study was to induce the children to report for treatment before flow rates dropped below PEFR values representing 60% of predicted normal scores. The children were randomly assigned to one of three experimental conditions. In the "script" condition the children could earn 25¢ worth of goods at the Center's co-op store if they met the criterion for reporting for treatment. In the "script plus graphing" condition, the children graphed their PEFR values each time criterion was reached, in addition to receiving 25¢ worth of goods. In the "graphing only" condition, the PEFR values were graphed but no goods were earned. Subjects in all three conditions were exposed to four experimental periods: baseline, treatment, return to baseline, and treatment. The experimenters found that the "script" and "script plus graphing" conditions were equally effective while "graphing only" produced little change. The results of the study are brought into question by the fact that half of the subjects were discharged or dropped from treatment before they completed all experimental periods. In addition, following the reversal period, the performance of several subjects deteriorated during the second treatment phase. The authors indicated that future research would be of interest to determine whether seeking treatment earlier actually reduces the severity and duration of asthma attacks. Such a reduction should result in fewer hospitalizations and less follow-up treatment and medication.

Although effective treatment is available for the symptomatic relief of asthma, the benefits of treatment can be nullified if the child is uncooperative or has difficulty following treatment protocols. Along these lines, Renne and Creer (1976) reported a study designed to teach children proper use of an intermittent positive pressure breathing apparatus (IPPB), a device to deliver bronchodilator medication to the patient's airways. The authors specified three behaviors (eye fixation, facial orientation, and diaphragmatic breathing) judged to be important to the appropriate use of the IPPB. The design was a multiple baseline across behaviors, using four children. "Tickets," which could be traded for gifts, were earned by the children for improved performance on the three target behaviors when the need for treatment arose. The results clearly showed a reduction of inappropriate responding and increased effectiveness of IPPB treatments. The initial results were replicated with two other children using nurses to carry out the treatment program. Renne and Creer recommended that appropriate medical personnel (inhalation therapists, nurses, etc.) be trained in operant technology. Such training would enable them to identify and remediate behaviors which interfere with effective treatment. They suggested that proper use of therapeutic equipment can result in greater benefits from treatment and may contribute to a decreased use of medications which produce undesirable side effects.

A number of studies have examined the impact of "conditioning" procedures (muscle relaxation, biofeedback, reciprocal inhibition) on objective and subjective measures of respiratory function in asthmatics. A frequently cited study by Moore (1965) compared three treatments (muscle relaxation, relaxation with suggestions, and reciprocal inhibition) for their effectiveness in providing subjective and objective improvement in asthmatics. Using a "balanced incomplete-block design," each of the 12 subjects (6 children and 6 adults) were exposed to two of three treatments. Each treatment consisted of 8 weekly sessions with a 1-week "rest" interval between treatments. Subjects in the muscle-relaxation treatment were taught progressive muscle relaxation and were instructed to practice at home twice a day for 5 minutes. In the relaxation-with-suggestion treatment, relaxation was taught, and, at weekly sessions, subjects were given "strong suggestions" that they would improve during the next week. In the reciprocal-inhibition treatment, relaxation was paired with exposure to three separate hierarchies, with each hierarchy graded in 10 steps from least to most disturbing. One hierarchy was based on elements of an asthma attack (e.g., "slight wheeze, a bit more wheezy," etc.). Another hierarchy was based on infectious or allergic factors (e.g., smoke-filled room). The third hierarchy was based on "psychodynamic formulations" (e.g., items related to the death of one child's mother). The hierarchies were individualized for each patient in order to incorporate idiosyncratic sensitivities and conditions relevant to their asthmatic condition. In all three treatments, Moore found significant improvement on the subjective measure (number of days per week that wheezing attacks occurred, as recorded by the patient). However, reciprocal inhibition yielded the only significant improvement on the objective measure (maximum peak flow values via Wright peak flow meter). Moore concluded that this was the case because reciprocal inhibition " . . . tackles the key reflex of conditioned bronchospasm. . . . "

Visser (1976) demonstrated that asthmatics can increase their vital capacity readings through an exhalation-biofeedback program, although medical records did not indicate greater clinical improvement for experimental subjects over control subjects. Feldman (1976) reported that, with asthmatic children, short-term biofeedback training was as effective as isoproterenol treatment in altering lower airway resistance. He suggested that some children may be able to use biofeedback to control airway reactivity completely or, at least, to obtain some symptomatic relief. Khan (1977) attempted to train asthmatic children to respond with bronchodilation when presented with stimuli that typically elicited bronchoconstriction; his procedures involved biofeedback and counterconditioning. The results were equivocal: one control group, in addition to the two experimental groups, improved in terms of the frequency, duration, and severity of asthma attacks. The effectiveness of frontalis muscle relaxation in improving peak expiratory flow rates in asthmatic children was investigated by Kostes, Claus, Crawford, et al. (1976). Subjects were assigned to a contingent feedback, noncontingent feedback, or control group. Children in the contingent feedback group received audio feedback which enabled them to monitor muscle activity and to reduce frontalis electromyographic activity. Children attended the sessions in pairs: one child from the noncontingent feedback group and one from the contingent feedback group. Children in the noncontingent group received feedback that reflected the measured muscle activity of the child with whom they were paired. The contingent feedback group showed significantly greater improvement in PEFR compared with the other groups. The results should be considered tentative, at best, as group assignment was apparently not random; in addition, as the authors indicate, the use of medication was not specifically controlled across groups. Danker, Miklich, and Creer (1975) unsuccessfully attempted to increase PEFR in two groups of asthmatic children by the use of operant conditioning techniques. The study can be criticized from a procedural standpoint, however. Subjects in one group received feedback and "points" for improving PEFR values, but the points did not have any exchange value and may not have functioned as conditioned reinforcers. Had the points had an exchange value, it is possible that operant conditioning would have been more successful in altering PEFR values. In a review of the treatment of asthma by conditioning procedures, Lukeman (1975) noted that there are few studies in the literature, and those that are reported involve a small number of patients and do not provide adequate follow-up measures. However, she did indicate that there has been some success in treating asthma at the "precipitant stage," and in treating disturbances " . . . produced by the presence of the asthma" (p. 167).

Bentley (1974) stressed the need for a "psychotherapeutic" approach to treating asthmatic children in residential settings. Such a procedure would involve tailoring therapeutic approaches to the child's "stage" of emotional maturity and development, with an emphasis on "talking things over" in times of crisis. She stresses the need for communication between staff and suggested that psychotherapy would make some children more amenable to milieu therapy. Similarly, Hindi-Alexander (1974) argues for treatment which deals with all aspects of asthma, including emotional aspects (e.g., excessive dependency on parents, anxieties and fears related to disease symptoms, and loss of valuable school time). Peshkin, a leading proponent of the need for "parentectomies," that is, placing intractable asthmatic children in residential settings, argued that such treatment produces dramatic changes in intractable asthmatics. He believes that residential treatment settings, in addition to providing comprehensive medical treatment, allow the child to escape the smothering efforts of "engulfing" parents and to develop self-reliance (Peshkin, 1968). Mascia (1974) suggested that in some cases it may be necessary to prescribe psychotropic drugs to manage the emotions, anxiety states, and behavior of asthmatic children. He indicated that these drugs should be prescribed only when "absolutely necessary" and in the "smallest effective dosages" (p. 74).

Hypnotic treatment has received some attention in the literature, although the designs are clinical case studies and do not involve experimental validation. Maher-Loughnan, Mason, MacDonald, et al. (1962) reported greater symptomatic improvement for hypnotherapy patients than for control patients. Improvement was measured using a daily diary of wheezing attacks kept by the patients (which the authors acknowledged could be subject to bias). No evidence of physical changes could be demonstrated in the study. Similarly, White (1961) presented 10 case studies in which subjective improvement following hypnosis was reported but in which no objective improvement was found using respiratory function measures (vital capacity, mean expiratory flow rate, and peak expiratory flow rates). White recommended that emotional difficulties should not be ignored, but that psychotherapy, including hypnosis, should proceed concurrently with pharmacological treatment. In a review of hypnotic treatment of asthma, Edwards (1964) noted that there are problems in interpreting results because the type of asthma being treated, the type of hypnotic treatment, and the fact that outcome measures have not been made explicit. He concludes that from the available evidence, the beneficial effects of hypnotherapy for asthmatics has not been demonstrated. He stresses the need for more controlled studies.

Several conclusions can be drawn from this literature. Psychological treatment should be considered adjunctive to the medical management of asthmatics. Biofeedback, reciprocal inhibition, and other conditioning procedures offer some promise in terms of symptom relief but should be carried out in controlled settings by qualified personnel with appropriate medical supervision. Appropriately controlled studies are needed to provide an evaluation of hypnotism as an approach to asthma. It is clear that, with asthma as with other childhood diseases, children can "profit" or derive a special status by using their symptoms to manipulate parents. Within reasonable limits, asthmatics should be treated as other children. Parents of asthmatic children can often benefit from behavioral management training to enhance the social and behavioral development of their children. The most promising of the studies reviewed involve the application of classical and operant conditioning paradigms; research in this area seems sufficiently promising to warrant further investigation with more subjects under more controlled experimental conditions.

Seizure Control

The term "epilepsy," used interchangeably with the term "recurrent convulsive disorder," has been defined as a " . . . variable symptom complex characterized by recurrent, paroxysmal attacks of unconsciousness or impaired consciousness, usually with a succession of tonic or clonic muscular spasms or other abnormal behavior" (Baird, 1975, p. 1380). Convulsive disorders have been estimated to occur in 1 or 2% of the general population (Cautela and Flannery, 1973). Convulsive disorders are considered to have a genetic or hereditary basis; however, it has been suggested that some seizures may be self-induced or maintained in part by the social attention that follows seizure behaviors (Baird, 1975; Robb, 1969). A number of studies have appeared in the literature over the last 10 years which explore the efficacy of operant and classical conditioning procedures in controlling seizures. A representative group of these studies will be reviewed. The reader should note that this literature is at best suggestive and mainly indicates areas for future research.

Forster (1969) proposed procedures to reduce "sensory-evoked" seizures. His procedures involved conditioning techniques specific to the type of sensory stimuli that elicit seizures. In two separate reports, Efron (1957a,b) suggested that conditioned inhibition to uncinate seizures can be developed by properly timed administration of olfactory stimuli. He reported the case of one patient who aborted seizures by smelling jasmine scent and other powerful unpleasant odors when she felt a seizure coming on. The olfactory stimuli were then paired with a visual stimuli (a bracelet) until the visual stimulus alone was effective in aborting seizures. Efron indicated that the presentation of the stimuli before the seizure climax yielded the most effective results. He also indicated that although his patient could abort seizures, the overall frequency of seizures did not decrease. Much of Efron's and Forster's reports involve theoretical discussions attempting to relate conditioning to physiological mechanisms operating in specific types of seizures.

Several studies have investigated the effectiveness of biofeedback and desensitization training in reducing or preventing seizures. Generalizing from animal studies which suggested that sensorimotor-rhythm biofeedback training produced resistance to seizures, Sterman, Macdonald, and Stone (1974) reported on four epileptic and four nonepileptic subjects who were given sensorimotor rhythm training. A biofeedback apparatus provided visual and auditory feedback for appropriate EEG signals, and the subjects were told to relax and think "positive thoughts." They reported significant reductions in electroencephalographic and clinical variables indicative of epileptic manifestations. They indicated that tonic-clonic and myoclonic seizures were effectively reduced. Johnson and Meyer (1974) reported on a 12-month biofeedback training regimen with an adult patient with grand mal seizures. The patient was trained in relaxation and then exposed to a phased electromyographic and electroencephalographic biofeedback training regimen. The patient was told to relax and stay calm during the day by practicing the techniques learned in the training sessions. According to the patient's own records, the frequency of seizures averaged 1.50 per month as compared to 2.79 per month prior to treatment. Three months after the training ended the patient reported not more than one seizure per month. Johnson and Meyer indicated that the patient could not suppress seizures once they occurred, but could effectively abort seizures by practicing relaxation prior to seizure climax. They speculated that the patient developed an "anti-stress response" to counter anxieties associated with preseizure sensations.

Cabral and Scott (1976) studied the effects of relaxation and biofeedback on three patients with resistant seizures. All three patients exhibited anxiety and phobic symptoms associated with their seizures.

Each patient was exposed to biofeedback and relaxation training while presented with anxiety-provoking stimuli or imagery. The total treatment time was 6 months, with an average follow-up period of 15 months. Both treatments produced improvement in EEGs for two patients, while the third patient improved with biofeedback training only. Seizures were reduced during treatment, but during the follow-up all patients showed an increase in seizures. Cabrall and Scott suggested that anxiety or phobias trigger seizures and that desensitization by relaxation had a direct effect on these precipitants. They suggested that the effectiveness of biofeedback training may be due to the patient's ability to control alpha rhythms which act directly on the epileptic process. The authors do acknowledge that, given the lack of experimental control, the effects obtained may be due to the passage of time or other nonspecific factors.

Ince (1976) reported elimination of petit mal seizures by desensitization procedures with a 12-year-old male who experienced numerous daily seizures at school and was quite fearful of attending school. Relaxation was taught to the child and hierarchies were constructed around anxiety-arousing situations (e.g., seizures at school or on the baseball field). The patient was systematically exposed to each hierarchy and was given an audio tape to help him practice relaxation at home. The desensitization procedures were then directly applied to the seizures. At the onset of a seizure, the patient was taught to initiate relaxation by covertly saying the word "relax" 10 times. Reports from the patient, his parents, and school personnel indicated that, 9 months after treatment was terminated, the child was seizure-free. Ince suggested that the cue word "relax" became a conditioned stimulus for relaxation. He indicated that the role played by the parents in maintaining the seizures was difficult to determine.

Reduction of grand mal seizures in an adult male through desensitization has been reported by Parrino (1971). Seizures with this patient were often precipitated by "emotionally laden stimuli;" therefore, hierarchies were developed around anxiety-provoking situations (e.g., socializing with other patients in the hospital unit when he was the focus of attention). In two weekly sessions, the patient was exposed to items from the hierarchy and was taught "self-desensitization," to be employed between sessions. All hierarchies were completed within 3 months. The frequency of seizures was gradually reduced to zero, and at a follow-up 5 months later, the patient was free of seizures and was not using medication. Parrino noted that as the patient improved, the topography of the seizures changed from gross motor movements to "tic-like" mannerisms. In general, the literature on biofeedback and desensitization presents equivocal results. Where positive results were obtained, it is difficult to attribute them to the experimental treatment because adequate controls were absent. There is, however, sufficient indication of potential effectiveness to warrant further investigation.

Several studies have suggested that seizures can be reduced through differential reinforcement, extinction, and aversive conditioning. Wright (1973a) reported on the implementation of shock to reduce self-induced seizures in a 5-year-old male retardate. The child induced seizures by moving his hands back and forth before his eyes and blinking while looking at a light source. The seizures were "trance-like," lasting up to 10 seconds each, with several hundred occurring per day. During five 1-hour daily sessions over a period of 3 days, the child was shocked each time he moved his hand before his eyes. By the 2nd day, the hand movements had been eliminated. Five months later, the child was seen over a 4-day period to reduce eye-blinking responses which induced seizures. These were decreased but not eliminated. At a follow-up interview 7 months later, the patient's mother reported that no seizures had occurred following hand movements, but that seizures did occur following blinking. No specific data were reported on the actual frequency of seizures before and after treatment.

Balaschak (1976) reported on a teacher-administered behavioral program which was effective in reducing seizures in an 11-year-old child. The child received positive attention from the teacher and other rewards for seizure-free time periods during the day. In addition, the teacher was in-structured to pay as little attention as possible to seizures. Teacher reports and records from the school nurse indicated a substantial reduction in seizure frequencies. The teacher discontinued the program following the child's return to school following an illness. A similar study involving teacher-administered contingencies was reported by Cautela and Flannery (1973).

Treatment of "psychogenic" seizures was reported by Gardner (1967) in the case of a 10-year-old female who exhibited seizure-like behaviors consisting of rhythmical head rolling with hair pulling; EEG and other physical tests were either negative or ambiguous. The parents were instructed to ignore seizures, other inappropriate behavior, and somatic complaints. They were instructed to reinforce appropriate behaviors, such as playing nicely with her siblings. Within 2 weeks, the parents reported seizure frequency of zero. The parents, as instructed, then returned to their previous response and within 24 hours a seizure occurred. The treatment plan was reinstated and, at the 1-year follow-up, the child had not exhibited a seizure. An obvious problem with this study is that no formal diagnosis of a convulsive disorder was made by a physician. In addition, as in the case with most of these reports, no experimental control or data collection was evident.

Zlutnick, Mayville, and Moffat (1975) conceptualized seizures as a climax in a chain of preseizure symptoms (such as headaches, tinnitus, and localized spasms). They reasoned that seizures might be prevented by intervening before the seizure climax occurred. They tested this hypothesis with five subjects, all of whom had at least one seizure per day and were formally diagnosed as epileptic by a neurologist. The treatment for four of the five subjects involved the following sequence contingent on preseizure activity (staring, lowered activity level, etc.): the experimenters shouted, "No," loudly and sharply, and the subject was grasped firmly by the shoulders and shaken once, vigorously. This "interruption" procedure yielded variable results across the four subjects, ranging from total elimination to transitory effects. The fifth subject was treated by a differential-reinforcement procedure which involved placing the subject's arms at his side and delivering social and primary reinforcers after 5 seconds of "hands down." A follow-up conducted 9 months later showed that this subject's seizure rate was at a near-zero level. The authors suggested that seizures can be modified by manipulating environmental variables before the seizure climax. They suggested further that close communication needs to be established and maintained between the medical and behavioral sciences. The Zlutnick et al. study is of interest because it is one of the few studies in this literature which employed an experimental design and method of data collection which was adequate. Of course, given the small number of subjects employed and the equivocal results obtained with some subjects, the need for replication is evident.

In summary, as with the asthma literature, the literature on behavioral control of seizures is suggestive and exploratory. Any attempt to employ the strategies described in the literature should occur under controlled medical conditions and only in conjunction with established anticonvulsant medication regimens. The literature in this area would be greatly enhanced if adequate experimental controls and systematic data collection were employed.

Symptom Substitution

Symptom substitution is a term well known to clinicians engaging in behavior therapy. The term itself stems from the position taken by psychodynamic theorists who hypothesize that the mere "symptomatic" treatment of a patient can have undesirable results, since doing so ignores the patient's "real" psychological problem (Bookbinder, 1962). Fortunately for the patient, the majority of practicing clinical psychologists (as opposed to theorists), as well as behavior therapists, are constantly examining their approaches to treatment to determine that they are, in fact, really meeting the needs of their clients. The hypothetical situation in which the behavior therapist blindly and unknowingly treats simple problems while overlooking profound pathology (as opposed to the situation in which the clinical psychologist always identifies *the* correct etiology and summarily treats it) simply does not exist. In actual practice, it is frequently difficult to identify at once whether the clinician is "behavioral" or not. As is pointed out in the two sections of this chapter which deal with enuresis and encopresis (two of the battlegrounds utilized extensively by the theorists), a thorough medical and psychological or social history is a prerequisite to any treatment program. When, in the opinion of the pediatrician, a particular family exhibits even moderate psychopathology, the family is best referred to a psychiatrist or psychologist prior to any attempt at intervention for the enuresis or encopresis. However, when the pediatrician does not detect psychopathology, then efficacious treatment procedures are available for use by the pediatrician or his associate.

There has been one major study which addressed the issue of symptom substitution with enuresis and one with encopresis. (At the option of the authors, the numerous case reports using very few subjects, which purport to support or refute the notion of symptom substitution, will not be discussed.)

ENURESIS

Baker (1969) studied a total of 90 children, 30 enuretics and 60 controls (randomly selected from each enuretic's classroom). The 30 enuretics were randomly assigned to one of three groups: behavior therapy treatment using a bed-wetting alarm; a wake-up treatment group where the parents were told to awaken their child every night at the same time for voiding; and a waiting-list control group.

The measures of adjustment included parent measures (Adjective Checklist, Behavior Problem Record), teacher ratings (adaptations of the Devereaux Elementary School Rating Scale and the Devereaux Child Behavior Rating Scale), and child measures (Draw-A-Person, Draw-Your-Family, Self-image Questionnaire, and the Neurotic Inventory).

Enuretics and controls did not differ significantly on any of the pretests. After treatment the behavior therapy group decreased their wetting from an average of 6 nights per week to 2 nights per week. The wake-up treatment group decreased from 6 nights per week to 3, and the waiting-list group remained unchanged. On each of the measures of adjustment, the treated enuretics were either the same on subsequent testing or showed some improvement over controls. Baker (1969) concluded that "the measures of adjustment did not show a worsening in adjustment subsequent [to treatment]; rather, other improvements were found" (p. 49).

ENCOPRESIS

Levine, Mazonson, and Bakow (1978) conducted a study with 46 patients to determine whether children who were cured of encopresis would substitute new symptoms and/or deteriorate following the "loss" of their incontinence. A 52-item behavioral inventory (School Age Behavior Symptom Inventory) was administered to each of the children. The three groups consisted of: cured encopretics, newly diagnosed encopretics, and a comparison group of age-matched children randomly selected from children without academic problems in a local school system. Statistically significant differences between new cases (uncured) and the comparison group were detected; on every measure (depressive, antisocial-aggressive, social-withdrawal, and somatacization), the cured encopretics were almost identical to the comparison group. The authors concluded that encopresis is a specific disorder that can safely be treated by the pediatrician without fear of or concern for symptom substitution.

SUMMARY AND CONCLUSIONS

Assuming that the pediatric clinician carefully evaluates each patient that he or she sees for clinical entities such as enuresis or encopresis, there is little more than theoretical conjecture to indicate that symptom substitution represents a legitimate concern. Of course, further work with these clinical problems as well as others in the area of behavioral pediatrics needs to be conducted using sound research practices. The large numbers of subjects and comparison groups utilized by Baker (1969) and Levine et al. (1978) represent the state of the art in this field and provide a standard for the clinical researcher interested in further investigation of symptom substitution.

Discussion

The present review of several major areas in the development of behavioral pediatrics suggests the feasibility of behavioral pediatrics in pediatric training programs, consistent with the recommendation of the 1978 Task Force on Pediatric Education. Unlike the situation that existed in 1930, when Anderson suggested that pediatrics increase its attention to growth and development, and unlike the state of the field in 1951, when the American Board of Pediatrics recommended that growth and development be given more emphasis in training programs, the foundation of research and clinical data necessary to support these recommendations now exists. What remains to be seen is whether or not pediatric training programs are able to recruit staff knowledgable enough in behavioral pediatrics to provide a rich and stimulating educational experience.

Although much of the work reviewed is preliminary (e.g., asthma, seizures, and anorexia nervosa), some of it represents a substantial improvement in the management of problems commonly seen in pediatric outpatient clinics (e.g., enuresis, encopresis, and noncompliance). The hallmark of behavioral medicine is its ability to document the efficacy of prevention and treatment programs, a task which *requires* an interdisciplinary alliance between the physician (in the present case, the pediatrician) and the behavioral scientist. The lack of experimental rigor which has so severely hampered the development of mental health services in the past has been remedied in part by investigators in behavioral medicine, for science cannot discover and disseminate research results without a reliable measurement technology. Progress in such areas as enuresis and encopresis, for example, did not really begin until Mowrer and Mowrer (1938) and Davidson (1958) risked taking a radical step by ignoring "underlying" (and thus *unobservable*) psychological processes. Since the initial efforts of the pioneers in the field, considerable advancement has been made in the treatment of these respective conditions. While the present authors would certainly recommend that each researcher and clinician be alert to the appearance of untoward side effects that come as a result of, or in spite of, specific treatment approaches, the problem of symptom substitution has been shown to be greatly exaggerated, freeing the field for further advancement along many new and exciting frontiers.

A lesson can be learned from the critics of behavioral medicine like Bruch (1974) who leveled sharp criticism at Agras et al. (1974) for their failure to look closely at patients years later to determine the durability of treatment effects, but that lesson is *not* that behavioral treatment programs possess unique perils. The lesson is that anytime legitimate scientific inquiry is compromised, regardless of the reasoning behind such compromise, the field of study is also compromised. Longitudinal research is expensive and frequently unrewarding, but contains the answers to many of the questions that researchers and clinicians are faced with almost daily. Anecdotal reports of long-term follow-up will not suffice. What is required in behavioral pediatrics as well as in behavioral medicine in general is a sound data base. The scientific method knows no favorites: raw data cannot tell whether the researcher is behaviorally or psychodynamically oriented.

The present authors are optimistic that there is a sufficient data base in behavioral pediatrics, so that now, almost 50 years after Anderson's call for a marriage between pediatrics and the behavioral sciences, such a marriage is not only possible but is well founded. Over the next decade, we expect a tremendous outpouring of data which will be of great benefit to the parents and children who have come to rely on the pediatric health care delivery system.

Acknowledgment

The authors gratefully acknowledge the editorial contributions of Ms. Suzanne Gleeson.

References

Agras, W. S., Barlow, D. H., Chapin, H. N., Abel, G. G., and Leitenberg, H. Behavior modification of anorexia nervosa. *Arch. Gen. Psychiatry*, 1974, *30*, 279–286.

American Board of Pediatrics. State of training requirements in growth and development. *Pediatrics*, 1951, *7*, 430.

Anderson, J. E. Pediatrics and child psychology. *J.A.M.A.*, 1930, *95*, 1015–1020.

Ayllon, T., Simon, S. J., and Wildman, R. W. Instructions and reinforcement in the elimination of encopresis: A case study. *J. Behav. Ther. Exp. Psychiatry*, 1975, *6*, 235–238.

Azrin, N. H., Sneed, T. J., and Foxx, R. M. Dry-bed training: Rapid elimination of childhood enuresis. *Behav. Res. Ther.*, 1974, *12*, 147–156.

Bachrach, A. J., Erwin, W. J., and Mohr, J. P. The control of eating behavior in an anorexic by operant conditioning techniques. In L. P. Ullman and L. Krasner (Eds.), *Case studies in behavior modification*. New York: Holt, Rinehart and Winston, 1965.

Baird, H. W. Convulsive disorders. In V. C. Vaughn, R. J. McKay, and W. E. Nelson (Eds.), *Nelson textbook of pediatrics*, (10th ed.) Philadelphia: W. B. Saunders, 1975.

Baker, B. L. Symptom treatment and symptom substitution in enuresis. *J. Abnorm. Psychol.*, 1969, *74*, 42–49.

Balaschak, B. A. Teacher-implemented behavior modification in a case of organically based epilepsy. *J. Consult. Clin. Psychol.*, 1976, *44*, 218–228.

Barnard, S. R. An experimental analysis of a parent-mediated behavioral treatment program for encopresis. Unpublished master's thesis, University of Kansas, Lawrence, 1978.

Bentley, J. A psychotherapeutic approach to treating asthmatic children in a residential setting. *J. Asthma Res.*, 1974, *12*, 21–25.

Bernal, M. E. Behavioral feedback in the modification of brat behaviors. *J. Nerv. Ment. Dis.*, 1969, *48*, 375–385.

Bianco, F. J. Rapid treatment of two cases of anorexia nervosa. *J. Behav. Ther. Exp. Psychiatry*, 1972, *3*, 223–224.

Blomfield, J. M. Bedwetting, prevalence among children aged 4–7 years. *Lancet*, 1956, *1*, 850.

Bollard, R. J., and Woodroffe, P. The effect of parent-administered dry-bed training on nocturnal enuresis in children. *Behav. Res. Ther.*, 1977, *15*, 159–165.

Bookbinder, L. J. Simple conditioning vs. the dynamic approach to symptoms and symptoms substitution: A reply to Yates. *Psychol. Rep.*, 1962, *10*, 71–77.

Brazelton, T. B. Anticipatory guidance. In S. B. Friedman (Ed.), *The pediatric clinics of North America*. Philadelphia: W. B. Saunders, 1975.

Bruch, H. Perils of behavior modification in treatment of anorexia nervosa. *J.A.M.A.*, 1974, *230*, 1419–1422.

Budd, K. S., Green, D. R., and Baer, D. M. An analysis of multiple misplaced parental social contingencies. *J. Appl. Behav. Anal.*, 1976, *9*, 459–470.

Cabral, R. J., and Scott, D. F. Effects of two desensitization techniques, biofeedback and relaxation, on intractable epilepsy: A follow-up study. *J. Neurol. Neurosurg. Psychiatry*, 1976, *39*, 504–507.

Cautela, J. R., and Flannery, R. B. Seizures: Controlling the uncontrollable. *J. Rehabil.*, 1973, *39*, 34–35.

Christophersen, E. R. Behavioral pediatrics for the pediatric clinician. In D. P. Hymovich and M. U. Barnard (Eds.), *Family health care*, 2nd ed. New York: McGraw-Hill, in press.

Christophersen, E. R., Barnard, J. D., Ford, D., and Wolf, M. M. The family training program: Improving parent-child interaction patterns. In E. J. Mash, L. C. Handy, and L. A. Hamerlynck (Eds.), *Behavior modification approaches to parenting*. New York: Brunner/Mazel, 1976.

Christophersen, E. R., and Rainey, S. Management of encopresis through a pediatric outpatient clinic. *J. Pediatr. Psychol.*, 1976, *1*, 38–41.

Christophersen, E. R., and Rapoff, M. A. Pediatric applications of behavioral technology in a medical setting. In J. Ferguson and B. Taylor (Eds.), *A comprehensive handbook of behavioral medicine*. New York: Spectrum Publications, in press.

Christophersen, E. R., and Rapoff, M. A. Enuresis treatment. *Issues in Comprehensive Pediatric Nursing*, 1978, *2*, 34–52.

Cohen, M. W. Enuresis. *Pediatr. Clin. North Am.*, 1975, *22*, 545–560.

Creer, T. L., Weinberg, E., and Molk, L. Managing a hospital behavior problem: Malingering. *J. Behav. Ther. Exp. Psychiatry*, 1974, *5*, 259–262.

Danker, P. S., Miklich, D. R., and Creer, T. L. An unsuccessful attempt to instrumentally condition peak expiratory flow rates in asthmatic children. *J. Psychosom. Res.*, 1975, *19*, 209–213.

Davidson, M. Constipation and fecal incontinence. *Pediatr. Clin. North Am.*, 1958, *5*, 749–757.

Davidson, M. D., Kugler, M. M., and Bauer, C. H. Diagnosis and management in children with severe and protracted constipation and obstipation. *J. Pediatr.*, 1963, *62*, 261–275.

Doleys, D. M., and Arnold, S. Treatment of childhood encopresis: Full cleanliness training. *Ment. Retard.*, 1975, *13*, 14–16.

Doleys, D. M., and Ciminero, A. R. Childhood enuresis: Considerations in treatment. *Pediatr. Psychol.*, 1976, *1*, 21–23.

Drabman, R. S., and Jarvie, C. Counseling parents of children with behavior problems: the use of extinction and time-out procedures. *Pediatrics*, 1977, *59*, 78–85.

Edwards, G. The hypnotic treatment of asthma. In H. J. Eysenck (Ed.), *Experiments in behavior therapy*. New York: Macmillan, 1964.

Efron, R. The conditioned inhibition of uncinate fits. *Brain*, 1957a, *80*, 251–262.

Efron, R. The effect of olfactory stimuli in arresting uncinate fits. *Brain*, 1957b, *79*, 267–281.

Ellis, E. F. Asthma. In V. C. Vaugh, R. J. McKay, and W. E. Nelson (Eds.), *Nelson textbook of pediatrics*, 10th ed. Philadelphia: W. B. Saunders, 1975.

Feldman, G. M. The effect of biofeedback training on respiratory resistance of asthmatic children. *Psychosom. Med.*, 1976, *38*, 27–34.

Forehand, R., and King, H. E. Noncompliant children: Effects of parent training on behavior and attitude change. *Behav. Modif.*, 1977, *1*, 93–108.

Forster, F. M. Clinical therapeutic conditioning in epilepsy. *Wis. Med. J.*, 1969, *68*, 289–291.

Friedman, S. B. *The pediatric clinics of North America*. Philadelphia: W. B. Saunders, 1975.

Gardner, J. E. Behavior therapy treatment approach to a psychogenic seizure case. *J. Consult. Psychol.*, 1967, *31*, 209–212.

Gaultieri, C. T. Imipramine and children: A review and some speculations about the mechanism of drug action. *Dis. Nerv. Syst.*, 1977, *38*, 368–375.

Geller, J. L. Treatment of anorexia nervosa by the integration of behavior and psychotherapy. *Psychother. Psychosom.*, 1975, *26*, 167–177.

Harris, L. S., and Purohit, A. P. Bladder training and enuresis: A controlled trial. *Behav. Res. Ther.*, 1977, *15*, 485–490.

Hawkins, R. P., Peterson, R. F., Schweid, E., and Bijou, S. Behavior therapy in the home: Amelioration of problem parent-child relations with the parent in a therapeutic role. *J. Exp. Child Psychol.*, 1966, *4,* 99–107.

Hindi-Alexander, M. The team approach in asthma. *J. Asthma Res.*, 1974, *12,* 79–88.

Ince, L. P. The use of relaxation training and a conditioned stimulus in the elimination of epileptic seizures in a child: A case study. *J. Behav. Ther. Exp. Psychiatry*, 1976, *7,* 39–42.

Johnson, R. K., and Meyer, R. G. Phased biofeedback approach for epileptic seizure control. *J. Behav. Ther. Exp. Psychiatry*, 1974, *5,* 185–187.

Kagan, J. The new marriage: Pediatrics and psychology. *Am. J. Dis. Children*, 1965, *110,* 272–278.

Kagan, S. G., and Weiss, J. H. Allergic potential and emotional precipitants of asthma in children. *J. Psychosom. Res.*, 1976, *20,* 135–139.

Kenny, T. J., and Clemmens, R. L. *Behavioral pediatrics and child development.* Baltimore: Williams & Wilkins, 1975.

Kent, R. A methodological critique of 'interventions for boys with conduct problems.' *J. Consult. Clin. Psychol.*, 1976, *44,* 297–299.

Khan, A. U. Effectiveness of biofeedback and counterconditioning in the treatment of bronchial asthma. *J. Psychosom. Res.*, 1977, *21,* 97–104.

Kostes, H., Claus, K. D., Crawford, P. L., Edwards, J. E., and Scherr, M. S. Operant reduction of frontalis EMG activity in the treatment of asthma in children. *J. Psychosom. Res.*, 1976, *20,* 453–459.

Lang, P. J. Behavior therapy with a case of nervous anorexia. In L. P. Ullmann and L. Krasner (Eds.), *Case studies in behavior modification.* New York: Holt, Rinehart and Winston, 1965.

Levine, M. D. Children with encopresis: A descriptive analysis. *Pediatrics*, 1975, *56,* 412–416.

Levine, M. D., and Barr, R. G. Clinical manual: Encopresis patient care data system. Unpublished manuscript, Children's Hospital Medical Center, Boston, Massachusetts, 1978.

Levine, M. D., Mazonson, P., and Bakow, H. Behavioral symptom substitution in children cured of encopresis. Presented at the annual meeting of the Ambulatory Pediatric Association, New York, April, 1978.

Lucas, A. R., Duncan, J. W., and Piens, V. The treatment of anorexia nervosa. *Am. J. Psychiatry*, 1976, *133,* 1034–1038.

Lukeman, D. Conditioning methods of treating childhood asthma. *J. Child Psychol. Psychiatry*, 1975, *16,* 165–168.

Maher-Loughnan, G. P., Mason, A. A., MacDonald, N., and Fry, L. Controlled trial of hypnosis in the symptomatic treatment of asthma. *Br. Med. J.*, Aug. 11, 1962, 371–376.

Mascia, A. V. Psychotropic agents in the management of chronic asthmatic children. *J. Asthma Res.*, 1974, *12,* 73–76.

McKendry, J. B. J., and Stewart, D. A. Enuresis. *Pediatr. Clin. North Am.*, 1974, *21,* 1019–1028.

McKendry, J. B. J., Stewart, D. A., Khana, F., and Netteg, C. Primary enuresis: Relative success of three methods of treatment. *Can. Med. Assoc. J.*, 1975, *113,* 953–955.

Meunier, P., Mollard, P., and Marechal, J. M. Physiopathology of megarectum: The association of megarectum with encopresis. *Gut*, 1976, *17,* 224–227.

Moore, N. Behavior therapy in bronchial asthma: A controlled study. *J. Psychosom. Res.*, 1965, *9,* 257–276.

Mowrer, O. H., and Mowrer, W. M. Enuresis—A method for its study and treatment. *Am. J. Orthopsychiatry*, 1938, *8,* 436–459.

Neisworth, J. T., and Moore, F. Operant treatment of asthmatic responding with the parent as therapist. *Behav. Ther.*, 1972, *3,* 95–99.

Neumann, M., and Gaoni, B. Preferred food as the reinforcing agent in a case of anorexia nervosa. *J. Behav. Ther. Exp. Psychiatry*, 1975, *6,* 331–333.

O'Dell, S. Training parents in behavior modification: A review. *Psychol. Bull.*, 1974, *81,* 418–433.

O'Leary, K. D., O'Leary, S., and Becker, W. S. Modification of a deviant sibling interaction pattern in the home. *Behav. Res. Ther.*, 1967, *5,* 113–120.

Olness, K. The use of self-hypnosis in the treatment of childhood nocturnal enuresis. *Clin. Pediatr.*, 1975, *14,* 273–279.

Parrino, J. J. Reduction of seizures by desensitization. *J. Behav. Ther. Exp. Psychiatry*, 1971, *2,* 215–218.

Patterson, G. R. Intervention for boys with conduct problems: Multiple settings, treatments, and criteria. *J. Consult. Clin. Psychol.*, 1974, *42,* 471–481.

Patterson, G. R. The aggressive child: Victim and architect of a coercive system. In E. J. Mash, L. A. Hamerlynck, and L. C. Handy (Eds.), *Behavior modification and families.* New York: Brunner/Mazel, 1976.

Patterson, G. R., Cobb, J. A., and Ray, R. S. A social engineering technology for retraining families of aggressive boys. In H. E. Adams and I. P. Unikel (Eds.), *Issues and trends in behavior therapy.* Springfield, Ill.. Charles C Thomas, 1973.

Patterson, G. R., and Gullion, M. E. *Living with children,* rev. ed. Champaign, Ill.: Research Press, 1968.

Patterson, G. R., Ray, R. S., Shaw, D. A., and Cobb, J. A. Manual for coding of family interactions, 1969 revision, Document #01234. New York: ASIS/NAPS, c/o Microfische Publications.

Patterson, G. R., and Reid, J. B. Intervention for families of aggressive boys: A replication study. *Behav. Res. Ther.*, 1973, *11,* 383–394.

Patterson, G. R., Reid, J. B., Jones, R. R., and Conger, R. E. *A social learning approach to family intervention: Families with aggressive children*, Vol. 1, Eugene, Ore.: Castalia Publishing Co., 1975.

Perlmutter, A. D. Enuresis. In T. P. Kelalis and L. R. King (Eds.), *Clinical pediatric urology.* Philadelphia: W. B. Saunders, 1976.

Peshkin, M. M. Analysis of the role of residential asthma centers for children with intractable asthma. *J. Asthma Res.*, 1968, *6,* 63–73.

Plachetta, K. E. Encopresis: A case study utilizing contracting, scheduling and self-charting. *J. Behav. Ther. Exp. Psychiatry*, 1976, *7,* 195–196.

Reid, J. B., and Patterson, G. R. Follow-up analyses of a behavioral treatment program for boys with conduct problems: A reply to Kent. *J. Consult. Clin. Psychol.*, 1976, *44,* 299–302.

Renne, C. M., and Creer, T. L. Training children with asthma to use inhalation therapy equipment. *J. Appl. Behav. Anal.*, 1976. *9,* 1–11.

Renne, C. M. Nau, E., Dretiker, K. E., and Lyon, R. Latency in seeking asthma treatment as a function of achieving successively higher flow rate criteria.

Paper presented at the Tenth Annual Convention of the Association for the Advancement of Behavior Therapy, New York, December 1976.

Robb, J. P. Clinical diagnosis in epilepsy. *Wis. Med. J.*, 1969, *68,* 292–296.

Roberts, M. W., McMahon, R. J., Forehand, R., and Humphreys, L. The effect of parental instruction-giving on child compliance. *Behav. Ther.*, in press.

Schnurer, A. T., Rubin, R. R., and Roy, A. Systematic desensitization of anorexia nervosa seen as a weight phobia. *J. Behav. Ther. Exp. Psychiatry*, 1973, *14,* 149–153.

Scrignar, C. B. Food as the reinforcer in the outpatient treatment of anorexia nervosa. *J. Behav. Ther. Exp. Psychiatry*, 1971, *2,* 31–36.

Starfield, B., and Mellits, E. D. Increase in functional bladder capacity and improvements in enuresis. *J. Pediatr.*, 1968, *72,* 483–487.

Sterman, M. B., Macdonald, L. R., and Stone, R. K. Biofeedback training of the sensorimotor electroencephalogram rhythm in man: Effects on epilepsy. *Epilepsia*, 1974, *15,* 395–416.

Task Force on Pediatric Education. *The future of pediatric education.* Denver, Colo.: Hirschfeld Press, 1978.

Taylor, P. D., and Turner, R. K. A clinical trial of continuous, intermittent and overlearning "bell and pad" treatments for nocturnal enuresis. *Behav. Res. Ther.*, 1975, *3,* 281–293.

Turnbill, J. W. Asthma conceived as a learned response. *J. Psychosom. Res.*, 1962, *6,* 59–70.

Visser, K. A. The effects of a biofeedback technique on asthmatics. *Diss. Abstr. Int.*, 1976, *37,* 994–B.

Wahler, R. G. Deviant child behavior within the family: Developmental speculations and behavior change strategies. In H. Leitenberg (Ed.), *Handbook of behavior modification and behavior therapy.* Englewood Cliffs, N.J.: Prentice-Hall, 1976.

Wahler, R. G. Oppositional children: A quest for parental reinforcement control. *J. Appl. Behav. Anal.*, 1969a, *2,* 159–170.

Wahler, R. G. Setting generality: Some specific and general effects of child behavior therapy. *J. Appl. Behav. Anal.*, 1969b, *2,* 239–246.

Wahler, R. G., Leske, G., and Rogers, E. S. The insular family: A deviance support system for oppositional children (Unpublished manuscript). Presented in part to the Banff International Conference on Behavior Modification, Banff, Alberta, Canada, March, 1977.

Wahler, R. G., Winkel, G. H., Peterson, E. F., and Morrison, D. C. Mothers as behavior therapists of their children. *Behav. Res. Ther.*, 1965, *3,* 113–134.

Werry, J. S., and Cohrssen, J. Enuresis—An etiologic and therapeutic study. *J. Pediatr.*, 1965, *67,* 423–431.

White, H. C. Hypnosis in bronchial asthma. *J. Psychosom. Res.*, 1961, *5,* 272–279.

White, M. L. Children's perceptions of contingency relationships in asthma. *Diss. Abstr. Int.*, 1975, *36,* 1465–B.

Wright, L. The pediatric psychologist: A role model. *Am. Psychol.*, 1967, *22,* 323–325.

Wright, L. Aversive conditioning of self-induced seizures. *Behav. Ther.*, 1973a, *4,* 712–713.

Wright, L. Handling the encopretic child. *Prof. Psychol.*, 1973b, *4,* 137–144.

Wright, L. Outcome of a standardized program for treating psychogenic encopresis. *Prof. Psychol.*, 1975, *6,* 453–456.

Wright, L., and Walker, E. Treatment of the child with psychogenic encopresis. *Clin. Pediatr.*, 1977, *16,* 1042–1045.

Zlutnick, S., Mayville, W. J., and Moffat, S. Modification of seizure disorders: The interruption of behavioral chains. *J. Appl. Behav. Anal.*, 1975, *8,* 1–12.

Chronic Pain*

WILBERT E. FORDYCE, PH.D.
Professor
Department of Rehabilitation Medicine
University of Washington School of Medicine
Seattle, Washington

JEFFREY C. STEGER, PH.D.
Assistant Professor
Department of Rehabilitation Medicine
University of Washington School of Medicine
Seattle, Washington

6

This chapter deals primarily with chronic pain observed in the clinical or medical setting. This type of pain and the experiences associated with it may relate to acute medical situations, psychiatric or emotional problems, and long-standing or chronic disabilities. Here chronic pain will be separated from both acute (recent onset) pain and experimental pain induced in laboratory settings.

The purpose of this chapter is to review behavioral methodology and strategies in the evaluation and treatment of chronic pain. No comprehensive overview of behavioral strategies is intended in this chapter and those interested in extensive descriptions of these classic techniques are referred to other sources (Bandura, 1969; Lazarus, 1972; Wolpe, 1969; Wolpe and Lazarus, 1966; Yates, 1970; Leitenberg, 1976.) Finally, while the focus will be on the learning aspects of an individual's experience of pain, it will not be limited to the individual alone. One must necessarily also be concerned with the impact of pain behavior on the immediate environment, and the extent to which antecedent and consequent events serve to effect each individual's perceptions and responses to pain.

The interest in behavioral management of chronic pain has increased steadily in the past decade. This is partially a result of the frequent ineffectiveness of traditional medical approaches where success rates for certain chronic pain problems (e.g., back pain) rarely exceed 60% and generally result in long-term success rates of less than 30% (Loeser, 1974). Similarily, discussions and descriptions of pain based solely on physiological or neurological factors fall short in their attempts to identify and account for all aspects of pain experienced in the clinical situation. This type of evidence, combined with the observation that placebo treatment alone can yield significant reduction in pain, has led investigators to adopt a more general and descriptive definition of pain which involves not only physiological sensations and mechanisms but behavioral and psychological components as well.

Pain has been referred to as complex and resisting definition. Weisenberg (1977) referred to pain as follows: "In some respects it is a sensation, in other respects it is an emotional-motivational phenomenon that

* Work for this chapter was supported in part by Rehabilitation Services Administration Grant 16-P-56818.

leads to escape and avoidance behavior" (p. 1009). This impression of pain as a primarily psychological experience is to some extent reiterated by Sternbach (1974) who reported that the word pain appears to be "an abstraction we use to refer to different feelings which have little in common except the quality of physical hurt, . . . a class of behaviors which operate to protect the organism from harm or to enlist aid in effecting relief" (p. 12). "Pain" then, appears to be generic in encompassing sensory, physiological, and behavioral components and is at once a sensation in response to a specific peripheral stimulation and the interaction of this response with a complex set of psychological and behavioral variables not easily described.

Further evidence suggesting the complexity of the concept of pain is provided in Beecher's reviews and articles where the psychological status of the patient appears to be the significant determinant of the efficacy of a pharmacological agent for reducing pain. For example, it was demonstrated that certain drugs, such as morphine, tend to work well for pain of a pathological origin (especially when this pain is associated with anxiety, not uncommon in a clinical situation), but these same drugs fail to work as well for experimentally produced pain (Beecher, 1972). Therefore, it has been suggested that one principle governing the action of medication and drugs is that certain pharmacological agents are effective only in the presence of a specific mental state (Beecher, 1972). A specific example of this hypothesis is presented by Sternbach (1968) who observed that pain tends to increase with anxiety. In addition, others have noticed that depression and anxiety are often significantly prevalent in patients reporting chronic pain (Merskey and Spear, 1967).

Further evidence of the significance of both emotional arousal and the secondary characteristics of the environment in which pain is imbedded is provided by Beecher's classic investigation. In this study, a comparison between the requests for narcotics for pain relief made by soldiers following wounds suffered in combat and those requested for narcotics made by hospitalized patients after comparable surgical wounds was made. It was discovered that only 25% of the wounded combat soldiers requested narcotics while greater than 80% of the hospital patients made similar requests for pain medication (Beecher, 1956). These studies indicate that cognitive set or expectancy, and individual's emotional state, and the negatively reinforcing or escape mechanisms (e.g., the secondary relief or gain provided a soldier allowed to leave the combat zone due to a wound) in the "pain environment" can all significantly effect the experience of pain.

Epidemiological factors may also interact with the physiology of the impingement of noxious stimulation upon an organism. For example, Tursky and Sternbach (1967) and Sternbach and Tursky (1965) demonstrated significant differences in reactions to electric shock in Yankees (Protestants of British descent with "phlegmetic, matter-of-fact orientation toward pain"), Irish subjects (described as inhibiting their pain expressions and sufferings), and Italians. A final anecdotal example of the cultural or learning history aspects of the experience of pain is provided by Christopherson (1966, p. 2) in describing a paragraph from a novel by Ruesch. In this description reference is made to the unexpected response of Eskimos in the face of anxiety and pain. Specifically, it has been reported that an Eskimo's response to pain is often to laugh, even when the stimulus involves a painful situation like having his arm ripped off by a polar bear. These studies and illustrations serve primarily to make the point that pain behavior or the response to pain can be influenced by a number of factors including mental set (cognitive expectancy) and the personality or anxiety state of the individual at a given time, and by such epidemiological variables as cultural upbringing (modeling).

Etiology of Pain

PHYSIOLOGY OF PAIN

To the neurophysiologist, pain is often conceptualized as some specific type of activity in the sensory system. Historically, the study of pain evolved from studies of the nature of pain in the human physiology. Von Frey initially proposed the specificity theory of pain in 1894 (Melzack and Wall, 1965). In this theory reference is made to specific receptors which result in the sensation of pain when stimulated. These receptors were believed to be free nerve endings which, upon stimulation, would only result in the sensation of pain. Therefore, pain was believed to have its own central and peripheral mechanisms, similar to those of other specific bodily senses.

Half a century later, scientific evidence surfaced in support of specificity theory. Bonica (1953) observed that there is a specific and unique experience of pain originating in the skin when appropriate stimulation is applied. In addition, this same author identified two sets of fibers which had stimulus-specific, as well as differentiated, conducting properties that clearly are involved in the transmission of pain. This research and the parsimony of this theory led to its popularity for many years.

Despite the productive qualities of the specificity theory, it could not account for certain bits of scientific information which appeared and seemed to contradict its implications. Some of the earlier evidence testing the accuracy of this theory occurred in experiments involving experimentally induced anxiety. In these studies, subjects with induced anxiety reported significantly higher intensities of pain (Hill, Kornetsky, Flanary, et al., 1952). These same experimenters demonstrated that morphine decreased pain much more effectively when the patient's anxiety was high, yet had little or no effect if that person's anxiety level was low. Another break in the connection between a specific pain stimulus-response chain conceptualization occurred in Beecher's observations of combat wounds at Anzio. In this situation, specificity theory would predict that each type of severe wound would automatically generate severe pain response, while this author reported little or no pain experienced by the soldiers who were being removed from this life-threatening situation (Beecher, 1956). Furthermore, Christopherson (1966) demonstrated that there are significant and identifiable differences in the magnitude of pain responses to identical pain stimuli as a function of a person's cultural identity. This evidence in itself is sufficient to seriously question the omniscience of specificity theory in explaining pain. Additionally, further inadequacies in this theory surface, when it is realized that surgical intervention aimed at disengaging the specific connection between the peripheral body damage site and the supposed central pain mechanism (for example, nerve cuts, frontal lobotomies) have not met with widespread positive effects in alleviating chronic pain. Clearly, then, while specificity theory does account adequately for certain aspects of pain perception, it does not entirely describe the complex mechanism of pain perception.

In view of these inconsistent findings, it is not surprising that at approximately the same time as Von Frey was proposing his specificity theory, another author was hypothesizing about pain in a supposedly contrasting and mutually exclusive way. This alternative conceptualization of pain was labeled the pattern theory and was originally proposed in 1894 by Goldschneider (Melzack and Wall, 1965). This formulation contended that the sensations of pain experience by an individual are primarily related to the transmission of nerve impulse patterns originating from and coded at the peripheral stimulation site. Therefore, it was felt that the pattern of stimulation resulting from a noxious event needed to be coded by the central nervous system, and this resulted in the experience of pain rather than a specific connection between pain receptors and the pain sites.

While pattern theory does not account for the physiological evidence of nerve fiber specialization (Bonica, 1953; Melzack and Wall, 1965), there is evidence to support some of its major axioms. For example, Livingston (1943) suggested that peripheral stimulation from body damage may set up a type of reverberating circuit in the spinal internucial pools which summate in their effects and account for the fact that rapid, repeated peripheral stimulation (e.g., pinpricks) leads to intense pain. That is, the stimulus-response relationship is obviously not 1-to-1 (as would be predicted from specificity theory), but a type of overall intense pain is experienced. Further evidence of pattern theory for pain perception was provided by Noordenbos (1959) who suggested that central summation of impulses may be prevented by the action of rapidly conducting fibers inhibiting transmission by the slower conducting fibers. These findings are supported by the studies of Melzack and Wall (1962) where it was demonstrated that skin receptors have specialized physiological properties by which they may transmit particular types and ranges of stimulation in the form of patterns of impulses. In this way, it can be seen that the pattern theory of pain allows for the existence of modulating or coding systems in the central nervous system (such as emotional state, prior experience, and alertness) which interact with the type of external stimulation to generate each person's pain experience.

The culmination of these theoretical trends and current state of the art appear to have occurred in the gate control theory (Melzack and Wall, 1965). This theory is summarized by Melzack (1968) as follows: "The theory proposes that (1) the substantia gelatinosa functions as a gate control system that modulates the amount of input transmitted from the peripheral fibers to the dorsal horn transmission (T) cells; (2) the dorsal column and dorsal lateral systems of the spinal cord act as a central control trigger, which activates selective brain processes that influence the modulating properties of the gate control system; and (3) the T cells activate neuromechanisms that constitute the action system responsible for both response and perception" (p. 362). This theory, then, proposes that pain phenomena are determined by the interaction between the above three systems, where effective closing of the gate results in pain *not* being experienced. In this system, the noxious stimulation of smaller A fibers results in rapidly transmitted and quickly experienced prickling pain where the gate could have little effect due to the short time delay. On the other hand, the slower C fiber impulses, which when stimulated can produce dull, diffuse, burning pain, can be affected by the closing of the gate, resulting in a decrease or elimination of the impact of such fibers on the pain perception. For this to happen, however, it has been hypothesized that activation of a system of nonpainful stimulation receptors (the large A fibers) is necessary. From this formulation it can be seen that both peripheral and central mediating factors can inhibit the transmission of slow pain impulses.

The gate control theory has been extremely useful in that it not only provided room for the evidence suggesting specific types of pain receptors (as well as allowing that pain stimulation and transmission may occur in patterns of sensations), but also allowed for the fact that central nervous system mediation is a significant factor in pain perception. Furthermore, this theory partially accounted for the types of fast-arising pain (e.g., cardiac pain, since the gate theoretically cannot close fast enough to inhibit all pain sensations) as well as the differential effects of time variables upon pain. That is, in addition to the stimulation of fast versus slow fibers, the gating effect is unstable, and the sequence of fiber stimulation can alter pain responses and perceptions. For example, movement can evoke renewed pain stimulation or rubbing adjacent skin areas (which activates large A fibers) can promote gate closure and thereby decrease pain. It is important to note that this last procedure, while consistent with the gate control theory of pain perception, is unlikely to yield a long-term benefit for chronic pain sufferers since continual stimulation of adjacent skin areas (despite its ability to provide competing stimulation for the central nervous system to process in lieu of pain) is unlikely to be maintained over a prolonged period of time.

This theory represented a major advance in the conceptualization of pain. Subsequent work on endorphins (endogenous morphine-like substances emanating from the brain) leads to alternative explanations for downward flowing pain inhibiting mechanisms and, therefore, calls into question some key details in gate control theory (Snyder, 1977). In addition, there are inherent limitations in the extent to which distraction, generation of competing stimuli and timing of sensations can be promoted as a way to decrease chronic pain problems. There are, however, strategies and tactics derived from the gate control theory which have an important role in pain management. These will be considered later. The major point is that this theory further supports the following formulations: (1) Pain is not a specific or discrete entity but rather a complex set of phenomena. (2) There is a loose link between specific noxious stimulation, peripheral to the central nervous system, and the sensation assumed to result from this stimulation, even when viewed physiologically. (3) Central nervous system and cerebral mediation are important ingredients in the perception of and responses to pain, opening the door for systematic perusal of past experience, attentional set, and other cognitive-behavioral variables which might impinge upon the central nervous system and, thereby, interact with one's perceptions and sensations of pain.

It is important to remember that these theories relate primarily to the sensations of pain and how these occur in man. There is no inference about and little reference to what people do in response to their sensations of pain. How one responds to pain sensations is an issue as important as the specific mechanisms transmitting and generating pain experiences.

PAIN AS BEHAVIOR

Sternbach (1968) has observed: "In order to describe pain, it is necessary for the patient to do something . . . in order for us to determine that he is experiencing pain" (p. 13). That is, there must be some form of pain behavior by which diagnostic inferences and treatment judgments can be made. A patient will signal the type of pain he or she is experiencing by describing the intensity, frequency, location, and type of pain experienced. In addition to these verbal cues available to the patient's environment as an indication of his or her pain, there is a myriad of nonverbal signs used to communicate pain experiences. These include grimaces, sighs, moans, limps, awkward or strained body positions, the use of a cane or crutch, and many other symbols associated in our society with discomfort or physical problems.

The susceptibility of verbal report to the many types of response bias has long been accepted and documented (Orne, 1962; Rosenthal, 1966). These findings and the scientific dedication to identifying the specific underlying cause of any reported sensation or experience (e.g., pain) have generally led to a focus upon the physiological mechanism underlying a report of pain, rather than upon the verbalization itself. However, a recent study demonstrated that verbal report measures of pain tend to yield significantly finer stimulus discrimination measures and are more systematically correlated to stimulus variation than are specific physiological measures (Hilgard, 1969). Therefore, it appears that bypassing verbal report measures in favor of purely physiological ones does not necessarily yield a more precise indication or measure of the extent of a person's problems. We have thus come full circle and in a sense are left with the notion that pain as a concept is a complex set of things and not simply a sensory event. Moreover, the behavioral components clearly play a major role.

ACUTE AND CHRONIC PAIN

The previous discussion is not intended to deny the importance of physiological components in the pain experience. One may choose to think of "pain" as a sensory phenomenon, but a pain problem necessarily includes many behavioral components. The significant extent to which pain problems embody behavior (independent of physiological sensation) emphasizes the importance of learning and conditioning principles as they apply to understanding and treating those problems. This behavioral emphasis becomes particularly apparent in chronic pain.

The discrimination between acute and chronic pain is important, since the acute type (e.g., a sprained ankle, a broken leg, a laceration) is often the result of specific and readily identifiable tissue damage. In this situation, a professional is usually consulted about the acute problem and upon following specific advice, the pain is relieved and does not persist beyond the expected period of recuperation (usually a relatively short time). Conversely, while chronic pain typically begins with an acute episode as mentioned above, professional advice and prolonged evaluation and treatment strategies have not resulted in significant reduction of pain. In fact, the pain problem can be exacerbated by multiple surgeries or extended narcotic prescriptions, as in the case of low back pain. In these cases, treatment based on a biomedical model has failed to solve the patient's problem and chronicity has begun.

An additional variable which differentiates acute from chronic pain is related to the type of anxiety experienced by the patients. Acute pain experiences generally are associated with increasing amounts of anxiety as the pain intensity increases, followed by a reduction in this anxiety once proper diagnosis and treatment begin. Reduction in anxiety, as previously discussed, generally results in a decrease in the pain sensation which is further alleviated by proper treatment. A similar cycle of anxiety (where anxiety decreases lead to perception of less pain) is seen in experimental pain situations where the subject knows that he or she need only endure the shock or discomfort for a finite and relatively short period of time, making toleration of this situation much easier.

The cycle is quite different for chronic pain patients in a clinical setting. In this situation, the initial anxiety associated with the pain experience persists and may eventually evolve into a feeling of helplessness and despair as the pain persists in spite of the health system's attempts to alleviate it. Without relief, the patient suffering from chronic pain begins to feel fatigued by constant pain and the relatively small amounts of sleep which result. In addition, he or she feels hopeless and frustrated, and cannot see an end to the suffering. With continuation of this scenario, the patient becomes increasingly frustrated and angry at the health care system or his or her immediate family, since no one has been able to provide a "cure" for the pain. Also by this time, typically it has been suggested that the pain may not be "real" and psychotherapy may be the only answer. To a person perceiving almost constant daily pain these suggestions are not anxiety-reducing.

The importance of the distinction between acute and chronic pain is further indicated by the work of Shealy and Maurer (1974). They analyzed the relative efficacy of transcutaneous nerve stimulation in treating chronic and acute pain. They found this particular treatment was 80% effective for the acute pain patients, but only 25% effective for the chronic pain patients. Given this type of result, it is not difficult to see how frustrated and helpless feelings can be readily generated in chronic pain patients.

Focusing upon tissue damage may be an effective and efficacious orientation in the treatment of acute pain, but this unidimensional approach appears to be much more problematic in dealing with chronic pain and may lead to fallacious conclusions. To further illustrate, causalgia (a burning pain associated with deformation of nerves by bullets or other high-velocity missiles) typically persists for months after the tissue damage has healed. This example may provide a useful model for chronic pain, since it implies that the pain sensations or experiences associated with the initial tissue damage are similar to those which persist and are like the sensations described by the patient in the absence of any prolonged or renewed tissue damage. This is likely a part of the cause behind many chronic pain patients' pleadings that "it really is hurting me, the pain is very real and I'm not making it up."

PSYCHOGENIC PAIN

After repeated treatment failures based solely on a biomedical model, the patient's medical history will have begun to grow. Often he or she will come to be labeled as a "crock," or otherwise rejected by the health care system with the implication that the failure of treatment is somehow the patient's fault. However, it is the system that has failed to provide adequate treatment and simultaneously failed to identify a specific "cause" for the origin of the persisting pain sensations. This generally leads to the patient's experiences of pain being labeled as psychogenic in nature.

The phrase "psychogenic pain" is used in a variety of ways with little concurrence among professionals about the specific intent of this label. In a broad sense, this labeling is an attempt to identify patients whose complaints of pain or whose "pain behavior" (Fordyce, Fowler, Lehmann, et al., 1968; Sternbach and Fordyce, 1975; Fordyce, 1976) are discrepant from the measurements taken concerning the physiological sensations and probable peripheral nociceptive stimuli existent in this patient. For example, if the patient presents him/herself to a physician complaining of severe neck pain and (following a comprehensive series of X-rays and medical procedures) no physiological evidence consistent with this report is found, it is assumed that the patient is "making up" or exaggerating the extent of the neck pain. Hence, the label "psychogenic pain" is applied. In this instance, therefore, strong reliance is placed upon the low stimulus-response correlation and the psychogenic label refers primarily to the large discrepancy between reported pain and the measured physiological causes for such pain (Fordyce, 1976). In this sense, it is a label and not an explanation.

Another use of the term psychogenic is more specific and perhaps more useful. In this formulation, emotional and psychological factors are assumed to be the primary cause of a patient's pain. Merskey (1968) hypothesized that this type of psychogenic pain occurs under three conditions: (1) during hallucinating experiences in schizophrenics; (2) due to muscle tension caused by psychological factors like obsessive fear or worry; and (3) in conversion hysteria. This conceptualization stems primarily from the observations that certain types of psychiatric illness are often associated with complaints of pain (Spear, 1967; Sternbach, 1974). While this useage of the phrase psychogenic pain attempts to explain the discrepancy between observed and measured stimuli for pain and the reported pain experience in some quantifiable terms (for example, levels of depression or certain personality variables), the experience of the patient is unknown. In fact, adding "psychogenic" to a pain diagnosis serves primarily to raise issues of philosophical cause and effect, or mind-body concepts, and does little to establish whether there is a cause-effect relationship between cortical or centrally mediated functions and the sensation of pain. This tautology regarding pain has been analyzed as follows: "the essence of the problem lies in assuming that there are real mental and physical events which can and do interact. In fact, there are simply phenomena which we describe in physical language or mental language; we delude ourselves to believe that because we can impose both mental and physical concepts on such an abstraction as 'pain,' that in fact, such a causative sequence exists" (Sternbach and Fordyce, 1975, p. 122). What does remain, in spite of any arbitrary labeling or complicated diagnostic workup, is the behavior of a patient reporting pain.

THE "DISEASE" MODEL OF PAIN

From the above discussion, it should be evident that a simplistic stimulus-response notion of clinical pain is inadequate. Such a view suggests that pain behavior is highly correlated with the evidence of tissue damage or physiological pain sensation transmission. Furthermore, either elimination of the stimulus or the interruption of the pain pathway should suffice to decrease pain experiences significantly. However, as previously noted, surgical results attempting to effect such a change have been generally disappointing in terms of their efficacy with chronic pain (Weisenberg, 1975, Section 7). Further evidence contraindicating the stimulus-response notion of pain is provided by Loeser (1977), who clinically identified examples of pain for which there was no apparent stimulus (e.g., central pain). Despite such evidence, the predominant treatment for chronic pain has continued to be based upon a pain stimulus-pain response formulation, which can be characterized as a biomedical or disease model approach to clinical pain treatment, as described by Fordyce and his colleagues (Fordyce et al., 1968; Fordyce, Fowler, Lehmann, et al., 1973).

A disease model of pain leads to treatment regimens focusing upon removing the inferred or observed underlying body damage factor with the expectation that the symptoms will then disappear. There is little emphasis placed upon treating symptoms per se, since it is assumed that the underlying pathological condition is the primary, if not sole, source of the symptom pattern. As noted, in the case of acute pain, this approach is relatively effective. Treating the underlying cause usually leads to an efficient and effective amelioration of the patient's pain (e.g., setting a leg in a cast and immobilizing it until the tissue damage is healed). The complications begin when either the diagnostic procedure fails to identify the correct body damage etiologic factors contributing to the symptoms of pain, or when the series of treatments actually decrease the "underlying pathology" but fail to relieve the patient of pain. This is most often the case with chronic pain patients. It implies the pain behaviors were only partially or not at all related to the identified tissue damage.

After several equally ineffective diagnostic and treatment procedures aimed at treating underlying pathological causes for his or her particular pain, the patient is often referred for psychiatric evaluation and perhaps for psychotherapy. A call for psychological intervention is generally based on the same disease model perspective; that there must be some underlying pathology (now assumed to be of a psychological nature) which needs to be treated in order for the pain symptoms to cease. While it is certainly true that some psychiatric and psychological strategies do focus upon emotional "causes" of pain (which can alleviate pain symptoms, especially muscle tension-related pain), there is a growing body of literature suggesting that patients with pain (whether labeled as "organic" or "psychogenic") are more similar in their psychological makeup than different (Woodforde and Merskey, 1972; Fordyce, Brena, DeLateur, et al., 1978; Sternbach, Wolf, Murphy, et al., 1973). These studies suggest that while people with chronic pain do tend to be more depressed and concerned about physiological symptoms than other pain patients; there are few differences between them in psychological measures, regardless of the evidence for underlying organic cause for their pain. It follows that reliance solely upon disease model concepts and attributing the pain behaviors to underlying pathological factors cannot suffice. Nor does it suffice to postulate as the only alternative explanation for the pain the effect of some psychic or emotional problem somehow manifested as "pain."

OPERANT VERSUS RESPONDENT PAIN

A more useful conceptualization of pain can be drawn from the differentiation between operant and respondent types of behavior. In chronic clinical pain, the "pain" must be understood in terms of behavior by which it is manifested. That behavior is subject to all of the laws of learning and conditioning. Respondent behavior occurs in response to a specific stimulus. Respondent behavior fits a stimulus response model because it occurs automatically when an adequate stimulus is presented; i.e., the behavior responds to the stimulus. Examples of respondent behavior include the knee jerk reflex, the eye blink in response to a puff of air, etc. Respondent pain behavior refers to pain behavior controlled by antecedent and specific nociceptive stimuli.

Operant behaviors, like respondent, can be produced by specific stimuli, but are also sensitive to the influence of factors occurring during and after the presentation of the stimulus. When an operant is followed systematically by either a reward or a punishment, the result is an increase or decrease, respectively, in the likelihood the behavior will occur in the future. One distinction, then, between operant and respondent behavior, is that while a respondent behavior's magnitude is dependent primarily upon the specific type and duration of the antecedent stimulus, an operant behavior can be increased in magnitude and frequency by systematic positive consequences following its occurrence. Similarly and in contrast to respondent behaviors, operants which are systematically followed by neutral or negative consequences (i.e., extinguished or punished) occur less frequently or with decreased magnitude of response. A problem of operant pain is one in which the pain behaviors can be said to have come under control of contingent environmental reinforcement. A problem of operant pain may evolve when the original respondent pain situation persists long enough under circumstances favorable to conditioning. The ever changing scientific knowledge surrounding physiological functions and self-control (especially related to biofeedback procedures demonstrating self-control of previously assumed automatic physiological functions) are continually demanding re-clarification of the distinction between operant and respondent types of behavior. More and more, behaviors originally thought to be insensitive to contingent reinforcement and therefore exclusively respondent, now are recognized as potentially operant because they can be conditioned.

Acquisition of Operant Pain

The following illustrations may help to clarify the respondent-operant distinction. A careless person backs suddenly into an open cupboard door and sharply strikes the occipital area. This may be followed immediately by a sharp pain, and gasping, grimacing, or moaning, as well as dizziness or visual blurring. These sensations slowly fade as the time passes. In this case, the pain is respondent; the pain behaviors occur automatically in response to a specific stimulus.

In a similar situation, another person, hurrying around as part of the morning ritual of preparing for work, inadvertently has a similar accident. But suppose this person's spouse has observed the incident and quickly expresses much attention and concern. A series of questions concerning the physiological status and well being follows and the victim receives the luxury of being driven to and from work on this particular day.

In both examples, there presumably will have been some amount of subjective distress or "pain." In both cases there also occurred some visible/audible pain behavior in response to the noxious stimulus of the bump on the head; i.e., there was some respondent pain behavior. In the first illustration, those respondent pain behaviors were not followed by systematic and pain contingent environmental reinforcement. The problem of respondent pain fades. In the second illustration, there were immediate and perhaps intense environmental reaction or consequences to the respondent pain behaviors. Those consequences were pain contingent; i.e., had the pain behaviors not occurred, the particular environmental consequences would not have occurred. The second example illustrates a situation having potential for conditioning a respondent pain problem to become an operant one. The likelihood that such would occur would be some complex function of the extent of the injury and therefore of the initial persistence of the respondent pain behaviors, of the potency or meaningfulness to the victim of the ministrations of the spouse, and of the persistence and militancy with which those spouse-arising consequences continue to occur as pain behaviors occur. Note also in the second illustration that the spouse made two kinds of intervention. One was to attend closely to pain behaviors. The second was to discourage the victim from full continuation of well behavior by insisting on driving the person to and from the job.

Pain behaviors can occur as direct and automatic responses to specific antecedent stimuli, thereby functioning as respondents. They may also occur independently of such antecedent stimuli, their persistence maintained by the positive or negative consequences to which they lead. It is of utmost importance to recognize, when confronted with chronic pain, that the pain behaviors observed can occur independent of physiological stimuli. They may be primarily under the control of a set of environmental contingencies outside the patient experiencing the pain. The implications of this possibility are pervasive. Adequate treatment of chronic pain often necessarily involves evaluation and eventually modification of the relevant environmental contingencies if lasting change is to be achieved.

"WELL" BEHAVIOR

An additional component of operant pain consists of the behaviors related to "well" role activities. Not only are the pain behaviors (e.g., moans, grimaces, limps) subject to operant learning principles, but the complement behaviors (i.e., "healthy" or nonpain behaviors) are equally prone to the effects of learning and conditioning principles. A chronic pain situation may involve not only the reinforcement of pain behaviors, but also nonreinforcement or punishment of well behavior.

The concept of development of alternative responses incompatible with sick behavior (e.g., activity, "well behavior," relaxation) have been demonstrated to be an effective way to combat depression (Lewinsohn, 1974), and anxiety (Wolpe, 1958), as well as pain (Fordyce et al., 1973). In any problem of chronic pain there may be, in addition to or instead of, respondent pain behaviors, either or both of two conditioning effects; (1) reinforced pain behavior; and (2) punished or nonreinforced well behavior.

TIME LIMITATIONS

A basic principle of conditioning is that learning and conditioning effects are time-limited. An operant behavior established or conditioned will be maintained only as long as reinforcing contingencies are applied. The rate and magnitude of reinforcement may diminish, but if the positive consequence is completely halted, the operant behavior will eventually extinguish. In the situation of chronic pain, this is both a blessing and a curse. Specifically, it is reassuring to know that one needs only to remove positively reinforcing consequences for pain behaviors to have them decrease in frequency and possibly disappear altogether. Conversely, this same principle applies for healthy behaviors. The cessation of effective positive consequences leads to a decrease in well behaviors.

This presents a particular dilemma if an individual patient's behavioral repertoire includes few socially reinforceable, health-oriented behaviors. Furthermore, this principle points up the necessity for in-depth analysis of the consequences built into the pain patient's environment. Those which reinforce pain behaviors or punish well behaviors will need to be altered if there is to be any chance for long-term decrease in pain behaviors.

DIRECT REINFORCEMENT

Direct positive reinforcement is one of the ways in which pain behaviors are often encouraged by the environment. Most people have suffered acute pain and noted that positive attention from some aspect of the environment is associated with their pain behavior. Sometimes such special attention occurs virtually only when there is pain or illness; i.e., it is pain-contingent, thereby increasing its reinforcing properties. As the duration of pain increases, there is more opportunity for pain behavior to be systematically followed by reinforcement. That is, the connection between complaints about pain and attentiveness (whether nagging or positive affection) occurs more often and the probability of conditioning pain behavior to produce an operant pain problem increases. For example, a husband may rarely comment about his wife's adequate housekeeping or excellent meal preparation, but display overt positive affection in the form of solicitude, rubbing her neck, or taking over arduous chores whenever she comments about discomfort. In this example, the woman's pain behaviors are receiving reinforcement and her well behaviors discouragement, within the same situation.

An additional source of direct reinforcement for operant pain behavior is the health care system. Genuine professional concern and attention can inadvertently encourage the continuance of pain complaints. This is particularly true when the patient does not have adequate social outlets and may be gaining much of his or her social contact through association with a health care facility. The attention or concern of a doctor, a consequence viewed by some as negative and indicative of ill health, may be positive and encouraging for other people. Contingent consequences may, in fact, be reinforcing for a given individual, even if they may seem onerous or aversive to others.

An even more potent pain contingent direct reinforcement of pain behaviors by physicians occurs when narcotics or potent analgesics are prescribed for long intervals on a *prn* or take-only-as-needed basis. That arrangement makes the consequences of medications, with whatever chemotherapeutic effects they have, pain contingent. The person must engage in some form of pain behavior in order to receive the medications. Clinical experience indicates a startling number of chronic pain patients who virtually cease to give evidence of any pain problems when they are helped to detoxify and to get rid of their medication habits.

Monetary compensation is another example of how pain behavior can be positively and directly reinforced. The patient on disability compensation is required to demonstrate disability to continue receiving monthly checks. Regardless of the initial cause for pain or disability, this situation has considerable potential for increasing the frequency and intensity with which a person expresses pain behaviors. It both directly reinforces pain behavior and diminishes the monetary aversiveness of being unable to work.

Another consequence for pain behavior which proves often to be an effective reinforcer is rest. A person experiencing pain in its respondent or acute stage, may find that increases in physical activity generate discomfort, while decreases in activity lead to lower pain levels. Lying down or resting is then a positively reinforcing event. The increased comfort positively reinforces the resting behavior, increasing the chances that it will occur in the future. This method of conditioning of pain behaviors seems particularly important and prevalent. In the initial stages of acute pain, rest is often an effective and appropriate treatment strategy because it reduces discomfort and minimizes movement and getting into exacerbating situations likely to increase the tissue damage. However, when pain persists and becomes chronic in nature, the therapeutic properties of rest, in terms of minimizing body damage, almost always diminish. Concomitantly, reduced physiological tonus and diminished effectiveness of well behavior are increased.

INDIRECT REINFORCEMENT (TIME-OUT)

Rest from noxious physical activity is related also to indirect reinforcement of pain behavior. In indirect reinforcement, pain behavior is frequently reinforced by allowing the patient to remove him/herself from a difficult or stressful situation. The situation may be physically tiring, for example, or it may consist of stressful interpersonal conditions such as a bad work situation which the patient finds aversive and would rather avoid. A complaint about pain may lead to staying home from a difficult job, time-out from engaging in sexual intercourse (which to some is aversive), avoiding arguments with a supervisor, or avoiding burdensome chores by remaining in bed.

Learning by indirect reinforcement is *avoidance conditioning*. This type of learning can be very resistant to change. For example, consider a male patient who has had a serious back injury for several years but who has adjusted to the discomfort and mild physical limitations imposed by this condition. Suppose he now changes jobs and encounters a new stressful job situation. Subsequently, a back strain may occur as happens to most of us in the course of normal living. The relief of prescribed rest experienced following a stay at home for the first day or two may have far reaching effects. That is, the following morning, independent of the actual discomfort experienced from the back strain, anticipating the work stress, this person may readily accept suggestions from his environment (e.g., a spouse) to take an extra day to recuperate and then another, and so on. The successful avoidance of an anxiety-producing or stressful situation at work will reinforce *any* behavior which facilitated the avoidance, in this case: the pain behavior.

Another common avoidance behavior relates to compensatory body positions adopted by people initially suffering from acute pain. For example, the person with a broken leg and resultant long casting interval, may initially have tenderness in the leg during ambulation. The pain encourages the patient to favor the leg during the healing process by generating a slight limp to avoid or minimize pain. In some individuals, the immediate reduction or avoidance of sharp pain from this new behavior is reinforcing enough that the limp becomes a habit not easily discarded. In addition, the patient's anticipation of pain discourages trying to walk without the limp. Finally, display of the limp may continue to elicit special attention and support from others. This example illustrates how pain behaviors serving as avoidance or escape mechanisms can generate longstanding habits which are highly perseverative.

MODELING

In addition to direct and indirect reinforcement, imitation or modeling effects can have a significant impact on chronic pain behavior. It has been shown that humans see or hear another's behavior and often will imitate some or all of that particular behavior (Bandura, 1965; Bandura and Walters, 1963).

Imitative behavior may occur with or without our awareness, as evidenced by language acquisition in infants. The importance of modeling effects in the acquisition of chronic pain is suggested by research demonstrating a tendency for individuals to imitate behavior which is reinforced and avoid behavior which is punished. Craig (1975), for example, has shown that modeling can influence "pain tolerance"; i.e., readiness to express distress. Parental or sibling responses to pain are potential learning situations for any child. Parents who readily and dramatically express pain behaviors in response to noxious stimuli and who respond to such behavior in others are likely to find that the child will imitate or model this response to noxious stimuli. The evidence suggesting significant cultural differences in the responses to pain almost certainly illustrates the effects of modeling.

OTHER FACTORS

It should be apparent from the preceding formulation of the acquisition and etiology of operant chronic pain, that the consequences of a long-standing and difficult pain problem are likely to be decreased activity, decreased social effectiveness, and decreased vocational effectiveness. The existence of clinical levels of depression is also observed in many chronic pain patients (Merskey and Spear, 1967; Sternbach, 1974). Behavioral conceptualizations of the etiology and treatment for depression have particular relevance to chronic pain, since they share the learning and conditioning framework as a basis for their treatment (Ferster, 1966; Lewinsohn and Atwood, 1968). These issues and others as they relate specifically to the treatment for chronic pain will be reviewed in the treatment section.

Review of Treatment Strategies for Chronic Pain

METHODOLOGICAL ISSUES

One of the most difficult issues in evaluating the effectiveness of any treatment strategy for chronic pain is selection of outcome criteria. The problem is essentially definitional. Among various approaches in the treatment of chronic pain, there appears still to be considerable confusion as to the nature of the problem being treated. The confusion seems to arise primarily through a blurring of the distinction between "pain" as a form of sensation, "suffering" as a negatively toned affective or feeling state, and "pain behavior"—the visible or audible manifestations of the patient's problem.† Clinicians typically use the term "pain" when in fact the phenomena they are observing and are using to arrive at judgements is mainly pain behavior. They are also making a three-stage inference when they do this, often without being aware of it. They are assuming first that the pain behaviors are direct reflections of underlying suffering which, in turn, is elicited by the sensation of "pain," which, finally, is elicited by nociception. Without doubt, there is a sensory system which, when stimulated, is capable of leading to the sensation of pain. But that sensation is not the clinical problem. "Pain," as a sensation, activates higher nervous centers which generate "suffering." But that, like "pain," remains a private experience not yet in the observable, confirmable, treatable domain of the clinician. "Suffering" leads to pain behaviors, previously defined.

The complicating element to the matter is that both "suffering" and "pain behavior," mediated by higher nervous centers, are subject to influence by a variety of factors, some quite foreign and unrelated to nociception and "pain." Prior experience, current affective states, and prevailing environmental contingencies all can and do influence both suffering and pain behavior. Moreover, pain behavior is quite capable of occurring in the absence of suffering.

As clinicians in the context of treating chronic pain, we deal with two sets of information. Foremost, we are confronted with and may observe and measure pain behavior. We may, as circumstances dictate, *infer* that those pain behaviors are an extension or reflection of underlying suffering, although there are alternative possibilities of which we must be mindful. We may also infer that the suffering has been elicited by the sensation of pain which, in turn, occurs because of nociception. Again, however, there are alternative possibilities. Aside from the direct observations of pain behavior, these conclusions are all inferential. The second set of information at hand for the clinician to consider is the medical history. The residual effects of previous trauma, effectiveness of prior treatment interventions for the reported pain problem, and "physical findings" derived from the current medical workup may be considered. That second set of information bears directly on the question of nociception. The information does not describe current nociception. The information may, with varying degrees of precision and reliability, provide a basis for *inferring* that there is currently nociceptive input. In essence, those kinds of data provide a basis for speculation as to the presence of nociception. They do not demonstrate or confirm either the presence of nociception or, if present, that no-

† This conceptualization is the work of John D. Loeser, M.D., Department of Neurological Surgery, University of Washington, Seattle, to whom a special note of gratitude is expressed. It represents, in the view of the authors, the clearest organization and conceptualization of the major dimensions of chronic pain yet formulated.

ception accounts for the observed pain behaviors. This is not to suggest that this speculation or inference is always highly questionable. Indeed, the evidence may be most compelling. However, it is still an inference or a speculation.

In problems of acute or recent pain onset, the linkage between the "physical findings" data and the pain behaviors is generally rather direct. The major exceptions are likely to relate to people with an extensive prior history of extended bouts of pain behavior.

In problems of chronic pain, the opportunity for other factors (e.g., prior experience, emotional or affective problems, and contingent environmental reinforcement) to have begun to exert influence on the pain behaviors is assured. How much that influence has distorted the linkage between speculated nociception and observed pain behavior remains to be clarified, principally by the kinds of behavioral analysis described in this chapter.

In acute pain, treatment aimed at removing or reducing nociception is often the desired point of attack. However, even then, the criterion of success ought to be pain behavior, or lack of it. Patient reports of alterations in amount of suffering are subject to many distortions and should be given limited credibility. In evaluating treatment of chronic pain, clearly the criterion should be changes in pain behavior.

The question often arises as to whether changes in pain behavior correlate with changes in nociception and (presumably) associated "pain" as a sensation. That is, if a treatment program has focused on changing pain behavior, will the "pain" remain, although now unexpressed behaviorally? The answer to the question can be neither confirmed nor disconfirmed, so this is a specious consideration. One can only describe and measure what patients do, while recognizing that what they say about suffering is a complex social communication linked to many parameters both within and without the organism.

It has been argued that ignoring the pain patient's feelings is an arbitrary approach derived from social learning theory but not necessarily essential to treatment. However, Hilgard and Hilgard (1975) found that immediately following the successful treatment of chronic pain, many patients reported hurting as much as they had before treatment started, yet these same patients were reportedly pain free 6 to 12 months later. Similarly, Fordyce et al. (1973) have shown that reports of hourly discomfort and ratings of interference with daily activities due to pain tend to remain the same or increase slightly over the course of treatment for many chronic pain patients. However, the outcome of treatment for this group of patients was positive for all other criteria (e.g., activity tolerance, uptime, medication use). It is difficult to assess whether these findings suggest that chronic pain patients' reports about continuing pain during successful treatment are simply an attempt to validate a continuing claim to pain, or whether this is one more example of attitude change occurring after behavior change. In either case, it appears that subjective reports of pain in chronic pain patients are not consistent with other measures of treatment outcome and progress.

If not verbal reports of pain, then what criteria can be used to evaluate the outcome in chronic pain treatment? As might be expected, criteria vary from treatment center to treatment center and from researcher to researcher. Nevertheless, there appear to be some generally accepted and useful guidelines. Observable and measurable criteria appear to have the most utility both in terms of evaluating the treatment's efficacy and in terms of providing the patient evidence of his or her improvement (despite "feeling" just as much pain). Such variables as uptime, number of miles walked in an hour, pounds lifted in a given body position, levels of muscle tension (measured by surface electromyography), amount of analgesic medication used per day, or hours of sitting tolerance can provide objective measures upon which to base outcome assessment decisions. Such measures avoid the complications of variable memory, response bias, positive and negative social desirability effects, and attempts to manipulate pain medication levels and provide the patient and therapist with a reliable determination of treatment progress. Perhaps, more importantly, these types of outcome criteria are more likely to generalize to actual life situations outside the treatment setting (e.g., work and avocational pursuits).

Most of the studies for the treatment of chronic pain have employed clinical case study designs, with no control groups and no placebo-control methodology. In addition, these studies have rarely separated different treatment elements, often combining several techniques in one package (e.g., physical therapy, occupational therapy, chemical management, psychotherapy, and physician reassurance and workup). Because of this, it is impossible to separate the essential ingredients or tease out the more important aspects of a given treatment program. To overcome these limitations, many of the clinical or research-oriented programs (e.g., at Minnesota and Washington) implement extended baseline periods in which patients keep records at home about their daily activities. In this way, an attempt is made to assess the effects of positive anticipation resulting from having been accepted into a reputedly effective program. In addition, long follow-up periods (2–5 years) are employed to minimize reporting bias and to measure the long-term effects of treatment more effectively. Since most chronic pain patients have had their problems for years, and since most placebo effects are short-lived, incorrect evaluation of outcome under these conditions becomes less likely. *Nevertheless, it is important to note that a systematic, controlled study of alternative approaches to similar pain problems has yet to be attempted.*

INPATIENT STRATEGIES

There are over 100 pain clinics in the United States, yet only a handful have published results concerning their efficacy. The inpatient strategies can be divided into two types: (1) "pure" behavioral or operant and (2) "mixed" behavioral and other. All of the inpatient treatment programs involve several aspects, including medication management, physical and occupational therapy, and supportive therapy. The difference between behavioral and mixed approaches is the extent to which the treatment involves strategies other than reinforcement for "well behavior" (e.g., group discussion with other patients, biofeedback for relaxation and placebo, family therapy not related to pain behavior management).

The prototype "pure" operant pain treatment program originated at the University of Washington Department of Rehabilitation Medicine. The program involves a 4- to 8-week inpatient period designed to increase gradually general activity level and socialization and to decrease medication usage and, ultimately, pain-related utilization of health services. This is accomplished through the use of quota systems of physical, occupational, and vocational activities which are part of a contingency plan. (A more detailed description of this treatment will be presented later in this chapter.) Using the approach, Fordyce et al. (1973) were able to obtain significant increases in uptime and activity level (exercises, walking, non-reclining time), and significant decreases in medication (narcotic and non-narcotic analgesics) usage. On the average, the changes were maintained at follow-up 22 months later.

In a similar treatment program in the Pain Clinic at the University of Minnesota Department of Rehabilitation Medicine, significant treatment gains were also observed following treatment in 75 to 80% of the patients (Roberts, in press). These gains were reported to have maintained in "most" of the patients for from 1 to 8 years (Anderson, Cole, Gullickson, et al., in press). One problem with the latter study, however, is the use of subjective outcome criteria (e.g., significant gains were viewed in terms of the patient leading a "normal life without pain medication"). Another inpatient operant-pain treatment center, Rancho Los Amigos Hospital in Downey, California, noted in a report on their program for treating chronic low back pain, that 70% of the patients indicated either some reduction in pain *or* an increase in activity level, with analgesic medication reduced to zero by the end of treatment for all patients. The decrease in medication was maintained in 58% of the patients at follow-up (10 months), with 74% not seeking further health care and 75% working or in a vocational training program (Cairns, Thomas, Mooney, et al., 1976). Although in most cases the post-treatment levels of functioning were significantly improved over the pretreatment levels, the above studies are limited by reliance upon subjective questionnaire data as the basis for follow-up evaluation.

An extension of these programs and a good example of the "mixed" approach exists at the Mayo Clinic. In this system, the average length of inpatient stay is about 3 weeks and treatment involves those aspects described in the "pure" programs as well as group exercises, organized group discussion among patients, and biofeedback and relaxation techniques to augment physical and occupational therapy. The results of this treatment approach were that 27 out of the 50 (54%) patients accepted into the program showed a moderate to marked improvement at post-treatment. These results may be a spuriously low estimate of the program's potential effectiveness, since 16 of the original patients dropped out of the program and of the 34 who completed treatment, 79% (27) showed improvement. Unfortunately, at 6 months follow-up only 50% of those who completed treatment had maintained their gains (Swanson, Floreen, and Swenson, 1976). Again, the criteria for outcome assessment are vague and are related to such subjective variables as attitude modification (remaining in the program and "generally accepting" the need to live with pain), changes in physical function (performing work-equivalent activities), and medication reduction; points were assigned to yield outcome "scores." While these measures are, at least, an attempt to specify outcome criteria, they leave far too much discretion to the raters.

A similar multidisciplinary approach lasting about 3 weeks has been evaluated by Newman, Seres, Yospe, et al. (1978). In this report, it was demonstrated that significant gains were maintained for chronic low-back patients in the reduction of analgesics and on four measures of physical functioning. An important aspect of the study is that follow-up occurred at 80 weeks and was done in the hospital by direct evaluation, thus minimizing the effects of biased verbal reports. As has been reported previously, these researchers also found that patients' verbalizations of pain did not change over the course of treatment, despite alterations in other behaviors.

Another mixed inpatient approach to the treatment of chronic pain, lasting 4 weeks, is situated on a neurological service and employs operant approaches, physical rehabilitation, and work-related procedures as well as group transactional and gestalt techniques (Greenhoot and Sternbach, 1974). Evaluation of treatment outcome for the 62 chronic-pain patients indicated that significant improvements in pain reports, medication use, and activity levels resulted. As has often been the case, however, at the 6-month follow-up, only medication use remained at the post-treatment level, with subjective pain reports and activity levels regressing toward pretreatment levels, although still significantly improved (Sternbach, 1974). Again, questionnaire data provided the data base for this analysis and no account was given for the one-third of follow-up patients who did not respond to the questionnaire.

A final example of the "mixed" inpatient approach to chronic pain treatment is evidenced by the Chronic Back Pain Management Program, Casa Colina Hospital for Rehabilitation in Pomona, California. In this setting, low-back pain patients are treated for an average of 6½ weeks with a variety of treatment modalities, designed around the theme of self-regulation. The treatment approach is similar to the one used at the Mayo Clinic in that it uses biofeedback for muscle tension reduction, group discussion among patients, and occupational and physical therapy. In addition, self-regulation techniques are taught using psychological counseling for stress management and assertion training, patient-regulated medication programs, and didactic presentations. A vocational planning service as well as individual and marital counseling are also provided. At the end of treatment, 57 of the initial 72 low-back pain patients demonstrated unimpaired physical movement and 59 of 72 were functioning successfully in vocational activities (Gottlieb, Strite, Koller, et al., 1977). Furthermore, using a clinical rating system based on physical functioning, clinical judgment, and vocational restoration, about 66% of the patients showed significant improvement, maintained at a 1-month follow-up. Given that 33% of the initially referred patients either dropped out of the program or were rejected by the staff on the basis of low level of involvement and that treatment involved many modalities in addition to self-control, it is difficult to evaluate the authors' claims that self-regulation plays a critical role in the treatment of chronic low-back pain. However, the use of operationalized outcome criteria (e.g., 1 point for walking less than 400 m, 4 points for walking over 1600 m, 3 points for 45 minutes sitting tolerance, 4 points for no pain-related medication intake other than aspirin) is a significant step in the direction of clarity and allows comparison with other programs with respect to the same variables. It is unfortunate that this approach was not uniformly applied across all outcome variables. Further operationalization of different outcome variables will be necessary if important psychological indicators are to be compared across treatment modalities and settings.

OUTPATIENT STRATEGIES

There are few critically evaluated studies on the effectiveness of outpatient treatment of chronic pain. Generally, the outpatient approaches consist of the same procedures as the inpatient, but implementation is in vivo using an intermediate such as the spouse. The difficulty of obtaining accurate and incorruptible observations of activity and medication on an outpatient basis puts this strategy at a greater risk of failure and may account for the paucity of studies in the area.

A recent and promising outpatient treatment strategy for chronic pain is labeled "cognitive-behavioral" (Turk, 1978). Typically, this approach is designed to reduce anxiety and covert self-statements concerning pain. In this way, it is hoped that indirect modification of pain perception and tolerance will occur and allow the patient to increase his or her activity levels and decrease medication use. Some outpatient treatment approaches for chronic pain have not been employed extensively enough to warrant discussion of efficacy. As can be gleaned from other chapters in this volume, however, chronic muscle tension pain (e.g., tension headaches, spasms) and vascular pain (e.g., migraine headaches) seem to respond well to outpatient biofeedback treatment and may not require the more intensive inpatient programs.

One of the most recent cognitive-behavioral techniques is "stress inoculation" (Meichenbaum and Turk, 1976). This outpatient technique combines didactic discussion about stress reactions, generation of alternative self-statements about one's ability to cope with stress, specific relaxation training, and in vivo application of newly learned stress coping mechanisms. While this approach has not been used with chronic pain patients to a large extent, stress inoculation incorporates many of the essential aspects of the effective inpatient chronic pain treatments (e.g., identifying antecedents of stress and pain, generating different self-statements or ways to cope with stress and pain, and practicing these coping skills in actual situations.

The use of stress inoculations appears particularly important on an outpatient basis, since less external structure and encouragement is available, and the patient is required to rely more on his or her own conceptualization of the treatment process. In one study of chronic tension headache pain, it was demonstrated that outpatient biofeedback treatment using stress inoculation was significantly more effective in reducing pain ratings and general feelings of anxiety and distress than self-monitored relaxation. An interesting aspect of this finding was that both treatments were equally effective in lowering muscle tension in these patients, but the cognitive orientation of the biofeedback treatment appeared to generate greater alleviation of symptoms (Steger and Harper, 1977). The above suggests that the reason inpatient programs have not consistently provided improvement in subjective pain ratings may be a failure to address the cognitive issues directly. Further research is needed before this issue can be resolved.

Based on this brief review, it can be seen that the theoretical and practical strategies in inpatient programs provide the common base for most approaches in the treatment of chronic pain. Graduated increments in activity, systematic fading of medications, in vivo practice in pain tolerance, and anxiety or muscle tension reduction are essential even in the outpatient setting. Since much of the outcome research has been carried out in the context of inpatient operant therapy, the treatment specifics of such a program will be presented in some detail. The following description does not purport to portray the ideal treatment approach, but merely indicates techniques which seem to have been effective.

Evaluation Phase

Chronic pain needs to be evaluated first within the framework of a disease model to check for respondent pain. If clearly identified, respondent pain should be treated within a medical context. A behavioral analysis should be undertaken if any of the following conditions exist: (1) medical assessment fails to reveal physical findings to account for the pain behavior displayed; (2) there are physical findings, but they are disproportionately small in comparison to the severity of the pain behaviors reported or observed; or (3) physical findings are only speculative or inferred.

It is important to note that a behavioral analysis of pain has nothing whatever to say about the extent to which the pain problem is respondent in nature. A behavioral analysis considers the viability of alternative explanations to a disease-model analysis. The primary purpose of such an assessment is to examine the extent to which the patient's pain behavior is controlled by environmental contingencies. Effective behavioral treatment strategies may also be identified by such a conceptualization. Even in a situation where the relationship between pain behavior and reinforcing consequences appears to be strong and pervasive, much or all of the pain behavior may, in fact, still be controlled to a significant degree by physiologically based variables.

The professional who is doing the initial evaluation should remember that, with few exceptions, the patient suffering from chronic pain has been a long-time "loser" in his or her dealings with the health care system. The fact of chronicity means that the health-care system has failed to solve the problem. In addition, as noted by Sternbach, Murphy, Akeson, et al. (1973) many chronic pain patients have such a small likelihood of future gainful employment and successful social adjustment that they are "chronic losers in life" (p. 136): i.e., they are only marginally capable of coping with life's demands except in the protected (although compromised) state of chronic illness. Moreover, many pain patients will have been told, directly or indirectly, that their pain is "in their head" or psychogenic. Such suggestions lead the chronic pain patient to adopt a distrustful attitude toward professionals in general. It is imperative that the interviewer be skillful in establishing an atmosphere of trust and candor, and not make the patient feel that he or she must prove that the pain is "real."

Since so many chronic pain patients view a behavioral assessment as a challenge to the authenticity of their pain, one must deal directly with this issue if accurate information is to be obtained. Clarifying the following points with the patient often helps: 1) Pain should not be considered as real or unreal, but as the experience one feels when one hurts. The assessment assumes that the pain is real and seeks to identify the factors which influence it. 2) Pain, like most other bodily functions and processes, is subject to the influence of learning and conditioning. Pain problems originate as a result of tissue damage, but can be maintained through conditioning (use of a Pavlovian conditioning example is often helpful). 3) Learning and conditioning effects are automatic and are not dependent upon emotional or personality factors. 4) If there is a significant amount of learned or conditioned pain, the patient may be suffering more than necessary and something usually can be done about that. Patients using many analgesics should be helped to understand that chronic and high levels of drug usage often interfere with normal activity and the physiological relearning processes needed to alter chronic pain patterns significantly.

Evaluation needs to identify the relationships between patient behavior (e.g., pain expressions and pain-related behavioral limitations) and environmental events or consequences resulting from this activity or inactivity. In addition to data obtained directly from the patient, highly useful information can be provided by the spouse, whose participation in evaluation should, with rare exceptions, be required. Patient and spouse are interviewed separately as well as conjointly. Data from the spouse provide additional perspective and information regarding the reliability of the correlation between patient behavior and environmental contingencies. With these general strategies and suggestions in mind, the following represent the major issues to be explored in the behavioral analysis of a chronic pain problem. A more detailed and extensive description is available from another source (Fordyce, 1976, Chapter 6).

TIME PATTERN

The core issue in analyzing a pain pattern involves the activities surrounding the patient and the sequence of these activities in relation to pain behavior. One must discriminate pain which occurs sporadically for varying intervals without relief and is followed by extended intervals of minimal pain from a pain pattern which is relatively steady. The former hardly could be under control of environmental contingencies unless it could be shown that environmental consequences change in correlated fashion with the onset and termination of pain episodes. A simple-minded illustration is a worker who hurts only on weekdays and is pain-free on weekends. In similar fashion, nocturnal patterns are important. Usually the environment "shuts down" at night—this includes the delivery of contingent reinforcement. If the pain does not shut down when the environment does, the problem is more likely respondent in character. However, reported pain-related activity at night always needs to be weighed carefully in terms of possible reinforcement factors. Awakening allegedly because of pain but then always taking medications, emptying one's bladder, or eliciting supportive behavior (such as a backrub) from one's spouse all illustrate potential pain-contingent reinforcement. Consistent time-delays of several hours between specific activities and the onset of pain suggests respondent pain. In general, a rule of thumb is that the longer the interval between the cessation of physical activity and the onset of pain, the less likely the pain is to have an operant component.

IDENTIFICATION OF PAIN BEHAVIORS

There should be specific identification of the sounds, grimaces, and body language used to communicate the experience of pain. A list of verbal and nonverbal behaviors which are consistently emitted to express pain will provide the basis for further analysis of antecedent and consequent events for pain behavior in the latter portion of the interview.

ENVIRONMENTAL RESPONSES TO PAIN BEHAVIORS

Direct reinforcement of pain behavior, indirect reinforcement of pain behavior (through avoidance of aversive activities), and discouragement of healthy activities need to be specified. The pain patient living alone is less likely to be reinforced directly and consistently by a companion's responses. In these cases, a closer scrutiny of the indirect reinforcing qualities of vocational or avocational consequences to pain behavior is indicated.

PAIN ACTIVATORS

This aspect of the assessment concerns activities or situations likely to exacerbate pain behaviors. It is important to obtain exact behavioral descriptions rather than generalities. For example, the response, "Any kind of movement," is insufficient and questioning should be continued until the patient specifies, for instance, "lifting and twisting movements but not bending" as more likely to generate pain. These pain-producing motions should then be related to meaningful activities which are curtailed because of the pain problem. Does the housewife who is vulnerable to "lifting and twisting but not bending" therefore limit or avoid significant amounts of housework? Similarly, does the male housepainter who reports that pain is increased by lifting his arms above his head, limit the amount of work he does? In this way, an estimate of the psychological cost-benefit ratio of pain to activity can be obtained. Also, the likelihood that a patient will increase physical activity above baseline levels can be estimated from a roster of physical activities which exacerbate pain, because the inquiry has identified behaviors previously in the repertoire and therefore more readily established or re-established.

PAIN DIMINISHERS

This portion of the assessment focuses on events or situations likely to decrease pain behaviors. Some activities or behavioral consequences can serve as reinforcers for pain behaviors because when they occur they have the effect of reducing distress.

The extent to which rest and time-out from usual activities consistently decreases pain is an important consideration. Patients who shift from one productive activity to another in order to reduce the pain experience are quite different from those who cease or markedly reduce productive activity and the meeting of responsibilities in favor of rest. In the former case, the probability that pain behavior is under control of environmental contingencies is low; in the latter case, it is somewhat higher, for rest or time-out from aversive events is pain-contingent.

The extent to which medication yields a decrease in pain is also important. The types of medication, quantity consumed, and the time patterns in which they are taken, are critical variables. Consistent and reliable information about medications is often difficult to obtain. Even when accurate reports on the specific type of prescribed medication are provided by the patient, omission of such pain-relieving substances as alcohol, "street" drugs, and home remedies often makes interpretation of medication-usage patterns difficult.

A major issue involving medication relates to habituation or addiction and the extent to which they are taken on a pain-contingent basis. Consistent patterns of medication ingestion (e.g., every 3 or 4 hours, day and night) over extended time periods indicate possible habituation and/or addiction. This situation markedly increases the likelihood that pain behaviors come under the control of medication habit patterns rather than physical causes; thus, the problem becomes one of operant rather than respondent pain. Not infrequently, chronic pain patients who become addicted to pain medications have been observed to display an almost total elimination of pain behaviors following completion of a de-conditioning or withdrawal program which led to minimal or zero consumption rates.

TENSION-RELAXATION

The objective here is to identify the extent to which increases and decreases in tension alter the experience of pain. An assessment is needed to identify whether self-hypnosis, relaxation training, or biofeedback may be appropriate adjuncts to behavioral treatment.

CHANGES IN ACTIVITY LEVEL AS A RESULT OF PAIN

The major issue here is to identify changes in the patient's and spouse's lifestyles after the onset of pain, obtaining a picture of the typical work and social or leisure activities of both patient and spouse across the span of the marriage in order to explore changes in these activities as a consequence of the pain problem. Both vocational and avocational activities are important. If, for example, vocational or homemaking activities have been compromised but not social or leisure activities (assuming rough equivalence in physical demands), the case for operant factors is considerably strengthened. Pain patients who report being unable to sit longer than 15 minutes at a time due to pain, but later sit for 2 to 3 hours in a movie or on a dock while fishing (despite their pain), illustrate the point. Impact of pain on sexual activity is often an important topic. It is not uncommon for significant sexual dysfunction to occur in conjunction with chronic pain; these problems usually require concomitant treatment before the pain problem can be resolved. Pain behavior may help a patient avoid engaging in what is, for him or her, aversive sexual activity.

ADDITIONAL DATA

Psychological or personality test profiles (particularly the MMPI, Minnesota Multiphasic Personality Inventory), tests of intellectual ability or vocational interests, and other data designed to provide a thorough picture of the pain patient can also help plan treatment. Obtaining an activity and medication diary from the patient prior to behavioral analysis provides simple and inexpensive data about actual activity levels. This format has been described previously in some detail by Fordyce (1976, Appendix A).

CONTRAINDICATIONS AND LIMITATIONS FOR AN OPERANT PAIN TREATMENT PROGRAM

Briefly, there are several variables which serve as contraindicators for operant pain treatment. One of these is the case in which neither social reinforcement nor rest appears to be an effective reinforcer. Other variables which work against success of an operant approach to chronic pain include: 1) A spouse who is uninvolved or unwilling to participate in the program, thereby minimizing the extent to which some of the potentially more significant environmental contingencies can be altered. 2) A patient who refuses to relinquish or to attempt to decrease medication use, when the extent of analgesic consumption suggests addiction or habituation. 3) Pain- or illness-contingent compensation payments which provide a reasonably comfortable existence for indefinite periods of time. The compensation issue should not be oversimplifed, however, for if there are remunerated activities which can be carried out with reasonable competence and gratification, treatment may be quite feasible regardless of the size of the monthly compensation check (Peck, Fordyce, and Black, 1978). 4) The extent to which psychological problems interfere with a patient's ability to engage in a consistent, self-monitored program will also limit the effectiveness of inpatient operant-pain treatment. For example, a severely psychotic patient for whom the core problem is not pain but an emotional or interactional kind of difficulty may generate sufficient complaints of pain to require help, but of a special kind. The core problem must be identified and treated and then the pain problem and its associated functional limitations. Devine and Merskey (1965) examined the frequency with which this mixture of pain complaints and psychological problems is encountered and found that 38% of those coming for help with pain could readily be identified as having significant psychiatric or psychological difficulties. Additional discussion of selection factors for identifying those for whom an operant approach is or is not indicated can be found in Fordyce (1976).

Treatment Phase

Let us consider treatment strategies designed to reduce pain behavior, to increase activity levels, and to retrain the family to provide pertinent environmental contingencies. Two additional treatment goals are important and will be considered first: They are (1) the reduction of excessive health care utilization behaviors—especially those which increase the risk of iatrogenic effects; and (2) the establishment and maintenance of effective well behavior. Reducing health care utilization is cost-effective, of course, and it also helps maintain function. Establishing or re-establishing well behavior is based on three assumptions. First, the antithesis of "sickness" (in this case, pain behavior) is not, inevitably, health or well behavior: the reduction of one is not automatically followed by an increase in the other. Secondly, people who have long been ill are often deficient in their ability to be well. If those gaps in well behavior are not remediated, the person will remain highly vulnerable to resumption of illness behavior soon after treatment. Thirdly, simply stated, people having something better to do seem not to hurt as much—whatever the reason they may have been hurting.

The potential conflict between other treatment approaches and the operant approach should be considered prior to initiating therapy. The difficulties can usually be reduced to two issues. The first concerns alternative treatments which may provide systematic professional activity or attention on a pain-contingent basis. An alternative treatment process should not begin because of a patient's display of pain behaviors nor be omitted due to their absence. A second and related issue involves the necessity for scheduling and orchestrating to take into account all elements of the pain program and the "other" treatments. Several types of problems can be managed at the same time—and often need be—but someone will be required to monitor treatment components to ensure that the pieces fit together and do not conflict or interfere with each other.

PATIENT AND SPOUSE ORIENTATION

After evaluation has established that a patient is an appropriate candidate for an operant program, it is essential that the patient and his or her family be presented with a clear explanation of the evaluation findings and treatment goals.

In general, the purposes of the orientation can be summarized as:

A. to explain how conditioning effects can become the reason pain behaviors persist beyond the healing time of the originating injury;

B. to identify treatment goals and specify activities that will be possible at the end of treatment (e.g., employment or no employment, full or part-time work, sexual activities—although perhaps limited to certain positions, etc.); and

C. to describe the procedures by which these treatment goals will be attained.

The following are suggestions for the orientation of a chronic pain patient and spouse which may contribute to more effective treatment.

PAIN AS A LEARNED BEHAVIOR. Note that the patient is experiencing and reporting more pain than is necessary, based on the physical findings, and that a significant amount of the suffering experienced is the result of learning or conditioning. This is not a matter of whether the pain is "real" or not; suffering is real. The heart of the matter is what maintains the suffering.

INCREASING ACTIVITY AND PHYSICAL ENDURANCE. Clarify that one goal of treatment is to increase gradually activities and physical tolerance, starting at or below current activity levels. One can next introduce the concept of working-to-quota rather than -to-tolerance. (In the operant approach, goals and treatment steps are, of course, based on physician recommendations concerning safe limits for each patient.)

PAIN MEDICATION AND THE PAIN COCKTAIL. One should explain thoroughly the reasons and methods for control of pain medications in an operant program. Explain to the patient and spouse that pain medications will be reduced gradually. Explain how and why this will occur. Reassure the patient that at no time will his or her medication be abruptly altered or discontinued, and that false or placebo medications will not be used. Explain that analgesics will be given on a time-contingent basis and that the active ingredients will be delivered in a color-and-taste-masking vehicle.

ATTENTION AND SOCIAL REINFORCEMENT. Special note should be made of the way in which staff will respond to expressions of pain. It is helpful to point out that everyone is sensitive to the reactions of others and that concerned staff around a pain patient often may have fallen into the trap of letting their responsiveness become pain-contingent, thereby providing inadvertent support for the behaviors they wish to help the patient diminish. An important aspect of treatment is to turn that around. One can point out that treatment staff will diminish attention and social support to pain behaviors and will respond instead to increases in exercise, activity, and effective involvement. A distinction should be drawn between ignoring pain behavior and being socially nonresponsive to it. Furthermore, if the patient feels that some significant pain-related development has occurred during the treatment program, discussion with his or her physician will always be possible.

STRENGTHENING WELL BEHAVIOR. Finally, one should explain that treatment focusing only upon reducing pain behaviors is insufficient to generate long-term improvement. It is essential to increase physical activity, exercise tolerance, and appropriate well behavior including, as indicated, vocational or social pursuits. It also is generally desirable to focus on the gaps in a person's social skills or "well behaviors" which need to be bridged to reach long-term treatment goals.

It is helpful to note that the initial phase of treatment is often difficult and how well it goes will depend on the involvement of the patient and on effective support by the family. Treatment can proceed only after both patient and spouse have considered all the issues (e.g., medication decreases, activity increases, return to employment, etc.) and have actively decided to participate in the program.

MANAGEMENT OF MEDICATION

PAIN MEDICATION. This section describes the management of pain medication for those patients who demonstrate addiction, habituation, or a history of previous heavy medication use.

The patient is instructed to bring his or her medications to the hospital when admitted. If injectable medications are being used, these are shifted to an oral form. For a period of 2 to 5 days, medication usage is prescribed on a *prn* or "as needed" basis, and the patient is instructed to take whatever amounts seem necessary. The only constraint in this procedure is medical prudence, to ensure that the patient does not ingest harmful amounts of medication.

A significant difference exists between a detoxification procedure and the deconditioning procedure to be explained in this section. If toxicity due to medication is evident, initial detoxification must be provided before an adequate evaluation of the pain problem can be made and a decision on preferred treatment-approaches reached. If the treatment choice is an operant approach, information from baseline observations prior to detoxification can be used as the starting point for a more deliberately paced deconditioning program. Details on methods and conversion tables describing equivalencies for shifts in medications can be found in Halpern (1974).

The key to an effective medication consumption *prn* baseline is an accurate account of the amount taken. What type of medication, the dosage level, the number of times taken per day, the interval between doses, and the total medication over a 24-hour period are required to determine the initial level of medication. Based on the initial baseline evaluation, a pain cocktail is prescribed. This cocktail consists of a color-and-taste masking vehicle (e.g., cherry syrup or glyceryl guaiagolate-robotussin) administered orally so that each dose consists of the active agents plus sufficient vehicle to total approximately 10 ml.

The success of the approach depends on exacting promptness in delivering the pain cocktail at the prescribed times during the first 24 to 48 hours of the regimen. Most heavy medication users have long experienced reluctance on the part of health care professionals to meet their medication needs. It is critically important to overcome that fear by meticulous adherence to the prescribed schedule during those first crucial hours. Furthermore, the patient needs to be reassured that the 24-hour total of medication will match or slightly exceed what he or she had been taking during the *prn* baseline period. Finally, it is imperative that the cocktail be administered at consistent time intervals around the clock; in this way the administration of the cocktail is time- rather than pain-contingent.

Fading Active Ingredients. There are two concerns in fading the active medications. One is to eliminate or decrease significantly the addictive or toxic agents; the other is to avoid side effects from acute or rapid withdrawal (e.g., seizures, severe emotional stress, acute respiratory embarrassment, or depression). Another objective is to provide opportunities for the patient to re-establish alternatives to excessive medication use, in a gradual and systematic way. Crash programs which replace active ingredients with methadone and fade the ingredients at the fastest possible rate may fail to provide for the relearning aspects of treatment.

From clinical experience, it takes approximately 7 to 10 weeks to bring relatively high medication levels down. Fading need not necessarily occur at the same rate for each medication. The general pattern is to change active ingredients approximately once every 7 to 14 days in equal decrements so that the amount of active ingredient in the cocktail will approach zero in 7 to 10 weeks. An example of pain cocktail is provided in Table 6.1.

It is the exceptional chronic pain patient for whom muscle relaxants or tranquilizers are of continuing help. Usually, when they have been consumed in conjunction with narcotics and/or barbiturates, they can be eliminated, following baseline observations. Depression can serve to reduce the effectiveness of a program. Regardless of whether the patient has been taking antidepressant medication, as observed in the evaluation process and from pretreatment diary data, it is often wise to add such a component to the pain cocktail. Amitriptyline (Elavil) and doxepin (Sinequan) are commonly used effective antidepressant ingredients. When used, they should also be given on a time-contingent basis. Antidepressant agents need not be tapered during the medication deconditioning treatment phase and can be maintained at therapeutic dosage levels throughout the treatment program. This should be periodically re-evaluated. Tapering of antidepressant medication should begin when the patient has started to engage in post-treatment target behaviors anticipated to be reinforcing.

Long-term Maintenance and Fading of Pain Cocktail Regimen. The consumption of active ingredients in the pain cocktail may not reach zero at the end of the inpatient treatment phase or may never

Table 6.1 Sample Pain Cocktail Regimen*

Inpatient days			Pain cocktail format
1–6		*Baseline:*	Patient reports preadmission pattern of "... one or two of the 50-mg tablets of Demerol two or three times a day, as needed, at home." *Physician orders to nurse:* "May have Demerol, *prn* pain, not to exceed three 50-mg tablets every 3 hours. Carefully record amount taken." *Analysis of baseline data:* Patient averaged 600 mg of Demerol per 24-hour period, at average of 3- to 4-hour intervals between requests.
7–9	*First cocktail*		
		℞ *to pharmacists:*	Demerol, 1920 mg Bevisol, Plebex, or other liquid B complex, 12 ml; cherry syrup qs 240 ml
		Sig:	Pain Cocktail, 10 ml po q3h, day and night, *not prn*
		Nursing order:	Pain cocktail, 10 ml po q3h, day and night, *not prn*
		Since contents of the pain cocktail are not on the label, a copy of the prescription must be kept in a separate pain cocktail book.	
10–12		Decrease each daily total by 64 mg, 1/10 or original amount. A 3-day ℞ is decreased by 64 × 3 or 192 mg.	
		℞ *to pharmacists:*	Demerol, 1728 mg Bevisol, Plebex, or other liquid B complex, 12 ml; cherry syrup qs 240 ml
		Sig:	Pain cocktail, 10 ml po q3h, day and night, *not prn*
		Nursing order:	Pain cocktail, 10 ml po q3h, day and night, *not prn*
13–15		℞ *to pharmacists:*	Demerol, 1536 mg Bevisol, Plebex, or other liquid B complex, 12 ml; cherry syrup qs 240 ml
		Sig:	Pain cocktail, 10 ml po q3h, day and night, *not prn*
		Nursing order:	Pain cocktail, 10 ml po q3h, day and night, *not prn*
16–18		℞ *to pharmacists:*	Demerol, 1344 mg Bevisol, Plebex, or other liquid B complex, 12 ml; cherry syrup qs 240 ml
		Sig:	Pain cocktail, 10 ml po q3h, day and night, *not prn*
		Nursing order:	Pain cocktail, 10 ml po q3h, day and night, *not prn*
19–21		℞ *to pharmacists:*	Demerol, 1152 mg Bevisol, Plebex, or other liquid B complex, 12 ml; cherry syrup qs 240 ml
		Sig:	Pain cocktail, 10 ml po q3h, day and night, *not prn*

Reprinted by permission from: Fordyce, W. *Behavioral methods for chronic pain and illness.* St. Louis, C. V. Mosby, 1976.

* The assistance of Barbara J. DeLateur, M.D., in preparing the pain cocktail regimen sample and the related discussion is gratefully acknowledged.

Table 6.1 (Continued)

	Nursing order:	Pain cocktail, 10 ml o q3h, day and night, *not prn*
22–24	℞ *to pharmacists:*	Demerol 960 mg Bevisol, Plebex, or other liquid B complex, 12 ml; cherry syrup qs 240 ml
	Sig:	Pain cocktail, 10 ml po q3h, day and night, *not prn*
	Nursing order:	Pain cocktail, 10 ml po q3h, day and night, *not prn*
37–39	℞ *to pharmacists:*	Demerol 0 mg Bevisol, Plebex, or other liquid B complex, 12 ml; cherry syrup qs 240 ml
	Sig:	Pain cocktail, 10 ml po q3h, day and night, *not prn*
	Nursing order:	Pain cocktail, 10 ml po q3h, day and night, *not prn*

(Maintain patient on vehicle for 2 to 10 days; if all is going well, inform patient and ask if continuation of vehicle is desired.)

reach zero, requiring the patient to maintain an indefinite pain cocktail regimen on an outpatient basis. Continued fading of medications on an outpatient basis is usually not difficult and tends to occur more frequently when there is a significant respondent element to the pain problem.

Chronic pain patients, like everyone, may occasionally have acute pain episodes, either respondent in nature as a result of some wound or trauma, or periodic resurgences of the operant pain problem. The referring physician should receive guidance on how to deal with such episodes. If some trauma, unrelated to the original pain problem, produces pain (e.g., wound, infection, sprain, etc.) and analgesics seem appropriate, administration should be on a time-contingent and time-limited basis. The number of days of medication should be based on the judgment of the physician as to the natural life of the wound or infection, etc., and its associated pain. Re-emergence of an operant pain problem can be handled in essentially the same way. A pain cocktail regimen can be reinstated, starting with a minimal amount of active ingredients and with a set schedule for fading to a termination point.

NON-PAIN MEDICATION MANAGEMENT. Many chronic pain patients are taking medications which are unrelated to the pain problems; e.g., hormones or vitamins. These can be handled independently from the pain cocktail procedure and delivered as prescribed in the usual fashion. The exceptions are tranquilizers or sedatives, which should either be eliminated or incorporated into the cocktail.

TERMINATION OF PAIN COCKTAIL AND SPECIAL PROBLEMS. The patient should be informed when active ingredients in the pain cocktail reach zero. It is generally advisable to wait for 1 or 2 days after this has occurred to allow adequate demonstration of functional performance in the absence of analgesics. Conditioning and its effects are potent. The ritual of medication usage may itself have significant conditioned properties for the patient. Each patient should, therefore, be offered the option of continuing with the cocktail (vehicle only, with no active ingredients) for a period of time, should that be desired. A fading regimen for the vehicle may then be worked out.

INCREASING EXERCISE AND ACTIVITY LEVELS

In contingency management treatment of pain, whether operant or respondent, exercise has a particularly important role. Exercise improves physiological tone and strength and can increase functional abilities. Exercise has the additional characteristic, in nearly all cases, of being incompatible with pain behavior. Activity levels usually diminish in response to competing pain behaviors. In addition, performing increased exercise tends to elicit more helpful responses from the environment than those elicited by displays of pain behavior. Family members who have been consistently discouraging activity or exercise have an opportunity to learn that activity is "safe" and can now rehearse ways for reinforcing activity rather than discouraging it. Finally, exercise and activity is well behavior in its own right.

Selection of Exercises. Among the criteria for selecting exercises are relevance to pain (i.e., the activity produces an increase in pain behavior following a few repetitions), contribution to physical conditioning, or rehabilitation for a specific functional weakness. Exercises should be measured in amount performed rather than time units (e.g., walking a set distance and not a number of minutes). Exercises should be visible, easily monitored, and relevant to post-treatment activities. Exercises are medically prescribed with medical and physical limits set for each patient individually. The following is a list of typical exercises and activities for low back pain patients:

Exercise	*Units of Measurement*
1. Riding a fixed bicycle	0.10 miles
2. Walking	50-m laps
3. Climbing and descending stairs	Flights of x steps each
4. Pelvic tilts	Repetitions
5. Hip extension	Repetitions
6. Hip abduction	Repetitions
7. Turkish knot tying while standing	Rows
8. Homemaking (cooking, sewing)	Time‡

These activities are prescribed either in physical therapy or occupational therapy, and comprise the majority of the patient's activity treatment while in the hospital.

Identifying Exercise Quotas and Increments. Once exercises have been chosen, baseline levels need to be identified. Twice-daily physical and occupational therapy sessions can begin for approximately 3 to 6 days. The patient is instructed to "work to tolerance" at each prescribed activity or exercise. "Tolerance" is explained as meaning that the activity should be performed without interruption until terminated by pain, weakness, or fatigue. It should be made clear that the patient is free to decide when to stop. Baseline trials should be observed by a therapist who records performance: e.g., number of repetitions. Baseline exercise or activity levels can be assessed on an outpatient basis as well, using the spouse or other person as observer and recorder. Following baseline evaluation, the exercise values obtained are reviewed and initial treatment quotas are established.

A primary objective of the initial treatment quota is to ensure success during early sessions of treatment. Initial quotas which fail to be reached or are followed immediately by increased displays of pain, weakness, or fatigue are, by definition, too high and need to be readjusted immediately. With patients who report significant pain without exercise, initial quotas are selected to avoid increases in pain. There is no set formula for initial quotas. One way is to average the baseline performance for each exercise and set the initial treatment quota approximately 10% below. The guiding principle in setting the initial quota is to select the highest value which the patient can meet. (Also, subsequent increments should be manageable without significant difficulty.) When in doubt, set a lower quota.

The patient is instructed that once initial baseline levels and initial quotas for exercise and activity have been set, he or she will be expected to engage in physical therapy twice daily and that these activities will be gradually and systematically increased. A judgment must be made as to how rapidly to increase the amount of exercise. There is no simple formula to compute this. The guiding principle is to increase at a pace that promises a high probability of success over many exercise trials. In the inpatient setting, ongoing observation by the therapists is helpful in setting realistic rates of increase; in the outpatient situation, rates of increment should be set very conserva tively and frequent monitoring or progress is essential to ensure accuracy and effectiveness.

Reinforcement for Exercise and Activity. The quota system provides rest con-

‡ A necessary compromise, but this activity is usually not begun until considerable treatment progress has occurred.

tingent upon and immediately following the exercise activity to be strengthened or increased. Rest intervals may usually be brief. Compliance is best encouraged through social reinforcement and other reinforcers available in the treatment setting.

One method to assist both inpatient and outpatient adherence is to display graphs of performance and quotas completed. With appropriate quotas and increments, the patient and spouse will see steady improvements in performance. A graph indicating initial baseline levels and several readjustments is provided in Figure 6.1 (from Fordyce, 1976). The visual representation of success is in itself encouraging.

FAILURE TO ACHIEVE QUOTAS. Patients will occasionally fail to meet quotas. For the first one to three consecutive failures, the therapist is instructed not to comment specifically but simply to record the amount the patient completed and make some matter-of-fact statement like, "Okay, see you this afternoon." Quotas are continued at the previous level during subsequent sessions. Under no circumstances should the therapist give the patient encouragement. If failure persists beyond the one to three consecutive times, the patient is told that quotas will be dropped below the failure threshold and recycled. Occasionally, failure will persist even after recycling and re-evaluation. In these instances, it is possible that too high a quota has been set for the patient and that reassessment is necessary. Ceilings should be set on all exercises. This is primarily a medical decision. For physical therapy exercises, typically, 20 to 25 repetitions is appropriate; with respect to walking, 1.5 to 2.0 miles twice a day is often a good upper limit.

Repeated and consistent failure, despite medical opinion that the ceiling for a particular exercise is not excessive, may indicate that the patient is simply not a good candidate for the operant approach. At this point, the patient can be given the choice of continuing training at the current quota or of terminating the program. If, after lowering the quotas to below the failure threshold, the patient continues to fail, treatment should be terminated, since it is apparent that the reinforcers available are not effective for that particular patient.

PROGRAMMING PAIN-RELATED TREATMENT PROCEDURES

The strategy for using other pain-related therapies is identical to the one described for non-pain medical procedures and med-

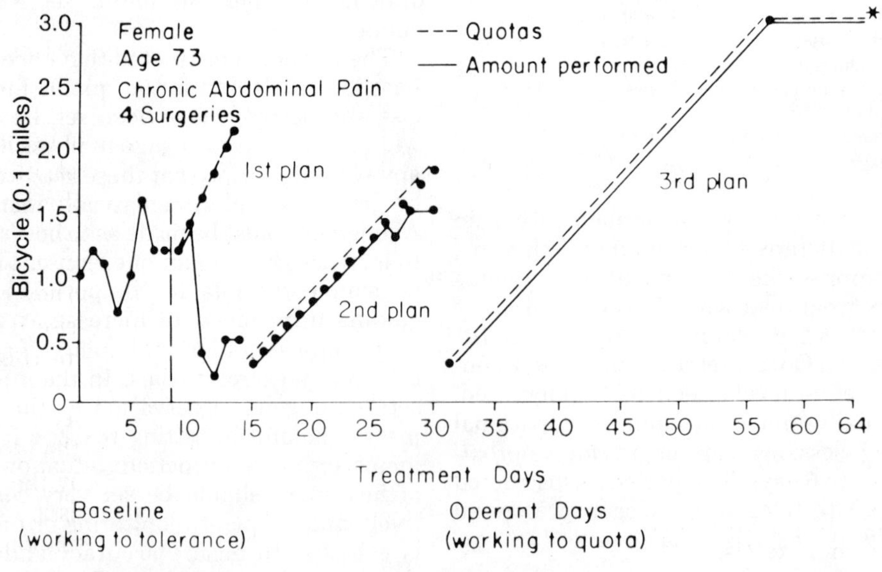

Figure 6.1. Quota adjustments to meet quota failures. (Reprinted by permission from Fordyce, W. *Behavioral methods for chronic pain and illness*. St. Louis: C. V. Mosby, 1976.)

ications for these conditions should be prescribed separately from the pain cocktail. Alternative pain-related treatment procedures may be considered (e.g., ethyl chloride spray, nerve blocks, heat or massage, transcutaneous stimulation, muscle relaxation training, or other procedures), and these are often less costly and less time-consuming than a fully programmed contingency-management approach. If successful, so much the better. If the approach provides significant help but not total relief (e.g., electromyographic biofeedback helps reduce headache pain but does not alleviate back pain sufficiently to allow increased activity level) then the operant program may need to be integrated with it. One underlying principle remains the same: specialized attention and medical procedures should not be prescribed on a pain-contingent basis, but when deemed necessary, should be provided in a time-contingent and consistent manner.

Conclusion

This chapter has reviewed major theories of etiology in chronic pain. It should be evident that pain, as a concept, clearly involves more than a sensory-receptor response system for nociceptive stimuli and physiological sensations. Pain also involves behavior and environmental consequences as well as attitudes and expectations based on prior experiences with pain. In the particular case of chronic pain, these variables—pain behaviors, environmental contingencies, and attitudes or expectations—often play major and even predominant roles in the manifestation of clinical pain. The importance of moving beyond the confines of a simple biomedical or disease conception of pain is also supported by the high incidence of continuing pain problems following standard treatment derived from the biomedical perspective.

Methods and a rationale for a multimodal, behaviorally based approach for treating and managing chronic pain have been set forth. The essential elements are:

1. Recognition that chronic pain rarely can be adequately understood or treated solely within the confines of a biomedical perspective;
2. Designation of comprehensive evaluation procedures encompassing medical, phychological, occupational, environmental, and behavioral assessment of the factors contributing to the current pain behavior;
3. Coordination of treatment which focuses on decreasing pain behavior as well as reliance upon medical services and on increasing well-behavior; and
4. Conduct of follow-up designed to encourage self-monitoring and environmental support for treatment gains.

Finally, further research is called for, to evaluate comprehensive treatment programs and to determine the effectiveness of various components. For example, it has been demonstrated that chronic tension-headache patients do not require intensive inpatient approaches, while chronic low-back pain patients may not respond well to an outpatient approach. The accurate assignment to different therapies will only be possible when research has been completed to provide information about the relative importance of components dealing with cognitive factors, physical exercise, anxiety and muscle tension reduction, in vivo pain-tolerance training, and psychotherapy as well as disease variables in different populations of chronic pain patients.

References

Anderson, T. P., Cole, T. M., Gullickson, G., Hudgens, A., and Roberts, A. H. Behavior modification of chronic pain: A treatment program by a multidisciplinary team. *J. Clin. Orthoped. Related Res.*, in press.

Bandura, A. Behavioral modifications through modeling procedures. In L. Krasner, and L. Ullmann (Eds.), *Research in behavior modification.* New York: Holt, Rinehart & Winston, 1965.

Bandura, A. *Principles of behavior modification.* New York: Holt, Rinehart & Winston, 1969.

Bandura, A., and Walters, R. *Social learning and personality development.* New York: Holt, Rinehart & Winston, 1963.

Beecher, H. K. Relationship of significance of wound to the pain experienced. *J.A.M.A.,* 1956, *161,* 1609–1613.

Beecher, H. K. The placebo effect as a non-specific force surrounding disease and the treatment of disease. In R. Janzen, W. D. Keidel, A. Herz, C. Steichele, J. P. Payne, and R. A. P. Burt (Eds.), *Pain: Basic principles, pharmacology, therapy.* Stuttgart, West Germany: George Thieme, 1972.

Bonica, J. J. *The management of pain.* Philadelphia: Lea & Febiger, 1953.

Cairns, D., Thomas, L., Mooney, V., and Pace, J. B. A

comprehensive treatment approach to chronic low back pain. *Pain,* 1976, *2,* 301–308.

Christopherson, V. Socio-cultural correlates of pain response. Final report of Project #1390, Vocational Rehabilitation Administration. Washington, D.C.: United States Department of Health, Education, and Welfare, 1966.

Craig, K. Social modeling determinants of pain processes. *Pain,* 1975, *1,* 375–378.

Devine, R., and Merskey, H. The description of pain in psychiatric and general medical patients. *J. Psychosom. Res.,* 1965, *9,* 311.

Ferster, C. Classification of behavioral pathology. In L. Krasner and L. Ullman (Eds.), *Research in behavior modification.* New York: Holt, Rinehart & Winston, 1966.

Fordyce, W. *Behavioral methods for chronic pain and illness.* St. Louis: C. V. Mosby, 1976.

Fordyce, W., Brena, S., DeLateur, B., Holcombe, S., and Loeser, J. Relationship of patient semantic pain descriptors to physician diagnostic judgments, activity level measures and MMPI. *Pain,* 1978, *5,* 293–303.

Fordyce, W., Fowler, R., Lehmann, J., and DeLateur, B. Some implications of learning in problems of chronic pain. *J. Chron. Disabil.,* 1968, *21,* 179–190.

Fordyce, W., Fowler, R., Lehmann, J., DeLateur, B., Sand, B., and Trieschmann, R. Operant conditioning in the treatment of chronic pain. *Arch. Phys. Med. Rehabil.,* 1973, *54,* 399–408.

Gottlieb, H., Strite, L., Koller, R., Madorsky, A., Hockersmith, V., Kleeman, M., and Wagner, J. Comprehensive rehabilitation of patients having chronic low back pain. *Arch. Phys. Med. Rehabil.,* 1977, *58,* 101–108.

Greenhoot, J., and Sternbach, R. Conjoint treatment of chronic pain. *Adv. Neurol.,* 1974, *4,* 595–603.

Halpern, L. Psychotropic drugs and the management of chronic pain. In J. J. Bonica (Ed.), *Advances in neurology: International symposium on pain,* Vol. 4. New York: Raven Press, 1974.

Hilgard, E. R. Pain as a puzzle for psychology and physiology. *Am. Psychol.,* 1969, *24,* 103–113.

Hilgard, E. R., and Hilgard, J. R. *Hypnosis in the relief of pain.* Los Altos, Calif.: Wm. Kaufmann, 1975.

Hill, H. E., Kornetsky, C. G., Flanary, H. G., and Wilder, A. Effects of anxiety and morphine on the discrimination of intensities of pain. *J. Clin. Invest.,* 1952, *31,* 473–480.

Lazarus, A. A. *Clinical behavior therapy.* New York: Brunner/Mazel, 1972.

Leitenberg, H. (Ed.). *Handbook of behavior modification and behavior therapy.* Englewood Cliffs, N.J.: Prentice-Hall, 1976.

Lewinsohn, P. Clinical and theoretical aspects of depression. In K. Calhoun, H. Adams, and K. Mitchell (Eds.), *Innovative treatment methods in psychopathology.* New York: Wiley, 1974.

Lewinsohn, P., and Atwood, C. Depression: A clinical-research approach. Paper presented at the Washington-Oregon Psychological Association joint meeting, Crystal Mountain, Wash., May 1968.

Livingston, W. K. *Pain mechanisms.* New York: The Macmillan Co., 1943.

Loeser, J. D. Dorsal rhizotomy: Indications and results. In J. J. Bonica (Ed.), *Advances in neurology: International symposium on pain,* Vol. 4. New York: Raven Press, 1974.

Loeser, J. D. Mechanisms of central pain. In M. Weisenberg (Ed.), *The control of pain.* New York: Psychological Dimensions, 1977.

Meichenbaum, D., and Turk, D. The cognitive-behavioral management of anxiety, anger, and pain. In P. Davidson (Ed.), *The behavioral management of anxiety, depression, and pain.* New York: Brunner/Mazel, 1976.

Melzack, R. Pain. In D. L. Sills (Ed.), *International encyclopedia of the social sciences,* Vol. 2. New York: Macmillan, 1968.

Melzack, R., and Wall, P. D. On the nature of cutaneous sensory mechanisms. *Brain,* 1962, *85,* 331–356.

Melzack, R., and Wall, P. D. Pain mechanisms: A theory. *Science,* 1965, *150,* 971–979.

Merskey, H. Psychological aspects of pain. *Postgrad. Med. J.,* 1968, *44,* 297–306.

Merskey, H., and Spear, F. G. *Pain: Psychological and psychiatric aspects.* London: Bailliere, Tindall & Cassell, 1967.

Newman, R., Seres, J., Yospe, L., and Garlington, B. Multidisciplinary treatment of chronic pain: Long-term follow-up of low-back pain patients. *Pain,* 1978, *4,* 283–292.

Noordenbos, W. *Pain.* New York: American Elsevier, 1959.

Orne, M. On the social psychology of the psychological experiment: With particular reference to demand characteristics and their implications. *Am. Psychol.,* 1962, *17,* 776–783.

Peck, C. J., Fordyce, W. E., and Black, R. G. The effect of the pendency of claims for compensation upon behavior indicative of pain. *Wash. Law Revi.,* 1978, *53,* 251–278.

Roberts, A. The behavioral treatment of pain. In J. M. Ferguson and C. B. Taylor (Eds.), *A comprehensive handbook of behavioral medicine.* New York: Spectrum, in press.

Rosenthal, R. *Experimenter effects in behavioral research.* New York: Appleton-Century-Crofts, 1966.

Shealy, C., and Maurer, D. Transcutaneous nerve stimulation for control of pain. *Surg. Neurosurg.,* 1974, *2,* 45–47.

Snyder, S. Opiate receptors and internal opiates. *Sci. Am.,* 1977, *236* (3), 44–56.

Spear, F. Pain in psychiatric patients. *J. Psychosoma. Res.,* 1967, *11,* 187–193.

Steger, J., and Harper, R. EMG biofeedback versus in vivo self-monitored relaxation in the treatment of tension headaches. Paper presented at the annual meeting of the Western Psychological Association, Seattle, April 1977.

Sternbach, R. A. *Pain: A psychophysiological analysis.* New York: Academic Press, 1968.

Sternbach, R. A. *Pain patients: Traits and treatment.* New York: Academic Press, 1974.

Sternbach, R. A., and Fordyce, W. Psychogenic pain. In J. J. Bonica (Ed.), *The management of pain,* 2nd ed., Philadelphia: Lea & Febiger, 1975.

Sternbach, R., Murphy, R., Akeson, W., and Wolfe, S. Chronic low back pain: Characteristics of the "low back loser." *Postgrad. Med.,* 1973, *53,* 135–138.

Sternbach, R., and Tursky, B. Ethic differences among housewives in psychophysical and skin potential responses to electric shock. *Psychophysiology,* 1965, *1,* 241–246.

Sternbach, R., Wolf, S., Murphy, R., and Wolfe, S. Aspects of low back pain. *Postgrad. Med.,* 1973, *53,* 226–229.

Swanson, D., Floreen, A., and Swenson, W. Program for managing chronic pain. II. Short-term results. *Mayo Clin. Proc.,* 1976, *51,* 409–411.

Turk, D. Cognitive-behavioral techniques in the management of pain. In J. Foreyt and D. Rathjen (Eds.), *Cognitive behavior therapy: Research and applications.* New York: Plenum, 1978.

Tursky, B., and Sternbach, R. Further physiological correlates of ethnic differences in responses to shock. *Psychophysiology,* 1967, *4,* 67–74.

Weisenberg, M. *Pain: Clinical and experimental perspectives.* St. Louis: C. V. Mosby, 1975.

Weisenberg, M. Pain and pain control. *Psychol. Bull.,* 1977, *84,* 1008–1044.

Wolpe, J. *Psychotherapy by reciprocal inhibition.* Stanford, Calif.: Stanford University Press, 1958.

Wolpe, J. *The Practice of behavior therapy.* New York: Pergamon, 1969.

Wolpe, J. and Lazarus, A. *Behavior therapy techniques: A guide to the treatment of neuroses.* New York: Pergamon, 1966.

Woodforde, J. and Merskey, H. Personality traits of patients with chronic pain. *J. Psychosom. Res.,* 1972, *16,* 167.

Yates, A. *Behavior therapy.* New York: Wiley, 1970.

Musculoskeletal and Stress-related Disorders*

7

JOHANN MARTIN STOYVA, PH.D.

Associate Professor of Psychology
Department of Psychiatry
University of Colorado Medical Center
Denver, Colorado

Since coordinated muscle activity is the sine qua non of behavior, it is not suprising that the modification of striate muscle system activity should be of great significance for behavioral medicine. There are both practical and theoretical reasons why this should be so. Since the striate musculature makes up almost 50% of body mass, it would seem likely to have powerful effects on the organism as a whole. Also, there is the obvious fact that the muscular activity is an inescapable part of adaptive behavior, and of the response to stress. Without it, there is no behavior. Moreover, there is a growing body of clinical evidence, much of it accumulated over the past several years, indicating that muscle relaxation is a powerful variable and one which can be clinically useful. Our own work with electromyographic (EMG) feedback as a means of inducing relaxation was triggered by reports in the older literature concerning the effects of progressive relaxation (Jacobson, 1938) and autogenic training (Schultz and Luthe, 1959). With both of these older techniques, essentially ways of training a "cultivated" low arousal condition, a number of successes with anxiety and stress-linked disorders have been reported. Similarly, in the behavior therapy technique of systematic desensitization, muscle relaxation has been utilized as a response incompatible with anxiety (Wolpe, 1973).

In the literature on EMG feedback, three major areas of clinical applications may be discerned: the use of EMG feedback in disorders involving localized muscular tension, its use with disorders in which a generalized relaxation response is called for, and its application in physical medicine. In physical medicine and rehabilitation a major emphasis has been upon recovering and retraining patterns of muscle activity following neurological disorder or accident. Each of these three foregoing areas, the status of clinical applications within it, and some special problems will be discussed in turn.

EMG Feedback in Disorders Involving Localized Muscle Tension

A disorder in which a considerable EMG feedback work has been conducted is with tension headache, also known as muscle contraction headache. This disorder is worth studying in a behavioral medicine context since: it is a very common affliction, its etiology is comparatively clear-cut, and it lends itself reasonably well to outcome measurements and a number of controlled clinical outcome studies are now available.

This type of headache, also known as "psychogenic" or "nervous" headache, is likely to arise at times of emotional conflict or psychological stress. The immediate

* This work was supported by National Institute of Mental Health Grants MH-25940 and MH-15596, and the National Institute of Mental Health Research Scientist Development Award K01-MH-43361.

cause of pain, as demonstrated in the experiments of Wolff (1968) and his associates, is thought to be the sustained contraction of muscles in the forehead, scalp, and neck. As indicated below, vasoconstriction of blood vessels in these regions may also contribute to the pain. The onset of pain is gradual and its duration can vary from hours to weeks. Typically, the pain is bilateral and often described as dull or "band-like;" the scalp may be sensitive to touch. Contrary to the case with migraine headaches scotomata are not present, nor is nausea a factor.

Most, but not all investigators, have noted elevated frontal EMG levels in tension headache patients. For example, in the mid-1950's, Sainsbury and Gibson (1954) reported that the resting level of frontal EMG activity was higher in tension headache patients than in normals. Similarly, in our study (Budzynski, Stoyva, Adler, et al., 1973), resting EMG levels in the patient group appeared to be at least twice those we typically observed in non-headache volunteers. More recently, Haynes, Griffin, Mooney, et al. (1975) reported that tension headache patients who reported a headache during a training session showed higher EMG levels (5.37 μV) compared to their *own* levels when headache was absent (4.19 μV). In a group of severe tension headache cases, Hutchings and Reinking (1976) found frontal EMG levels to be dramatically higher than in non-headache controls. Similarly, Phillips (1977) found headache sufferers to have significantly higher frontal EMG levels than controls.

There is also evidence of vasoconstriction component in tension headache. Dalessio (1972), in summarizing several studies, states that a moderate amount of vasoconstriction by itself does not lead to pain. However, if vasoconstriction occurs in a contracted muscle, pain can occur. Dalessio further states that sustained muscle contraction by itself can be painful, but if, in addition, there is vasoconstriction of the relevant nutrient arteries, then the resultant pain from muscle contraction may be much greater.

EMG FEEDBACK IN TENSION HEADACHE

Since there was strong evidence that striate muscle contraction was central to the etiology of tension headache, we reasoned that if patients could be taught relaxation of the head and neck area, their headaches should diminish. A pilot study with five patients showed that the training seemed to be effective in reducing the frequency and severity of headaches (Budzynski, Stoyva, and Adler, 1970). During their laboratory sessions, these patients learned to reduce frontal EMG activity with the aid of an EMG feedback device. Its essential operation was as follows: surface electrodes were utilized to detect EMG activity in the frontal area. The patient would then hear a feedback signal consisting of a stream of clicks. A rapid click rate indicated high muscular tension; a diminishing click rate indicated that a shift toward relaxation was occurring. The task of the patient was to relax as thoroughly as possible (with the aid of the information feedback provided by the clicks).

With EMG feedback training and muscle relaxation, these patients not only learned to produce lowered EMG activity (frontalis monitored) but showed associated reduction in headache activity. Follow-up results over a 3-month period indicated that for the five patients, headache activity remained at a low level, especially if they continued to practice relaxation for a short time every day. An interesting collateral observation was that many patients, when they felt tension headache beginning to develop in a stress situation, learned to abort the headache by deliberately relaxing their upper body musculature.

Since our pilot observations looked highly favorable, we initiated a controlled-outcome study (Budzynski et al., 1973) in order to guard against the possibility that our pilot results were mainly attributable to either placebo or suggestion effects. The experimental design involved one treatment group and two control groups. The six patients in the experimental group received accurate information feedback as to their frontal EMG levels. Over a 9-week period, they received two EMG feedback sessions per week. The six patients in the "pseudo-feedback" group were given the same number of laboratory sessions of relaxation training, but instead of true feedback they listened to feedback signals which had been tape-recorded from the experimental group. To help in applying the relaxation response to everday life, all patients in both the experimental and pseudo-feedback group were told to do the relaxation training at home or at work twice a day. The six subjects in the second control group received no treatment at all.

All persons chosen for the study suffered from frequent tension headaches and had been afflicted for an average of 7 years or more. Patients in all three groups kept daily records of headache activity (a rating scale of intensity recorded on an hour-by-hour basis) during the baseline period, the training period, and for a 3-month follow-up period. In roughly 25% of the patients there was a pronounced decline in headache activity during the baseline period. Although their headaches later returned, the patients showing this placebo-like effect were not included in the controlled study.

RESULTS

The main observations were as follows:

1. In the feedback group, frontal EMG levels fell to less than 40% of baseline values. In the pseudo-feedback group, levels remained at about 80% of baseline values.
2. Headache levels showed a significant decline in the experimental group, but not in either of the two control groups. It is worth emphasizing that although *both* the feedback and the pseudo-feedback groups practiced relaxation twice a day at home, only the feedback group showed a significant reduction in headache activity.
3. Feedback patients showed a sharply reduced usage of tranquillizers and headache medications, as assessed at the end of the 3-month follow-up period. Such a reduction was not characteristic of the pseudo-feedback patients.

In summary, patients in the treatment group showed markedly reduced frontal EMG levels, diminished headache activity and greatly reduced drug usage.

CURRENT STATUS OF RELAXATION TREATMENTS FOR TENSION HEADACHE

Since the completion of the two foregoing investigations, many further studies concerning the application of relaxation training to tension headache have been published. To summarize these: the weight of evidence strongly supports the conclusion that relaxation training produces clinically useful reductions in tension headache pain. There is some debate, however, as to how relaxation may be best produced. One way of achieving the requisite relaxation is by means of EMG feedback, usually from the frontal area. Another method, but one which needs further study on representative clinical populations, may be the use of various "verbal-instruction" methods for producing relaxation.

EMG FEEDBACK STUDIES

Wickramasekera (1972) reported a study with five patients in which a 3-week baseline was followed by 3 weeks of non-contingent or sham feedback. The latter, in turn, was followed by 12 weeks of genuine feedback of frontal EMG. Although the patients thought they were receiving real feedback during the sham feedback phase, their frontal EMG levels and headache activity did *not* decrease until the genuine feedback was introduced. During this genuine feedback phase there were significant decreases in both headache activity and frontal EMG in all patients. Interestingly, there was no significant placebo effect simply from receiving sham "biofeedback."

A second study by Wickramasekera (1973) employed a similar design with the exception that the baseline period of 3 weeks was followed by a 3-week period of verbal relaxation instructions taken from Wolpe and Lazarus. This period, in turn, was followed by 3 weeks of frontal EMG feedback training. The five patients showed a slight decrease in headache activity and frontal EMG levels during the verbal relaxation phase, but a sharp drop in both measures during the final biofeedback phase. A follow-up of 9 weeks' duration showed that headache activity had remained at minimal levels during this time.

The conclusion drawn from this study was that the frontal EMG training was more powerful than were verbal relaxation instructions for the reduction of muscle-contraction headache. This conclusion was supported in a more extensive study by Hutchings and Reinking (1976). Eighteen chronic tension headache patients were randomly assigned to one of three treatment conditions: "Wolpe-Jacobson" verbal relaxation instructions, frontal EMG feedback training, or combined "Wolpe-Jacobson" instructions plus frontal EMG feedback. A 28-day baseline and subsequent 28-day training period were followed by a 28-day follow-up. Each patient received 10 1-hour training sessions and kept daily records of headache activity. The statistical analysis showed that whereas all groups decreased in headache activity, the two EMG feedback groups were significantly better than the "Wolpe-Jacobson" verbal instruction group. The authors concluded that frontal EMG feedback-assisted procedures appeared to be the method of choice in tension headache therapy.

Reduction of tension headache pain also occurred in an experiment chiefly designed to test the efficacy of frontal EMG feedback with chronic anxiety (Raskin, Johnson, and Rondestvedt, 1973). All 10 patients were afflicted with chronic anxiety; four of them also suffered from tension headache. Although anxiety reduction was reported to be only moderate, it is worth noting that all four of the patients with muscle contraction headache showed decrements in headache pain.

Finally, a recent paper by Phillips (1977) describes a controlled study of EMG feedback in tension headache and in cases of mixed tension-migraine headaches. Treatment subjects received frontal EMG feedback. Control patients were in a pseudo-biofeedback condition in which they listened to the taped feedback of a successful biofeedback session. They were told that monotonous auditory stimuli were relaxing and would help them to clear their minds of stressful thoughts.

Biofeedback proved superior in producing decrements in resting muscle tension levels, headache intensity, and medication frequency. Pseudo-feedback produced little change. Phillips also notes that the correlation of muscle tension level and headache intensity was high only for the pure tension headache cases. In the mixed tension-migraine cases these correlations were low, some even being negative. The mixed tension-migraine cases, moreover, failed to benefit much from the training.

STUDIES UTILIZING NON-BIOFEEDBACK INDUCTION OF RELAXATION

Although EMG feedback appears to be a powerful procedure for the alleviation of tension headache, not all investigators regard it as the preferred method of relaxation. Lance (1973), the Australian neurologist, maintains that all cases of tension headache will remit with systematic relaxation training if the patient is sufficiently conscientious in his practice. It should be noted, however, that this statement is based on a series of individual cases, not on a controlled study.

Haynes et al. (1975) compared frontal EMG feedback with a specially prepared relaxation program. Patients in both conditions showed significant reduction in a headache compared to a no-treatment control group. Moreover, the feedback group did not differ significantly from the relaxation group in headache reduction. In both treatment groups, improvement was maintained 5 to 7 months after training.

Chesney and Shelton (1976) compared the separate and combined effects of muscle relaxation and biofeedback in the treatment of muscle contraction headache. Four different conditions were utilized: a muscle relaxation group, an EMG biofeedback group, a group which involved a combination of relaxation training and frontal EMG feedback, and a no-treatment condition. Nearly all of the subjects were college undergraduates. Duration of headache history was not given; nor was there any quantification of EMG levels. In this experiment, the biofeedback condition was not significantly better than the no-treatment condition. However, both the muscle relaxation treatment and the combined muscle relaxation and biofeedback treatment were equally more effective than the no-treatment condition with respect to headache frequency and duration. As regards headache severity, it was only the combined treatment which was significantly more effective than the no-treatment control.

Cox, Freundlich, and Meyer (1975) compared frontal EMG feedback with a placebo capsule and the verbal relaxation procedure of Bernstein and Borkovec (1973). Mean age of their patients was 39 years and average duration of headache history was 11 years. Treatment involved two sessions a week for a total of eight sessions. The placebo subjects were administered a green and white capsule at their weekly individual (hourly) sessions. They were told it was a peripherally acting time-release muscle relaxant known to be effective. Both the biofeedback and the verbal relaxation conditions were found to be equally superior treatments to medication placebo in reducing headache activity and frontal EMG levels.

In summarizing the available studies, one can say that the data clearly demonstrate the usefulness of relaxation training in tension headache. EMG feedback is one useful method. Verbally instructed relaxation appears to be another. It should be pointed out that the verbal methods of inducing relaxation are probably more cost-effective than biofeedback since they do not involve expensive electronic equipment and readily lend themselves to group training techniques. On the other hand, it is worth sounding a note of caution, lest we fall into some unnecessary errors. It will be recalled that some quite sophisticated approaches to relaxation such as progressive relaxation and autogenic training have been in existence at least since the 1930's, yet their impact on psychology and psychiatry was for a long time fairly modest. Probably an important reason for this was that, despite their apparent simplicity, these techniques are not very easy to learn well—at least not just from reading a book, and without physiological monitoring it is difficult for both the therapist *as well as the patient* to tell if the latter is learning anything or not. The biofeedback techniques, despite their esoteric flavor, should act to standardize relaxation training and to make it more reliable. At the very least, the feedback instruments will be important as monitoring and checking devices.

MISCELLANEOUS DISORDERS OF LOCALIZED MUSCULAR TENSION: CASE STUDIES

In addition to tension headache, several other disorders involving comparatively localized muscle tension have been treated with EMG feedback. Haynes (1976), for example, reports working with a 25-year-old woman suffering from chronic dysphagia (difficulty swallowing because of constriction of the throat muscles) who was treated with 20 sessions of frontal EMG feedback and home relaxation practice. The patient monitored her difficulty swallowing during meals for 2 months before treatment, during treatment, and after treatment. A significant decrease in swallowing difficulty was associated with frontal EMG feedback training. Improvement was maintained at a 6-month follow-up.

A case of blepharospasm was reported by Peck (1977). This disorder is an eye tic characterized by involuntary clonic and tonic spasms of the eyelids and surrounding muscles. Eye closure, facial spasms, and interference with sight dependent activities can occur. Peck's patient, a 50-year-old woman, was treated with 17 sessions of frontal EMG feedback. Electrodes were placed on the patient's left frontalis and lower orbicularis oculi muscles. In addition to her two baseline sessions, the patient was given two placebo sessions in which she listened to white noise. Although she was told that this would divert her attention from the spasms and thus reduce their frequency, no reduction occurred until EMG feedback training was introduced. Spasm rate dropped from approximately 1600 per 20-minute session during the baseline phase to roughly 15 blinks during the last three treatment sessions.

Levee, Cohen, and Rickles (1976) utilized visual EMG feedback with a woodwind musician who suffered from tics and high levels of tension in his throat and facial muscles. These difficulties had progressed to the point where they interfered with his ability to perform as a professional musician. EMG feedback training was initiated for the muscles showing chronically high tension levels. After 20 sessions the patient showed dramatic reductions in tension levels of throat and facial muscles along with increased proficiency as a musician. It should be emphasized that in the treatment of this man—*as typically occurs in practice—biofeedback was not used as an isolated procedure.* Since the patient had a severe addiction problem, he was first detoxified from alcohol and Dexamyl. Then, after a brief period of psychotherapy, he commenced biofeedback training.

STRESS-RELATED DENTAL DISORDERS

Although dentistry is not generally thought of as a behavioral science area, several common dental disorders have been treated with EMG feedback. These include temporomandibular joint syndrome (TMJ) and bruxism; in both of these an exaggerated reaction to stress can be a prominent etiological factor.

TMJ pain syndrome is defined as a functional disorder of the masticatory system. The most common sympton is a dull, aching pain in the periauricular area, frequently radiating to the ear, face, head and as far as the neck and shoulders. Carlsson and Gale (1977) worked with 11 individuals suffering from TMJ pain of many year's standing. The patients were trained in tension awareness and relaxation by means of EMG feedback from the masseter muscle. At a follow-up examination 4 to 15 months after termination of treatment, 8 of 11 patients were totally symptom-free or significantly better; one patient was slightly better, and there was no effect for two patients. Earlier work with relaxation training for TMJ pain has been described by Gessel and Alderman (1971).

EMG feedback has similarly been employed with bruxism (tooth-grinding), also thought to be stress-related. Solberg and Rugh (1972) used a portable feedback device with 15 bruxist patients. Two-thirds improved significantly while wearing the device.

A recent book by Rugh, Perlis, and Disraeli (1977), *Biofeedback in Dentistry,* is of special interest to behavioral medicine for its description of techniques for assessing stress reactions in everyday life. In addition to interview and questionnaire techniques, Rugh has utilized portable EMG units for monitoring muscle tension responses in real-life situations. It can be expected that such *in vivo* physiological monitoring will become a fertile path of inquiry concerning etiology, diagnosis, and treatment of psychosomatic and stress-linked disorders.

EMG Feedback in the Induction of Generalized Relaxation

A second important area of application lies with disorders in which EMG feedback is used to produce a generalized relaxation response. In this type of application, biofeedback intervention acts in an *indirect* way; that is, the striate muscle relaxation produced by EMG feedback leads to either autonomic or central nervous system (CNS) effects which, in turn, beneficially affect the symptom in question. Examples of disorders in which biofeedback has been utilized in this way include chronic anxiety, sleep-onset insomnia, and essential hypertension. Some pertinent studies will be briefly described; then questions pertaining to the mechanisms thought to be involved will be discussed.

CHRONIC ANXIETY

Recent evidence shows that EMG feedback training can be helpful for chronic anxiety patients. Given the typically refractory nature of this affliction, these results are quite encouraging. Raskin et al. (1973) found frontal EMG feedback training in combination with daily practice of relaxation to be moderately useful for several patients suffering from severe chronic anxiety. Their 10 patients had been troubled by severe anxiety symptoms for a least 3 years, and previous therapeutic efforts by those same investigators—treatment with individual psychotherapy and medication—had not been successful. After considerable biofeedback training, patients proved able to achieve relaxation to a criterion point of 2.5 μV or less on frontal EMG levels. One patient showed dramatic lessening of all his anxiety symptoms. Three other patients found relaxation to be useful in controlling previously intolerable situational anxiety.

In a controlled study, Townsend, House, and Addario (1975) compared chronically anxious patients given EMG feedback training to a matched control group treated with group psychotherapy. In the feedback group, there were significant decreases in EMG levels, mood disturbance, trait anxiety—and, to a lesser extent, state anxiety—that did not occur in the psychotherapy group.

LaVallée, Lamontagne, Pinard, et al. (1977) compared EMG feedback-assisted relaxation with diazepam (Valium)-treated patients. Placebo control conditions were also included. All active treatment groups showed reduced anxiety after treatment, but the Valium—treated patients (with or without EMG feedback) did less well than other subjects on anxiety measurements, medication usage, and home practice of relaxation. The authors conclude that EMG feedback treatment without Valium had a more prolonged therapeutic effect for chronically anxious patients than did the tranquilizing medication.

In this laboratory, we have worked with a number of chronically anxious patients on a case-by-case basis over the past 8 or 9 years (Budzynski and Stoyva, 1975). Our observations indicate that pervasive anxiety patients are able to master a relaxation response if they persist in their biofeedback training. It should be stressed, however, that this step is only a beginning. Once relaxation has been mastered, it is useful to add other interventions such as systematic desensitization, assertive training, modeling, and role-playing. In other words, the patient must not only learn to relax, he must also learn to reshape his coping responses.

INSOMNIA

Sleep-onset insomnia is another disorder for which some useful results have been reported with relaxation training. Unfortunately, most of the reports on insomnia have not utilized the arduous but critical step of all-night EEG monitoring. Such monitoring was, however, included in the four following experiments. Hauri (1978) has reported negative results with EMG-assisted relaxation training. Although his patients (who suffered from insomnia of long standing) stated verbally that they were falling asleep more easily, this improvement was not reflected by reduced sleep latencies as measured by EEG criteria (Note 1). Positive results, however, have been reported by Freedman and Papsdorf (1976a), by Coursey, Frankel, and Gaarder (1976), and Borkovec (1975). The first two experiments employed primarily frontal EMG feedback; Borkovec (1975) used a modified form of progressive relaxation.

ESSENTIAL HYPERTENSION

Several studies suggesting that muscle relaxation can be useful in the management of essential hypertension have been reported. Various types of relaxation training have been employed. For example, Jacobson (1970) reported that cases of moderate essential hypertension respond successfully to progressive relaxation—pressures decrease to within normal range. Klumbies and Eberhardt (see Luthe, 1969, Vol. 2, pp. 70–72), using autogenic training with a group of young adult essential hypertensives, have reported decreases of 35 mm Hg systolic and 18 mm Hg diastolic over a 4-month period. In a Canadian study (Smith, Black, Vanderwel-Johnston, et al., 1975) in which a variant of autogenic training was employed, pressure decrements of 15 mm Hg systolic were reported in a hypertensive group. Control patients, who received direct feedback of blood pressures per se, failed to show any significant decrement. Patel (1975) in several studies has noted favorable results using a combination of feedback-assisted relaxation and a yogic relaxation exercise. Moeller (1973) using techniques of EMG feedback-assisted relaxation developed in this laboratory has also reported significant decrements in pressure. Brady, Luborsky, and Kron (1974), utilizing a metronome-assisted type of relaxation, reported that three out of four hypertensive patients showed significant decreases in blood pressure. Further, when these patients stopped their daily practice of relaxation, their pressures again began to climb. Resumption of daily training again brought about a decrease in pressures.

Some conflicting results have also been reported. Surwit and Shapiro (1977) failed to show significant decreases in blood pressure over a 5-week training period. This lack of training effect was true for each of the three hypertensive groups employed: a group receiving blood pressure feedback through the constant cuff pressure method, an EMG feedback group, and a relaxation group. The discrepancy between this study and the studies described above underscores the need for determining what the causal links might be between muscle relaxation and blood pressure. With this knowledge we should be able to decide which cases of essential hypertension might benefit from systematic relaxation training and which would not. It should be emphasized that essential hypertension—sometimes called "high blood pressure of unknown origin"—is a very broad classification, and consists of those cases having no identifiable organic basis (such as restriction of renal circulation). The diagnosis is basically a residual category. Consequently, it seems unlikely that the same causal mechanisms are involved in every case or that relaxation training will be helpful for every patient. An eminently reasonable endeavor, therefore, is to try to identify some subgroup of hypertensives who respond favorably to relaxation training (Note 2).

ISSUES IN THE GENERALIZATION OF RELAXATION

In the three foregoing disorders—anxiety, insomnia, and essential hypertension—EMG feedback has been utilized for its *indirect* effects. Fundamentally, it is assumed that the relaxation brought about will have autonomic or CNS effects that will help alleviate the symptom in question. It can be seen that this type of EMG feedback application brings up the whole question of the relations between the striate muscle system and the autonomic nervous system (Gellhorn, 1967).

As the author has argued elsewhere (Stoyva, 1976), in using EMG feedback to induce a generalized relaxation response, several related questions arise. These questions form a logical series of steps:

1. For a *particular muscle group,* does EMG feedback result in greater muscular relaxation than do various control conditions?
2. Is there *generalization* of relaxation from the trained muscle to those which are not receiving EMG feedback?
3. Does muscular relaxation affect other bodily systems?
4. What are the *long-term consequences* of the regular daily practice of muscular relaxation? For example, does it produce a shift in the direction of parasympathetic responding? This last question will not be taken up in the present chapter (for a brief discussion, see Stoyva, 1976, p. 383).

The available evidence concerning the first three issues will be presented. Parenthetically, it may be noted that the use of feedback procedures has conceptual as well as practical advantages. With respect to the rather global word "relaxation," for example, biofeedback methodology encourages an analysis of this term into its components—both with respect to the training sequence involved and in studying the effects on various bodily systems.

Feedback Training in a Particular Muscle Group. To date, a great deal of empirical support has accumulated for the contention that EMG feedback is superior to various control conditions when the object is to produce relaxation of a particular muscle (Budzynski and Stoyva, 1969, 1973: Reinking and Kohl, 1975; Coursey, 1975; and others).

Recently, Alexander, White, and Wallace (1977) have raised the issue of whether EMG feedback is really necessary in order to produce a good degree of relaxation. Perhaps non-feedback techniques are just as efficient. These investigators found that verbally instructed (young normal) subjects reached as good a degree of relaxation as did the subjects receiving EMG feedback (relaxation was assessed by frontal EMG levels). Special efforts were made toward motivating control subjects to perform normally.

While it is certainly a worthwhile development to be able to cultivate relaxation without biofeedback apparatus—we want techniques that are not only effective but economical—there are several questions worth raising about this topic: (a) Are the results with verbal relaxation instructions readily replicable? (b) Is retention of the response good, especially under stressful conditions? (c) What are the results with a clinical population? For any relaxation technique, a point of key interest is its usefulness with a population in which difficulty in relaxing is a prominent part of the symptom structure. The answers to these questions will require careful comparative studies among the various techniques which have been utilized to produce relaxation (Additionally, we will need studies which examine the various components of relaxation such as frequency of practice, striate muscle relaxation per se versus cognitive strategies such as the repetition of certain phrases, the cultivation of passive volition, and so forth.)

It is also worth pointing out, as Jacobson (1929) did some time ago, that simply telling the tense individual "to relax" is no guarantee of success. Instead, as Jacobson emphasized, it is important that the individual be taught a set of relaxation skills.

GENERALIZATION TO OTHER MUSCLES. Some controversy has arisen regarding the second issue mentioned above, i.e., if feedback training brings about relaxation in one muscle, does this relaxation generalize to other untrained muscle groups? Unfortunately, the evidence on this point is not yet as clear as we would like.

In our laboratory, generalization to other muscles typically seems to occur; at the very least, the untrained muscles do not go in the wrong direction. For example, in a study conducted some time ago (Stoyva and Budzynski, 1974, pp. 273–274), we examined whether some muscles are better than others for promoting general bodily relaxation. In this experiment, we ran 21 college age male volunteers under one of the following three conditions: (a) one group received variable-rate auditory clicks from the frontalis; (b) a second group received variable rate clicks from the forearm extensor; (c) the control group, received tape recorded clicks produced by the frontalis feedback subjects.

The results showed that only the frontal EMG feedback subjects declined on *both* frontal and forearm EMG levels. According to these data, when the frontalis is low, the forearm is also likely to be low, but the converse relationship does not hold. Subjects receiving forearm feedback decreased substantially on forearm EMG levels, but remained virtually the same on frontal EMG levels.

Opinion on the generalization issue, however, has been less than unanimous. An experiment by Alexander (1975) indicates an absence of generalization. In this study, feedback of frontal EMG activity was utilized in normal subjects. EMG activity was simultaneously recorded from sites on the frontalis, the forearm extensor muscles, and the extensors of the lower leg. Although EMG levels declined significantly at the frontalis location, such a change failed to occur at the forearm and lower leg sites. Oddly enough, forearm EMG levels even showed a significant *increase* over the 5 training days. This was true for both experimentals and controls.

Shedivy and Kleinman (1977) have similarly reported a failure of generalization when frontal EMG feedback was utilized. They recorded EMG activity simultaneously from a frontal site and the semispinalis and splenius capitus muscles. Frontal EMG showed a significant decline. But EMG activity from the semispinalis and splenius muscles not only failed to decrease but actually increased significantly.

What are we to conclude from these conflicting observations? Several interpretations may be proposed:

1. Generalization does not occur. The experiments of Alexander (1975) and Shedivy and Kleinman (1977) would support this position.

2. Generalization of relaxation does occur, but it is very limited in extent. The observations of Freedman and Papsdorf (1976a,b) may be offered in support of this interpretation. In these studies, it was noted that when frontal feedback was given, a significant decline occurred in levels of both frontal and masseter EMG activity, but not in forearm extensor activity.

3. Generalization occurs, but the extent of it varies considerably depending both upon the individual and on the conditions of the experiment. Certainly anyone who has himself worked with frontal EMG feedback is aware that low frontal EMG levels seem to occur only when other facial muscles are also at a very relaxed level and eye movements have ceased (Basmajian, 1976). Moreover, Basmajian (1976) also remarks that with low frontal EMG activity the entire upper body is simultaneously relaxed.

If this third interpretation is correct (which is the one we favor), then we are left with the question of *specifying the conditions which promote the occurrence of generalization.* One such condition is the *set* of the subject. Has he or she been instructed as to how to use his or her relaxation skill? That is, once he or she has learned to relax a particular muscle well, are there instructions to employ this skill on other untrained muscles as well?

Other contextual aspects of the experiment are also important. For example, have steps been taken to make the subject feel at ease? One suspects that sometimes the experimental setting can appear forbidding or oppressively complicated, a circumstance not likely to promote extensive relaxation.

In any case, as the writer already proposed (Stoyva, 1976), the matter of generalization can really be broken down into two issues: (a) Does generalization to other muscles occur *automatically*? It is this question to which the above studies have been addressed. (b) Even if generalization does not occur automatically, perhaps it can be *made to occur*. A few words on this topic are in order.

To begin with, there is no reason why feedback training should be limited to the frontalis muscle. For example, subjects may receive feedback from widely separated muscle groups, either simultaneously or sequentially (Note 3). An instance of the latter can be seen in the study of Sittenfeld, Budzynski and Stoyva (1976). Here, the object was to teach subjects to produce the theta rhythms characteristic of low arousal. When this rhythm is dominant the individual is almost asleep. It was found that the most effective method of teaching subjects to augment theta was to use muscle relaxation training *prior* to initiating theta training. Thus, as a means of beginning the shift to low arousal, subjects were first given four sessions of EMG training. The intial session consisted of auditory forearm EMG feedback. This was followed by three sessions of auditory frontal EMG feedback. It should be stressed that while they were receiving auditory frontal EMG feedback, the subjects continued receiving a degree of information feedback regarding forearm activity. This was in the form of visual feedback. As long as his forearm remained relaxed, the subject would see a green light. If he tensed up and exceeded his criterion level, then the light turned red. Following their four EMG training sessions, subjects next received four sessions of theta EEG feedback. Finally, there were two post-baseline sessions in which no feedback of any kind was given. When pre-baseline and post-baseline levels of various parameters were compared, it could be seen that not only had frontal EMG levels dropped dramatically, but forearm EMG values had remained at extremely low levels (averaging $<1.0\ \mu V$). Moreover, theta levels—measured by pulses from a resetting integrator—rose to 50% above baseline levels. These results support the conclusion that the striate muscle and cortical systems, at least in the relaxed, pre-sleep condition, are likely to move in the same low arousal direction.

In sum, it seems reasonable to conclude that a degree of generalization does occur. The important remaining practical problem will be how to maximize this effect. One approach, as in the above Sittenfeld et al. (1976) experiment, is to train subjects on more than one muscle group—either simultaneously or sequentially (for procedural details, see Budzynski, Stoyva, and Peffer, in press). Further, it should be noted that biofeedback is by no means a static enterprise. Innovations can be expected. For example, several laboratories, including our own, are experimenting with a "wrist-to-wrist" electrode placement (in which an active electrode is placed on each wrist). This configuration appears sensitive to EMG activity in the arms, shoulder girdle and neck regions. Respiratory and heart rate activity are also reflected in the character of the auditory feedback signal. Thus, if a subject learns to produce low EMG activity at both frontal and "wrist-to-wrist" locations, it should result in an extensive relaxation response.

DOES MUSCLE RELAXATION AFFECT OTHER BODILY SYSTEMS? A related, and more fundamental question, is how muscle relaxation might affect other bodily systems. Let us first make note of several observations which indicate that such generalization to other systems frequently does occur. Then let us consider what the available evidence is concerning the mechanisms responsible for these effects.

Examples of Generalization to Other Systems. As early as 1923, Jacobson (1938, p. 368) noted that in patients suffering from spastic esophagus—a condition which makes it difficult to swallow—the spasticity was eliminated after the patient utilized a progressive relaxation response. In other words, striate muscle relaxation led to relaxation of esophageal smooth muscle. The method of observing the esophagus was the fluoroscopic technique in which patients were X-rayed after swallowing radio-opaque barium paste.

More recently, Connor (1974) found that when he gave subjects only a brief training in progressive relaxation, they showed smaller skin conductance and heart rate responses when exposed to a stressful stimulus than did the controls. In this laboratory, Budzynski (1969) noted that muscle relaxation produced a lessened ability to discriminate temporally paired flashes of light—a sign of decreased cortical arousal (Venables and Wing, 1962). As already mentioned, muscle relaxation training is a useful prelude to the induction of EEG theta rhythms, a drowsy condition (Sittenfeld et al., 1976). Indeed, subjects with high baseline muscle tension levels were only able to learn the subtle response of theta enhancement after receiving training in muscle relaxation.

A recent pertinent experiment by DeGood and Chisholm (1977) involved a comparison of frontal EMG feedback and parietal alpha EEG feedback. In essence, frontal EMG affected alpha levels, but the converse was not true. Thus, as frontal EMG levels *decreased* (in the EMG feedback condition) alpha levels significantly *increased.* However, in the alpha feedback condition, an increase in alpha did not lead to a significant decrement in frontal EMG. Also, it was observed that when frontal EMG levels decreased, subjects simultaneously showed significant decreases in heart rate and respiration rate, and increases in alpha levels. Of five measures, only finger pulse volume failed to shift in the expected direction.

Evidence is also available to show that when EMG levels are *increased,* other systems move in an ergotropic direction (to use Hess's term). Thus, Lynch, Schuri, and D'Anna (1976) noted a close association between muscular exercise and cardiovascular effects. Subjects performed two isometric exercises at three levels of exertion. The two muscle groups involved were located either in the hand *or* the foot. In the case of each exercise condition, there were significant increases in heart rate and respiration, as well as significant decreases in finger pulse amplitude and skin temperature. The authors, moreover, conclude that in autonomic conditioning experiments, even moderate contractions of muscles at some distance from the site of recorded autonomic activity, may be producing the autonomic changes. For example, muscle contractions could be producing increases in heart rate and decreases in skin temperature and relaxation might have the opposite effects. These results are similar to those reported some years ago by Pinneo (1961), who noted a variety of activational responses as subjects vigorously grasped a hand dynamometer.

POSSIBLE MECHANISMS

In view of the many observations which support the idea that muscle relaxation has effects on other systems, which are characteristically in the direction of low arousal, it becomes important to determine what the responsible mechanisms might be. Since the observed effects are quite extensive in nature, our supposition is that multiple mechanisms are probably involved. Some of these may be of a direct mechanical nature. One example would be the action of the leg muscles upon blood pressure in leg veins, for example. Other mechanisms of a indirect nature probably involve effects on the CNS. These changes in CNS activities, in turn, have autonomic consequences which are probably mediated by the hypothalamus, the "head ganglion" of the autonomic nervous system (Gellhorn and Kiely, 1972). Listed below are four possible mechanisms through which muscle relaxation might exercise effects upon other systems such as the autonomic nervous system and the CNS.

Direct Effects. Perhaps striate muscle relaxation has a direct effect on certain autonomic responses. One instance would be the action of muscle activity on blood flow in the legs. Thus, it is known that striate *muscle activity* influences the efficiency of venous return from the arms and legs; the leg muscles exert a rhythmic action upon the leg veins. This pumping, or more accurately a venous "milking" action, alternately increases and decreases pressure on the wall of the vein, and venous return to the heart is accelerated (see Folkow and Neil, 1971, pp. 409–410).

Nutrient Demands of Active versus Resting Muscle. The nutrient requirement of resting muscle is only a fraction of that utilized by the same muscle during strenuous exercise. For example, at rest, only 20% of total oxygen consumption is utilized by skeletal muscle. However, during vigorous exercise, 90% or more of total oxygen is consumed by the muscle system (see Folkow and Neil, 1971, pp. 399–401).

These observations suggest that relaxation of the striate muscle system, as occurs in the resting individual, should lead to a reduced load on the various organs comprising the cardiovascular system—such as heart, lungs and blood vessels.

PROPRIOCEPTIVE EFFECTS ON HYPOTHALAMIC NUCLEI. As Hess (1954) and others (e.g., Dempsey, 1951) have pointed out, the somatic and autonomic nervous systems are intimately linked at the level of central representation. Although the two systems are clearly separated at peripheral sites, the opposite is true in the CNS. For example, under hypothalamic stimulation, the two systems act together. Thus, with stimulation of the posterior hypothalamus, there is a simultaneous sympathetic outflow and behavioral activation—as in a rage response. In order to emphasize the integrated action of muscle and autonomic systems, Hess coined the terms "ergotropic" and "trophotropic." Thus, a rage response would classify as an "ergotropic" reaction, since there is sympathetic discharge along with muscle activity.

A specific model designed to account for the multiple effects of muscle relaxation has been proposed by the neurophysiologist Gellhorn who builds on the work of Hess. A major impetus to Gellhorn's formulation of this model was his noting of similarities in the physiological consequences of progressive relaxation, autogenic training, and certain forms of meditation.

In the model advanced by Gellhorn and Kiely (1972), they first cite the work of Hess concerning the distinction between ergotropic and trophotropic systems. Gellhorn and Kiely propose that the *balance* between ergotropic and trophotropic systems may be altered in two fundamentally different ways: (a) a *direct stimulation* of ergotropic or trophotropic "centers" in the hypothalamus or other cerebral areas; (b) by *indirect stimulation* of the two systems. The latter may be accomplished either by altering input from the cerebral cortex, or by changing afferent input impinging on the reticular formation and hypothalamus. Particularly effective in changing proprioceptive input are discharges from the muscle system. Gellhorn (1958) has previously shown, in animal preparations, that reduction of proprioception through curare-like drugs greatly reduces the ergotropic responsiveness of the hypothalamus and diminishes hypothalamic-cortical discharges. The loss of muscle tone produced by these drugs promotes drowsiness and sleep. In other words, there is a shift toward trophotropic activity. Similar results have been reported by Hodes (1962). When he injected Flaxedil (a curare-like drug) into the veins of cats, their EEGs quickly showed signs of drowsiness and sleep. In interpreting the signs of sleep observed in his cats, Hodes suggested that the probable mechanism involved was a *feedback system from muscle receptors to sites in the central nervous system.*

Gellhorn and Kiely (1972) suggest that it is this hypothalamic mechanism which accounts for many of the similarities among progressive relaxation, autogenic training, Wolpe's systematic desensitization procedure, and certain techniques of meditation. In each, muscular relaxation results in reduced proprioceptive input to the hypothalamus, a diminution of hypothalamic-cortical discharges, and a dominance of the trophotropic system through reciprocal innervation.

CORTICAL TRIGGERING OF ACTIVATION. Muscle relaxation probably affects the CNS in another important way. It may, through feedback loops in the nervous system, produce CNS changes which act to prevent the triggering of any (generalized) activation pattern, including the defense-alarm reaction.

Ample evidence has accumulated from psychophysiological and psychosomatic research over the past quarter century that the defense-alarm reaction, an activation pattern, can be cortically triggered. The neuroendocrinologist, Mason (1972), even maintains that in the case of man it is chiefly *psychological influences* which are responsible for eliciting the hormonal reactions to stress—as opposed to the more "purely" physical agents of the type cited by Selye (1956).

Actually, there is quite a bit of evidence suggesting that muscle relaxation acts to produce CNS changes incompatible with the elicitation of an activation response. When the condition of muscle relaxation is examined from an experiential viewpoint, its salient features are these: The individual is in a markedly non-striving condition; what remains of his mental activity is very much "present-centered," and active, problem-oriented thinking has disappeared.

EEG evidence suggests a similar conclusion. For example, Sittenfeld et al. (1976) noted that when levels of frontal EMG activity became very low (3.50 μV or less with filter bandpass at 95–1000 Hz), then the occurrence of sleep-onset theta rhythms was highly probable. It is also worth noting that, many years ago, Jacobson (1938) maintained that when facial and laryngeal EMG activity dropped to extremely low levels (zero or close to zero EMG values), then the individual was asleep. The reader will also recall the observations of Hodes (1962). In each of 24 Flaxedil-treated cats the EEG showed a shift from alert waking pattern to synchronized patterns (slow waves and "spindles") characteristic of sleep 15 or more minutes after the injection.

These various observations support the inference that extensive muscle relaxation is closely associated with lowered cortical arousal. It is quite conceivable that a cortical condition of lowered arousal may act to prevent the elicitation of the individual's defense-alarm reaction, regardless of any more direct effects exerted by muscle relaxation. Such a phenomenon could be expected to have widespread physiological consequences since it would affect the various components of the defense-alarm reaction, a response which has been implicated in various stress-related disorders (Alexander, 1950; Folkow and Neil, 1971; Selye, 1956; Wolff, 1968).

Parenthetically, it should be noted if the foregoing mechanism is the chief way in which muscle relaxation operates, then other means of producing a change in consciousness may be similarly useful in aborting an activation response. These other means could include acquisition of biofeedback control over parameters such as alpha EEG, skin temperature, and the electrodermal response—all of which seem to involve a shift to a relaxed, non-striving condition, and which are associated with reduced sympathetic activity.

Furthermore, it could be expected that a variety of attention-shifting or attention-absorbing devices might be just as useful as biofeedback techniques in preventing cortical triggering of activation. These, depending on the individual, could be as diverse as meditation, observing nature, listening to concerts, being in the company of friends, engaging in various games, and so forth.

Applications in Neuromuscular Rehabilitation

A third group of disorders to which EMG feedback techniques have been applied lies in the area of neuromuscular rehabilitation. Applications in this area typically occur in a physical medicine or neurology setting and can be conveniently viewed as separate from the psychosomatic work already described.

In addition to its use in relaxation training, a topic which has been dealt with in some detail already, there are at least two other ways in which EMG feedback may be utilized. One is to use EMG feedback as a means of the controlling very fine units of electromyographic activity, such as the modification of single motor unit firing (Basmajian, 1974). The first reports describing the use of external EMG feedback in the control of single motor unit activity were those of Harrison and Mortenson (1962) and Basmajian (1963). Over the past decade, these original reports have been followed up extensively by Basmajian (1974) and his associates.

A second use of EMG feedback in physical medicine has been to bring about improvement or recovery of function in neuromuscular disorders. Of particular interest here are cases of peripheral nerve-muscle damage, and central nervous system dysfunctions such as stroke and torticollis. A valuable discussion of this work may be found in the review by Inglis, Campbell, and Donald (1976).

DISORDERS OF THE CENTRAL NERVOUS SYSTEM

Spasmodic Torticollis. This condition, also known as "wry neck," is characterized by episodic spasms of the neck muscles. These spasms cause an involuntary and apparently uncontrollable twisting of the head to a distorted and uncomfortable position on one side. The etiology of spasmodic torticollis remains obscure. One school of thought regards it as a consequence of basal ganglia dysfunction. Others think the disorder is a conversion hysterical phenomenon. Since EMG feedback techniques have shown a measure of success, and since conventional physiotherapy procedures have not been particularly successful in treating this disorder, further investigation of biofeedback approaches is clearly warranted.

An early treatment approach, and one of considerable historical interest, was the investigation of Meige and Feindel (1907) who had the patient use a mirror as a means of training himself both in producing movement and in eliminating it. By observing his reflection, the patient could be quickly informed of any mistakes in his execution of a given exercise; in other words, the mirror provided visual feedback of bodily movements.

In recent years, Cleeland (1973) has utilized a combination of EMG feedback training and aversive conditioning in the treatment of torticollis. By means of surface electrodes EMG activity from the sternocleidomastoid muscle was presented to the patient as an auditory signal, a tone of varying pitch. The patient's task was to keep the tone at a low frequency by relaxing the muscle. In addition, the patient received a mildly aversive shock which was triggered by rising EMG activity in the neck muscle.

Frequency of spasmodic activity in the neck showed a marked decrease during the actual training sessions in 8 of the 10 patients. Most of the patients, furthermore, showed improvement which lasted beyond the laboratory training period. At the end of the follow-up period (mean of 19 months), 6 patients had maintained substantial improvement.

Encouraging results have also been reported by Brudny, Grynbaum, and Korein (1974) who used a somewhat different training technique. Not only did patients receive EMG feedback from the muscle producing the torticollis, they were also instructed to exercise by contraction of the muscles on the other side of the neck. This helped patients to maintain equal muscle outputs on both sides of the neck. The authors reported that 7 of 9 patients were greatly helped by the training and were able to control their spasms voluntarily in the absence of EMG feedback.

In view of the fairly intractable nature of torticollis, the foregoing reports are clearly encouraging. However, as Inglis et al. (1976) pointed out, these studies leave many questions unanswered. In particular, suitable control groups need to be utilized. Other issues, such as the role of electric shock, need to be examined. Does it function as an aversive stimulus or as an additional form of feedback? Fundamentally, though, one suspects that a really high degree of therapeutic success with this disorder will not occur until we acquire a precise knowledge of the mechanisms responsible for it.

STROKE. Stroke, which is typically the result of a cerebrovascular accident, can produce many impairments of function, including a variety of disorders of muscular control. A major impairment is hemiplegia. Here there is a disturbance of voluntary movement on one side of the body with an ensuing paralysis. Generally, there are associated disturbances in muscular tone; sometimes this is reflected in spasticity, at other times in flaccidity.

The first report describing the use of EMG feedback with the rehabilitation of voluntary movement of stroke hemiplegia was by Marinacci and Horande (1960). Curiously, though, despite the encouraging nature of the results, even Marinacci (1968) himself does not appear to have followed them up to any extent. One case treated with EMG feedback was a 64-year-old man suffering from left-sided hemiplegia. When needle electrodes were inserted into the muscles of his left deltoid, no voluntary nerve impulses were apparent. The investigators then placed an electrode into the intact right deltoid and the patient was shown how his muscle activity on this normal side could produce auditory feedback. Surprisingly, when the EMG electrodes were again inserted into the paralyzed left deltoid muscle, the investigators noted that the patient was able to activate from 10 to 15% of motor units where previously there had been a complete absence of such activity. Other muscles of the left hand such as the triceps, the extensors and flexors, and the hand muscles were treated with the same procedure. In less than an hour, the patient was able to develop something like 20% function in the muscles of the previously paralyzed arm.

More recently, Johnson and Garton (1973) worked with a group of 11 hemiparetic patients afflicted with foot dorsiflexion paralysis (foot-drop). Both auditory and visual feedback were utilized. After first inserting electrodes into the paralyzed tibialis anterior muscle, both visual and auditory feedback were provided. Training sessions were 30 minutes a day over a 3-day period. Following this, patients were given portable EMG units equipped with surface EMG electrodes for extensive home practice. Outcomes for the 11 patients were as follows: three patients improved so much that they could walk without their short leg braces; four showed moderate improvement; the remaining patients failed to show much evidence of improvement.

In New York, Brudny and his associates have treated hemiparesis by means of auditory and visual EMG feedback techniques. Surface EMG electrodes were utilized. Recently, Brudny, Korein, Grynbaum, et al. (1976) summarized their results with the biofeedback in 45 cases of hemiparesis. Thirty-nine of these cases involved paralyses of the arm. At follow-up times, which ranged from 3 months to 3 years, 20 of these 39 patients had retained significant gains in arm function.

It will be noted that the previous reports were uncontrolled studies. A recent investigation which did, however, utilize a control group was described by Basmajian, Kukulka, Narayan, et al. (1975). Twenty patients suffering from chronic foot-drop after stroke were randomly divided into two groups of 10. The control subjects received conventional physiotherapy for three 40-minute sessions a week for 5 weeks. Over the same span of time, the experimental group received an equal number of sessions. The first part of each session consisted of 20 minutes of standard physiotherapy exercises. The second 20 minutes consisted of biofeedback training with a miniature EMG muscle trainer (Kukulka and Basmajian, 1975). Following treatment, the increase in both strength and range of motion in the biofeedback group was almost twice as great as in the conventional physiotherapy control group. Four patients in the biofeedback group achieved and retained conscious control of dorsiflexion; three of these patients were later able to walk without the use of a short leg brace. Such evidence of marked improvement was much less apparent in the control group.

Cerebral Palsy. Cerebral palsy is a disorder involving sensorimotor dysfunction arising from brain damage that has generally occurred before or around the time of birth. Patients typically suffer from disorders of posture and gait and stereotyped abnormal patterns of movement, and they show both spastic and flaccid paralyses as well as characteristic involuntary, athetoid (twisting) movements.

It should be noted that the application of feedback methodology to cerebral palsy need not be limited to electromyographic activity. For example, Harris, Spelman, and Hymer (1974), in an attempt to restore or supplement defective proprioceptive feedback so as to normalize movements in their patients, developed one device for the control of head posture and another for assessing limb position. The guiding idea behind the development of these devices was the hypothesis of Harris (1971) that a possible basis for the athetoid movements in cerebral palsy was "inappropriception." This term refers to a faulty kinesthetic monitoring based on defective or disordered proprioceptive feedback. The aim of Harris, Spelman, and Hymer (1974) was to develop electronic sensory aides that would provide these children with external feedback of a kind that would carry correct information about their posture and movements.

All of the 18 children using the head control device improved considerably in head stability. It was also noted that all of the children using the limb position monitor showed a decrease in tremor and improvement in the smoothness and accuracy of arm movements. Range of motion at the elbow joint also increased. There also seemed to be considerable generalization of these improvements to other settings.

Another approach to cerebral palsy has utilized EMG feedback as a means of producing relaxation. The work of Finley, Niman, Stanley, et al. (1976) began with an attempt to use sensorimotor (SMR) feedback with cerebral palsy patients. What Finley *et al.* (1976) noted, however, was that with these patients muscle activity of the head and face was at such a high level that it was not possible to detect SMR. Consequently, as a means of reducing unwanted EMG activity before commencing SMR training, they provided one patient with frontal EMG feedback. The patient proved able to effect substantial reductions in frontal EMG activity. Surprisingly, the child then seemed improved in many respects, according to his parents. This unexpected observation led to work with five additional patients. With the six patients described in the initial report, frontal EMG levels on the average decreased from 28.9 to 13.0 μv. The children were tested before and after the EMG feedback training on a number of measures. Typically, the patients were improved in terms of both fine and gross coordination, they showed less tremor and many could even articulate words more clearly. One interesting observation was that some of these patients became better at detecting their own muscular sensations. For example, one patient reported:

> After the third session, I was still becoming aware of tension in my body that I hadn't been aware of before. There were muscles that had been in a constant state of tension during most of my waking life. . .and. . .when I began to learn to relax these muscles for the first time, I began to experience sensation. Coming out of the third session, I noted slight changes in my coordination. I noticed more of the feeling of separation in the muscles in my hand. I found that if I would take a few seconds to relax before I did something like handling a cup of coffee, I could do it with more ease and coordination. I found that if I would stop a few seconds and recall the feelings of relaxation that I experienced during the feedback session, I could usually become truly relaxed in a very short period of time and after that I would usually have better coordination in whatever I was doing (Finley *et al.*, 1976, p. 180).

SPINAL CORD INJURIES. Several cases have been reported in which EMG feedback has been utilized with patients suffering from spinal cord injuries. Central to this use of EMG feedback has been the assumption that some pathways still remain for the transmission of neural impulses. According to Fernando (1978), such patients can be evaluated for treatment by using EMG monitoring as a means of determining whether the lesion is complete or incomplete (i.e., is there any residual electromyographic activity or not?). Subsequently, EMG feedback can be used to enhance the EMG activity which remains. Not only can it be used to bring about desired movements but to inhibit spasticity as well.

Some of the case reports in the literature are those of Seymour and Bassler (1977), Fernando (1976), and Toomin and Johnson (1974). In these studies, EMG feedback was initially employed as a tool to determine which muscles were still innervated and was then subsequently used to enhance activity in these muscles. Since, in these various studies, other therapeutic programs were used in addition to EMG feedback, it is difficult to evaluate precisely the results that were due to feedback *per se*. Nonetheless, it is worth noting that the EMG monitoring and feedback procedures helped both patients and therapists to locate target muscles which originally had not shown any signs of function.

PERIPHERAL NERVE DAMAGE

Another area of neuromuscular rehabilitation deals with patients suffering from peripheral nerve damage. An early account of EMG feedback used therapeutically with such patients was that of Marinacci and Horande (1960). These investigators recorded EMG impulses from impaired muscles and then converted the output to auditory signals which, in turn, provided the patient with feedback information about his muscle activity. This technique appeared to be an effective means of restoring voluntary motor control in many of their patients.

In their paper, Marinacci and Horande described a series of five patients suffering from Bell's palsy, that is, facial paralysis caused by damage or impaired function of the seventh cranial nerve. A description of one patient, a 19-year-old man suffering from a right-sided Bell's palsy, will serve to illustrate their technique. The initial step was to detect some electromyographic activity in the paralyzed side of the patient's face. He was then shown how the intact side of his face could control an EMG feedback signal. Next, he was provided with auditory feedback from the partially paralyzed side. Training was carried out twice a week for a 6-month period. Over the course of that time, the amplitude of motor unit signals increased approximately fourfold. At his last session, the patient had recovered about 40% function of the right orbicularis and frontalis.

These same investigators also reported on a series of post-poliomyelitis patients suffering from residual paralyses. This disorder, a lower motor neuron dysfunction, involves damage to the anterior motor horn cell in the spinal cord. Many of these patients showed improvement even though their paralyses had been of considerable duration. Marinacci and Horande (1960) concluded that where some minimal muscle function remains, it can be increased with feedback training, even in cases where other methods of therapy such as physical treatment, electrical stimulation, and reconstructive surgery have failed.

Another report describing treatment of a peripheral neuromuscular disorder was that of Jacobs and Felton (1969). They utilized EMG feedback to assist muscle relaxation in a group of patients who experienced difficulty in relaxing the trapezius muscle after having suffered neck injury. In this controlled study, 10 patients with injuries were compared to a group of 10 normal subjects. In the first half of the session, when no feedback was provided, the patients with neck injuries had much more difficulty than the control subjects in relaxing the trapezius muscle group. It was most interesting to note, however, that in the second half of the session, when visual feedback was provided, the EMG levels of the experimental subjects quickly reached the same level as those achieved by the normal group.

CONCLUSIONS ABOUT REHABILITATION

It can be fairly said that the biofeedback developments in rehabilitation are indeed most encouraging. Particularly exciting are the cases where recovery of function has occurred in disabilities of many year's duration. Moreover, many types of symptoms have been treated such as spasticity, flaccidity, and movement disorders. Biofeedback technology may be regarded as a natural and logical extension of the training and re-education efforts that occupy a central place in physical medicine. It seems likely, too, that for the most part, biofeedback procedures will be incorporated into regular physical medicine settings where the need for sophisticated diagnosis and the use of additional medical treatments can be effectively coordinated into the treatment program as a whole.

Despite these encouraging developments, however, there is clearly room for much additional work. A very high incidence of the studies cited have been either case reports or uncontrolled group-outcome investigations. Often there has been little precise description concerning the condition of the patients. Many of the reports have suffered from sketchy descriptions not only of the presenting problem, but of the intervention technique itself and subsequent assessments of improvement. One would want to know something about the type of lesion, the presence of sensory or cognitive deficits in addition to motor ones, the age of the patient, the time since the accident occurred, and the nature of the symptom treated—whether it was spasticity, flaccidity, or clonus.

In view of the promising results to date, the need for additional controlled experiments is quite important. It will be necessary to control for nonspecific factors such as improved motivation, and the possibility of spontaneous recovery (especially if the lesion has been of recent origin). Convincing control conditions will have to be utilized so that it can be determined how much of the effect is attributable to biofeedback intervention per se. Eventually, comparisons with standard physiotherapy techniques will have to be made in order to determine whether biofeedback techniques are more efficacious or not. More attention will have to be paid to the characteristics, physiological and psychological, of the patients who are likely to benefit. It can be presumed that, as with most treatment techniques, there will be marked individual differences in response to biofeedback.

Finally, it should be noted that it is unrealistic to expect high levels of therapeutic success until the origins of a particular disorder are precisely understood. In physical medicine, for example, the mechanisms involved in cerebral palsy and in torticollis remain obscure. As the etiology of these afflictions becomes better known, the place of biofeedback interventions should also become more clear. The same statement no doubt holds true for the other disorders discussed in this chapter as well.

General Conclusions

Finally, a word or two needs to be said about relaxation in general and the place of

EMG feedback in its induction. Over the past 10 years, EMG feedback has emerged as the clinical workhorse of the biofeedback area; and, by now, there is a network of evidence from many sources that relaxation techniques are useful in a great many disorders of a psychosomatic (psychophysiological) nature. This evidence derives from progressive relaxation (Jacobson, 1938), from autogenic training (Luthe, 1969), from certain meditation techniques and their variants (Benson, 1975), as well as from the EMG feedback procedures outlined in this chapter.

Given that there are various relaxation techniques now in existence, it should occasion no surprise if some argument occurs as to which is most effective. Although important, this is basically a technical question which will be resolved over time. It should not be allowed to obscure a more basic issue in the clinical application of biofeedback and behavioral procedures. Historically, the first issue has been to find out whether there is any effect at all with the use of a particular biofeedback or behavioral techniques for a given disorder. Once we see an effect, then we can pursue the other questions: How can the effect be maximized? Will it survive the scrutiny of controlled studies? Are there alternative procedures for inducing relaxation which are just as effective as EMG feedback but more economical? And lastly a major question: What are the causal mechanisms involved? Specifically, how does the biofeedback intervention impinge upon the pathophysiological mechanisms thought to be involved in the disorder? It is worth noting that within the history of medicine, effective and rational therapies have rarely emerged until a clear understanding of causation was at hand. (Note 4).

Notes

1. Hauri (1978) did, however, observe favorable results with sensorimotor rhythm feedback. The learning of sensorimotor rhythm was significantly associated with improvement in laboratory sleep. Hauri also makes the valuable suggestion that the type of biofeedback training provided should be tailored to the deficiency shown by the particular insomniac. For example, EMG feedback training would be given to the patient showing signs of high arousal, but not to the one who is already relaxed. Some experimental data in support of this idea are reported by Hauri.
2. The matter of individual differences in response to biofeedback or relaxation treatments is a very important one. Thus, in the case of hypertension, for example, it seems likely that some individuals might respond very strongly. Who are they; can they be identified? In most disorders in which biofeedback treatment can be attempted, individuality of response will probably turn out to be a key phenomenon. Thus, biofeedback may prove useful for *some* cases of essential hypertension, *some* cases of insomnia, *some* types of anxiety and so forth. Over the next decade, we can expect to see more light shed on this matter.
3. It should be emphasized that there is no reason to confine EMG feedback training to the frontalis muscle—although this laboratory has sometimes been accused of advocating just such an approach. Actually, for many years we have strongly recommended a "shaping of low arousal" technique which typically involves feedback training at several sites (Stoyva and Budzynski, 1974, as well as earlier publications).
4. An attempt to provide a rationale for the use of biofeedback in stress-related (functional) disorders is elaborated in a recent paper by the author (Stoyva, 1977). A model is presented which is based upon an earlier one proposed by Sternbach. The model is essentially psychophysiological in nature and involves a psychological triggering of the defense-alarm reaction. Key concepts are response-stereotypy under stress, and the gradual failure of recovery mechanisms. On the basis of the model, it is proposed that biofeedback intervention may be useful at one or more of four points: (1) in reducing aberrant activity under resting conditions; (2) in reducing excessive responding under stress conditions; (3) in speeding recovery to resting (unstressed levels); or, (4) through action on the CNS, in preventing the defense-alarm reaction from being triggered at all. A useful feature of the model is that it emphasizes the importance of looking at the aberrant response, not just under resting conditions, but also during a stress episode and in the period following stressful stimulation, i.e., in the recovery phase.

References

Alexander, A. B. An experimental test of assumptions relating to the use of electromyographic biofeedback as a general relaxation technique. *Psychophysiology,* 1975, *12,* 656–662.

Alexander, A. B., White, P. D., and Wallace, H. M. Training and transfer of training effects in EMG biofeedback assisted muscular relaxation. *Psychophysiology,* 1977, *14,* 551–559.

Alexander, F. *Psychosomatic medicine.* New York: Norton & Co., Inc. 1950.

Basmajian, J. V. Control and training of individual motor units. *Science,* 1963, *141,* 440–441.

Basmajian, J. V. *Muscles alive: Their functions revealed by electromyography,* 3rd ed. Baltimore: Williams & Wilkins, 1974.

Basmajian, J. V. Facts vs. myths in EMG biofeedback. *Biofeedback Self-Regulation,* 1976, *1,* 369–371.

Basmajian, J. V., Kukulka, C. G., Narayan, M. G., and

Takebe, K. Biofeedback treatment of foot-drop after stroke compared with standard rehabilitation technique: Effects on voluntary control and strength. *Arch. Phys. Med. Rehabil.,* 1975, *56,* 231–236.

Benson, H. *The relaxation response.* New York: William Morrow & Co., 1975.

Bernstein, D. A., and Borkovec, T. D. *Progressive relaxation training: A manual for the helping professions.* Champaign, Ill.: Research Press, 1973.

Borkovec, T. D. Progressive relaxation treatment of sleep disturbance. Paper presented at the second annual meeting of the American Association for the Advancement of Tension Control, Chicago, October, 1975.

Brady, J. P., Luborsky, L., and Kron, R. E. Blood pressure reduction in patients with essential hypertension through metronome-conditioned relaxation: A preliminary report. *Behav. Ther.,* 1974, *5,* 203–209.

Brudny, J., Grynbaum, B. B., and Korein, J. Spasmodic torticollis: Treatment by feedback display of the EMG. *Arch. Phys. Med. Rehabil.,* 1974, *55,* 403–408.

Brudny, J., Korein, J., Grynbaum, B. B., Friedmann, L. W., Weinstein, S., Sachs-Frankel, G., and Belandres, P. V. EMG feedback therapy: Review of treatment of 114 patients. *Arch. Phys. Med. Rehabil.,* 1976, *57,* 55–61.

Budzynski, T. H. Feedback-induced muscle relaxation and activation level. Unpublished doctoral dissertation, University of Colorado, Denver, 1969.

Budzynski, T. H., and Stoyva, J. M. An instrument for producing deep muscle relaxation by means of analog information feedback. *J. Appl. Behav. Anal.,* 1969, *2,* 231–237.

Budzynski, T. H., and Stoyva, J. M. An electromyographic feedback technique for teaching voluntary relaxation of the masseter. *J. Dent. Res.,* 1973, *52,* 116–119.

Budzynski, T. H., and Stoyva, J. M. EMG-Biofeedback bei unspezifischen and spezifischen Angstzustanden. In H. Legewie and L. Nusselt (Eds.), *Biofeedback-Therapie: Lernmethoden in der Psychosomatik, Neurologie and Rehabilitation,* (Fortschritte der Klinischen Psychologie, Vol. 6). München: Urban & Schwarzenbery, 1975, pp. 163–185.

Budzynski, T. H., Stoyva, J. M., and Adler, C. S. Feedback-induced muscle relaxation: Application to tension headache. *Behav. Ther. Exp. Psychiatry,* 1970, *1,* 205–211.

Budzynski, T. H., Stoyva, J. M., Adler, C. S., and Mullaney, D. J. EMG biofeedback and tension headache: A controlled outcome study. *Psychosom. Med.,* 1973, *35,* 484–496.

Budzynski, T. H., Stoyva, J. M., and Peffer, K. E. Biofeedback techniques in psychosomatic disorders. In E. Foa and A. Goldstein (Eds.), *Handbook of Behavioral Interventions.* New York: Wiley, in press.

Carlsson, S. G., and Gale, E. N. Biofeedback in the treatment of long-term temporomandibular joint pain: An outcome study. *Biofeedback Self-Regulation,* 1977, *2,* 161–171.

Chesney, M. A., and Shelton, J. L. A comparison of muscle relaxation and electromyogram biofeedback treatments for muscle contraction headaches. *J. Behav. Ther. Exp. Psychiatry,* 1976, *7,* 221–225.

Cleeland, C. Behavioral techniques in the modification of spasmodic torticollis. *Neurology,* 1973, *23,* 1241–1247.

Connor, W. H. Effects of brief relaxation training on autonomic response to anxiety evoking stimuli. *Psychophysiology,* 1974, *11,* 591–599.

Coursey, R. D. Electromyograph feedback as a relaxation technique. *J. Consult. Clin. Psychol.,* 1975, *43,* 825–834.

Coursey, R. D., Frankel, B., and Gaarder, K. EMG biofeedback and autogenic training as relaxation techniques for chronic sleep-onset insomnia. *Proceedings of the Biofeedback Research Society,* Seventh Annual Meeting, Colorado Springs, Col., 1976.

Cox, D. J., Freundlich, A., and Meyer, R. G. Differential effectiveness of electromyograph feedback, verbal relaxation instructions, and medication placebo with tension headaches. *J. Consult. Clin. Psychol.,* 1975, *43,* 892–898.

Dalessio, D. J. *Wolff's headache and other head pain.* New York: Oxford University Press, 1972.

DeGood, D. E., and Chisholm, R. C. Multiple response comparison of parietal EEG and frontalis EMG biofeedback. *Psychophysiology,* 1977, *14,* 258–265.

Dempsey, E. W. Homeostasis. In S. S. Stevens, (Ed.), *Handbook of experimental psychology.* New York: Wiley, 1951.

Fernando, C. K. Audio-visual reeducation in neuromuscular disorders. Paper presented at the meeting of the Biofeedback Research Society, Colorado Springs, Colo., February 1976.

Fernando, C. K. The use of biofeedback in physical medicine and rehabilitation. Task Force study section report prepared for the Biofeedback Society of America, May 1978.

Finley, W. W., Niman, C., Standley, J., and Ender, P. Frontal EMG biofeedback training of athetoid cerebral palsey patients. *Biofeedback Self-Regulation,* 1976, *1,* 169–182.

Folkow, B., and Neil, E. *Circulation* New York: Oxford University Press, 1971.

Freedman, R., and Papsdorf, J. D. Biofeedback and progressive relaxation treatment of sleep-onset insomnia: A controlled, all-night investigation. *Biofeedback Self-Regulation,* 1976a, *2,* 253–271.

Freedman, R., and Papsdorf, J. Generalization of frontal EMG biofeedback training to other muscles. *Biofeedback Self-Regulation,* 1976b, *1,* 333 (Abstract).

Gellhorn, E. The influence of curare on hypothalamic excitability and the electroencephalogram. *Electroencephalogr. Clin. Neurophysiol.,* 1958, *10,* 697–703.

Gellhorn, E. *Principles of autonomic-somatic integrations: Physiological basis and psychological and clinical implications.* Minneapolis: University of Minnesota Press, 1967.

Gellhorn, E., and Kiely, W. F. Mystical states of consciousness: Neurophysiological and clinical aspects. *J. Nerv. Ment. Dis.,* 1972, *154,* 399–405.

Gessel, A. H., and Alderman, M. M. Management of myofascial pain dysfunction syndrome of the temporomandibular joint by tension control training. *Psychosomatics,* 1971, *12,* 302–309.

Harris, F. A. Inapproprioceptions: A possible sensory basis for athetoid movements. *Phys. Ther.,* 1971, *51,* 761–770.

Harris, F. A., Spelman, F. A., and Hymer, J. W. Electronic sensory aids as a treatment for cerebral palsied children: Inappropriocepetion, Part II, *Phys. Ther.,* 1974, *54,* 354–365.

Harrison, V. F., and Mortenson, O. A. Identification and voluntary control of single motor unit activity in the tribialis anterior muscle. *Anat. Rec.,* 1962, *144,* 109–116.

Hauri, P. Biofeedback techniques in the treatment of serious, chronic insomniacs. *Proceedings of the Biofeedback Society of America;* Ninth Annual Meeting, Albuquerque, N.M., 1978.

Haynes, S. N. Electromyographic biofeedback treatment of a woman with chronic dysphagia. *Biofeedback Self-Regulation,* 1976, *1,* 121–126.

Haynes, S. N., Griffin, R., Mooney, D., and Parise, M. Relaxation instructions and biofeedback in the treatment of muscle-contraction headaches. *Behav. Ther.,* 1975, *6,* 672–678.

Hess, W. R. *Diencephalon: Autonomic and extraphramidal functions.* New York: Grune & Stratton, 1954.

Hodes, R. Electrocortical synchronization resulting from reduced proprioceptive drive caused by neuromuscular blocking agents. *Electroencephalogr. Clin. Neurophysiol.,* 1962, *14,* 220–232.

Hutchings, D. F., and Reinking, R. H. Tension headaches: What form of therapy is most effective? *Biofeedback Self-Regulation,* 1976, *1,* 183–190.

Inglis, J., Campbell, D., and Donald, M. W. Electromyographic biofeedback and neuromuscular rehabilitation. *Can. J. Behav. Sci.,* 1976, *8,* 299–323.

Jacobs, A., and Felton, G. S. Visual feedback of myoelectric output to facilitate muscle relaxation in normal persons and patients with neck injuries. *Arch. Phys. Med. Rehabil.,* 1969, *50,* 34–39.

Jacobson, E. *Progressive relaxation.* Chicago: University of Chicago Press, 1929.

Jacobson, E. *Progressive relaxation,* 2nd ed. Chicago: University of Chicago Press, 1938.

Jacobson, E. *Modern treatment of tense patients.* Springfield, Ill.: Charles C Thomas, 1970.

Johnson, H. E., and Garton, W. H. Muscle re-education in hemiplegia by use of electromyographic device. *Arch. Phys. Med. Rehabil.,* 1973, *54,* 320–325.

Kukulka, C. G., and Basmjian, J. V. Assessment of an audio-visual feedback device used in motor training. *Am. J. Phys. Med.,* 1975, *54,* 194–208.

Lance, J. W. *The mechanism and management of headache,* 2nd ed. London: Butterworth & Co., 1973.

LaVallée, Y. J., Lamontagne, Y., Pinard, G., Annable, L., and Tétreault, L. Effects of EMG feedback, diazepam and their combination on chronic anxiety. *J. Psychosom. Res.,* 1977, *21,* 65–71.

Levee, J. R., Cohen, M. J., and Rickles, W. H. Electromyographic biofeedback for relief of tension in the facial and throat muscles of a woodwind musician. *Biofeedback Self-Regulation,* 1976, *1,* 113–120.

Luthe, W. (Ed.). *Autogenic therapy,* Vols. 1–4. New York: Grune & Stratton, 1969.

Lynch, W. C., Schuri, U., and D'Anna, J. Effects of isometric muscle tension on vasomotor activity and heart rate. *Psychophysiology,* 1976, *13,* 222–230.

Marinacci, A. A. *Applied electromyography.* Philadelphia: Lea & Febiger, 1968.

Marinacci, A. A., and Horande, M. Electromyogram in neuromuscular re-education. *Bull. Los Angeles Neurol. Soc.,* 1960, *25,* 57–71.

Mason, J. W. Organization of psychoendocrine mechanisms. In N.S. Greenfield & R.A. Sternback (Eds.), *Handbook of psychophysiology.* New York: Holt, Rinehart & Winston, 1972, pp. 3–91.

Meige, H., and Feindel, E. Tics and their treatment. London: Appleton, 1907.

Moeller, T. A. Effects of EMG feedback and relaxation training in essential hypertensives. Unpublished doctoral dissertation, Nova University, Fort Lauderdale, Fla., 1973.

Patel, C. Randomised controlled trial of yoga and biofeedback in management of hypertension. *Lancet,* July 19, 1975, 93.

Peck, D. F. The use of EMG feedback in the treatment of a severe case of blepharospasm. *Biofeedback Self-Regulation,* 1977. *2,* 273–277.

Phillips, C. The modification of tension headache pain using EMG biofeedback. *Behav. Res. Ther.,* 1977, *15,* 119–129.

Pinneo, L. R. The effects of induced muscle tension during tracking on level of activation and on performance. *J. Exp. Psychol.,* 1961, *62,* 523–531.

Raskin, M., Johnson, G., and Rondestvedt, J. W. Chronic anxiety treated by feedback-induced muscle relaxation. *Arch. Gen. Psychiatry,* 1973, *28,* 263–267.

Reinking, R. H., and Kohl, M. L. Effects of various forms of relaxation training on physiological and self-report measures of relaxation. *J. Consult. Clin. Psychol.,* 1975, *43,* 595–600.

Rugh, J., Perlis, D., and Disraeli, R. (Eds.). *Biofeedback in dentistry.* Phoenix, Ariz.: Semantodontics, 1977.

Sainsbury, P., and Gibson, J. F. Symptoms of anxiety and tension and the accompanying physiological changes in the muscular system. *J. Neurol., Neurosurg. Psychiatry,* 1954, *17,* 216–224.

Schultz, J. H., and Luthe, W. *Autogenic training: A psychophysiological approach in psychotherapy.* New York: Grune & Stratton, 1959.

Selye, H. *The stress of life.* New York: McGraw-Hill, 1956.

Seymour, R. J., and Bassler, C. R. Elctromyographic biofeedback in treatment of incomplete paraplegia. *Phys. Ther.,* 1977, *57,* 1148–1150.

Shedivy, D. I., and Kleinman, K. M. Lack of correlation between frontalis EMG and either neck EMG or verbal ratings of tension. *Psychophysiology,* 1977, *14,* 182–186.

Sittenfeld, P., Budzynski, T. H., and Stoyva, J. M. Differential shaping of EEG theta rhythms. *Biofeedback Self-Regulation,* 1976, *1,* 31–46.

Smith, S. L., Black, A. H., Vanderwel-Johnston, C., and Cott, A. Successful behavioral treatment for hypertension: A study of methods and predictors. Paper presented at the annual meeting of the Canadian Psychiatric Association, Calgary, Alberta, Canada, September, 1975.

Solberg, W. K., and Rugh, J. D. The use of biofeedback devices in the treatment of bruxism. *S. Calif. Dent. Assoc. J.,* 1972, *40,* 852–853.

Stoyva, J. M. Self-regulation and the stress-related disorders: A perspective on biofeedback. In D. I. Mostofsky (Ed.), *Behavior control and modification of physiological activity.* Englewood Cliffs, N.J.: Prentice-Hall, 1976.

Stoyva. J. M. Why should muscle relaxation be clinically useful? Some data and 2½ models. In J. Beatty and H. Legewie (Eds.), *Biofeedback and behavior: NATO conference series.* New York: Plenum, 1977.

Stoyva, J. M. and Budzynski, T. H. Cultivated low arousal—an anti-stress response? In L. V. DiCara (Ed.), *Recent advances in limbic and autonomic nervous systems research.* New York: Plenum, 1977.

Surwit, R. S., and Shapiro, D. Biofeedback and meditation in the treatment of borderline hypertension. In J. Beatty and H. Legewie (Eds.), *Biofeedback and behavior: NATO conference series.* New York: Plenum, 1977.

Toomin, H., and Johnson, H. E. Electromyometer feedback in paraplegia: A case study in neuromuscular reeducation. *Proceedings of the Biofeedback Research Society,* Fifth Annual Meeting, Colorado Springs, Colo., 1974, p. 27 (abstract).

Townsend, R. E., House, J. F., and Addario, D. A comparison of biofeedback-mediated relaxation and group therapy in the treatment of chronic anxiety. *Am. J. Psychiatry,* 1975, *132,* 598–601.

Venables, P. H., and Wing, J. K. Level of arousal and the subclassification of schizophrenia. *Arch. Gen. Psychiatry,* 1962, *7,* 114–119.

Wickramasekera, I. Electromyographic feedback training and tension headache: Prelminary observations. *Am. J. Clin. Hypn.,* 1972, *15,* 83–85.

Wickramasekera, I. Temperature feedback for the control of migraine. *J. Behav. Ther. Exp. Psychiatry,* 1973, *4,* 343–345.

Wolff, H. G. In S. Wolf (Ed.), *Harold G. Wolff's "Stress and disease,"* 2nd ed. Springfield, Ill.: Charles C Thomas, 1968.

Wolpe, J. *The practice of behavior therapy.* New York: Pergamon Press, 1973.

Sexual Dysfunction*,†

JOSEPH LOPICCOLO, PH.D.

Professor of Psychiatry
Department of Psychiatry and Behavioral Science
State University of New York
Stony Brook, New York

DOUGLAS R. HOGAN

Department of Psychology
State University of New York
Stony Brook, New York

8

Introduction and Historical Overview

Until relatively recently, the mainstream of American psychiatry and psychology held to a basically psychodynamic and psychoanalytic view concerning the etiology and treatment of sexual dysfunctions. While behavioral psychotherapy techniques and other nondynamic approaches had been reported in the literature since the early 1950's, these reports did not have a significant effect on prevailing therapeutic practice. It was only the publication of Masters and Johnson's *Human Sexual Inadequacy* in 1970 which changed the field. Masters and Johnson's report of a basically behavioral treatment paradigm was couched in nonbehavioral and indeed atheoretical language, causing some anguish among behavior therapists who felt, rightly or wrongly that "their" techniques had been appropriated by Masters and Johnson. It remains an undisputed fact, however, that the publication of *Human Sexual Inadequacy* marked a major turning point in the history of our conceptualization of sexual dysfunction. What follows is a brief synopsis of this history.

THE TRADITIONAL PSYCHOANALYTIC APPROACH

The traditional analytic approach to sexual dysfunction is well known (Blum, 1949) and will not be presented in any detail here. Within analytic theory, failure to accomplish the childhood developmental tasks associated with the resolution of the Oedipal complex has remained the major etiological factor in sexual dysfunctions (Rosen, 1977; Fenichel, 1945; Freud, 1905). Thus, erectile failure is seen as a result of failure to differentiate forbidden incestuous sex with mother from sex with other women; as a result of a fear that father (or other men) will castrate the patient for taking a woman; as a castration anxiety reaction to the female genitals, and so forth. Similarly, orgasmic dysfunction in women is conceptualized as reflecting a failure to resolve penis envy; as failure to transfer sexual excitability from the clitoris to the vagina; as a failure of identification with mother during resolution of the Oedipal complex, and a host of other similar formulations. All of these formulations stress the central role of very early parent-child interactions

* Preparation of the chapter was supported in part by a grant from the National Institute of Mental Health, United States Public Health Service.

† This chapter was co-authored equally by Douglas R. Hogan and Joseph LoPiccolo.

around the instinctual Oedipus complex as the major etiological factor in producing failure of sexual functioning many years later in adulthood.

The analytic approach to treatment follows logically from this formulation. Treatment consists of re-enacting the Oedipal situation in the transference relationship with the analyst, and thus finishing in a healthy way the developmental tasks which were not accomplished in childhood.

Critiques of analytic theory, especially with regard to sexuality, are too numerous to bear repetition here. At a theoretical level, analytic theory was, of course, developed at a period when knowledge of the basic physiology of sexual response was nonexistent. Thus, a number of Freud's inspired insights into the nature of sexuality have since become insupportable in the light of advances in our biological knowledge. The most obvious example of analytic theoretical speculation since contradicted by empirical research concerns the famous and crucial distinction between clitoral and vaginal orgasm. The Kinsey, Pomeroy, Martin, et al. (1952) sociological data and the Masters and Johnson (1966) physiological data on female sexuality obviously have made this particular aspect of analytic theory extremely dubious at best. There have been repeated attempts to incorporate such new data into analytic theory, as witness Bergler and Kroger's *Kinsey's Myth of Female Sexuality* (1954) and Sherfey's *The Nature and Evolution of Female Sexuality* (1973), but such attempts have done little to further the development of new and effective treatment techniques.

It is at the level of this question of therapeutic effectiveness that the analytic approach to sexual dysfunction is most vulnerable. In the few empirical studies that have been conducted, analytic therapy simply does not work very well for sexual problems (Lorand, 1939; Moore, 1961), and even its most ardent supporters admit that the length of time required for a successful analysis is simply prohibitive (Bergler, 1951).

The basis for the low effectiveness of analytic therapy for sexual dysfunction probably lies in the analyst's passive and nondirective role. If one considers that many cases of sexual dysfunction are caused by a lack of knowledge about sexual response and techniques, an active and directive role of the therapist in providing education and skill training for the patient is obviously indicated. Focusing on a woman's childhood is not likely to lead her to have orgasm if her sexual partner is unaware of the role of the clitoris in female orgasm.

"COMMON SENSE" REMEDIES FOR SEXUAL DYSFUNCTION

Partially as a result of the failure of analytic therapy to provide effective and practical treatments for sexual dysfunction, clinicians working with patients with sexual concerns in the past developed a wide variety of essentially folk medicine remedies. While some of these procedures are somewhat effective and have been incorporated into behavioral treatment programs, the majority of the techniques are of little demonstrable value beyond placebo effects.

For premature ejaculation, one commonly advocated folk remedy is advising the patient to think distracting, anti-erotic thoughts about work, financial problems, and so forth during intercourse. Another approach involves having the patient wear a condom—or even two or three condoms—to cut down on penile sensitivity. A similar approach is to have the patient use a skin anesthetic cream on the penis before beginning sexual activity. Still another procedure is to have the patient masturbate immediately before engaging in sexual relations with his partner, as latency to ejaculation is inversely proportional to recency of the last previous ejaculation. The use of alcohol or sympathetic blocking agents (e.g., phenothiazenes) to delay ejaculation has also been widely recommended. While all of these procedures have some effectiveness in delaying ejaculation, they also reduce the sexual encounter to a joyless, non-pleasurable, performance oriented experience for the man. Some of these procedures also have the potential for turning a relatively simple premature ejaculation case into a more complicated case of erectile failure.

For erectile failure, folk remedies have been even less successful than for premature ejaculation. Approaches have included suggesting that the male patient have an affair with a more exciting sexual partner, the use of alcohol as an antianxiety agent, and the use of various penile appliances such as a rubber band around the base of the penis, splints, and so forth. Another medical approach to impotence has been the administration of testosterone. In general, research tends to indicate that if the male has normal endogenous plasma testosterone levels, as is true of virtually all erectile failure cases, administration of exogenous testosterone has no effects on erection, beyond a predictable placebo effect (Jarvik and Brecher, 1977).

Folk medicine and common sense approaches to female sexual dysfunctions have a similarly poor record of effectiveness. For female orgasmic dysfunction, probably as a reflection of double standard morality and the chauvinism of male professionals, the most common advice has been for the woman to simply meet her husband's needs, to fake orgasm, and to not be concerned about her own lack of response.

The record for treatment of vaginismus is similarly bleak. Ignoring the fact that vaginismus is a spastic contraction of the vaginal musculature, the common treatment of vaginismus has been hymenectomy or surgical enlargement of the vaginal opening. Both of these procedures are generally ineffective, as they do nothing to reduce the involuntary contraction of the vaginal musculature.

BEHAVIORAL APPROACHES TO SEXUAL DYSFUNCTION

"Behavioral approaches" refers to a type of therapy in which the therapist actively and directly educates the patient about sexual physiology and sexual techniques, restructures maladaptive behavior patterns and cognitions regarding sexuality, and uses anxiety-reduction and skill-training techniques to improve the patient's functioning. The history of the application of behavioral techniques to sexual dysfunction is a long one which much predates the rise of formal behavior therapy. In the late 18th century, a British physician, Sir John Hunter (cited in Comfort, 1965) described a treatment program for erectile failure which is very similar to the program described by Wolpe (1958) and by Masters and Johnson (1970). Hunter emphasized having the patient couple agree to forego intercourse for a fortnight, but to lie in bed naked every night during this period and hug and caress each other, thus eliminating performance anxiety. More recently, hypnotherapists such as von Schrenk-Notzing (1895) at the turn of the century, used direct sex education and instruction in sexual techniques to successfully treat sexual dysfunction. However, the rise of psychoanalysis effectively suppressed development of these techniques until the re-emergence of behaviorism in the late 1950's and early 1960's.

A major breakthrough in our conceptualization of sexual dysfunction occurred with the application of systematic desensitization to sexual problems. Salter (1949) and Wolpe (1958) conceptualized sexual dysfunctions as conditioned anxiety responses to the sexual situation. Engaging in a graduated hierarchy of sexual behaviors while forbidding the goal of orgasm or erection, sometimes coupled with muscle relaxation, proved quite effective in many cases.

Another behavioral technique used in this period was assertive training (Salter, 1949; Wolpe, 1958; Lazarus, 1965). In this approach, socially and sexually inhibited patients were given modeling and behavior rehearsals to increase their communication skills.

Although Ellis' (1962) rational-emotive therapy is not usually conceptualized as behavioral, rational-emotive therapy techniques for sexual dysfunction do include skill training, education, and anxiety reduction through restructuring irrational cognitions about the catastrophic nature of sexual dysfunction. Thus, Ellis' early work stands as one of the pioneering efforts in application of behavioral techniques to sexual dysfunction.

OTHER DIRECTIVE APPROACHES

Before the rise of direct "sex therapy" with the publication of *Human Sexual Inadequacy* in 1970, there were two therapists who had described very effective quasi-behavioral treatment techniques for sexual dysfunction. For treatment of premature ejaculation, Semans (1956) described his technique of repeated pauses during penile stimulation as nearly 100% effective. This technique became the basis for the Masters and Johnson program (1970) for premature ejaculation. Hastings (1963) described simple retraining programs designed to instruct couples in effective sexual techniques, such as concurrent clitoral manipulation for coitally inorgasmic women. What is remarkable is the lack of impact these works had on prevailing therapeutic practices.

SEX THERAPY

Following the publication of Masters and Johnson's *Human Sexual Inadequacy* in 1970, a number of other accounts of behavioral or quasi-behavioral approaches to treatment of sexual dysfunction have appeared (Kaplan, 1974; Hartman and Fithian, 1972; LoPiccolo and Lobitz, 1972; Lobitz and LoPiccolo, 1972). These accounts all differ greatly in the degree to which behavioral terminology is used and in the theoretical framework that is presented. However, if differences in language are ignored, all of these reports seem to describe fairly similar treatment procedures (LoPiccolo, 1977a). While there are unique elements in various programs, the reduction of performance anxiety (often through implicit counterconditioning and cognitive behavior therapy), sex education, skill training in communication and sexual technique, and attitude change procedures remain elements common to both "behavior therapy" and "sex therapy" approaches to sexual dysfunction. What *is* missing in sex therapy is the sort of careful evaluation of stimulus-response links, environmental contingencies, and operant functional analyses which characterize much of the more rigorous behavioral literature. This lack of evaluation points to another lack in "sex therapy" procedures: the lack of a coherent and consensually accepted classification scheme for diagnosis of sexual dysfunction.

Classification of Sexual Dysfunctions

CURRENT STATUS

At the present time, there is no well accepted system of classification of sexual dysfunctions. Each research center studying dysfunctions has its own terminology, and the categories described by different researchers overlap rather than correspond. In addition, the various centers often use the same term in different ways. For example Wolpe's (1969) category of "frigidity" apparently includes two of Kaplan's (1974) categories ("general sexual dysfunction" and "orgastic dysfunction"), while Kaplan uses the terms "frigidity" and "general sexual dysfunction" equivalently, and Masters and Johnson (1970) have no category corresponding to "general sexual dysfunction." Also, Masters and Johnson's categories of "primary" and "situational" orgasmic dysfunction do not correspond to Kaplan's categories of the same names, and Kaplan's and LoPiccolo's (1977a) "secondary orgasmic dysfunction" are not equivalent.

Furthermore, the meaning of the term "sexual dysfunction" itself changes over time, so that classes of people who would not have been diagnosed as "dysfunctional" 10 or 20 years ago would be considered dysfunctional now, and other classes of formerly dysfunctional people are no longer considered dysfunctional. For example, formerly neither Masters and Johnson (1970) nor Kaplan (1974) described a male dysfunction involving lack of sexual desire, but by 1977 Kaplan described a "highly prevalent" disorder termed "hypoactive sexual desire" (Kaplan, 1977). Conversely, women who were unable to reach orgasm during coitus were considered dysfunctional in 1970 (Masters and Johnson, 1970) but were considered normal in 1974 (Kaplan, 1974). Premature ejaculation was a "disease" in 1887 (Gross, 1887, cited by Spiess, 1977), a "superior" biological trait in 1948 (Kinsey, Pomeroy, and Martin, 1948), and a sexual "dysfunction" in 1970 (Masters and Johnson, 1970).

These inconsistencies reflect three underlying factors: (1) the concept of sexual "dysfunction" is not value free, and values vary over time and across individuals; (2) systems of classification are constructed for different purposes, and consequently, different systems will reflect the differing needs of those who construct them; and (3) all of the current systems of classifications are typological, and typologies have severe inherent limitations.

CULTURAL AND INDIVIDUAL VALUES. The concept of "sexual dysfunction" implies a concept of "normal sexual functioning." However, "normal sexual functioning" cannot be objectively defined (except in a statistical sense). Consequently, the definition of normality will always depend on the sexual attitudes, values, and behaviors of a particular society in a specific historical period and of the individual who is defining the term. Thus, society's view of female sexual functioning will determine whether or not the lack of coital orgasms is normal and healthy or dysfunctional, and the definition of "normal," "hyperactive," and "hypoactive" sexual desire will depend on such factors as the frequency of sexual intercourse in the society, the society's belief as to what constitutes normal and abnormal frequency, and the individual investigator's beliefs and values (LoPiccolo and Heiman, 1978a; Strupp and Hadley, 1977).

The inconsistencies in these definitions are increased by the fact that there is no single, consistent view in our society at any single time as to what constitutes normal (or abnormal) sexual functioning, and attitudes toward sex have been rapidly changing in this society in the last 20 years (LoPiccolo and Heiman, 1978a).

The fact that the terms "normal sexual functioning" and "sexual dysfunction" are value laden does not imply that they are invalid concepts. However, it does imply that these terms will always be highly relative concepts and that they will continue to change over time. A useful system of classification must take these considerations into account.

Purposes of Classification. Systems of classification can be constructed for a single purpose or for multiple purposes (Spitzer and Wilson, 1975). Investigators in the area of psychiatric nosology (Kanfer and Saslow, 1969; Spitzer, Sheehy, and Endicott, 1977; Spitzer and Wilson, 1975) have listed a number of possible purposes: (1) communication between researchers and clinicians in the area; (2) understanding the disorder (etiology, maintaining variables, process of the pathology); (3) prediction (behavior in various situations, prognosis with and without treatment); and (4) selection of appropriate treatment.

No single system can optimally fulfill all of these purposes, and any system must constantly be revised as new information is obtained. These facts in part account for the alterations in nosologies of sexual dysfunctions over time and across investigators. Unfortunately, most investigators in the area of sexual dysfunctions do not state the purposes of their nosologies, and seem to assume that they have discovered and listed a set of categories that exist in nature, rather than realizing that they have constructed a set of concepts for specific purposes. This has led to reification of these concepts and consequent confusion. The solution to this problem is for investigators to state explicitly the purposes of their classificatory systems.

Limitations of Typologies. All of the present systems of classifying sexual dysfunctions divide the dysfunctions into discrete types. Bandura (1968) and Hempel (1965a) point out several inherent shortcomings in such typologies. First, individual cases are often distributed along various continua and do not fit neatly into discrete classes. Thus, diagnosticians are often presented with borderline cases that are difficult to classify and, if a class is broad enough, the cases within that class will often only remotely resemble one another (Note 1). These problems are illustrated by the example of orgasmic dysfunction in women, where situational orgasmic dysfunction gradually shades off into normal sexual functioning on one side and absolute orgasmic dysfunction on the other (Kaplan, 1974), producing many unclassifiable borderline cases. In addition, situational orgasmic dysfunction includes so many different types of cases (e.g., women unable to reach orgasm except in masturbation, those who can reach orgasm with a lover but not with their husband, and those who can only reach orgasm with a vibrator or through cunnilingus) that prognosis and treatment choice are not clearly determined by knowledge of the typological classification.

Second, often one individual will fit into two or more categories. For example, Cooper (1968a) reports on a series of cases of male dysfunction where individuals would often report low sex drive, erectile failure, and premature ejaculation. All of Masters and Johnson's (1970) vaginismus cases also reported orgasmic dysfunction (although not all of Kaplan's (1974) cases did).

Third, typologies do not allow quantification, which precludes the possibility of establishing functional relationships between variables. Consequently, only gross behavioral prediction is usually possible.

Finally, sexual dysfunctions often reflect

complex, dynamic, interacting systems of variables (Hogan, 1978; Kaplan, 1974). These variables can include multiple sexual dysfunctions in a single relationship (premature ejaculation and female orgasmic dysfunction often coexist, as do erectile failure and vaginismus), marital factors (such as hostility), and psychological factors (e.g., performance anxiety). The sexual dysfunction and the maintaining variables can be connected through complex feedback loops in systems that change over time (Hogan, 1977; Kaplan, 1974). Typologies of individuals cannot adequately describe such systems, and typologies of systems would prove to be unwieldy because of the infinite number of such systems and their tendency to change over time.

MULTIDIMENSIONAL CLASSIFICATION

Bandura (1968) and Hempel (1965a) have suggested multidimensional classification as an alternative to typologies. Sets of variables for which each individual could be given a quantitative score could be selected for the specific purpose of the classification. Thus, each case would be classified by a dimensional profile consisting of a set of numbers referring to these variables or dimensions. The dimensions should be selected on theoretical and empirical grounds, and should constantly be refined through empirical research. Eventually it may be possible to establish functional relationships connecting weighted scores on these dimensions to relevant variables such as response to specific interventions.

For example, Cooper (1969c) has found a number of variables to be significantly correlated with positive outcome following behavioral treatment of erectile failure, retarded ejaculation, and premature ejaculation, including short duration, heterosexual sex drive (Note 2), intermittent success (rather than persistent failure) in coitus, satisfactory premarital coitus, presence of love for the wife, male marital happiness, normal personality (both spouses), motivation for therapy, and the wife's cooperation in therapy. Cooper (1970) also investigated prognostic indicators in coitally inorgasmic women undergoing behavior therapy, and found short duration, strong sex drive (operationally defined), premarital coitus, premarital orgasm, positive attitudes toward sex, love for the husband, normal personality in the patient, emotional arousal in coital situations, pleasurable sexual fantasies and dreams, positive attitudes toward partner's genitalia, positive attitudes toward sexual techniques and experimentation, self-referral, and a number of other factors associated with positive treatment response.

Nowinski (1977) is currently examining a set of operationally defined variables taken from social learning theory, systems theory, communication theory, and Gestalt therapy, in order to see whether treatment response can be predicted. Any variables that are significantly correlated with outcome can then be used in a multidimensional classificatory system.

Variables which may prove particularly relevant in such research are frequency of various sexual behaviors; levels of marital discord; anxiety level in response to specific sexual activities, ability to communicate feelings, sexual desires, and sexual aversions directly, concurrent levels of specific types of psychopathology (e.g., depression), attitudes (e.g., disgust, liking) toward various sexual behaviors, and motivation to change.

KAPLAN'S TYPOLOGY AND DSM-III

At the present time, Kaplan's (1974, 1977) typology is the most comprehensive classificatory system of sexual dysfunctions. A modified version of her system with slightly different terminology has been included in a 1977 draft of the third edition of the American Psychiatric Association's *Diagnostic and Statistical Manual of Mental Disorders* (DSM-III) (Spitzer et al., 1977).

Kaplan (1974, p. 250) defines sexual dysfunctions as " . . . psychosomatic disorders which make it impossible for the individual to have and/or enjoy coitus." Dysfunctions can involve the disruption of any of the three phases into which Kaplan (1974, 1977) divides the sexual response. The first phase is sexual *desire*. Kaplan defines *hypoactive sexual desire* as inhibited sexual desire, while *hyperactive sexual desire* is an abnormally intense sexual desire (Kaplan, 1977). The second phase is *excite-*

ment, consisting of vasocongestion and erection in the male, and vasocongestion, genital swelling, and lubrication in the female. Inhibition of this phase produces *erectile dysfunction* (also termed "erectile failure" or "impotence") in the male and *general sexual dysfunction* in the female. Erectile failure is the inability of the male to achieve or maintain an erection of sufficient firmness or for a sufficient length of time to perform intercourse. General sexual dysfunction is a lack of sexual arousal, vasocongestion, and lubrication. The final phase is *orgasm*, consisting of reflex muscular contractions. Disorders of this phase include *premature ejaculation* and *retarded ejaculation* (also termed "ejaculatory incompetence" and "ejaculative impotence") in the male and *orgastic dysfunction* in the female. Kaplan defines "premature ejaculation" as the inability of the male to exert voluntary control over his ejaculatory reflex, so that once he reaches the plateau phase of sexual arousal he ejaculates rapidly and reflexly (Kaplan, 1974; Kaplan, Kohl, Pomeroy, et al., 1974) (Note 3). Retarded ejaculation is the inhibition of the ejaculatory reflex (Kaplan, 1974) resulting in a delayed ejaculation or the inability to ejaculate. Orgastic dysfunction is the corresponding inhibition of orgasm in the female.

Two other dysfunctions do not fit neatly into Kaplan's triphasic system. *Vaginismus* involves an involuntary spasm of the muscles surrounding the vaginal introitus (Kaplan, 1974), and thus prevents penile penetration. *Dyspareunia* is painful intercourse (Masters and Johnson, 1970), and while it is more often found in women, can also be found in some male patients (Note 4).

Kaplan further subdivides the dysfunctions along two independent dimensions, a temporal dimension (primary-secondary) and a situational dimension (absolute-situational). The term "primary" refers to a dysfunction which has always existed in the individual, starting with the first sexual experiences, while "secondary" means that the individual has functioned at least once successfully, but at the time of the diagnosis is dysfunctional. "Absolute" refers to a disorder that is present at the time of diagnosis in all sexual situations (i.e., involving all types of self-stimulation or partner stimulation, with all partners), while "situational" refers to a dysfunction present in some sexual situations but not in others (Note 5).

Although Kaplan's system is the most comprehensive of the existing typologies, it suffers from all of the limitations discussed above, and consequently, it has little utility for research purposes. It is useful in terms of helping clinicians communicate, but even here there are problems, because most of the diagnoses are very gross and contain a large variety of unspecified subtypes. A number of subtypes of erectile failure, premature ejaculation, and situational orgasmic dysfunction have been described by Ansari (1975), Cooper (1968a,b), and Masters and Johnson (1970), which have different etiologies, symptomatologies, and prognoses from other subtypes within the same category. Because of this, knowledge of the diagnosis imparts only limited information to the clinician. Thus, there is a need for careful assessment of each individual case before treatment is begun.

Assessment of Sexual Dysfunction

The aim of assessment procedures is generally three-fold: to produce a diagnosis or description of the problem, to clarify etiology of the problem, and to suggest an appropriate treatment regimen for the problem. Unfortunately, assessment procedures for sexual dysfunction fall short of all three goals in varying degree. While this failure is more or less true of other psychotherapeutic endeavors, the field of sexual dysfunction has an obvious and unique handicap. Both social stigma and personal embarrassment (of both patients and therapists) make the gathering of truthful and complete data about a couple's sexual relationship inordinately difficult.

CURRENT STRATEGIES FOR ASSESSMENT

Attempts to assess sexual dysfunction generally fall into three categories, which differ in the method of data collection:

DIRECT OBSERVATIONS OF SEXUAL BEHAVIOR, VIDEOTAPING OF SEXUAL BEHAVIOR, AND "SEXOLOGICAL" EXAMS. One obvious approach to assessment of sexual dysfunction is to simply observe the patient couple during their sexual relationship, either by having the therapist present (Hartman and Fithian, 1972) or by videotaping the patient couple (Serber, 1974), with the tape later viewed by the therapist.

Another variety of direct observation technique is the "sexological exam" (Hartman and Fithian, 1972). In this procedure, the therapist stimulates the breast and genitals of the opposite sex patient, for the purpose of assessing and demonstrating physiological responsiveness.

While such procedures may seem to offer the advantage of direct, nondistorted recording of actual sexual behavior, there are a number of issues which rather convincingly argue against their use. First, of course, is the issue of stimulus control and reactivity of sexual behavior to the stimulus situation. It seems unlikely that most couples with a sexual dysfunction will be unaffected by being observed, videotaped, or stimulated by their therapist. Thus, the behavior elicited in these situations may have little generalizability to the target stimulus situation—the couple interacting alone in the privacy of their own bedroom. Similarly, such assessment procedures would probably simply be unacceptable to the majority of dysfunctional couples seeking treatment. Finally, the ethical problems in patient-therapist sexual contact, and the possibility for exploitation of the patient, are obvious (LoPiccolo, 1977b).

Sex History Interviews. A major element in many sexual treatment programs is the sex history interview (Masters and Johnson, 1970; Kaplan, 1974; Hartman and Fithian, 1972). The format of such an interview is usually that of an extended face-to-face semi-structured interview, conducted separately with each patient, by a therapist of the same sex. The content of such an interview varies considerably from program to program, with some history interviews routinely taking as much as 7 hours to complete.

The utility of such extensive history taking has not been empirically demonstrated, and is open to question in terms of the most efficient use of therapeutic time. Certainly, many of the questions asked in the more extensive interviews have minimal clinical utility, in that treatment procedures remain the same regardless of the varying nature of the patient's answer. Such extensive history interviews may, however, serve a useful rapport building function, in that the therapist demonstrates great interest in the patient. Extensive histories may also allay the therapist's and, to a lesser degree, the patient's anxiety, by providing a seemingly coherent explanation for the cause of the sexual problem.

A good example of a relatively complete yet brief and treatment relevant sex history interview is provided by LoPiccolo and Heiman (1978b).

Paper and Pencil Self-report Inventories. There have been relatively few attempts to develop valid psychometric inventories with content specific to sexual dysfunction. Such inventories have more typically focused on issues such as masculinity-femininity (Goldberg, 1971), sex guilt (Mosher, 1968), or heterosexual-homosexual orientation (Feldman and McCulloch, 1971).

A few symptom-specific sexual dysfunction inventories have been offered in the literature (El-Senoussi, 1964; Derogatis, 1976), but these instruments tend to be developed on logical (as opposed to empirical) grounds. That is, without consideration of the statistical issues of validity and reliability during the test construction process, these inventories have either not been demonstrated to be empirically useful, or, as in one case, have actually been shown to be invalid (Beutler, Karacan, Anch, et al., 1975). Perhaps the two best paper and pencil inventories are the Sexual Arousal Inventory (Hoon, Hoon, and Wincze, 1976) and the Sexual Interaction Inventory (LoPiccolo and Steger, 1974). The Sexual Arousal Inventory is specific to females only and is a measure of the arousal a woman experiences in response to various sexual activities. The Sexual Interaction Inventory attempts to describe a couples' sexual relationship in terms of frequency and enjoyment of specific sexual activities and communication between the sexual partners about these activities. While both of these inventories are statistically valid, neither of them provides symptom-specific descriptions of particular sexual dysfunctions, nor do they clarify etiology. Both instruments do provide guidelines for treatment, in that they identify arousal deficits, problem behaviors, and so forth for therapeutic focus.

There are two obvious problems with all such self-report paper and pencil inventories. First, they are highly reactive, in that asking couples in great detail about their sexual relationship undoubtedly has some behavior change effects. Secondly, such inventories are extremely susceptible to social desirability, defensiveness, and simple falsification by the respondent (Jemail, 1977). Thus, the relationship between what patients report on such inventories and what actually goes on in their bedroom is open to question.

THE NEED FOR MULTIDIMENSIONAL ASSESSMENT

None of the strategies discussed above really offers an adequate assessment scheme for sexual dysfunction. Sexual dysfunction does not exist in a vacuum, but is related to a large number of historical, behavioral, personal, relationship, and physiological factors. An evaluation of each of the following factors needs to be conducted for an adequate assessment of a sexually dysfunctional patient couple:

HISTORY. Within the reservations noted above, an examination of the sexual history of the patient is needed to provide the best plan for successful treatment. A woman with a history of terrifying incestual sexual molestation as a child, for example, needs very different therapy than an inorgasmic woman with an unremarkable sexual history.

CURRENT BEHAVIOR. Through questionnaires, interviewing, or perhaps some observational strategy, an understanding of the actual sexual behavior a couple engages in is obviously crucial. If the therapist does not know just what the patients *do* sexually, it is impossible to plan a therapeutic course of prescribed "homework" sexual assignments, as will be discussed in a later section of this chapter.

ATTITUDINAL AND COGNITIVE FACTORS. How do the patients think about their sexual dysfunction? Do they have negative attitudes toward sex, or religious beliefs which must be considered? Attitude change and cognitive restructuring are major elements in treatment, and an accurate picture of the patient's cognitive structuring of their sexuality is therefore crucial.

PSYCHODYNAMIC AND INTRAPSYCHIC DEFENSES. Although treatment of sexual dysfunction is basically a cognitive behavior therapy type of procedure, the role of intrapsychic defenses cannot be ignored in many cases. Some males with erectile failure, for example, seem to be struggling with the issue of an unacceptable and therefore consciously denied homosexual orientation. While denying the existence of an instinctual and biologically determined Oedipal complex and sequence of psychosexual development, the therapist should acknowledge that patients *do* have intrapsychic defense mechanisms for dealing with stress. Failure to consider these anxiety defenses often leads to therapeutic failure. Such failed cases are often labeled "resistant," as the patients failed to complete behavioral homework assignments. A consideration of the patients' anxiety and defensive structure can lead to such "resistant" clients being able to follow through on homework assignments.

INTERPERSONAL SYSTEMS. The importance of considering the role of the sexual dysfunction in the couples' broader emotional relationship cannot be overemphasized. For some couples, the dysfunction plays a very functional role in the maintenance of their emotional relationship and life style. A dysfunction may be a means of avoiding intimacy, of expressing hostility, of maintaining control in the relationship, or of retaliating for other grievances in the relationship. A failure to assess such factors typically leads to failed cases, with the puzzled therapist concluding, "These people don't really seem to want to change." Indeed, the couple may want very badly to overcome their dysfunction, but may be unable to do so until the needs which are now being expressed through the dysfunction are resolved in some more direct and adaptive way.

PSYCHIATRIC STATUS. At the present time, there is only very sparse evidence that the behavioral treatments for sexual dysfunctions are applicable to patients with a significant degree of overt psychopathology. Certainly, the effect of depression on inhibiting sexual drive and expression is well known, and assessment for depression should be included in multidimensional assessment. Overtly psychotic or overwhelmingly anxious patients are possibly also best screened out and referred for less symptom focused therapy at assessment, although some clinical programs do report success with such cases (Lobitz, 1977).

BIOLOGICAL FACTORS. Despite the fact that the large majority of sexually dysfunctional patients are organically intact, it is becoming clear that there are a large number of biological processes which can be implicated in sexual dysfunction. The differentiation between biogenic and psychogenic etiology of sexual dysfunction is especially crucial in male erectile failure cases and female dyspareunia cases. Organic factors do not, at the present stage of our knowledge, seem as clearly implicated in premature ejaculation or female orgasmic dysfunction.

A complete evaluation of the patient's biological status requires consideration of a number of parameters not included in routine physical examinations. Obviously, complete and thorough pelvic examinations by a consultant urologist or gynecologist are indicated. Beyond this, tests for thyroid function, endocrine status (especially testosterone), and glucose tolerance should probably be routine, especially in low sex drive and erectile failure cases. An examination for neuropathy and peripheral vascular function is also indicated, with penile pulse and blood pressure especially important in erectile failure cases. In differentiating organic from psychogenic erectile failure, measurement by penile plethysmograph of nocturnal erection during REM sleep has been found to be a valid and highly useful measure (Karacan, 1978). Similarly, vaginal plethysmography shows great promise in the diagnosis of female arousal deficits (Heiman, 1978).

Etiology

METHODOLOGY

In order to determine specific etiological factors leading to sexual dysfunctions, a researcher would need to compare groups of dysfunctional patients with a normal control group and discover which variables were differentially associated with the dysfunctions. Control groups of dysfunctional and nondysfunctional psychiatric outpatients would also have to be examined in order to determine which of these variables were specifically associated with sexual dysfunctions and which were associated with psychopathology in general. To date, no major study (Note 6) has been conducted to examine relevant variables employing appropriate control groups. Instead, researchers have taken sex histories from patients and made the illogical assumption that when certain "abnormal" factors were present in the histories, these factors had caused the dysfunction. In fact, many of these alleged etiological factors may be present in the normal population at the same frequency. Even if it is shown (through controlled research) that these factors are found at a higher incidence in dysfunctional patients, the direction of causation will still be uncertain. The dysfunction may actually have caused the "etiological factor," both the dysfunction and the "etiological factor" may have been caused by a third variable (Neale and Liebert, 1973), or the dysfunction and "etiological factor" may be interacting in a dynamic system through positive feedback loops (Kaplan, 1974).

Another methodological problem is that information obtained through retrospective self-reports is notoriously unreliable, and etiological variables corresponding to the theoretical system of the interviewer are frequently elicited (Bandura, 1969). Thus, Ellis (1971) discovers irrational self-statements, Masters and Johnson (1970) find frequent cases of restrictive religious upbringing, and Wolpe (1969) finds conditioned anxiety. Because of these methodological problems, the variables to be discussed below must be considered only tentative etiological factors.

AN INTERACTIONAL/SYSTEMS MODEL

Kaplan (1974) presents a multicausal/interactional etiological model in which a large number of potential interacting factors are presented. Hogan (1978) has combined the approaches of Davison and Neale (1974), Ellis (1962, 1971), Kaplan (1974), Lazarus (1974), Masters and Johnson (1970), and Wolpe (1958, 1969) into an interactional/systems model. In this model, the various etiological variables, maintaining variables, and sexual dysfunctions are seen as interacting elements in dynamic systems (von Bertalanffy, 1968; Watzlawick, Weakland, and Fisch, 1974). The concepts of cause and effect become highly relative, and the idea of linear causation is supplemented by that of systems operating in cyclical fashions through positive and negative feedback loops.

The high level of sexual functioning that is currently considered "healthy" by sex therapists requires that a considerable number of factors be present to an optimum degree (Kaplan, 1974). These factors include psychological, anatomical, physiological, marital, and environmental variables. The absence or insufficiency of any of these factors (or conversly, the presence of the pathological opposites of these factors) can inhibit sexual functioning.

No attempt will be made here to present an exhaustive list of specific etiological factors; rather, the major categories of factors will be listed with a few examples from each (Note 7).

Anatomical and physiological factors interfering with the sexual response can lead to dysfunctions. For example, illness can affect the sexual response through the nonspecific factors of pain, fatigue, and exhaustion (Kaplan, 1974). Diseases affecting the central nervous system (e.g., multiple sclerosis), the vascular supply to the penis (e.g., local thrombotic disease), or the androgen level (e.g., feminizing tumors) can cause dysfunctions, as can anatomical abnormalities of the genitals (Kaplan, 1974; Masters and Johnson, 1970). Surgery and drugs can also create sexual problems: episiotomy scars can lead to dyspareunia, central nervous system depressants (e.g., alcohol, barbiturates) can lead to low sex drive, anticholinergic medication to ejaculatory problems (through blocking of neurotransmitters at the synapses) (Kaplan, 1974) (Note 8).

The major psychological factor implicated in the etiology of sexual dysfunctions is anxiety. Wolpe (1969) believes that anxiety conditioned to sexual situations inhibits sexual response, and Kaplan (1974) and Masters and Johnson (1970) stress the role of performance anxiety. Cooper (1969a) presents data in support of these hypotheses. Depression (Kaplan, 1974; Kiev and Hackett, 1968), hostility (Cooper, 1968b), guilt (Kaufman, 1967), and irrational thoughts about sex (Ellis, 1971) are also believed to cause dysfunctions. Finally, Masters and Johnson (1970) present data indicating that one dysfunction can lead to another dysfunction; for example, premature ejaculation can lead to erectile problems.

The role of psychiatric problems (with the exception of anxiety and depression) is less clear. Sexual dysfunctions may coexist with neurosis and psychosis, but it has not been determined whether there are significant relationships between specific psychiatric illnesses and sexual dysfunctions, and if so, whether the dysfunction is a symptom of the illness, a defense against decompensation, or involved in some other relationship with the illness. Kaplan (1974) believes that dysfunctions can play a number of roles in psychiatric problems, but there is little solid knowledge available on this issue.

Marital problems, such as dissatisfaction (McGovern, et al., 1975), lack of trust, love or communication, and power and control conflicts (Kaplan, 1974) have been implicated as etiological factors, especially in the case of situational orgasmic dysfunction (McGovern, et al., 1975). Environmental problems involving the early familial environment and/or the current environment can also lead to dysfunctions. For example, Masters and Johnson (1970) found a large number of cases with strict religious upbringings, and Kaplan (1974) cites job pressure as a possible factor.

Lack of skill and knowledge are often found in dysfunctional cases. Women with orgasmic dysfunction are often married to men who are unskilled lovers (Kaplan, 1974; LoPicolo, 1977a), and Ellison (1972) found a high degree of sexual misinformation in a series of vaginismus cases. However, these two factors appear to be on the decline as sexual knowledge becomes more available through the mass media.

A final factor that has been cited as an etiological variable is homosexual orientation (Lazarus, 1963; Masters and Johnson, 1970). However, if a homosexual is forced by society into a heterosexual relationship in which he cannot function sexually, it seems to be inappropriate to call it a case of "sexual dysfunction." Large numbers of heterosexuals would probably have difficulty functioning homosexually, but no clinician would state that heterosexual orientation is a cause of homosexual dysfunction. The underlying (and no doubt correct) assumption is that few heterosexuals would want to function homosexually, but many homosexuals would like to function heterosexually. However, this leads to an extremely narrow view, in that socio-political problems become disguised as medico-psychological problems. If society were equally tolerant of homosexuality and heterosexuality, there would probably be many fewer homosexuals presenting at sex therapy clinics with opposite-sexed partners.

There are probably other cases of unconventional sexual preferences that are disguised as sexual dysfunctions. For example, a case of "orgasmic dysfunction" was seen by one of the authors in which the wife stopped having orgasms after marriage when the husband stopped spanking her as part of foreplay. When the therapist "gave them permission" to engage in spanking, the woman quickly became orgasmic again.

The Treatment of Sexual Dysfunctions

Behavior therapy and social learning theory have contributed most of the effective techniques that now comprise sex therapy (Hogan, 1978; LoPiccolo, 1977a). Before Wolpe's (1958) introduction of the behavioral technique of systematic desensitization, the treatment of sexual dysfunctions was lengthy, expensive, and ineffective (LoPiccolo, 1977b). With the introduction of behavioral anxiety-reduction and skill-training techniques, success rates converging on 70–80% began to be reported following fairly brief interventions (Laughren and Kass, 1975). However, despite the domination of the sex therapy field by behavior therapy, other therapeutic approaches are useful as adjunct techniques. Cognitive therapy (Ellis, 1962, 1971), general systems theory (von Bertalanffy, 1968; Kaplan, 1974), communication theory (Watzlawick, Beavin, and Jackson, 1967), humanistic/existential therapy (Lobitz, LoPiccolo, Lobitz, et al., 1976), psychodynamic theory (Kaplan, 1974), and Gestalt therapy have contributed conceptualizations and techniques which appear to be helpful at a clinical level.

Eight classes of components of sex therapy will be discussed below: sex education; anxiety-reduction techniques; skill training; sensory, cognitive, and attitude-change procedures; behavior change techniques; marital therapy; psychodynamic techniques; and medical/physical procedures. In addition, several modalities of therapy will be examined.

METHODOLOGICAL ISSUES

The majority of studies on the treatment of sexual dysfunction are uncontrolled case reports or series of case studies (Hogan, 1977, 1978; LoPiccolo, 1977c). Many of the studies that include control groups have employed deficient or inappropriate control groups (Note 9). For example, Obler (1973) compared desensitization to traditional therapy for a mixed group of dysfunctions. However, the desensitization patients were treated individually by the researcher, while the traditional therapy patients were treated in a group by clinicians who were unaware of the design or purpose of the experiment, thus confounding two critical variables (treatment modality and therapist variables) with type of therapy. Munjack, Cristol, Goldstein, et al. (1976) compared behavior therapy to a waiting list control group, but the control subjects were on the waiting list for half the time of the therapy program. Schneidman and McGuire (1976) compared two behavior therapy groups with a waiting list control group in the treatment of primary orgasmic dysfunction. Masturbation therapy was an important element of their therapy. However, the majority of the control group subjects had masturbated before therapy, while the experimental subjects had not. Thus, the control group may have been composed of women who were much less likely to reach orgasm than were the treated subjects, which would inflate the success rates artificially.

The two basic requirements of experimental design are: (1) a control group which differs from the experimental (or treatment) group on only the variable that is being studied; and (2) random assignment of subjects to the two groups (Campbell and Stanley, 1963; Neale and Liebert, 1973). When subjects are not randomly assigned to groups, subject differences or interactions between subject and treatment variables, rather than pure treatment effects, may be responsible for any post-treatment differences. When the treatment and control groups differ on more than one variable, it is not possible to determine which of the two was responsible for any changes following therapy. Each of the three studies cited above violated one of these two requirements. These examples are especially interesting because all three involved *behavioral* techniques, and the use of the experimental method is often cited as a fundamental aspect of behavior therapy (Rimm and Masters, 1974).

The complexity of experimental design is increased in the case of sex therapy, where treatments usually consist of packages rather than individual techniques. For example, Masters and Johnson (1970) combined skill training, counseling, sex education, and anxiety-reduction techniques in their therapy package, and made the untenable assumption that since patients were helped by the entire package, each of the components of the package is necessary (Masters and Johnson, 1970).

In order to determine conclusively the effectiveness of any specific technique employed as a component of a treatment package, a factorial experiment with untreated and nonspecific treatment control groups is required (Paul and Bernstein, 1973). No such studies have been conducted on the treatment of sexual dysfunctions. Because of these limitations in experimental design, in most cases only tentative conclusions can be drawn about the effectiveness of specific techniques. However, certain procedures, especially anxiety-reduction techniques (e.g., desensitization) and sexual skill training, are well supported by empirical evidence.

TREATMENT TECHNIQUES

SEX EDUCATION. When clients are deficient in sexual knowledge, sex education is an important element of therapy. Such education includes facts about sexual anatomy and physiology (e.g., the location and function of the clitoris), information on sexual behavior (e.g., the normality of masturbation and oral-genital sex), and correcting misconceptions about such things as the necessity of simultaneous orgasms or coital orgasms.

Sex education is not an effective technique when divorced from behavioral techniques. Lazarus (1961), for example, found sex education combined with insight therapy to be less effective than systematic desensitization in the treatment of erectile failure. However, it is a useful adjunct to behavior therapy (Barbach, 1974) and is sufficient by itself to reverse what Lazarus (1971) terms "pseudoinadequacies"—sexual problems due entirely to ignorance or misinformation, when no real behavioral problems or psychopathology exist.

ANXIETY-REDUCTION TECHNIQUES. *Desensitization.* Anxiety-reduction techniques are a major component of sex therapy. Wolpe's systematic desensitization and in vivo desensitization have been used for all of the sexual dysfunctions (Hogan, 1978) with success rates averaging about 75 and 82%, respectively (Laughren and Kass, 1975). However, the majority of the studies that have been reported combine desensitization with other techniques such as skill training, so these success rates are inflated. Desensitization appears to be highly effective when the dysfunction is largely caused and maintained by anxiety; when skill deficits or marital conflicts are involved, it must be supplemented by appropriate techniques.

Desensitization involves exposing the client to a hierarchy of sexual scenes which elicit progressively greater degrees of anxiety. The scenes can be presented in imagination (systematic desensitization), via videotapes (video desensitization), or in reality, with the client actually engaging in the sexual activities at home with his or her spouse (in vivo desensitization). While the scene is presented to or engaged in by the client, relaxation can be induced through the techniques of progressive relaxation (systematic desensitization), hypnosis (hypno-desensitization; Lazarus, 1973), or injections of methohexital sodium (Brevital, Brietal), a fast acting barbiturate (Brevital desensitization).

Wolpe (1958, 1969) believes that the technique works on the principal or reciprocal inhibition: parasympathetically mediated responses such as relaxation or sexual arousal inhibit the incompatible sympathetically mediated response of anxiety. Other explanations have included counterconditioning (without Wolpe's neurological explanation) (Mischel, 1968), cortically mediated counterconditioning (Bandura, 1969); and the use of relaxation as a skill to cope with anxiety (Goldfried, 1973). At the present time this controversy has not been resolved (Rimm and Masters, 1974). In addition to anxiety reduction, video and in vivo desensitization probably also promote sexual functioning through (unplanned) sexual skill training via modeling (video desensitization) and instruction and feedback from the partner (in vivo desensitization).

Desensitization techniques have been shown to be effective in reducing anxiety in all types of sexual dysfunction, and in many cases have completely restored sexual functioning. The evidence consists of both case studies (see Hogan, 1978; Laughren and Kass, 1975 for reviews of this literature) and controlled experiments and quasi-experiments (Asirdas and Beech, 1975; Auerbach and Kilman, 1977; Husted, 1972; Obler, 1973; Wincze and Caird, 1976). However, the literature also suggests that the effects of desensitization are often limited to anxiety reduction (Husted, 1972; Kockott, Dittmar, and Nusselt, 1975). In cases where the dysfunction is due in part to skill deficits, treatment effects will be maximized to the extent that sexual skill training is included either implicitly, as is often true in video and in vivo desensitization, or explicitly (Asirdas and Beech, 1975; Kockott, Dittmar, and Nusselt, 1975; Kohlenberg, 1974; Mathews, Bancroft, Whitehead, et al., 1976; Wincze and Caird, 1976).

In vivo desensitization is the most commonly used variant of the technique in clinical practice, because it allows the therapist to alter the clients' sexual behavior directly through therapist and partner instruction and feedback. It is often supplemented by films or videotapes when the client experiences high levels of anxiety or is particularly unskilled in sexual technique. Imaginal exposure to the scenes, and anxiety-reducing agents such as progressive relaxation, hypnosis, and methohexital sodium, are also useful with an extremely anxious client (Brady, 1971; Fuchs, Hoch, Paldi, et al., 1973; Hogan, 1978; Husted, 1972; Kaplan, 1974).

An effective variation of desensitization for cases of vaginismus involves the insertion of progressively larger dilators or fingers into the vagina until it can dilate sufficiently to accommodate a penis (Ellison, 1972; Fuchs et al., 1973; Kaplan, 1974; Masters and Johnson, 1970).

Implosion and Guided Imagining. Two other anxiety-reduction techniques, implosion and guided imagining, have been employed to treat sexual dysfunctions. Implosion involves having the client imagine scenes that produce a maximum amount of anxiety, rather than a minimum amount, as in the case of desensitization. In addition, the scenes involve unrealistic and psychodynamic elements, and the technique is believed to work on the basis of extinction rather than counterconditioning (Stampfl and Levis, 1967). Frankel (1970) reports a successfully treated case of orgasmic dysfunction and general sexual dysfunction.

In guided imagining, the client imagines a continuous sexual scene rather than a hierarchy of discrete scenes, as in the case of desensitization. Wolpin (1969) believes that it works via extinction and positive reinforcement for imagining the scenes. Guided imagining has been used to treat erectile failure (Wolpin, 1969), and, in conjunction with hypnosis, to treat erectile failure (Dittborn, 1957; Hussain, 1964), vaginismus, dyspareunia, and frigidity (Hussain, 1964; Leckie, 1964).

Masters and Johnson's Program. Masters and Johnson (1970) have reported a treatment program that has been used with a variety of dysfunctions with a failure rate of only 18.9% at post-treatment and 20% at a 5-year follow-up. Although Masters and Johnson do not explain their program on the basis of behavioral principles, it resembles in vivo desensitization in that the couple is assigned a series of graduated sexual activities to be carried out at home. Dengrove, in fact, has described their program as "typically Wolpeian" (Dengrove, 1971b, p. 112), and Laughren and Kass (1975) consider it to be a form of in vivo desensitization.

It is clear that the Masters and Johnson program does borrow heavily from Wolpe, but it is an error to consider it to be pure in vivo desensitization. It differs in a number of ways from Wolpe's approach, such as (1) the 2-week stay in St. Louis, which removes the couple from its normal environment; (2) 2-week intensive therapy instead of the more widely spaced sessions in desensitization; (3) an emphasis on treating the couple's relationship rather than the individual client; (4) the use of cotherapists; (5) explicit communication training; (6) sexual skill training; and (7) an emphasis on obtaining pleasure in addition to anxiety reduction (Mathews et al., 1976). No experimental study has directly compared the effectiveness of Masters and Johnson's program to in vivo desensitization, but the evidence cited above suggests that the explicit sexual skill training found in Masters and Johnson's program may add to the effectiveness of a pure anxiety-reduction technique.

SKILL TRAINING. Behavior therapists (Bandura, 1968) have pointed out the necessity of distinguishing between behavioral inhibitions and behavioral deficits. If a client has learned a certain skill, but anxiety prevents him from exercising it, he is said to have a behavioral inhibition. If the client has never learned the skill, and is thus unable to perform it even if he is perfectly relaxed, he is said to have a behavioral deficit. In cases of sexual dysfunction the two often coexist, so that the patient is both deficient in sexual and social skills and inhibited in expressing them. To the extent that a client is deficient in sexual skills, skill training must be incorporated as part of the treatment.

Sexual and social skills have been taught in a variety of ways in the treatment of sexual dysfunctions, including bibliotherapy (Barbach, 1974; LoPiccolo, 1977a; Mikulas and Lowe, 1974); modeling of responses by the therapist, films, videotapes, and slides (LoPiccolo, 1977a; Wincze and Caird, 1976; Wolpe, 1973; Yulis, 1976); behavioral rehearsal (LoPiccolo and Lobitz, 1972; Yulis, 1976); and feedback from the therapist and from the sexual partner (LoPiccolo, 1977a; Masters and Johnson, 1970; Serber, 1974).

The skills most commonly taught are specific sexual skills, such as techniques of stimulating the client's sexual partner (LoPiccolo, 1977a; Masters and Johnson, 1970), self-stimulation (LoPiccolo and Lobitz, 1972), and in cases of premature ejaculation, the highly effective squeeze (Masters and Johnson, 1970) and pause (Semans, 1956) techniques. Communication skills have also been emphasized by many sex therapists, including communication of sexual likes and dislikes, feedback during sexual activity, techniques of initiating and refusing sex, and communication of nonsexual feelings (Kaplan, 1974; Lobitz and LoPiccolo, 1972; LoPiccolo, 1977a; Masters and Johnson, 1970; Prochaska and Marzilli, 1973; Snyder, LoPiccolo, and LoPiccolo, 1975). In spite of the apparent clinical utility of communication training and the emphasis placed upon it by sex therapists (including the authors), the only experimental study investigating the effectiveness of communication training found no differences on a series of dependent variables between patients receiving communication training and those not receiving such training (Husted, 1972). Since clinical practice contradicts the experimental findings in this area, further research, employing different target behaviors, assessment instruments, and communication techniques, is needed.

A final skill often taught by sex therapists is assertiveness, which is useful in helping clients establish sexual relationships, initiate sex, refuse sex, ask for specific types of sexual stimulation, and express dislike for certain types of sexual activities (Dengrove, 1967; Lazarus, 1971; Salter, 1961; Wolpe, 1973; Wolpe and Lazarus, 1966). Yulis (1976) found that assertiveness training increased the likelihood of generalization of treatment gains to sexual partners not involved in therapy in cases of premature ejaculation.

SENSORY AWARENESS, COGNITIVE THERAPY, AND ATTITUDE-CHANGE PROCEDURES. Lazarus (1974) has stressed the importance of considering a number of different modalities in psychotherapy, including sensations, imagery, and cognitions. Sex therapists have intervened in each of these modalities in the treatment of sexual dysfunctions. Kaplan (1974) instructs clients to concentrate on the physical sensations experienced during sexual activities in order to both increase sexual arousal and to distract themselves from interfering, obsessive thoughts. Heiman, LoPiccolo, and LoPiccolo (1976) teach clients to relax through a method of sensory awareness (developed by Weitzman), when anxiety is interfering with arousal.

Ellis (1962, 1971) uses an approach called rational-emotive therapy in which the client is instructed to replace irrational, anxiety-provoking thoughts about performance and failure with rational thoughts. LoPiccolo and his colleagues (Lobitz et al., 1976; LoPiccolo, 1977a) help their clients change negative attitudes about sex through such methods as bibliotherapy and therapist self-disclosure (about sexual behavior) and teach clients to relabel anxiety, tension, and coldness as "sexual arousal" when they have been mislabeling their sexual sensations. The use of sexual fantasy has been advocated by Kaplan (1974) for increasing patients' sexual arousal and reducing distracting thoughts. Finally, the technique of direct thought stopping has been used to stop obsessive performance concerns (Garfield, McBrearty, and Dichter, 1969) and to stop ejaculation in a case of premature ejaculation (Ince, 1973). These techniques are usually employed as adjuncts to more behavioral techniques, and no experimental research has been conducted on their effectiveness.

Behavior Change Techniques. A number of procedures are used in the treatment of sexual dysfunctions to alter directly the frequency of certain target behaviors. Clients are instructed to engage in or refrain from certain behaviors by most sex therapists (Kaplan, 1974; LoPiccolo, 1977a; Masters and Johnson, 1970). Operant techniques are also used, such as client self-monitoring of sexual behavior, positive reinforcement of the client's behavior change by the sexual partner and by the therapist, and refundable penalty deposits from which clients are fined if they do not carry out homework assignments (Lobitz and LoPiccolo, 1972). In addition, Lobitz and LoPiccolo (1972) have clients participate in the planning of homework assignments and in writing out maintenance programs at the end of therapy in order to maintain treatment gains.

Marital Therapy. Sexual dysfunctions are often embedded in dysfunctional marriages (Kaplan, 1974; McGovern et al., 1975). In some of these cases it is possible to bypass the marital conflicts, but it is often necessary to resolve the nonsexual problems in the marriage before the sexual ones are amenable to treatment (Kaplan, 1974). This is especially true in some cases of erectile failure and situational and secondary orgasmic dysfunction (Snyder, et al., 1975).

Psychodynamic Techniques. Kaplan (1974) presents an interesting integration of behavioral and psychodynamic techniques in the treatment of sexual dysfunction. She concentrates on the current sexual behaviors of the couple until client resistance requires her to deal with dynamic material. Although there are no data to support the adjunct use of psychodynamic techniques, the authors have found it clinically useful to conceptualize sexual dysfunctions in terms of psychodynamics and systems theory while employing behavioral interventions. The usefulness of psychodynamic theory appears to increase with complex cases in which skill deficits and conditioned anxiety are not paramount.

Medical/Physical Procedures. In evaluating the effectiveness of pharmacological, surgical, and other physical procedures in treatment of sexual dysfunction, the clinical literature tends not to include the appropriate double blind placebo studies. Thus, the effects of many of these procedures cannot be separated from placebo effects, which can, of course, be very powerful (Shapiro, 1971; Silbergeld, Manderscheid, and Soeken, 1976). Assuming the patients are physiologically within normal limits, the mechanism for genuine therapeutic effects (beyond placebo effects) of such pharmacologic or surgical procedures is unclear at best (Note 10).

Pharmacotherapy. A wide variety of pharmacological agents have been used with varying degrees of success to raise level of sexual drive, delay ejaculation, induce orgasm, or heighten the intensity of orgasm.

One genuinely effective type of pharmacological therapy is the use of antidepressant medication for mildly to moderately depressed sexually dysfunctional patients. The effect of depression in suppressing libido is well documented, and a course of antidepressant medication is indicated for patients with low sex drive *and* with symptoms of clinical depression (Winokur, 1963). There is no evidence that the use of antidepressant medication is helpful in non-depressed cases of low sex drive. There is also no good evidence to indicate superiority of one particular class of antidepressant medication, in terms of effects on sex drive and sexual functioning.

A less effective use of psychopharmacological agents is the use of phenothiazenes or other antianxiety agents to delay ejaculation in premature ejaculation cases. Ejaculation is primarily sympathetically ennervated, and inability to ejaculate at all is a reported side effect of some antisympathetic phenothiazenes (LoPiccolo, 1977a). However, evidence for clinical effectiveness of antianxiety drugs such as methohexital (Kraft and Al-Issa, 1968; Friedman, 1968) in treatment of premature ejaculation is weak at best. Given the major sedating effects of phenothiazenes, their use in treatment of premature ejaculation is not recommended.

A somewhat more effective use of antianxiety agents is in cases of erectile failure or orgasmic dysfunction related to severe anxiety. Here there is better evidence that use of tranquilizing drugs (Brady, 1966, 1971; Friedman, 1968; Kraft, 1969a,b) or alcohol (Dengrove, 1971a) can be a somewhat useful adjunct to other behavioral treatment techniques.

As previously noted, exogenous administration of testosterone does not seem useful in treatment of erectile failure in men with normal endogenous plasma testosterone levels (Jarvik and Brecher, 1977). Exogenous testosterone does seem to have a genuine effect of raising sex drive and orgasmic capacity in hormonally normal women, but only in very large doses where clitoral hypertrophy and a host of undesirable virilizing side effects occur, thus making clinical use impractical (Kennedy, 1973).

There is a small and primarily anecdotal literature which indicates inhalation of epinephrine or amyl nitrate can induce orgasm and also heighten the sensations of orgasm in both men and women (Jarvik and Brecher, 1977). These effects apparently depend on the sympathetic arousal and the peripheral vasodilation produced by these agents. Again, controlled studies are lacking, and potentially dangerous side effects (e.g., cardiovascular failure) contraindicate the routine therapeutic use of such agents.

The effects of alcohol on sexual response have been a subject of discussion for centuries, as witness the door porter's comment on alcohol in *Macbeth* "Lechery, sir, it provokes and unprovokes; it provokes the desire but takes away the performance," (Act II, Scene I). Retrospective questionnaire data generally indicate that alcohol enhances subjective enjoyment of sex (Athanasiou, Shauer, and Tavris, 1970). Although alcohol has been prescribed as a treatment for anxiety-related erectile failure, as noted above, physiological evidence for genuine tension-reducing effects of alcohol is unconvincing (Cappell and Herman, 1972). Beyond an initial very small facilitative effect on erection (probably through general peripheral vasodilation), increasing doses of alcohol have been shown to have a linearly increasing effect of interfering with erection. Furthermore, the cirrhotic liver damage associated with chronic alcoholism has been shown to be associated with depleted plasma testosterone, feminized body structure, lack of sex drive, and erectile failure in men (Wilson, 1977). Such changes are not always reversible, even after years of sobriety.

A large but almost entirely anecdotal literature exists on the effects of "recreational" drugs on sexual functioning. Cannabis (marijuana and hashish) does seem to facilitate both arousal and orgasm, and has been used in treatment of orgasmic dysfunction, with some success. LSD has been reported to both facilitate and to block sexual arousal, and the same effects have been reported for cocaine. Opiates such as heroin and morphine have been used in India for centuries to prolong erection and delay ejaculation, but have been shown to lead to loss of sex drive, lowered serum testosterone levels, and erectile failure as well (Jarvik and Brecher, 1977). Again, it is impossible to separate placebo effects from genuine pharmacological effects in these anecdotal reports.

The search for a genuine aphrodisiac, to induce sexual desire, seems to be a cultural and historical universal in human societies. The list of substances which have been identified as aphrodisiacs is almost endless, and ranges from substances with suggestive shapes (e.g., rhinoceros horn) to urethral irritants (e.g., cantharides or Spanish fly). There is some suggestion in recent animal experimental literature that dopamine facilitates sexual arousal and function, and serotonin has an opposite effect (Gessa and Tagliamonte, 1974), which matches clinical reports of increased sexual drive produced by agents such as L-dopa, *p*-chlorophenylalanine, and apomorphine (Jarvik and Brecher, 1977). However, the possible therapeutic use of such substances must await much further research.

Surgical Procedures. Currently, there are two surgical procedures which are being used for treatment of male erectile impotence. Obviously, before subjecting the patient to surgical intervention, an accurate diagnosis of organic as opposed to psychogenic etiology should be made, preferably by the use of plethysmographic monitoring of nocturnal penile tumescence (Karacan, 1978). Furthermore, a differential diagnosis should be made between cases involving a failure of penile blood flow and those involving neurological or endocrine factors. Finally, all even minimally doubtful cases should be given a trial in psychotherapy, as a final diagnostic screening (Renshaw, 1978).

One promising surgical procedure has recently been developed for erectile failure caused by failure of penile blood flow (Britt, Kemmerer, and Robison, 1971; Gaskell, 1971). In this procedure, adequate penile blood flow is reestablished through transplant of the inferior epigastric artery. This procedure is as yet very new, and adequate outcome data have not been reported. Clinical reports, however, indicate a good prognosis for recovery of normal erection and ejaculation.

A less completely successful surgical intervention is the use of an implanted penile prosthesis. These prostheses, either a rigid plastic rod (Small-Carrion device) or an inflatable hydraulic system (Bradley-Scott device), make the flaccid penis sufficiently rigid for intercourse to take place. However, true functioning with arousal, pleasure, and ejaculation is not restored. Thus, the devices are indicated only in men with neuropathy or endocrinological pathology which is not reversible, and only when the patients will be satisfied with this level of functioning. This point needs emphasis, as patients often believe that the prosthesis will produce true erection and ejaculation (Renshaw, 1978).

For female sexual dysfunction there are at present no surgical interventions which could be considered to be of proven effectiveness. There has been mention of the freeing of adhesions between clitoral shaft and hood, or indeed the circumcision of the clitoral hood, as treatment for female orgasmic dysfunction (Barbach, 1975). Since the clitoris retracts under the hood during high plateau levels of arousal (Masters and Johnson, 1966), the rationale for circumcision seems to be contradicted by normal physiology. The rationale for freeing of adhesions is more physiologically sound, as friction between clitoral hood and shaft (caused by the penis displacing the labia) is a factor in coital orgasm (Masters and Johnson, 1966). Painful deposits of smegma or adhesions could interfere with this process, but the vast majority of inorgasmic women do not have such adhesions. Again, placebo effects probably account for reported effects of removal of clitoral adhesions.

Recently, there have been reports in the popular literature of a surgical procedure to induce coital orgasm by narrowing the vaginal opening, tucking the clitoris and labia into the introitus, and cutting the pubococcygeal muscle to displace the vagina so that penile thrusting can be in a plane which leads to penile-clitoral contact. There are no objective data on this process to date, and it raises serious issues of pelvic floor support, complications of delivery in the event of subsequent pregnancy, and also seems simply illogical: clitoral stimulation during intercourse can be accomplished simply through the use of concurrent manual manipulation.

Physical Therapy Procedures. Jogging, yoga, breathing exercises, and a wide variety of other physical training procedures have all been advocated for treatment of sexual dysfunction. While anything that leads to an increased sense of physical well-being probably contributes to sexual function, there is no evidence for specific effects of such treatments.

There is one physical training procedure that does seem to be genuinely useful in treatment of female orgasmic dysfunction. This procedure is voluntary contractile exercise of the pubococcygeal musculature which surrounds the vagina. Originally developed by Kegel (1952) for treatment of urinary stress incontinence, it was soon discovered that a serendipitous side effect of strengthening these muscles was the occurrence of orgasm in previously inorgasmic women. The Kegel exercises have since become a part of most sex therapy programs for inorgasmic women, and indeed a major component of some programs (Kline-Graber and Graber, 1975).

THERAPY MODALITIES

Sex therapy has been conducted in a variety of modalities: individual therapy, conjoint therapy, and group therapy, with one therapist, two therapists, and minimal therapist contact.

Masters and Johnson (1970) emphasize the necessity of conjoint therapy and cotherapy, but both of these features appear unnecessary. Many patients have been treated successfully without their spouses participating in treatment (Franks and Wilson, 1974; Hogan, 1977, 1978; Laughren and Kass, 1975), and one experiment found no difference in effectiveness between individual and conjoint therapy (Husted, 1972). Individual therapists have often successfully treated patients without the aid of a cotherapist (Franks and Wilson, 1974; Hogan, 1977, 1978; Kaplan, 1974; Laughren and Kass, 1975). The one experimental study on the subject found that overall, with three different types of therapy (systematic desensitization plus counseling, directed practice plus counseling, modelled on Masters and Johnson's program, and directed practice with minimum therapist contact), patients receiving cotherapy did no better than those seen by single therapists. However, there was a nonsignificant increase in the effectiveness of the Masters and Johnson type therapy when cotherapists were used rather than single therapists (Mathews et al., 1976).

Bibliotherapy with minimal therapist contact has been effective in the treatment of premature ejaculation (Mikulas and Lowe, 1974; Zeiss, 1977) and a mixed group of dysfunctions (Mathews et al, 1976). Group therapy has been successful in cases of primary orgasmic dysfunction (Barbach, 1974; McGovern, Kirkpatrick, and LoPiccolo, 1976; Schneidman and McGuire, 1976), general sexual dysfunction (Lazarus, 1968), premature ejaculation (Kaplan et al., 1974; McGovern et al., 1976), and a heterogeneous group (Leiblum, Rosen, and Pierce, 1976). These two modalities can be very efficient and economical, and are probably most useful in the simpler sexual dysfunctions (primary orgasmic dysfunction and premature ejaculation) where clear-cut instructional programs are available (Kaplan et al., 1974).

FUTURE RESEARCH

Future research in the area of treatment would be most useful if it were aimed at answering the questions of which treatment components and therapy modalities are most effective, efficient, and economical with which specific types of dysfunctions and clients. Complex interactions probably exist between all of these factors, and factorial designs with waiting list control groups are necessary (Note 10). An emphasis on various skill-training techniques (especially communication training), brief therapy, minimal therapist contact, group therapy, and the poorly understood area of low sex drive are particularly germane. In addition, approaches combining and comparing component techniques drawn from different theories (e.g., social learning theory, systems theory, and psychodynamic theory) would be very interesting. Finally, further research on patient samples drawn from different populations (e.g., the physically handicapped, the aging, psychiatric patients, working class patients, minority group members, and homosexual clients) is important.

Applications of Behavioral Sex Therapy Procedures to Special Populations

Until very recently, there has been a tendency to screen out patient applicants whose sexual dysfunction was occurring in a context of physical illness or psychiatric disturbance. Currently there is considerable interest in working with such patients, and with other special populations, such as the aged.

SEXUAL REHABILITATION OF CHRONICALLY ILL PATIENTS

In working with chronically ill patients, the clinician must consider just what level of sexual functioning is physiologically possible for the patient. Irreversible cord injury, diabetic neuropathy and vasculopathy, and severely restricted cardiovascular output are examples of conditions which will, in varying degree, limit the level of sexual response which can be obtained by the patient. It is important, however, not to assume that the organic disease is necessarily the maintaining cause of a sexual dysfunction. Physicians often tend to ignore the sexual concerns of medically ill patients, and not to recognize the role of anxiety in producing sexual dysfunction in physically ill patients. Thus, for example, a post-coronary male may have erectile failure not due to restricted pelvic blood flow, but secondary to anxiety about his sexual functioning after a heart attack.

CARDIAC PATIENTS. Excellent recent reviews of sexual response in post-coronary patients are provided by Wagner (1977) and Friedman (1978). Research has shown that many coronary patients have a loss of sex drive and begin to experience erectile failure during their recovery. These problems are associated with a low frequency of sexual activity and continue even after the patient has undergone an otherwise successful rehabilitation and has resumed a normally active life in all other areas. A major concern of such patients seems to revolve around the possibility of sudden death during sexual activity. In actuality, the cardiac cost of marital sexual intercourse has been found to be rather low, roughly equal to climbing one or two flights of stairs. Clinical lore to the contrary, the male superior position does not seem to require greater cardiac output than a male supine position (Friedman, 1978).

Treatment for the post-coronary patient with sexual concerns needs to include some elements beyond the procedures previously discussed in this chapter. An exercise program to increase cardiac output, the use of prophylactic nitroglycerin to prevent (or treat) pain during intercourse, and the instruction to avoid sex after large intake of food or alcohol, are all indicated. An exercise stress test ECG is useful both in ensuring that the patient can tolerate the cardiac cost of sexual activity, and to reassure the patient about this. Antihypertensive and diuretic medications sometimes have the side effect of interfering with erection, and it may be necessary to prescribe alternative medications if erectile failure occurs in response to the initially prescribed medication.

DIABETIC PATIENTS. It is well established that a significant percentage of diabetic males will eventually experience erectile failure (Ellenberg, 1971). This erectile failure is strongly associated with diabetic neuropathy, and occurs even in patients who are well managed with diet control and insulin. In contrast, the effects of diabetes on female sexual response seem to be minimal (Ellenberg, 1977).

Diabetic erectile failure tends to have a slow and gradual onset, with sex drive remaining intact. Neurological, vascular, and nocturnal penile tumescence examinations need to be conducted before concluding that erectile failure in a diabetic man is organic and irreversible. There have been reports in the literature that standard sex therapy procedures are successful in restoring erectile capacity to some diabetics (Renshaw, 1978). For cases where such psychotherapy is unsuccessful, behavioral counseling emphasizing the use of non-intercourse methods of sexual pleasuring is indicated. In cases where the patients are unsatisfied by such oral and manual stimulation techniques, referral for implant of a penile prosthesis may be indicated, as previously discussed.

RENAL FAILURE PATIENTS. Around one-half of patients with end-stage kidney disease will have erectile failure. Renal dialysis only slightly reduces the incidence of erectile failure in such patients. However, many dialysis patients with erectile failure will have erectile capacity restored after a successful kidney transplant (Abram, Hester, Sheridan et al., 1975). The physiological basis for the erectile failure is not known, and psychological factors, especially depression, probably play some role in the loss of erectile function. In working with such cases, the clinician should again try a course of behavioral sex therapy before routinely assuming that the loss of function is exclusively physiological. Advising dialysis patients about non-coital techniques of sexual gratification is indicated, both to reduce performance anxiety and to help alleviate depression about loss of sexual function.

SPINAL CORD-INJURED PATIENTS. There is an extensive literature on the topic of sexual functioning in cord-injured patients. An excellent review of this literature is provided by Higgins (1978). As is the case for the diseases discussed above, assessment of the level of physiological response which is possible following injury, and then helping the patients to find a satisfying pattern of sexual activity within these limits, are the major elements of rehabilitation.

SEXUAL DYSFUNCTION IN PSYCHIATRIC PATIENTS

In the past, patients with any significant degree of psychopathology, except for marital distress, have been routinely excluded from sex therapy. There is a considerable change in this attitude now taking place, and clinicians are beginning to treat both neurotic and psychotic patients who have coexistent sexual problems. Indeed, the few studies that have been done tend to show remarkably little effect of psychiatric status upon sexual functioning, except in the cases of depression (Winokur, 1963). There are even some programs which are now treating hospitalized psychotic patients, with initially promising results (Lobitz, 1977).

OTHER SPECIAL POPULATIONS

THE AGED. There are relatively few changes in sexual response with aging, and the changes that do occur are not necessarily incompatible with a highly active and satisfying sex life. In the aging male, it takes longer and more intense stimulation to produce erection and to reach ejaculation. These changes, of course, can be entirely positive. This slowing of response occurs in women also, which means that adequate vaginal lubrication takes longer to develop. Males will not have as firm and rigid an erection in age as in youth, and may not be able to ejaculate on every occasion. The role of the clinician in working with elderly patients should be to explain these normal changes, and to ensure that the patients do not develop anxiety reactions which can lead to sexual dysfunction. For example, a man who has always had an erection rapidly may note that he is not getting an erection early in a session with his wife, become anxious, and discontinue the session before the erection has a chance to develop. Thus, many sexually dysfunctional elderly patients are dysfunctional not because of physiological changes in aging per se, but because of their reaction to these changes. Good reviews of sex and aging are provided by Martin (1977) and by Van Keep and Gregory (1977).

SEXUALITY DURING PREGNANCY AND POST PARTUM. There is evidence that some women experience a decrease in sex drive and in orgasmic capacity during the last trimester of pregnancy (Solberg, Butler, and Wagner, 1973) and the post partum period (Haspels, 1977). Physical discomfort, fear of injury to the baby, and awkwardness in coitus seem to be the reasons women identify for such changes (Solberg et al., 1973). In cases where this change in interest has occurred and is causing distress, the patients should be instructed in techniques of manual and oral-genital stimulation as an alternative to coitus, and in the use of comfortable coital positions (e.g., side to side). There is no evidence that coitus injures the fetus or mother, and many obstetricians now feel that coitus can be continued virtually until delivery and resumed as soon after delivery as is physically comfortable.

Conclusion

CONTRIBUTIONS AND LIMITATIONS OF BEHAVIOR THERAPY IN THE TREATMENT OF SEXUAL DYSFUNCTIONS

Behavior therapy and social learning theory have contributed more to the treatment of sexual dysfunctions than any other theoretical approach. These contributions have been in three major areas: (1) providing a simple and useful model of reality, which has allowed researchers to focus on the critical variables involved in the treatment of dysfunctions; (2) an emphasis on the experimental method; and (3) providing effective and efficient techniques.

MODEL OF REALITY. Social learning theory has constructed a model of reality by adopting a methodological rule of simplicity, limiting the number of variables under consideration, limiting the type of variables studied to those that are observable, and insisting on operational definitions of these variables.

The parsimony rule requires that when a number of explanations can account for a phenomenon, the simplest one is adopted. This principle eliminates excess theoretical concepts which, while often appealing in their elegance, actually add nothing to a simpler explanation based on fewer constructs. Thus, many complex psychodynamic explanations can be replaced by simpler ones based on conditioning and learning principles. By eliminating these excess constructs, attention can be focused on a fewer number of variables, and consequently the probability of discovering the variables controlling a given behavior is increased, which leads in turn to more effective treatments.

In addition to limiting the number of variables under consideration, social learning theory deals with variables that are maximally observable. Hypotheses are verifiable to the extent that their critical variables are observable; thus, etiological explanations based on performance anxiety are much more verifiable than those based on castration anxiety and unresolved Oedipal conflicts. Because of this, social learning theory evolves as old hypotheses are continually superseded by more adequate ones, while psychodynamic explanations tend to persist because they are impossible to refute. The emphasis on operationism (Note 11) also helps pin down concepts to observable events, which further increases the objectivity and testability of the theory.

These factors together increase the power of social learning theory. Once an investigator has restricted the variables under study to a limited number of relevant, observable factors, he is able to gain considerable control over the target behavior in question. In contrast, an investigator who devises techniques based on a more general theory consisting of many unobservable, nonoperationalized constructs will have little chance of stumbling upon the relevant controlling variables. These factors are in part responsible for the dramatic improvement in treatment effectiveness and efficiency that resulted when sex therapy researchers switched from psychodynamic theory to social learning theory.

EXPERIMENTAL METHOD. The second major advance in sex therapy research involves the gradual replacement of investigation based solely on the case study method with that based on the experimental method. For years psychoanalysis and psychodynamic psychotherapy were employed in the treatment of sexual dysfunctions with no real evidence of effectiveness. Once behavior therapists began reporting objective data from experimental studies, the ineffective dynamic techniques were quickly replaced by effective behavioral ones. If behavior therapists had relied on uncontrolled case studies, their arguments would have been much less convincing.

EFFECTIVE AND EFFICIENT TECHNIQUES. The third major contribution, effective and efficient techniques, is largely a result of the other two contributions. Twenty years ago, clients suffering from sexual dysfunctions could look forward to years of expensive psychotherapy with a minimal chance for a successful outcome. The picture has changed completely, so that now the majority of clients presenting with sexual dysfunctions can be helped to some degree in a matter of months.

A MULTIDIMENSIONAL CONCEPTUALIZATION OF SEXUAL DYSFUNCTIONS AND THEIR TREATMENT

Some of the very factors which make behavior therapy so effective in the treatment of sexual dysfunctions also put limitations upon its usefulness. In the early stages of development of the field, the narrowly focused high-power approach was necessary. However, now that some of the basic techniques are fairly well established (e.g., anxiety-reduction and skill training), the viewpoint must be widened to include other variables. Including these new variables in sex therapy will not produce the dramatic results first obtained with behavior therapy, but it may help in those cases in which the current behavioral techniques are ineffective.

A multidimensional approach includes, in addition to behaviors, eliciting stimuli, and reinforcing stimuli: (1) personality and psychiatric status, which are almost completely ignored by the behavioral approach, but which are important in fitting the technique to the individual patient; (2) psychodynamics and defenses, which appear, at least at a clinical level, to be important in many sexual dysfunctions; (3) cognitive variables, such as those emphasized by Ellis; (4) interpersonal systems, especially marital relationships, which often have a great impact on sexual functioning; (5) biological factors, which are known to affect sexual functioning, but which are usually considered error variance by behaviorists; (6) subtle communication variables, which are difficult to describe in behavioral terminology; and (7) an existential view of the client's position, which can capture many phenomena totally outside of the behavioral world view. The combination of the effective techniques and sophisticated research strategies of the behavior therapists with the wider focus of a multidimensional conceptualization should lead to even more effective treatments for sexual dysfunctions.

Notes

1. The usual approach to dealing with this problem has been to divide the categories into subtypes (Ansari, 1975; Cooper, 1968a, 1969b; Masters and Johnson, 1970). However, this leads to ever lengthening lists of diagnoses which soon become unmanageable.
2. All of the couples treated were heterosexual. If a therapist treats homosexual couples, a homosexual sex drive would no doubt be related to successful outcome.
3. Other investigators define "premature ejaculation" differently. See Kaplan (1974), LoPiccolo (1977a), and Masters and Johnson (1970) for discussions of this issue.
4. *Psychogenic* dyspareunia is even less often found in males; therefore, throughout this chapter, "dyspareunia" will refer to female dyspareunia unless otherwise stated.
5. In comparing reports from different investigators, it is important to keep in mind that LoPiccolo (1977a) and Masters and Johnson (1970) define these terms differently than does Kaplan. LoPiccolo's and Masters and Johnson's "primary" equals Kaplan's "primary absolute"; LoPiccolo's "secondary" is equivalent to Masters and Johnson's "situational," and includes both Kaplan's "situational" and "secondary."
6. Ansari (1975) and Cooper (1968b,c) have compared dysfunctional patients to control groups, but the number and types of variables studied were extremely limited.
7. For a thorough review of etiological factors, see Amelar and Dubin (1968), Ansari (1975), Cooper (1968a,b,c; 1969a,b), Dengrove (1968), Ellis (1971), Ellison (1972), Friedman (1973), Kaplan (1974), Kaufman (1967), Lazarus (1963), Masters and Johnson (1970), McGovern, Stewart, and LoPiccolo (1975), Ovesey and Meyers (1968), and Twombly (1968).
8. Erectile failure and dyspareunia are often due to physical or physiological factors, and patients presenting with these problems should always receive physical examinations. This is true even if an obvious psychogenic component is present, since psychological factors can interact with organic and physiological ones to cause the dysfunction (Kaplan, 1974).
9. For discussions of experimental methodology in psychotherapy research in general, see Campbell and Stanley (1963), Kiesler (1971), and Neale and Liebert (1973); for experimental methodology in sex therapy research, see Hogan (1977) and LoPiccolo (1977c).
10. Placebo control groups are logically necessary in order to draw firm conclusions, but in the authors' opinion they are usually unethical.
11. "Operationism" is here used in a broad sense which includes chains of reduction sentences (Hempel, 1965b), rather than in the narrow sense originally advanced by Bridgman (1953).

References

Abram, H., Hester, L., Sheridan, W., and Epstein, G. Sexual functioning in patients with chronic renal failure. *J. Nerv. Ment. Dis.*, 1975, *160*, 220–226.

Amelar, R. D., and Dubin, L. Sex after major urologic surgery. *J. Sex Res.*, 1968, *4*, 265–274.

Ansari, J. M. A. A study of 65 impotent males. *Br. J. Psychiatry*, 1975, *127*, 337–341.

Asirdas, S., and Beech, H. R. The behavioral treatment of sexual inadequacy. *J. Psychosom. Res.*, 1975, *19*, 345–353.

Athanasiou, R., Shauer, P., and Tavris, C. Sex. *Psychol. Today*, 1970, *4*, 37–52.

Auerbach, R., and Kilman, P. R. The effects of group systematic desensitization on secondary erectile failure. *Behav. Ther.*, 1977, *8*, 330–339.

Bandura, A. A social learning interpretation of psychological dysfunctions. In P. London and D. Rosenhan (Eds.), *Foundation of abnormal psychology*, New York: Holt, Rinehart, and Winston, 1968, pp. 293–344.

Bandura A. *Principles of behavior modification*. New York: Holt, Rinehart, and Winston, 1969.

Barbach, L. G. Group treatment of preorgasmic women. *J. Sex Marital Ther.*, 1974, *1*, 139–145.

Barbach, L. G. *For yourself: The fulfillment of female sexuality*. New York: Doubleday, 1975.

Bergler, E. *Neurotic counterfeit-sex*. New York: Grune & Stratton, 1951.

Bergler, E., and Kroger, W. *Kinsey's myth of female sexuality: The medical facts*. New York: Grune & Stratton, 1954.

von Bertalanffy, L. *General system theory: Founda-*

tions, developments, applications. New York: George Braziller, 1968.

Beutler, L., Karacan, I., Anch, A., Salis, P., Scott, F., and Williams, R. MMPI and MIT discriminators of biogenic and psychogenic impotence. *J. Consult. Clin. Psychol.,* 1975, *43,* 899–903.

Blum, S. A study of the psychoanalytic theory of psychosexual development. *Genet. Psychol. Monogr.,* 1949, *39,* 3–99.

Brady, J. P. Brevital-relaxation treatment of frigidity. *Behav. Res. Ther.,* 1966, *4,* 71–77.

Brady, J. P. Brevital-aided systematic desensitization. In R. D. Rubin, H. Fensterheim, A. A. Lazarus, and C. M. Franks (Eds.), *Advances in behavior therapy: Proceedings of the third conference of the association for advancement of behavior therapy.* New York: Academic Press, 1971, pp. 77–83.

Bridgman, P. W. The logic of modern physics. In H. Feigl and M. Brodbeck (Eds.), *Readings in the philosophy of science.* New York: Appleton-Century-Crofts, 1953, pp. 34–46.

Britt, D. B., Kemmerer, W. T., and Robison, J. R. Penile blood flow determination by mercury strain gauge plethysmography. *Invest. Urol.,* 1971, *8,* 673–677.

Campbell, D. T., and Stanley, J. C. *Experimental and quasi-experimental designs for research.* Chicago: Rand McNally, 1963.

Cappell, H., and Herman, C. Alcohol and tension reduction: A review. *Q. J. Stud. Alc.,* 1972, *33,* 33–64.

Comfort, A. *The anxiety makers.* Camden, N.J.: T. Nelson and Sons, 1965.

Cooper, A. J. A factual study of male potency disorders. *Br. J. Psychiatry,* 1968a, *114,* 719–731.

Cooper, A. J. Hostility and male potency disorders. *Compr. Psychiatry,* 1968b, *9,* 621–626.

Cooper, A. J. "Neurosis" and disorders of sexual potency in the male. *J. Psychosom. Res.,* 1968c, *12,* 141–144.

Cooper, A. J. A clinical study of "coital anxiety" in male potency disorders. *J. Psychosom. Res.,* 1969a, *13,* 143–147.

Cooper, A. J. Clinical and therapeutic studies in premature ejaculation. *Compr. Psychiatry,* 1969b, *10,* 285–295.

Cooper, A. J. Disorders of sexual potency in the male: A clinical and statistical study of some factors related to short-term prognosis. *Br. J. Psychiatry,* 1969c, *115,* 709–719.

Cooper, A. J. Frigidity: Treatment and short-term prognosis. *J. Psychosom. Res.,* 1970, *14,* 133–147.

Davison, G. C. and Neale, J. M. *Abnormal psychology: An experimental clinical approach,* New York: Wiley, 1974.

Dengrove, E. Behavior therapy of the sexual disorders. *J. Sex Res.,* 1967, *3,* 49–61.

Dengrove, E. Sexual responses to disease processes. *J. Sex Res.,* 1968, *4,* 257–264.

Dengrove, E. Behavior therapy of impotence. *J. Sex Res.,* 1971a, *7,* 177–183.

Dengrove, E. Book review of *Human sexual inadequacy. Behav. Ther.,* 1971b, *2,* 112–113.

Derogatis, L. R. Psychological assessment of sexual disorders. In J. Meyer (Ed.), *Clinical management of sexual disorders.* Baltimore, Williams & Wilkins, 1976.

Dittborn, J. Hypnotherapy of sexual impotence. *Int. J. Clin. Exp. Hypn.,* 1957, *5,* 181–192.

Ellenberg, M. Impotence in diabetes. *Ann. Intern. Med.,* 1971, *75,* 213–219.

Ellenberg, M. Sex and the female diabetic. *Med. Aspects Human Sexuality,* 1977, *11,* 30–38.

Ellis, A. *Reason and emotion in psychotherapy.* New York: Lyle Stuart, 1962.

Ellis, A. Rational-emotive treatment of impotence, frigidity and other sexual problems. *Profess. Psychol.,* 1971, *2,* 346–349.

Ellison, C. Vaginismus. *Medical Aspects of Human Sexuality,* August 1972, 34–54.

El-Senoussi, A. *The male impotence test.* Los Angeles: Western Psychological Services, 1964.

Feldman, M. P., and MacCulloch, M. J. *Homosexual behavior: Therapy and assessment.* New York: Pergamon, 1971.

Fenichel, O. *The psychoanalytic theory of neurosis.* New York: Norton, 1945.

Frankel, A. S. Treatment of multisymptomatic phobia by a self-directed, self-reinforced technique. *J. Abnorm. Psychol.,* 1970, *76,* 496–499.

Franks, C. M., and Wilson, G. T. (Eds.). *Annual review of behavior therapy: Theory and practice.* New York: Brunner/Mazel, 1974.

Freud, S. *Three essays on the theory of female sexuality.* New York: Avon, 1962. (First published in 1905.)

Friedman, D. The treatment of impotence by Brietal relaxation therapy. *Behav. Res. Ther.,* 1968, *6,* 257–261.

Friedman, G. Sexual adjustment of the post-coronary male. In J. LoPiccolo and L. LoPiccolo (Eds.), *Handbook of sex therapy.* New York: Plenum, 1978.

Friedman, M. Success phobia and retarded ejaculation. *Am. J. Psychother.,* 1973, *27,* 78–84.

Fuchs, K., Hoch, Z., Paldi, E., Abramovici, H., Brandes, J. M., Timor-Tritsch, I., and Kleinhaus, M. Hypno-desensitization therapy of vaginismus: Part I. "In vitro" method. Part II. "In vivo" method. *Int. J. Clin. Exp. Hypn.,* 1973, *21,* 144–156.

Garfield, Z. H., McBrearty, J. F., and Dichter, M. A case of impotence successfully treated with desensitization combined with in vivo operant training and thought substitution. In R. D. Rubin and C. M. Franks (Eds.), *Advances in behavior therapy, 1968.* New York: Academic Press, 1969, pp. 97–103.

Gaskell, P. The importance of penile blood pressure in cases of impotence. *J. Can. Med. Assoc.,* 1971, *20,* 1047–1050.

Gessa, G. L. and Tagliamonte, A. Possible role of brain serotonin and dopamine in controlling male sexual behavior. *Adv. Biochem. Psychopharmacol.,* 1974, *11,* 217–228.

Goldberg, R. R. A historical survey of personality scales and inventories. In P. McReynolds (Ed.), *Advances in psychological assessment.* Vol. 2. Palo Alto, Calif.: Science and Behavior Books, 1971.

Goldfried, M. R. Systematic densensitization as training in self-control. In M. R. Goldfried and M. Merbaum (Eds.), *Behavior change through self-control.* New York: Holt, Rinehart and Winston, 1973, pp. 248–256.

Hartman, W. E., and Fithian, M. A. *The treatment of sexual dysfunction.* Long Beach, Calif.: Center for Marital and Sexual Studies, 1972.

Haspels, A. A. The postpartum period. In J. Money and H. Musoph (Eds.), *Handbook of sexology.* New York: Elsevier-North Holland, 1977.

Hastings, D. W. *Impotence and frigidity.* Boston: Little, Brown and Company, 1963.

Heiman, J. Uses of psychophysiology in the assessment and treatment of sexual dysfunction. In J. LoPiccolo and L. LoPiccolo (Eds.), *Handbook of sex therapy.* New York, Plenum, 1978.

Heiman, J., LoPiccolo, L., and LoPiccolo, J. *Becoming orgasmic: A sexual growth program for women.* Englewood Cliffs, N.J.: Prentice-Hall, 1976.

Hempel, C. G. Fundamentals of taxonomy. In C. G. Hempel, *Aspects of scientific explanation and other essays in the philosophy of science.* New York: The Free Press, 1965a.

Hempel, C. G. The theoretician's dilemma: A study in the logic of theory construction. In C. G. Hempel, (Ed.), *Aspects of scientific explanation and other essays in the philosophy of science.* New York: The Free Press, 1965b.

Higgins, G. Aspects of sexual response in spinal cord injured adults. In J. LoPiccolo and L. LoPiccolo (Eds.), *Handbook of sex therapy.* New York: Plenum, 1978.

Hogan, D. R. Sex therapy, *Society,* 1977, *14,* 38–42.

Hogan, D. R. The effectiveness of sex therapy: A review of the literature. In J. LoPiccolo and L. LoPiccolo (Eds.), *Handbook of sex therapy.* New York: Plenum, 1978, pp. 57–84.

Hoon, E. F., Hoon, P. W., and Wincze, J. The S.A.I.: An inventory for the measurement of female sexual arousal. *Arch. Sexual Behav.,* 1976, *5,* 208–215.

Hussain, A. Behavior therapy using hypnosis. In J. Wolpe, A. Salter, and L. Reyna (Eds.), *The conditioning therapies: The challenge in psychotherapy.* New York: Holt, Rinehart and Winston, 1964, pp. 54–61.

Husted, J. R. Effect of method of systematic desensitization and presence of sexual communication in the treatment of sexual anxiety by counterconditioning. In *Proceedings of the 80th Annual Convention of the American Psychological Association.* (Honolulu, Hawaii), 1972, *7,* 325–326.

Ince, L. P. Behavior modification of sexual disorders. *Am. J. Psychother.,* 1973, *27,* 446–451.

Jarvik, M. E., and Brecher, E. M. Drugs and sex: Inhibition and enhancement effects. In J. Money and H. Musaph (Eds.), *Handbook of sexology.* New York: Elsevier-North Holland, 1977.

Jemail, J. A. *Response bias in assessment of marital and sexual adjustment.* Unpublished Ph.D. thesis, State University of New York at Stony Brook, 1977.

Kanfer, F. H., and Saslow, G. Behavioral diagnosis. In C. M. Franks (Ed.), *Behavior therapy: Appraisal and status.* New York: McGraw-Hill, 1969, pp. 417–444.

Kaplan, H. S. *The new sex therapy.* New York: Brunner/Mazel, 1974.

Kaplan, H. S. Hypoactive sexual desire. *J. Sex Marital Ther.,* 1977, *3,* 3–9.

Kaplan, H. S., Kohl, R. N., Pomeroy, W. B. Offit, A. K., and Hogan, B. Group treatment of premature ejaculation. *Arch. Sexual Behav.,* 1974, *3,* 443–452.

Karacan, I., Advances in the psychophysiological assessment of male erectile impotence. In J. LoPiccolo and L. LoPiccolo (Eds.), *Handbook of sex therapy.* New York: Plenum, 1978.

Kaufman, J. Organic and psychological factors in the genesis of impotence and premature ejaculation. In C. W. Wahl (Ed.), *Sexual problems: Diagnosis and treatment in medical practice.* New York: The Free Press, 1967, pp. 133–148.

Kegel, A. H. Sexual function of the pubococcygeus muscle. *West. J. Obstet. Gynecol.,* 1952, *60,* 521.

Kennedy, B. J. Effect of massive doses of sex hormones on libido. *Med. Aspects Human Sexuality,* 1973, *7,* 67–80.

Kiesler, D. J. Experimental designs in psychotherapy research. In A. E. Bergin and S. L. Garfield (Eds.), *Handbook of psychotherapy and behavior change: An empirical analysis.* New York: Wiley, 1971, pp. 36–74.

Kiev, A., and Hackett, E. The chemotherapy of impotence and frigidity. *J. Sex Res.,* 1968, *4,* 220–224.

Kinsey, A. C., Pomeroy, W. B., and Martin, C. E. *Sexual behavior in the human male.* Philadelphia: W. B. Saunders, 1948.

Kinsey, A. C., Pomeroy, W. B., Martin, C. E., and Gebhard, P. H. *Sexual behavior in the human female.* Philadelphia: W. B. Saunders, 1952.

Kline-Graber, G., and Graber, B. *Woman's orgasm.* New York: Bobbs-Merril, 1975.

Kockott, G., Dittmar, F., and Nusselt, L. Systematic desensitization of erectile impotence: A controlled study. *Arch. Sexual Behav.,* 1975, *4,* 493–500.

Kohlenberg, R. J. Directed masturbation and the treatment of primary orgasmic dysfunction. *Arch. Sexual Behav.,* 1974, *3,* 349–356.

Kraft, T. Behavior therapy and target symptoms. *J. Clin. Psychol.,* 1969a, *25,* 105–109.

Kraft, T. Desensitization and the treatment of sexual disorders. *J. Sex Res.,* 1969b, *5,* 130–134.

Kraft, T. and Al-Issa, I. The use of methohexitone sodium in the systematic desensitization of premature ejaculation. *Br. J. Psychiatry,* 1968, *114,* 351–352 (Abstract).

Laughren, T. P., and Kass, D. J. Desensitization of sexual dysfunction: The present status. In A. S. Gurman and D. G. Rice (Eds.), *Couples in conflict: New directions in marital therapy.* New York: Aronson, 1975, pp. 281–302.

Lazarus, A. A. Group therapy in phobic disorders by systematic desensitization. *J. Abnorm. Soc. Psychol.,* 1961, *63,* 504–510.

Lazarus, A. A. The treatment of chronic frigidity by systematic desensitization. *J. Nerv. Ment. Dis.,* 1963, *136,* 272–278.

Lazarus, A. A. The treatment of a sexually inadequate man. In L. P. Ullman and L. Krasner (Eds.), *Case studies in behavior modification.* New York: Holt, Rinehart and Winston, 1965, pp. 243–245.

Lazarus, A. A. Behavior therapy in groups. In G. M. Gazda (Ed.), *Basic approaches to group psychotherapy and group counseling.* Springfield, Ill.: Charles C Thomas, 1968, pp. 149–175.

Lazarus, A. A. *Behavior therapy and beyond.* New York: McGraw-Hill, 1971.

Lazarus, A. A. "Hypnosis" as a facilitator in behavior therapy. *Int. J. Clin. Exp. Hypn.,* 1973, *21,* 25–31.

Lazarus, A. A. Multimodal behavior therapy: Treating the "BASIC ID." In C. M. Franks and G. T. Wilson, (Eds.), *Annual review of behavior therapy: Theory and practice*. New York: Brunner/Mazel, 1974, pp. 679–690.

Leckie, F. H. Hypnotherapy in gynecological disorders. *Int. J. Clin. Exp. Hypn.*, 1964, *12,* 121–146.

Leiblum, S. R., Rosen, R. C., and Pierce, D. Group treatment format: Mixed sexual dysfunctions. *Arch. Sexual Behav.*, 1976, *5,* 313–322.

Lobitz, W. C. The treatment of sexually dysfunctional psychotic couples. Paper presented at annual meeting at the American Psychological Association, San Francisco, August, 1977.

Lobitz, W. C. and LoPiccolo, J. New methods in the behavioral treatment of sexual dysfunction. *J. Behav. Ther. Exp. Psychiatry,* 1972, *3,* 265–271.

Lobitz, W. C., LoPiccolo, J., Lobitz, G., and Brockway, J. A closer look at simplistic behavior therapy for sexual dysfunction: Two case studies. In H. J. Eysenck (Ed.), *Case studies in behavior therapy.* London: Routledge and Kegan Paul, Ltd., 1976, pp. 237–272.

LoPiccolo, J. Direct treatment of sexual dysfunction in the couple. In J. Money and H. Musaph (Eds.), *Handbook of sexology.* New York: Elsevier/North Holland, 1977a.

LoPiccolo, J. From psychotherapy to sex therapy. *Society,* 1977b, *14,* 60–68.

LoPiccolo, J. Methodological issues in research and treatment of sexual dysfunction. In R. Green and J. Winer (Eds.), *Methodological issues in sex research.* Washington, D.C.: United States Government Printing Office, 1977c.

LoPiccolo, J., and Heiman, J. The role of cultural values in the prevention and treatment of sexual problems. In D. Qualls, J. Wincze, and D. Barlow (Eds.), *The prevention of sexual disorders: Issues and approaches.* New York: Plenum, 1978a.

LoPiccolo, L. and Heiman, J. Sexual assessment and history interview. In J. LoPiccolo and L. LoPiccolo (Eds.), *Handbook of sex therapy.* New York: Plenum, 1978b.

LoPiccolo, J., and Lobitz, W. C. The role of masturbation in the treatment of orgasmic dysfunction. *Arch. Sexual Behav.,* 1972, *2,* 163–172.

LoPiccolo, J., and Steger, J. The sexual interaction inventory: A new instrument for assessment of sexual dysfunction. *Arch. Sexual Behav.,* 1974, *3,* 585–595.

Lorand, S. Contribution to the problem of vaginal orgasm. *Int. J. Psychoanal.,* 1939, *20,* 432–438.

Martin, C. E. Sexual activity in the aging male. In J. Money and H. Musaph (Eds.), *Handbook of sexology.* New York: Elsevier-North Holland, 1977.

Masters, W. H., and Johnson, V. E. *Human sexual response.* Boston: Little, Brown, and Company, 1966.

Masters, W. H., and Johnson, V. E. *Human sexual inadequacy.* Boston: Little, Brown, and Company, 1970.

Mathews, A., Bancroft, J., Whitehead, A., Hackman, A., Julier, D., Bancroft, J., Gath, D., and Shaw, P. The behavioral treatment of sexual inadequacy: A comparative study. *Behav. Res. Ther.,* 1976, *14,* 427–436.

McGovern, K., Kirkpatrick, C., and LoPiccolo, J. A behavioral group treatment program for sexually dysfunctional couples. *J. Marriage Family Counsel.,* October, 1976, 397–404.

McGovern, K., Stewart, R., and LoPiccolo, J. Secondary organismic dysfunction. I: Analysis and strategies for treatment. *Arch. Sexual Behav.,* 1975, *4,* 265–272.

Mikulas, W. C., and Lowe, J. C. Self-control of premature ejaculation. Paper presented at the annual meeting of the Rocky Mountain Psychological Association, Denver, 1974.

Mischel, W. *Personality and assessment.* New York: Wiley, 1968.

Moore, B. E. Frigidity in women. *Am. Psychoanal. Assoc. J.,* 1961, *9,* 571–584.

Mosher, D. L. Measurement of guilt in females by self-report inventories. *J. Consult. Clin. Psychol.,* 1968, *32,* 690–695.

Munjack, D., Cristol, A., Goldstein, A., Phillips, D., Goldberg, A., Whipple, K., Staples, F., and Kanno, P. Behavioral treatment of orgasmic dysfunction: A controlled study. *Br. J. Psychiatry,* 1976, *129,* 497–502.

Neale, J. M., and Liebert, R. M. *Science and behavior: Introduction to methods of research.* Englewood Cliffs, N.J.: Prentice-Hall, 1973.

Nowinski, J. K. Predictors of treatment outcome: Factors that maintain sexual inadequacy. Unpublished manuscript, State University of New York at Stony Brook, 1977.

Obler, M. Systematic desensitization in sexual disorders. *J. Behav. Ther. Exp. Psychiatry,* 1973, *4,* 93–101.

Ovesey, L., and Meyers, H. Retarded ejaculation: Psychodynamics and psychotherapy. *Am. J. Psychother.,* 1968, *22,* 185–201.

Paul, G. L., and Bernstein, D. A. *Anxiety and clinical problems: Systematic desensitization and related techniques.* Morristown, N.J.: General Learning Press, 1973.

Prochaska, J. O., and Marzilli, R. Modifications of the Masters and Johnson approach to sexual problems. *Psychother. Theory Res. Prac.,* 1973, *10,* 294–296.

Renshaw, D. Impotence in diabetics. In J. LoPiccolo, and L. LoPiccolo (Eds.), *Handbook of sex therapy.* New York: Plenum, 1978.

Rimm, D. C., and Masters, J. C. *Behavior therapy: Techniques and empirical findings.* New York: Academic Press, 1974.

Rosen, I. The psychoanalytic approach to individual therapy. In J. Money and H. Musaph (Eds.), *Handbook of sexology.* New York: Elsevier-North Holland, 1977.

Salter, A. *Conditional reflex therapy.* New York: Creative Age Press, 1949.

Salter, A. *Conditioned reflex therapy, the direct approach to the reconstruction of personality,* 2nd ed. New York: Creative Press, 1961.

Schneidman, B., and McGuire, L. Group therapy for nonorgasmic women: Two age levels. *Arch. Sexual Behav.,* 1976, *5,* 239–247.

Schrenck-Notzing, A. von (1895). *The use of hypnosis in psychopathea sexualis, with special reference to contrary sexual interest.* New York: Julian Press, 1956.

Semans, J. H. Premature ejaculation: A new approach. *S. Med. J.,* 1956, *49,* 353–357.

Serber, M. Videotape feedback in the treatment of couples with sexual dysfunction. *Arch. Sexual Behav.,* 1974, *3,* 377–380.

Shapiro, A. K. Placebo effects in medicine, psychotherapy, and psychoanalysis. In A. E. Bergin and S. L. Garfield (Eds.), *Handbook of psychotherapy and behavior change.* New York: Wiley, 1971.

Sherfey, M. J. *The nature and evolution of female sexuality.* New York: Vintage, 1973.

Silbergeld, S., Manderscheid, R. W., and Soeken, D. R. Issues at the clinical-research interface: Placebo effect control groups. *J. Nerv. Ment. Dis.,* 1976, *163,* 1126–1133.

Snyder, A., LoPiccolo, L., and LoPiccolo, J. Secondary orgasmic dysfunction. II: Case study. *Arch. Sexual Behav.,* 1975, *4,* 277–283.

Solberg, D. A., Butler, J., and Wagner, N. Sexual behavior in pregnancy. *N. Engl. J. Med.,* 1973, *288,* 1098–1103.

Spiess, W. F. J. *The Psycho-physiology of premature ejaculation: Some factors related to ejaculatory patency.* Unpublished doctoral dissertation, State University of New York at Stony Brook, 1977.

Spitzer, R. L., Sheehy, M., and Endicott, J. DSM-III: Guiding principles. In V. M. Rakoff, H. C. Stancer, and H. B. Kedward (Eds.), *Psychiatric diagnosis.* New York: Brunner/Mazel, 1977, pp. 1–24.

Spitzer, R. L., and Wilson, P. T. Nosology and the official psychiatric nomenclature. In A. M. Freedman, H. I. Kaplan, and B. J. Sadock (Eds.), *Comprehensive textbook of psychiatry,* 2nd ed., Vol. I. (2nd ed.) Baltimore: Williams & Wilkins, 1975, pp. 824–845.

Stampfl, T. G., and Levis, D. J. Essentials of implosive therapy: A learning theory based psychodynamic behavioral therapy. *J. Abnorm. Psychol.,* 1967, *72,* 495–503.

Strupp, H. H., and Hadley, S. W. A tripartite model of mental health and therapeutic outcomes: With special reference to negative effects in psychotherapy. *Am. Psychol.,* 1977, *32,* 187–196.

Twombly, G. H. Sex after radical gynecological surgery. *J. Sex Res.,* 1968, *4,* 275–281.

Van Keep, P. A., and Gregory, A. Sexual relations in the aging female. In J. Money and H. Musaph (Eds.), *Handbook of sexology.* New York: Elsevier-North Holland, 1977.

Wagner, N. N. Sexual behavior and the cardiac patient. In J. Money and H. Musaph (Eds.), *Handbook of sexology.* New York: Elsevier-North Holland, 1977.

Watzlawick, P., Beavin, J., and Jackson, D. *Pragmatics of human communication.* New York: Norton, 1967.

Watzlawick, P., Weakland, J. H., and Fisch, R. *Change: Principles of problem formation and problem resolution.* New York: Norton, 1974.

Wilson, T. Alcohol and human sexual behavior. *Behav. Res. Ther.,* 1977; *15,* 239–252.

Wincze, J. P., and Caird, W. K. The effect of systematic desensitization and video desensitization on the treatment of essential sexual dysfunction in women. *Behav. Ther.,* 1976, *7,* 335–342.

Winokur, G. Sexual behavior: Its relationship to certain effects and psychiatric diseases. In G. Winokur (Ed.), *Determinants of human sexual behavior.* Springfield, Ill.: Charles C Thomas, 1963.

Wolpe, J. *Psychotherapy by reciprocal inhibition.* Stanford, Calif.: Stanford University Press, 1958.

Wolpe, J. *The practice of behavior therapy,* 1st ed. New York: Pergamon Press, 1969.

Wolpe, J. *The practice of behavior therapy,* 2nd ed. New York: Pergamon Press, 1973.

Wolpe, J., and Lazarus, A. A. *Behavior therapy techniques.* New York: Pergamon Press, 1966.

Wolpin, M. Guided imagining to reduce avoidance behavior. *Psychother. Theory Res. Prac.,* 1969, *6,* 122–124.

Yulis, S. Generalization of therapeutic gain in the treatment of premature ejaculation. *Behav. Ther.,* 1976, *7,* 355–358.

Zeiss, R. A. Self-directed treatment for premature ejaculation: Preliminary case reports. *J. Behav. Ther. Exp. Psychiatry,* 1977, *8,* 87–91.

Hypertension

STEWART AGRAS, M.D.

Professor of Psychiatry and
Director of the Laboratory for the Study of Behavioral Medicine
Department of Psychiatry and Behavioral Sciences
Stanford University School of Medicine
Stanford, California

ROLF JACOB, M.D.

Research Fellow
Department of Psychiatry and Behavioral Sciences
Stanford University School of Medicine
Stanford, California

9

Although pharmacologic methods form the backbone of the current approach to the treatment of essential hypertension, it is becoming increasingly clear that certain behavior change procedures can influence blood pressure, both directly and indirectly. Thus, for example, relaxation and biofeedback procedures directly influence blood pressure, while enhancing adherence to the medical regimen provides an indirect influence via increased accuracy of drug ingestion.

Although the above topics form the content of this chapter, some emergent areas of behavioral influence upon hypertension should not be forgotten. Thus, altering diet to lower salt intake, decreasing weight, and increasing exercise, may all lower blood pressure (Boyer and Kasch, 1970; Freis, 1976; Reisin, Abel, Modan, et al., 1978). These topics will not be discussed here, either because they have been covered elsewhere, or because not enough research exists to allow for a detailed consideration.

For the most part, the behavioral procedures to be discussed in this chapter have not yet been absorbed into clinical practice. Thus, implications of the findings presented, both for clinical management of the hypertensive patient and for future research will be highlighted.

Clinical Aspects of Hypertension

The frequency distributions of systolic and diastolic blood pressure in the general population, although slightly skewed to the right, are continuous and unimodal, showing no evidence of a segregation into "normotensive" and "hypertensive" subpopulations (Smith, 1977a). Thus, any dividing line between elevated and normal blood pressure is somewhat arbitrary. Although actuarial data indicate that longevity in adults is progressively reduced the more blood pressure exceeds 100/60 mm Hg (systolic/diastolic; Engelman and Braunwald, 1977, pp. 185–188), the diagnosis of hypertension is usually given to people whose blood pressure is 160/95 mm Hg or above, with 140-159/90–94 mm Hg being labeled as "borderline" hypertension (Smith, 1977a). Using these criteria, 15% of adult whites and 27% of blacks, or 24 million

Americans, have hypertension. In addition, 17 million Americans have borderline hypertension. "Mild" hypertension is a term sometimes used for the diastolic blood pressure range of 95–104 mm Hg. "Malignant" or "accelerating" hypertension is diagnosed if diastolic pressure is increasing rapidly in excess of 120–130 mm Hg. This constitutes a medical emergency, and such patients should be hospitalized.

Hypertension or borderline hypertension can have different causes, such as renal disease, malfunction of certain endocrine organs (adrenals, parathyroid glands), coarctation of the aorta (a constriction of the aortic arch), pregnancy, or oral contraceptive medication. Hypertension with an identifiable cause is called "secondary" hypertension. In about 80% of cases, however, no such cause can be found (Bech and Hilden, 1975). To these patients, a diagnosis of "essential" hypertension is given. People with essential hypertension who display elevations of their blood pressure only temporarily are sometimes called "labile" hypertensives. Such lability often represents the beginning stages of the disorder.

Patients with newly detected hypertension should be given a medical workup to rule out specific causes. Such a workup should be done by a physician and includes an inquiry for symptoms characteristic of causes of secondary hypertension, physical examination, and laboratory tests such as urinanalysis for protein, blood and glucose, blood creatinine or urea, serum potassium level, hematocrit and an electrocardiogram (Moser, 1977). If signs or symptoms of secondary hypertension are detected (and in certain other cases, e.g., age less than 30, or unsatisfactory response to drug therapy), a more extensive workup is required.

Prospective collaborative studies have shown that pharmacotherapy leads to a significant reduction of certain complications of hypertension (Veterans Administration Cooperative Study Group on Antihypertensive Agents, 1967, 1970, 1972). The higher the pretreatment pressure, the larger the benefits from medication. In 73 treated patients with diastolic pressures between 115 and 130 mm Hg, the incidence of severe complications was only two over a 1½ year period as compared with 27 for the 70 patients treated with placebo. (These complications included sudden death, advanced retinal changes, renal malfunction, strokes, myocardial infarction, congestive heart failure, and malignant hypertension.) In patients with diastolic pressure of 90–114 mm Hg, the estimated risk of developing a complication over a 5-year period was reduced from 55% to 18% by treatment. However, patients with mild hypertension, unless they were over 50 years old or already had cardiovascular or renal abnormalities, derived relatively little benefit from medication. This lower payoff for drug therapy for mild hypertension was confirmed in a recently completed 10-year controlled intervention trial (Smith, 1977b). In this study, cardiac abnormalities on the electrocardiogram or on x-rays were more common in the placebo group (53.1% vs. 23.8%), but the major complications of death, myocardial infarction, and stroke occurred as frequently in the pharmacologically treated group as in the control group. In addition, a larger number of patients in the treatment group dropped out because of drug intolerance (9.8% vs. 2%).

For borderline hypertension, the above findings may indicate that a favorable treatment effect for pharmacotherapy is even less clearly established. However, the overall mortality of these patients exceeds the age-adjusted mortality of the general population by at least 100% (Julius, 1977). Thus, a place may exist for the development of alternative or adjunctive treatments for hypertension under the following conditions: (1) for those in the borderline or mildly hypertensive range and (2) as an adjunctive treatment for those in higher ranges who do not respond well to pharmacotherapy. It is in this light that we should consider the newer behavioral approaches to hypertension. However, before describing the various behavioral procedures, it seems reasonable to consider some of the methodological problems which beset work in this field and which limit the interpretation of many of the studies to be described in subsequent sections of this chapter.

Methodology

As we consider some of the methodological problems associated with research on the behavioral treatment of hypertension, the reader will encounter themes already raised in other contexts throughout this volume, namely, the problems of experimental design and of choosing a sensitive and relevant dependent variable.

EXPERIMENTAL DESIGN

The considerations applying to outcome research in general also apply to research on the behavioral treatment of hypertension. The main reason for doing the research is to answer the question: Is the treatment likely to be effective in the future with other patients? To answer this question, a second question is asked: Is the relationship between treatment and result a causal one? Having established a causal relationship, we often conclude that the treatment effect can be replicated. However, even if a study demonstrates a causal relationship beyond reasonable doubt, the conclusion that the treatment will work in the future may not always be justified. Thus, if a study selected patients with some special characteristic, the results may not be generalizable to patients without this characteristic. For example, the results of a study on hypnotic relaxation with subjects selected for hypnotizability may not be generalizable to a less narrowly selected sample. The effect of transcendental meditation on hypertensives who pursued this practice on their own initiative may be different from the effect on hypertensives who were referred to meditation for treatment of their high blood pressure. (For the latter example, compare Benson, Rosner, Marzetta, et al., 1974a,b with Pollack, Weber, Case, et al., 1977.) The result of a study which used subjects not identified as hypertensives, but whose blood pressure was above a certain cutoff point during a screening examination, is not a good predictor of the result one might get with hypertensives, since, in the former case, a larger proportion of the treatment effect will be caused by regression to the mean (Peters, Benson, and Peters, 1977).

To answer the question whether the result is caused by the treatment, alternative explanations must be ruled out. If blood pressure is used as the dependent variable, these alternative explanations may include spontaneous fluctuations in blood pressure with regression to the mean, environmental changes, expectation effects, change of salt intake and other dietary changes, change in life style, or change in adherence to medication (unless that was the target behavior studied). In order to rule out these alternative explanations, one approach, of course, is to include one or several control groups in the study. The control group equals the treatment group in regard to the confounding variable, but not the treatment itself. For example, the "attention placebo" control group is designed to be equal to the treatment in regard to expectation effects but not in regard to the crucial treatment variable. When assigning patients to treatment or control groups, one has to make sure that no systematic differences will arise in the personal characteristics of the members of the two groups. As the reader probably knows, random assignment, perhaps combined with matching or blocking, can achieve this end. One person-variable that should not be ignored is pretreatment pressure, since a relationship between average pretreatment pressure and average decrease of blood pressure after relaxation therapy or placebo treatment has been found (Jacob, Kraemer, and Agras, 1977). The higher the average pretreatment pressure, the larger the reduction of blood pressure. Thus, if the treatment and control groups are not equivalent in regard to pretreatment pressure, the results will be confounded.

Another design that can establish a causal relationship between treatment and result is the single-subject experiment (Hersen and Barlow, 1976). While this design is optimal for establishing the effect of treatment in the particular individual being studied, it is less suited to give us information on how the treatment would work with other individuals, unless the experiment has been replicated with different individuals.

Although one of these two designs—control group design or single-subject experiment—is needed to establish a causal relationship between treatment and result, most studies have employed simpler designs, such as single-group designs or group designs with a nonrandomly selected comparison group. We will explore the problems with these designs as we discuss individual studies.

DEPENDENT MEASURES

The prime motive for treating hypertension is to reduce the incidence of medical complications later in life. Thus, the best proof of treatment effectiveness would be to demonstrate a reduction in the occurrence of these complications. This crucial information is available only for pharmacotherapy, as described above, and is not available for the behavioral methods. Second best, of course, is to use blood pressure itself as an indicator of outcome. However, to reduce the risk of medical complications, blood pressure should probably be lowered throughout the day, rather than only in the treatment situation. Thus, measures of blood pressure should be obtained in such a way that they reflect generalization outside the treatment session. One way to obtain such measures is to record blood pressure 24 hours a day. This is cumbersome, but not impossible (Bachmann, Zerzwy, Riess, et al., 1970; Hinman, Engel, and Bickford, 1962; Littler, Honour, Sleight, et al., 1972). However, we are not aware of any studies using behavioral methods which have demonstrated a treatment effect in this way. Another way to study generalization is to measure blood pressure only occasionally, but still outside of treatment.

The effect of expectations on part of the patient or on the part of the assessor on the measurement should be minimized. For example, in one study, the measure of blood pressure was that obtained at the patient's regular clinic visit, recorded by staff who were not aware of which treatment the patient had been assigned to (Taylor, Farquhar, Nelson, et al., 1977). In other studies, a "random-zero" blood pressure cuff has been used (Garrow, 1963), a device which adds a random constant to the blood pressure levels measured, thus making it less likely that expectations of the assessor would influence measurement (Benson et al., 1974a,b; Patel and North, 1975).

The least convincing indicator of treatment effect is the decrease in blood pressure occurring within a treatment session, while the patient is engaging in the treatment procedure. Yet, this is the measure most often reported in biofeedback experiments. At best, measures obtained during a session can be used to demonstrate subtle immediate effects of the treatment, for example, when comparing two treatments or when investigating the mechanism of a treatment. In addition, when a new treatment is evaluated, the demonstration of a reduction of within-session blood pressure can serve as an encouragement to proceed to demonstrate the treatment effect with a measure that reflects generalization as well.

We will now proceed to see how these general considerations apply to research on relaxation therapy, biofeedback, or adherence to medication.

RESEARCH ON RELAXATION THERAPY AND BIOFEEDBACK. The methods with direct effect on blood pressure which we will consider here are biofeedback and relaxation therapy. The methodology for the two treatments is similar in several respects, so we will use a hypothetical biofeedback treatment course as an example for both. Figure 9.1 depicts this hypothetical biofeedback treatment. Baseline blood pressures are obtained at the patient's regular clinic during his or her visit there (Visits 1–4). After the baseline clinic measurements, a series of sessions are held in the biofeedback laboratory. In these sessions blood pressure is determined repeatedly. One such determination is often called a trial. Since reporting data for each trial separately would be excessively space consuming, results of several trials are often combined into trial blocks, each consisting of, say, five trials. In the treatment sessions (Visits 6–8), the patient is given feedback on his or her blood pressure (● in Figure 9.1) with the exception of the first trials, which constitute the "on arrival" baseline pressures for the session. In the control sessions (baseline and follow-up), the patient receives no feedback at any time during the session. After the end of treatment, the patient can be followed by checking blood pressure during his or her regular clinic visits (Visits 10–13).

As discussed above, two fundamentally different measures can be employed to report outcome of treatment: changes in blood pressure across sessions (visits) and within session changes. Of the former, it seems that the pre-post difference in clinic measures (for example, the average of Visits

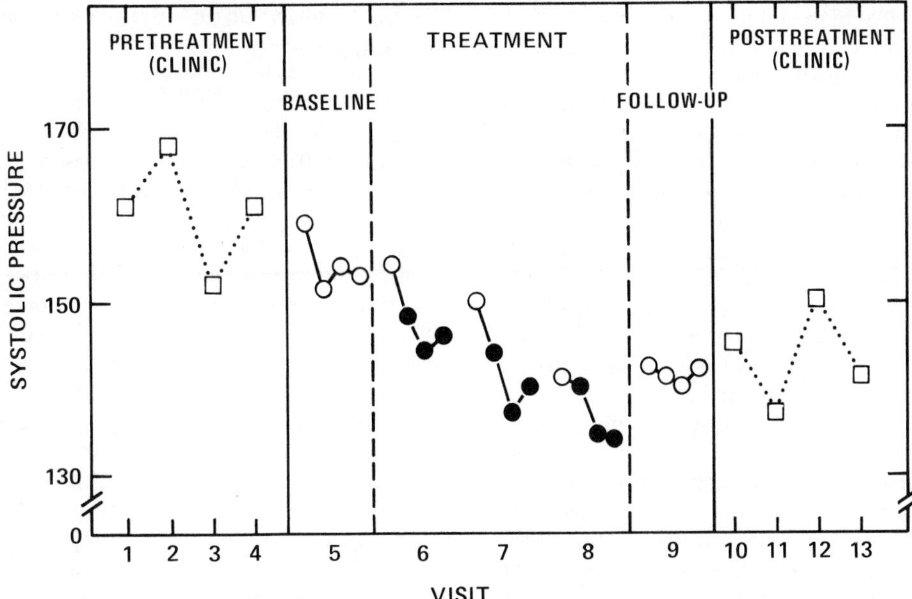

Figure 9.1. Results of a hypothetical blood pressure feedback treatment program to illustrate various possible outcome measures. □, pressures obtained outside the laboratory; ● and ○, pressures obtained inside the laboratory. Pressures obtained while subject is receiving feedback: solid symbols; no feedback: open symbols.

1–4 subtracted from the average of Visits 10–12) reflect the greatest degree of generalization. A second choice is to compare the pressures obtained during baseline and follow-up or during the first and last treatment sessions (Visit 5 vs. Visit 9; Visit 6 vs. Visit 8, see Figure 9.1). This measure, however, gives us less information about generalization, since it was taken in the treatment environment. Still, by definition, changes across sessions, even if in the same environment, reflect a greater degree of generalization than within-session change scores (for example, the difference between on-arrival pressure and the pressure of the last trial block of the session), since the patients are actually engaging in the treatment while the latter measure is taken.

ADHERENCE RESEARCH. Measurement poses a most difficult problem for a low-frequency behavior such as medication taking, since the preferred method, direct observation, is not usually possible. There are four main ways to measure the taking of antihypertensive agents: pill count, self-monitoring, blood pressure measurement, or detection of the drug or a chemical marker in blood or urine. Each has its own problems and limitations. Pill count, the only direct measure of adherence, relies on the patient to return unused medication, allowing the number of pills apparently consumed to be compared with the number prescribed. Obviously, pills can be lost or taken from another bottle. Moreover, since the count is usually performed over an interval of several weeks, daily variation in adherence behavior is not measured.

Self-monitoring, using a calendar or other especially designed recording form, allows for an examination of finer variations in medication taking. However, it is susceptible to error from forgetting, particularly if the amount taken is filled in many hours or days after the fact. Both pill count and self-monitoring are probably affected by experimenter demand of high adherence, a problem which has been circumvented in some experiments by keeping patients unaware of the fact that their pills are being counted. Finally, self-monitoring may be reactive in the sense of positively affecting medication taking, since this procedure provides performance feedback, which has been found to influence a variety of behaviors. Both pill count and self-monitoring are preferable to more global assessment methods, such as interview or physician judgement, both of which have been shown to be grossly inaccurate (Park and Lipman, 1964; Caron and Roth, 1968).

Detection of a drug or its metabolite or a chemical marker in blood or urine is at first glance appealing. However, such methods measure adherence over a very short time due to the rapid excretion of the substance. Moreover, in most cases it is a simple binary measure—present or absent—rather than a parametric measure. Thus, patients could take their medication only in the few days preceding a visit and be considered as excellent compliers. Comparisons between pill count and detection of chemical substances as measures of adherence are not proper, since they refer to different time intervals, e.g., 24 hours in one case and several weeks in the other. Thus, it is not surprising that such comparisons show low correlations. Most studies, however, suggest that the pill count may overestimate adherence by between 10 and 50% (Joyce, 1962; Maddock, 1967).

As we have seen, blood pressure is the most commonly used measure in the treatment of hypertension. However, it is an indirect measure of medication taking, since a multitude of other variables affect blood pressure, such as varying biological responses to medication, physiological variables, variations in salt intake, weight, exercise, and emotional state. Moreover, blood pressure measurements may not be very responsive to decreases in medication taking, since it has been shown that blood pressure can remain unchanged for several months after discontinuation of the medication in patients who have taken medication for a long time (Page and Dustan, 1962; Thurm and Smith, 1967). On the other hand, if blood pressure is not decreased by an adherence procedure in a large enough group of patients, then we must conclude that such a strategy is not useful.

Given this problem in measurement, the solution is to provide multiple measures such as pill count, drug excretion, and blood pressure in most experiments.

Other behaviors involved in adherence to antihypertensive agents pose less of a problem than medication taking. Thus, appointment keeping can be monitored accurately and track kept of dropouts from clinical programs or experiments.

Methods with Direct Effect on Blood Pressure

RELAXATION THERAPY

We define relaxation therapy here as any method in which reduction of muscular tension is emphasized. A number of methods fit this description, including progressive relaxation (Jacobson, 1939), a metronome-conditioned relaxation (Brady, Luborsky, and Kron, 1974), psychological relaxation (Stone and DeLeo, 1976), biofeedback-assisted relaxation (Patel, 1973), certain types of meditation (Benson et al., 1974a,b), yogic exercises (Datey, Deshmukh, Dalvi, et al., 1969), and autogenic training (Luthe and Schultz, 1969, pp. 69–76). Although reduction of muscle tension is emphasized in these methods, empirical findings concerning the role of muscular relaxation itself are sparse and conflicting. Thus, on reanalyzing data presented by Jacobson (1939) we found that there was a correlation of 0.71 between reduction of biceps muscle tension and fall in systolic pressure during relaxation in a group of 10 normotensive subjects (Jacob et al., 1977). On the other hand, in another study, no association was found between reduction of blood pressure and decrease in frontalis muscle tension (Masi, Moore, and Weston, 1976).

Beside reduction of muscular tension, the different methods of relaxation therapy have other features in common. One such component is mental focusing. This implies a deliberate direction of attention to a constant or repetitious external, internal, or self-generated stimulus. In progressive relaxation, mental focusing occurs when the subject concentrates on the state of relaxation or tension of a particular muscle, or upon the rhythm of breathing. In metronome-conditioned relaxation, the beat of a metronome provides an additional focus of attention. In meditation and autogenic training, self-generated mental phrases or sounds are used. In hypnotic relaxation, special care is taken to facilitate mental focusing on the instructions by using verbal patterns thought to be more "suggestive." In one study it was found that adding hypnotic suggestions of deep inner relaxation, heaviness, drowsiness, and relaxation of internal organs, including the heart and blood vessels, resulted in further reduction of blood pressure (Deabler, Fidel, Dillenkoffer, et al., 1973). Unfortunately, we cannot take this result as evidence for the importance of mental focusing, since the effect of hypnosis, in that study, was confounded with passage of time. The observed further reduction of blood pressure could have been due to the subjects merely having relaxed longer. Thus, we have little data pertaining to the role of mental focusing in relaxation therapy.

A third component common to all relaxation therapies is the expectation effect or task awareness. This factor should not be ignored, since, in all studies of relaxation therapy with hypertensives, the subjects have probably known what they were being treated for. This effect is made even more salient with the recent finding that hypertensive subjects can raise or lower their blood pressure as a result of instructions alone (Redmond, Gaylor, McDonald, et al., 1974). We can obtain a rough estimate of expectation effects by studying the results of various placebo treatments of hypertension. For example, the "electrone gun," an impressive electronic gadget with strange sparks and lights which could be directed to different parts of the patient's body, led to an average reduction of 27/18 mm Hg, from 197/119 mm Hg before treatment (Goldring, Chasis, Schreiner, et al., 1956). A placebo given intramuscularly led to reduction of 22/13 mm Hg from 182/112 mm Hg before treatment, whereas the reduction obtained with oral placebo was 12–14/4–6 mm Hg in two groups of patients with pretreatment pressures of 181/109 and 183/108 mm Hg, respectively (Grenfell, Briggs, and Holland, 1962). Comparing these different results is made difficult by the fact that, for systolic pressure, a positive relationship over studies between the average reduction of blood pressure and average pretreatment pressure was found not only for relaxation but also for placebo treatment (Jacob et al., 1977). If we take this regression into consideration, it seems that the placebo procedure with the most pronounced effect on systolic pressure was intramuscular injections, and the procedure with the largest effect on diastolic pressure was the "electrone gun."

Attention-control groups used for comparisons with relaxation therapy have shown changes of varying magnitude. In one study in which the control patients were instructed to come to the laboratory three times a week to "rest" on a couch for 30 minutes, the average reduction was 0.5/2.1 mm Hg from 163/99 mm Hg before treatment (Patel, 1975a). In another control group receiving similar but somewhat less intensive treatment, the reduction was 8.9/4.2 mm Hg from 168.9/100.6 mm Hg (Patel and North, 1975). A decrease of 2.8/1.8 mm Hg from 141/92 mm Hg was obtained with "nonspecific therapy," a treatment which involved the patient's daily monitoring of stressful events and discussing them with one of the experimenters in about six sessions of nondirective therapy (Taylor et al., 1977). While it may seem that these changes were smaller than for the placebo studies presented in the preceding paragraph, it should be kept in mind that the placebo studies had higher pretreatment pressures and were selected because they had shown the largest effects.

Although in some cases we cannot make comparisons because of differences in pretreatment pressures, on the whole it seems that larger treatment effects have been reported for relaxation therapy than for different placebo therapies or control treatments. Thus, we may conclude that task awareness is probably not a sufficient condition to account for the effects obtained with relaxation therapy. However, we cannot rule out task awareness as a *necessary* condition, since the experiment of treating a group of hypertensives with relaxation procedures who are unaware of what they are being treated for has not been done. Thus, it is advisable to heighten expectation effects in clinical applications of relaxation therapy, for example, by presenting a rationale that the patient accepts and is motivated by, and by using whatever other technique that therapists may have found useful to increase their patients' hope for a positive outcome.

The most important component of relaxation therapy may be regular practice. Patients are usually asked to practice for 15 to 30 minutes once or twice daily. Some therapists also instruct their patients to relax as often as possible during daily activities, to relax briefly before answering the telephone or when looking at their watch (Patel and North, 1975). However, only one study has evaluated the importance of regular practice (Brady et al., 1974). After a baseline of 2 to 4 weeks, during which three subjects came to the laboratory 5 days a week to have their blood pressure recorded, daily relaxation sessions were given for 4 weeks. During this treatment phase, the subjects attended the clinic twice daily, once for relaxation training and once for measurement of their blood pressure. After 4 weeks of treatment, baseline conditions were reinstituted for 4 weeks. A fourth subject went through the same phases except that both recording and practice occurred at home. For this subject and for one of the other three subjects, a second treatment phase was instituted after the second baseline. The results showed a significant decrease from the last ten baseline sessions during the treatment phase for three of the subjects. When the subjects stopped practicing during the second baseline phase, diastolic pressure rose significantly for the subjects who had displayed a decrease during treatment. For the two subjects who went through a second treatment phase after baseline, a significant reduction of diastolic pressure was again noted. This experiment suggests that if the practice of relaxation is stopped, blood pressure will return to pretreatment levels. No clear data are available at this point, however, to answer the question whether a longer program would result in a less reversible outcome. Thus, it seems advisable to emphasize regular practice as an important component in clinical applications of relaxation therapy with hypertensives.

The importance of regular practice does *not* imply, however, that additional benefits can be expected from prolonging the length of individual sessions. On the contrary, psychosis-like experiences have been reported in some individuals who have practiced meditation for prolonged sessions (Benson, Kotch, and Crasweller, 1977). Other side effects of relaxation therapy, particularly of meditation, may include derealization experiences and altered reality testing, but only two published cases have come to our attention (French, Schmid, and Ingalls, 1975; Kennedy, 1976). Another risk is that of the patient prematurely stopping medication (Taylor et al., 1977), but this is not a direct effect of relaxation treatment. Nonetheless, while encouraging patients to practice regularly and often, they should be cautioned against prolonging the sessions beyond the time prescribed and against stopping their prescribed medication.

In the following sections we will discuss studies that evaluated various relaxation procedures and provide separate sections for progressive relaxation, meditation, and combination methods. The results of each study are listed in Table 9.1. This table also provides an estimate of the expected treatment effect ($\hat{\Delta}_R$) for a relaxation group with equivalent pretreatment pressure, based on the regression found between pretreatment pressure and treatment effect, as calculated in a later section of this chapter (Note 1). The residual ($\Delta - \hat{\Delta}_R$) indicates how far the result of the study deviated from the expected value. Parentheses around the estimated values and deviations indicate that these groups either did not receive relaxation therapy or were not used in the calculation of the regression for other reasons (see below).

A positive sign for the deviation ($\Delta - \hat{\Delta}_R$) indicates that the result was better than expected, and a negative sign indicates, of course, that it was not as good as expected.

PROGRESSIVE MUSCULAR RELAXATION. In this method, the patient is taught to let individual muscles or muscle groups become relaxed. In the initial phases of practice, the patient is made aware of the contrast between the feelings of tension and relaxation by first deliberately tensing a muscle or muscle group, focusing on the feeling of tension, and then letting go and allowing the muscles to relax. This tension-relaxation cycle is then applied to other muscle groups. When the patient has developed an ability to tense and let go of tension in all the muscle groups, the tension relaxation cycle can be applied to larger combinations of muscles, and is eventually dispensed with.

To generalize the benefits of relaxation, instructions in differential relaxation may be given. While engaged in activities during which the muscles are kept tense, patients are instructed to become aware of tension and allow the muscles to relax. For example, attention might be focused upon the trapezius (shoulder) muscles while driving in order to allow them to relax. Or patients might pay attention to their rate of breathing while waiting at a red light, letting the breathing become slower as they become more and more relaxed. (For a more detailed account of the techniques of progressive muscular relaxation, see Bernstein and Borkovec, 1973.)

The first study of progressive relaxation with hypertensives was performed by Jacobson (1939), who reported the blood pressures of three "trained" and one "partly trained" hypertensive subjects before and during a relaxation session. Systolic pressure fell an average of 13 mm Hg from 172 mm Hg before relaxation, and diastolic pressure by an average of 9 mm Hg from 94 mm Hg. This study was truly pioneering, but did not fulfill the stricter methodological criteria of our time for an outcome study of behavioral treatment: subject-selection procedures were not reported, no experimental controls were provided, and blood pressures were measured while the subjects were engaging in treatment, thus not providing information regarding generalization of treatment effects.

The study on the effect of metronome-conditioned relaxation reviewed above (Brady et al., 1974), by virtue of its A-B-A(-B) design, was one of the first controlled studies of the effect of progressive relaxation on hypertension. However, while this study effectively pinpointed one component of relaxation therapy, it did not control for expectation effects. A more recent study (Taylor et al., 1977) controlled for expectancy effects in subjects who were undergoing medical treatment for hypertension by randomly assigning them to one of three groups: relaxation, nonspecific therapy (described above), and medical treatment only. The reductions of systolic blood pressure, after 8 weeks of treatment, were reported as significantly larger for relaxation therapy than for the other two treatments. A similar trend was noted for diastolic pressure, although the magnitude of these differences did not reach the 5% significance level ($p = 0.054$). After 6 months, the relaxation group still displayed a greater reduction of blood pressure compared with the other two groups, although the differences were no longer statistically significant.

MEDITATION. In this section we will describe studies using certain meditative techniques such as transcendental meditation, which has generated the greatest amount of research in this area. Transcendental meditation usually involves two daily 20-minute sessions in which the subject sits in a relaxed erect posture in a quiet place, adopts a passive mental attitude, and focuses attention on the thought of a specific mental sound or syllable (mantra).

The first research evaluating transcendental meditation as a treatment method for hypertension was performed by Benson and his co-workers (1974a,b). In these studies, subjects were recruited at introductory lectures given by the Transcendental Meditation Society, and the onset of meditation practice was delayed until a series of blood pressures had been obtained over a 5-week period. The first study included only subjects who were not on antihypertensive medication (Benson et al., 1974a). These 22 patients obtained an average reduction of blood pressure of 7.0/3.9 mm Hg from 146.5/94.6 mm Hg before treatment. Most of this reduction occurred during the first 30 days of practice, whereas no significant changes had occurred during the 5-week preinstructional control period. The second study included only patients who were on antihypertensive medication, and a special effort was made to keep medications constant during the meditation trial (Benson et al., 1974b). Again, a statistically significant reduction of blood pressure was noted during treatment, amounting to an average of 10.6/4.9 mm Hg from a mean pretreatment level of 145.6/91.9 mm Hg.

More recently, two studies attempting to replicate these findings yielded less impressive results (Blackwell, Haneson, Bloomfield, et al., 1976; Pollack et al., 1977). Both had designs similar to that of Benson et al., except that the subjects were not recruited at the introductory lecture but were referred to meditation as a treatment for their high blood pressure. In the first study (Blackwell et al., 1976), self-recordings of the patient's blood pressure at home were obtained in addition to clinic measurements. Although, according to our calculations, neither home nor clinic measurements showed statistically significant treatment effects for the whole group of seven patients, the authors reported, using pre-post comparisons *within* a given subject,

Table 9.1
Summary of Results in Studies of Relaxation Therapy*

Source	Treatment	*N*	Systolic (mm Hg) Pre	Systolic $-\Delta$	Systolic $-\hat{\Delta}_R$	Systolic Difference $(-\Delta) - (-\hat{\Delta}_R)$	Diastolic (mm Hg) Pre	Diastolic $-\Delta$	Diastolic $-\hat{\Delta}_R$	Diastolic Difference $(-\Delta) - (-\hat{\Delta}_R)$
Jacobson, 1939	Relaxation	4	171.8	130	(25.7)	−12.7	94.3	9.3	7.3	2.0
Brady et al., 1974	Relaxation	4					90.1	3.4	4.8	−1.4
Taylor et al., 1977	Relaxation	10	149.8	13.6	(11.0)	2.6	96.2	4.9	8.5	−3.5
	Nonspecific therapy	10	141.0	2.8	(5.1)	−2.3	92.0	1.8	(5.9)	−4.1
	Medication only	11	145.9	1.1	(8.4)	−7.3	96.3	−0.3	(8.5)	−8.2
Redmond et al., 1974	Relaxation	5	143.8	5.7†	(7.0)	−1.3	102.8	7.8†	12.5	−4.7
Shoemaker and Tasto, 1975	Relaxation	5	136.4	6.8	(2.0)	4.8	90.4	7.6	5.0	2.6
	Blood pressure feedback	5	132.2	−0.6	(−0.8)	0.2	89.8	1.2	(4.6)	−3.4
	Control	5	133.8	−1.6	(0.3)	−1.3	90.4	−1.2	(5.0)	−6.2
Walsh et al., 1977	Relaxation	13	142.0	3.0	(5.8)	−2.8	93.6	6.5	6.9	−0.4
	Pulse wave velocity feedback	11	151.0	13.0	(11.8)	2.0	94.5	7.9	(7.4)	0.5
Benson et al., 1974a	Meditation	22‡	146.5	7.0	8.8	−1.8	94.6	3.9	7.5	−3.6
Benson et al., 1974b	Meditation	14‡	145.6	10.6	8.2	2.4	92.0	4.9	5.9	−1.0
Blackwell et al., 1976	Meditation	7‡	138.8	4.2	3.6	0.6	97.9	1.6	9.5	−7.9
Pollack et al., 1977	Meditation	20‡	155.0	11.0	14.5	−3.5	96.2	4.0	8..5	−4.5
Stone and DeLeo, 1976	Meditation	14‡	141.3	9.0	5.3	3.7	90.3	8.1	4.9	3.2
Datey et al., 1969										
Group without medication	Combination	10‡	184.5	37.0	34.2	2.8	109.0	23.0	16.2	6.8
Group not controlled with medication	Combination	15	167.3	9.3	(22.7)	−13.4	105.0	9.3	13.8	−4.5
Group well controlled with medication	Combination	22	136.8	1.6	(2.3)	−0.7	86.4	0.9	2.5	−1.6
Patel, 1975 (1973)	Combination	20	159.1	14.5	(17.2)	−2.7	100.1	14.1	10.8	3.3
	Control	20	163.1	0.5	(19.9)	−19.4	99.1	2.1	(10.2)	−8.1

* N, number of subjects in one group. $-\Delta$, decrease; $-\hat{\Delta}_R$, predicted decrease by relaxation therapy from regression on pretreatment pressure; $-\hat{\Delta}_R$ values with parentheses were not used in the regression calculation.

† Difference between "on arrival" pressure sessions 1 and 5.

‡ Criteria fulfilled (see Footnote 1).

§ Senior citizens only.

¶ Mean of last four sessions; percentage of baseline pressure of each individual.

‖ Hypnotizable subjects.

Table 9.1 (*cont.*)

Source	Treatment	*N*	Systolic (mm Hg)				Diastolic (mm Hg)			
			Pre	$-\Delta$	$-\hat{\Delta}_R$	Difference $(-\Delta) - (-\hat{\Delta}_R)$	Pre	$-\Delta$	$-\hat{\Delta}_R$	Difference $(-\Delta - (-\hat{\Delta}_R)$
Patel and North, 1975	Combination	17‡	167.5	26.1	26.1	3.3	99.6	15.2	10.5	4.7
	Control	17	168.9	8.9	(23.8)	−14.9	100.6	4.2	(11.2)	−7.0
	Control after Rx	16‡	176.6	28.1	28.9	−0.8	104.3	15.0	13.4	1.6
Patel and Carruthers, 1977	Combination	22‡	164.5	18.6	20.8	−2.2	101.1	11.2	11.4	−0.2
Dowdell, 1977	Combination	10§	158.0	(16.0)	(16.5)	−0.5	85.0	9.0	1.7	7.3
Deabler et al., 1973	No medication and relaxation	6	163.0	10.5%			96.0	10.6%		
	Relaxation + hypnosis			16.0%				16.3%		
	Medication and relaxation	9	158.0	13.0%¶			95.0	5.8%¶		
	Relaxation + hypnosis			16.4%¶				10.2%¶		
	Control	6	155.0	3.0%¶			95.0	0.1%¶		
Friedman and Taub, 1977	Hypnosis	13‖	142.5	12.5	(6.1)	6.4	93.1	9.6	6.6	3.0
	Hypnosis + blood pressure feedback	10‖	139.8	2.8	(4.3)	−1.5	91.8	2.8	(5.8)	−3.0
Friedman and Taub, 1977	Blood pressure feedback	13	146.5	6.9	(8.8)	−1.8	95.8	7.0	(8.2)	−1.2
	Control	12	139.9	2.4	(4.4)	−2.0	94.7	2.6	(7.6)	−5.0

that clinic systolic and diastolic pressures decreased significantly in four patients, no significant changes occurred in two patients, and a significant increase of diastolic pressure occurred in one patient.

In the second replication study, 20 subjects were followed for 6 months (Pollack et al., 1977). Systolic pressure was significantly reduced during the first 3 months of treatment. During the last 3 months, however, the average systolic pressure was no longer significantly different from baseline. Moreover, the reduction obtained in diastolic pressure failed to reach significant levels at any time during the study. The authors concluded that it was unlikely that transcendental meditation contributed directly to the lowering of blood pressure. It is tempting to speculate that the smaller effect seen in the two latter studies compared to those by Benson and coworkers had some relationship to subject selection procedures. As discussed in the methodology section above, subjects who are recruited at an introductory transcendental meditation lecture are probably more enthusiastic and have greater expectations of success than a less selected sample of hypertensives.

Whereas the studies described so far employed transcendental meditation as the treatment, other meditative techniques have also been used. One such technique was described by Stone and DeLeo (1976). This method, labeled "psychological relaxation," was derived from Buddhist meditation and involved the patients sitting erect in a comfortable chair, letting their muscles relax, and counting breath cycles in arithmetic progression. Each session lasted 10 to 15 minutes, and two sessions were held each day, one before breakfast and one before retiring. Fourteen patients were treated, and the effects compared to corresponding measures on five (nonrandomly assigned) comparison patients whose blood pressure was measured once a month during the 6-month duration of the experiment. The treatment group exhibited a significant decline of both systolic and diastolic pressure compared with its own baseline, and the post-treatment systolic and diastolic pressures were also reported to be significantly lower than those of the control group. It was also found that the changes of mean arterial pressure were correlated with changes of plasma dopamine-β-hydroxylase, an enzyme which supposedly reflects the level of sympathetic activity. The authors concluded that reduction of peripheral adrenergic activity was an important contributor to the effect of relaxation therapy. However, a more recent study from our laboratory failed to replicate these findings (Brauer, Horlick, Nelson, et al., 1978).

BIOFEEDBACK-ASSISTED RELAXATION AND OTHER COMBINATIONS. In this section we will describe studies which employed combinations of the procedures of muscular relaxation and meditation or used electronic equipment, such as electromyographic feedback or feedback of skin resistance, to augment relaxation. Research on feedback of blood pressure itself will be covered under a separate heading, since it can be argued that this method involves mechanisms different from those involved in facilitating relaxation (Pickering, Brucker, Frankel, et al., 1977).

One of the first large-scale applications of relaxation therapy to the treatment of hypertension employed a yogic exercise called "Shavasan" (corpse posture; Datey et al., 1969). This was a pioneering study, and the treatment method was described in some detail, so we will quote the description of Datey et al. of the technique here:

> The patient lies in a supine position, lower limbs 30 degrees apart and the upper making an angle of 15 degrees with the trunk, with the forearms in the midprone position and fingers semiflexed. The eyes are closed with eyelids drooping. The patient is taught slow, rhythmic diaphragmatic breathing with a short pause after each inspiration and a longer one at the end of each expiration. After establishing this rhythm, he is asked to attend to the sensation at the nostrils, the coolness of the inspired air and the warmth of the expired air. These procedures help to keep the patient inwardly alert and to forget his usual thoughts, thus becoming less conscious of the external environment, thereby attaining relaxation. The patient is asked to relax the muscles so that he is able to feel the heaviness of different parts of his body. This is achieved automatically once the patient learns the exercise. The exercise is performed for 30 minutes.... Most patients learn the exercise correctly in about 3 weeks.... After patients learn the exercise correctly, the respiratory rate is usually between 4 and 10 per min (pp. 325–333).*

This method can be conceptualized as a combination of muscular relaxation and meditation, with mental focusing on the breathing movements and their associated sensations at the nostrils. The patients were advised to come to the clinic daily until they had mastered the technique, and then weekly in order to check their blood pressure and the correct execution of the exercise.

Three different groups were treated. Group I, 10 patients who had received no medication other than placebo for 1 month prior to treatment, achieved a reduction of 36/23 mm Hg from 184.5/109 mm Hg before treatment. This is the largest reduction ever reported for a group of hypertensives treated with relaxation therapy. In Group II, consisting of 22 patients whose blood pressure was considered adequately controlled with medication, the dosage was reduced to 32% of the original amount in 13 of the patients. In Group III, composed of 15 patients on medication, but not adequately controlled, medication dosage was reduced to 29% in six of the patients, but had to be increased slightly in two patients. Overall, 62.5% of the patients with "essential" hypertension and 42% of the patients with "renal" hypertension were reported to derive benefit from the treatment.

A similar treatment, with added feedback of skin resistance and of muscle tension, was developed by Patel and tested in a

* Reprinted by permission from Datey, K. K., Deshmukh, S. N., Dalvi, C. P., and Vinekar, S. L. "Shavasan": A yogic exercise in the management of hypertension. *Angiology*, 1969, *20*, 325–333.

series of studies (Patel, 1973, 1975a,b; Patel and North, 1975; Patel and Carruthers, 1977). In the first study, patients attended three ½ hour individual sessions per week over a period of 3 months. In each session patients were instructed to lie on an examination couch, pay attention to their breathing, and, when this became regular, mentally go over various parts of their bodies and let them become more and more relaxed. For mental focusing, the patient could choose between different phrases to repeat to himself, such as "relaxed, relaxed." In addition, auditory feedback was given of the patient's skin resistance. The patient was to influence the tone in such a way that skin resistance would be increased, this being a sign of decreased sweat-gland activity, and, therefore, of decreased sympathetic activity. In addition to the clinic visits, the patient was to practice relaxation twice daily at home. The "generalizing" instructions mentioned in a previous section were also given, particularly to those patients who found it hard to adhere to a regular practice schedule during follow-up (Patel, 1977). Twenty patients received treatment. The result was a reduction of blood pressure by 26/16 mm Hg from 159/100.1 mm Hg before treatment. Medication was reduced by 33 to 60% in seven patients and discontinued in five patients. This study precipitated a lively discussion as evidenced by letters to the editor of the journal, *Lancet.* One important point raised was that the study did not control for expectation or placebo effects (Pickering, 1973).

In the second study, Patel attempted to answer this point by adding a comparison group, selected in such a way that it would be matched to the original treatment group for sex and age (Patel, 1975a), while following the treatment group during a 12-month period. Members of the comparison group were asked to attend the clinic three times per week for 3 months and rest on a couch for ½ hour (without receiving instructions in relaxation) and have their blood pressure taken. They were then followed monthly for 9 months. Of course, this comparison group did not control for factors that may have acted on the treatment group before the formation of the control group, and, because of the nonrandom group assignment, it also did not control for individual differences other than the matching variables. After 3 months of control "treatment," the comparison group exhibited an increase of medication dosage of 5.5% and a small (nonsignificant) decline of blood pressure. During the remaining 9 months of follow-up, the blood pressure level of the comparison group remained essentially at the pre-"treatment" level. Importantly, the treatment group maintained its treatment gains throughout the 12-month treatment period. This is the longest follow-up of relaxation therapy of hypertension reported in the literature.

The third outcome study included treatment and control groups of 17 patients each (Patel and North, 1975). The group assignment was random this time and medication was kept constant throughout the experiment. Treatment was the same as before, with added features of group sessions before the actual practice sessions, in which the rationale for the treatment was given and in which the patients could discuss their problems with the investigator or with each other. Practice sessions occurred twice weekly for 6 weeks. During some of the sessions, electromyographic feedback was given instead of feedback of skin resistance. After completion of treatment, the patients were followed biweekly for 3 months. The changes of blood pressure during treatment observed in this study were of similar magnitude to those of the initial study.

As in the previous study, members of the control group came to the clinic to rest on the examination couch and have their blood pressure taken, the visits being scheduled as frequently as those for the treatment group. During this "treatment," the control group exhibited a significant decrease of blood pressure, but this decline was significantly smaller than that of the treatment group (8.9/4.2 mm Hg vs. 26.1/15.2 mm Hg, cf. Table 9.1). After 6 months, members of the control group were given relaxation therapy identical to that of the treatment group. This resulted in a significant treatment effect, comparable in magnitude to that of the initial treatment group.

A subsample of the patients underwent a series of stress tests. Treated patients were found to have significantly shorter recovery times from their pressor response to the exercise and cold pressor test than the controls (Patel, 1975b).

The findings of Patel's earlier studies were again replicated in a recent study which focused more broadly on coronary risk-factor reduction and included normotensive groups in addition to one hypertensive group of 22 patients (Patel and Carruthers, 1977). In the latter, a reduction of blood pressure of 18.6/11.2 mm Hg from 164.5/101.1 mm Hg was noted.

COMPARISON BETWEEN DIFFERENT RELAXATION THERAPIES

Since several different types of relaxation therapy have been used to treat hypertension, the question arises whether there is a difference in their effectiveness. One way to make this comparison is to compare the magnitude of the treatment effects reported in different studies. In making these comparisons, however, it is necessary to take into account the regression of reduction of blood pressure on pretreatment pressure (Jacob et al., 1977). Since more studies have appeared since the latter paper appeared and because we wanted to base the analysis on measures as free from within-session effects as possible, we repeated the regression analysis for the present chapter (Figures 9.2 and 9.3) (Note 1).

For systolic pressure, the regression coefficient of 0.67 was significantly different from zero ($p < 0.001$). As can be seen in Figure 9.2, with the exception of two treatment groups (Jacobson, 1939; Datey et al., 1969, Group III), all treatment groups maintain a close proximity to the regression line. For diastolic pressure, the regression coefficient of 0.61 was again significantly greater than zero ($p < 0.001$), but the spread around the regression line is greater than for systolic pressure (Figure 9.2).

Little is known whether person-variables other than initial pressure can be used to predict outcome of relaxation therapy for a group of hypertensives. Old age does not appear to be a hindrance. In a recent study, 10 hypertensive senior citizens with a mean age of 71 years obtained an average reduction of blood pressure of 16/9 mm Hg from 158/85 mm Hg before treatment (Dowdall, 1977).

Comparing the results of various treatment modalities, it appears that studies utilizing combination treatments displayed the largest treatment effects but also tended to have the largest pretreatment pressures. Thus, the effect of treatment modality is confounded with the effect of pre-

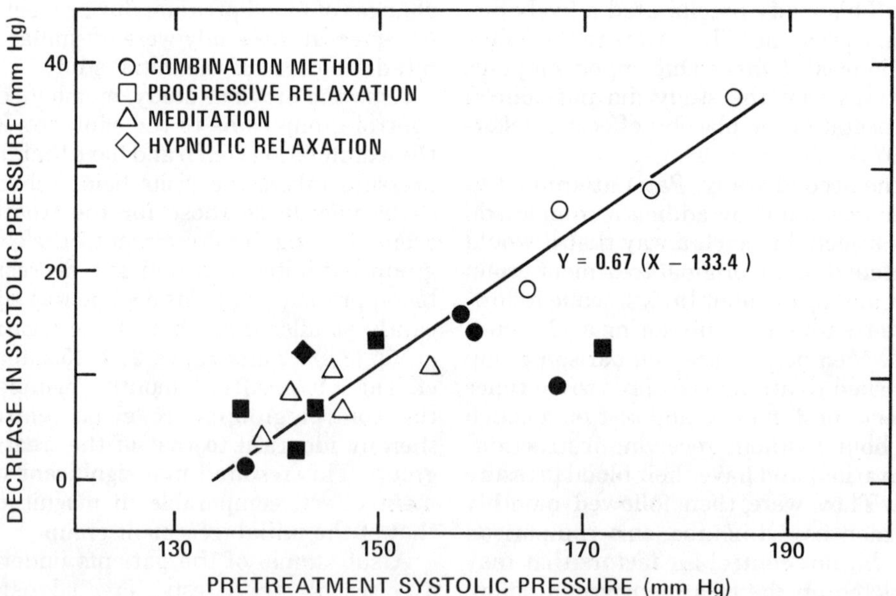

Figure 9.2. Average decrease of systolic pressure as a function of average pretreatment systolic pressure. Open symbols: criteria fulfilled; solid symbols: criteria not fulfilled.

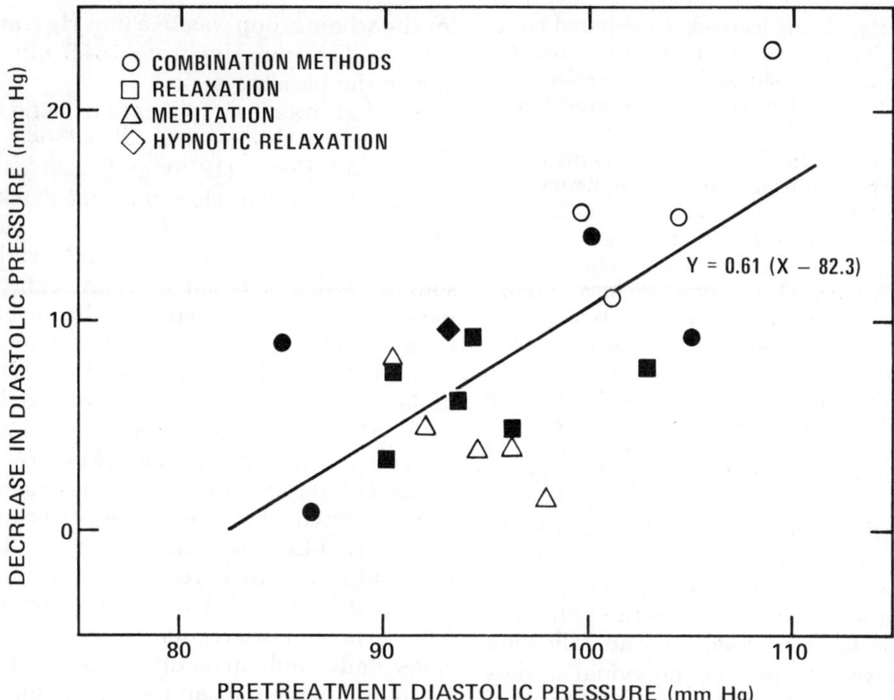

Figure 9.3. Average decrease of diastolic pressure as a function of average pretreatment diastolic pressure. Open symbols: criteria fulfilled; solid symbols: criteria not fulfilled.

treatment values. Firm conclusions regarding the relative values of different treatments must be deferred until the results of studies comparing treatments on a randomized basis are available.

BLOOD PRESSURE FEEDBACK

In biofeedback training, a biological function is measured, and the patient is provided almost immediate knowledge of the outcome of this measurement. By virtue of this feedback, the subject may be able to exert voluntary control over the function. In the case of blood pressure feedback, the measurement device most often used is a sphygmomanometer with a built-in microphone. When the blood pressure cuff is placed around the upper arm the microphone located over the brachial artery picks up the beat of the pulse (Korotkoff sounds), which can be heard when the cuff is inflated to a level between systolic and diastolic pressure. To obtain frequent measurements, the cuff needs to be inflated quite often, for example, once per minute. This may be uncomfortable for the patient, because of ischemic forearm pain. Recently, a less intrusive indirect measure of blood pressure has been developed in the measurement of pulse-wave velocity, and this approach was used in one study which we will describe later (Walsh, Dale, and Anderson, 1977).

The following excerpt describes one of the early cases of treatment with feedback of blood pressure. It was selected because it gives a picture of the clinical process that one may encounter (Miller, 1972).

> This intelligent 33-year-old [woman] had had a stroke producing brain stem damage (a complication) approximately 4 months before she entered the [hospital] for rehabilitation of disabling motor deficits. There, [we] gave her training in voluntary control over her high blood pressure. A special device indirectly recorded diastolic blood pressure automatically on a beat-to-beat basis and sounded a tone that served as a reward by signalling to her that she had achieved the correct change of her blood pressure.... First, we rewarded her for a small decrease and then changed to reward for a small increase so that she could again succeed in producing another decrease. We also hoped that the contrast of successive reversals would help to teach her voluntary control.
>
> At first she was able to produce changes of only

> 5–6 mm Hg. As she learned, we required larger changes. Then, in order to be sure that the change was not produced by any transient maneuver of skeletal muscles we required her to hold it. . . .
> In spite of daily medication with 750 mg of the antihypertensive drug Aldomet (alpha-methyldopa) plus 100 mg of . . . Hydrodiuril, her diastolic pressure averaged 97 mm Hg during the 30 days in the hospital before training started. During this period, the pressure was variable but there was no appreciable trend. When training started her pressure came down. . . . After her blood pressure had come down to normal, she was taken off medication. During the three days while the effects of Aldomet were wearing off, her pressure rose but then decreased to an average level of 76 mm Hg . . . (pp. 247–249).†

In this connection we would again like to caution against discontinuation of antihypertensive medication during biofeedback or relaxation training, unless the patient is very closely supervised. In the following sections we will describe individual studies on feedback of blood pressure, highlighting interesting modifications of technique, assessment of generalization of treatment effect, or improvement in study design. Table 9.2 summarizes the findings of each study, and the treatment effect is displayed graphically in relation to the relaxation regression line in Figures 9.4 and 9.5.

FEEDBACK OF SYSTOLIC PRESSURE. Although some workers argue that diastolic feedback is to be preferred to systolic feedback (Elder, Leftwich, and Wilkerson, 1974), most investigators have employed the latter. In this section we will briefly review studies in which systolic feedback was used.

The first report of reduction of blood pressure in hypertensives during feedback training was an uncontrolled study by Benson, Shapiro, Tursky, et al. (1971). Seven patients were seen daily for 5 to 16 control sessions, followed by 8 to 33 treatment sessions. With a moving criterion level, it was possible to shape successively larger decreases of systolic pressure within a treatment session. On completion of treatment, the average reduction of systolic pressure for the whole group was 16.5 mm Hg (range: −0.9 to 33.8 mm Hg) from 164.9 mm Hg during the baseline period.

A rather drastic simplification of the biofeedback technique was developed by Kristt and Engel (1975) and used as an adjunct to regular electronic feedback of blood pressure. This technique was based on patients listening to their own Korotkoff sounds. Using a blood pressure cuff, the patients inflated the cuff to the level of their systolic pressure, at which point, by definition, the Korotkoff sounds were audible. Then the patients were asked to make these disappear, which, of course, happened only if systolic pressure decreased. After an initial 4-week assessment, during which the five patients recorded their own blood pressures at home, they were admitted to a research ward for 3 weeks of intensive biofeedback practice. They attended two regular biofeedback sessions daily and, in addition, learned the Korotkoff sound disappearing technique. After discharge, the patients practiced Korotkoff sound disappearing 4 to 30 times daily and again monitored their home blood pressure. Comparing pre and post home pressures, there was an average decline of 18.5/7.5 mm Hg from 162.5/94.5 mm Hg before treatment.

Another simplified feedback system was described by Blanchard, Young, and Haynes (1975), consisting of a closed-circuit TV system with the camera focused on a piece of graph paper on which the therapist plotted the systolic pressures obtained at each trial. Thus, the patients were provided with feedback as to their blood pressure by looking at a graph displayed on the TV monitor. Comparing the first and second baselines (which is the measure least confounded with within session effects), the average decline of systolic pressure for the four subjects was 17.4 mm Hg from 154.1 mm Hg during the first baseline.

An interesting measure of generalization of treatment effect was reported by Goldman, Kleinman, Snow, et al. (1974, 1975) and Kleinman, Goldman, Snow, et al. (1977). Prompted by earlier research, which suggested that patients with moderate to severe hypertension have impaired brain function (Apter, Halstead, and Heimburger, 1951; Reitan, 1954), the authors tested

† Adapted from *Current Status of Physiological Psychology*, D. Singh and C. T. Moran (Eds.). Copyright © 1972 by Wadsworth Publishing Company, Inc. Reprinted by permission of the publisher, Brooks/Cole Publishing Company, Monterey, Calif.

a group of hypertensives on the category subtest of the Halstead-Reitan Neuropsychological Test Battery for Adults (Goldman et al., 1974). The category test, which assesses the ability of the subject to form concepts and change mental sets, consists of a series of tasks requesting the subject to choose one of four objects according to an organizing principle, such as size or shape. After each choice, the subject is given immediate feedback ("correct" vs. "incorrect"). The 14 patients tested, with systolic pressure of 173 ± 24 mm Hg (mean ± 1 standard deviation) and diastolic pressure of 118.1 ± 16.5 mm Hg, obtained an error score on the category test of 73.9 ± 33.1, as compared with the cutoff point of 51 considered suggestive of cerebral impairment. Moreover, a significant correlation was found between diastolic pressure and the error score on the test (Pearson's $r = 0.52$), which remained significant even when the effects due to age or IQ had been partialed out ($r = 0.57$ and 0.51, respectively). On the other hand, no significant correlation was found between level of systolic hypertension and the error score.

Having established the association between diastolic hypertension and brain dysfunction as measured by errors on the category test, the authors now proceeded to see if test performance would improve when the hypertension was treated with feedback of systolic pressure (Goldman et al., 1975). Seven of the original subjects received biofeedback training, consisting of nine weekly 2-hour sessions and home practice of at least ½ hour per day. Following training, five of the seven patients showed improvements on a repeat category test, and a statistically significant correlation was found between improvement on the test and decrease of blood pressure (rho = 0.82 for systolic and 0.78 for diastolic pressure). The study also included a comparison group of four hypertensive subjects who received three weekly 2-hour blood pressure monitoring sessions, but these subjects were not retested on the category test.

Since the finding of a correlation between decrease of blood pressure and reduction of errors on a repeat category test appeared promising, the authors did a second study, utilizing a similar design but, in addition, obtaining home pressures (Kleinman et al., 1977). Eight subjects participated in this study. In the laboratory, the average decline of blood pressure was 6/8 mm Hg from 149/93 mm Hg. Home pressures decreased 8/9 mm Hg from 155/98 mm Hg. Reduction of systolic pressure again correlated significantly with improvement on the category test, but the correlation for diastolic pressure was nonsignificant.

The results of these two studies are intriguing and should be followed by better controlled studies. Since both the test and the treatment involved the patient receiving feedback (of errors or of blood pressure, respectively), a confounding variable, such as the "ability to learn from feedback," rather than recovery of the brain from the adverse effect of hypertension, could have caused the observed correlation.

The studies described so far have either presented new treatment methods or attempted to assess generalization of treatment effects. However, the designs of these studies did not provide adequate controls for confounding variables such as practice or expectation effects. Although a control group of four subjects was employed in the Goldman et al. (1975) study, the members of this group were seen for only three sessions, compared with nine sessions for the treatment group. An interesting control procedure was used by Richter-Heinrich et al. and reported in a series of publications (Knust and Richter-Heinrich, 1975; Richter-Heinrich, Knust, Muller, et al., 1975; Richter-Heinrich, Knust, Lori, et al., 1976; Richter-Heinrich, Knust, and Lori, 1977). The control group received false feedback, which was identical to the true feedback given to member of the feedback group. Unfortunately, it is unclear if the assignment to treatment vs. control group was randomized. Comparing earlier with later reports, it appears that new subjects were added to the treatment group without additional subjects being assigned to the control group. In the first report (Knust and Richter-Heinrich, 1975), 10 subjects in the feedback group (all hospitalized patients who were in the beginning stages of hypertensive disease) decreased their systolic pressure by 16 mm Hg from 145 mm Hg after only four sessions. However, this treatment effect did not generalize outside the biofeedback situation, as routine blood

Table 9.2
Summary of Results for Studies of Blood Pressure Feedback

Source	Treatment*	N	Systolic (mm Hg)		Diastolic (mm Hg)		Number† of Sessions		Average Decrease Within Sessions (mm Hg)		Remarks
			Pre	−Δ	Pre	−Δ	Mean	(Range)	Systolic	Diastolic	
Benson et al., 1971	S	7	164.9	16.5			21.7	8–24	4.8		
Kristt and Engel, 1975	S	4(−5[1])	162.5[1]	18.2[1]	94.5[1]	7.5[1]	52.0		11.0[2]		1. Home blood pressure (N = 4) 2. Average of last 4 lowering sessions
Blanchard et al., 1975	S	4	154.1	17.4[1]			7.8	5–9[2]			1. Baseline$_1$ − Baseline$_2$ 2. First training period
Goldman et al., 1975	S	7	167.0	8.0	109.0	15.0	9		7.0		
Kleinman et al., 1977	S	8	155.0	8.0	97.0	8.0	9		4.4	4.1	Home pressures
Knust et al., 1975	False feedback	10	145.7	11.6			4		1.1		Subjects at the beginning stages of hypertension Within session values recalculated from % reported in Figure 9.3 (Knust et al., 1975).
	S	10	145.0	16.0			4				Ward pressures
			142.0	−2.0							
Schwartz et al., 1973	D	7			102.0	0.0		10–15		5.0	
Elder et al., 1973	D + Reinforcement	5(−6)	154.4	19.8	102.2	19.0	7				Pretreatment values based on the subjects who remained at follow-up
	D	4(−6)	156.3	5.8	111.5	9.0					
Elder et al., 1975	D + Reinforcement	22	146.7	7.8	84.4	2.4	9.2	9–10			Spaced and massed practice combined

* S, systolic feedback; D, diastolic feedback; P, pulse wave velocity feedback.
† When no number specified: all S's received the same number of sessions (range = 0).

Table 9.2 (*cont.*)

Source	Treatment*	N	Systolic (mm Hg)		Diastolic (mm Hg)		Number† of Sessions		Average Decrease Within Sessions (mm Hg)		Remarks
			Pre	−Δ	Pre	−Δ	Mean	(Range)	Systolic	Diastolic	
Shoemaker et al., 1975	SD	5	132.2	−0.6	89.8	1.2	6		0.8	2.5	
	Relaxation	5	136.4	6.8	90.4	7.6	6		9.6	6.7	
	Control	5	133.8	−1.6	90.4	−1.2	6		0.8	0.6	
Friedman and Taub, 1977	SD	13	146.5	6.9	95.8	7.0	7				Nonrandom group assignment. See Table 9.1 for results for the other 3 groups
Walsh et al., 1977	P	11	151.0	13.0	94.5	7.9	5		4.8	4.1	Period I only.
	Relaxation	13	142.0	3.0	93.6	6.5	5		3.4	2.4	Period I only.

pressure measurements on the hospital ward remained essentially unchanged. Additional findings reported in these publications were that a larger treatment effect was seen in patients with moderate as opposed to high anxiety, and that the treatment effect appeared more quickly in patients who were on a tranquilizing medication as opposed to placebo.

FEEDBACK OF DIASTOLIC PRESSURE. One of the early attempts to use diastolic rather than systolic pressure feedback with a group of hypertensives was not successful (Schwartz and Shapiro, 1973, pp. 139–142): no decline of average diastolic pressure of seven subjects occurred over 10 biofeedback sessions.

In contrast to these negative findings, the results of two studies by Elder and his coworkers, in which diastolic feedback was combined with social reinforcement, appear to at least equal those obtained with systolic feedback (Elder, Ruiz, Deabler, et al., 1973; Elder and Eustis, 1975). The first of these studies is also one of the best controlled experiments on biofeedback treatment for hypertension. Eighteen hospitalized patients were randomly assigned to three groups of six subjects each. Group I was a no-feedback control group. Members of Group II were given feedback of reduction in their diastolic pressure. Members of Group III received not only feedback but also contingent praise from the experimenter. All three groups went through the following conditions: one baseline session, seven feedback sessions (two sessions per day), and one no-feedback follow-up session. The results of the study were that the feedback-plus-praise group achieved a significantly greater decrease of diastolic pressure than the other two groups. The feedback-only group showed intermediary results.

The praise-plus-feedback strategy that had proven successful in this study was applied in a later study to a group of outpatients (Elder and Eustis, 1975). This study also attempted to answer the question of optimal scheduling of training. Two different training schedules were used: massed and spaced. The massed-practice schedule involved 10 daily sessions, whereas the spaced schedule involved two sessions per week for 2 weeks, followed by one session per week for 2 weeks, 2 biweekly sessions, and a final session after 1 month (total of nine sessions). Eighteen patients were assigned to spaced practice, and four patients, the last ones admitted to the study, were assigned to massed practice. Comparing baseline pressures with those of the last training session, the overall reduction for both groups was 7.8/2.4 mm Hg. On within-session measures, the four patients receiving massed practice had results superior to those receiving spaced practice.

COMPARISON BETWEEN BLOOD-PRESSURE BIOFEEDBACK, AND RELAXATION THERAPY

Three studies have attempted to answer the question whether blood pressure feedback is more effective than relaxation therapy. In the first, 15 subjects were matched for diastolic pressure and assigned to one of three groups: control (blood pressure measurements), progressive relaxation, and feedback of both systolic and diastolic pressure (Shoemaker and Tasto, 1975). The biofeedback system required the patients to inspect, via a mirror, graphs of their pulse oscillations and their relationship to two criterion lines representing systolic and diastolic pressure. For each group, three baseline sessions, six treatment sessions, and three post-treatment sessions were held. The results indicated that subjects in the relaxation group showed a significantly greater decline of blood pressure than the other two groups combined, both over treatment sessions and over trials within sessions. Thus, the overall result indicated a superiority of relaxation therapy. One could argue, however, that the results of this study were not really representative of biofeedback, since the feedback display might have been difficult to interpret, and the rate of feedback was only once every $16^1/_2$ minutes.

The second study compared feedback of systolic and diastolic pressure with hypnotic relaxation and with biofeedback and hypnosis combined (Friedman and Taub, 1977). The experimental design also included a measurement-only comparison group. Unfortunately, the assignment to groups was not completely random: patients who were highly hypnotizable were consistently assigned to either hypnotic relaxation or the biofeedback-hypnosis combination. After a baseline session, seven training sessions were given (two per week). Hypnosis resulted in significantly larger reduction of diastolic pressure compared with measurements only and the biofeedback-hypnosis combination. The hypnosis-only and biofeedback-only groups were the only ones exhibiting a significant reduction at 1-month follow-up. While the effect of treatment modality in this study was confounded with person-variables (hypnotizability), the study does indicate that the effect of biofeedback was not strong enough to overcome these variables. Moreover, as the authors pointed out, adding biofeedback to hypnosis detracted from, rather than added to, the effect of hypnosis in highly hypnotizable subjects. Perhaps actively attending to the biofeedback display was incompatible with the more passive kind of attention typical for hypnotic relaxation.

In the third study, the effect of progressive relaxation was compared with the effect of feedback of pulse-wave velocity (Walsh *et al.*, 1977). Since pulse-wave velocity is a less obtrusive measure of blood pressure than the cuff method, one might expect that more specific effects of feedback would result. Twenty-four patients were matched for age and randomly assigned to feedback or relaxation. Indeed, the feedback group showed a significantly larger within-session decrease of diastolic pressure. However, across sessions the two techniques were equally effective in reducing systolic and diastolic pressure. In a second phase of the experiment, the two treatments were combined in both groups, but no further reduction of blood pressure took place across sessions.

We may obtain another estimate of the relative merits of relaxation vs. biofeedback of blood pressure by comparing the results of biofeedback with the results predicted by the regression of reduction of blood pressure on pretreatment level for relaxation therapy. If biofeedback were more effective, the decline of blood pressure reported should be consistently greater than those predicted for relaxation therapy. Figures 9.4 and 9.5 show this relationship for systolic and diastolic pressures, respectively. For systolic pressure, five studies fall above the relaxation therapy regression line (indicating superior results) and seven fall below. For diastolic pressure, four biofeedback points fall above and six below the

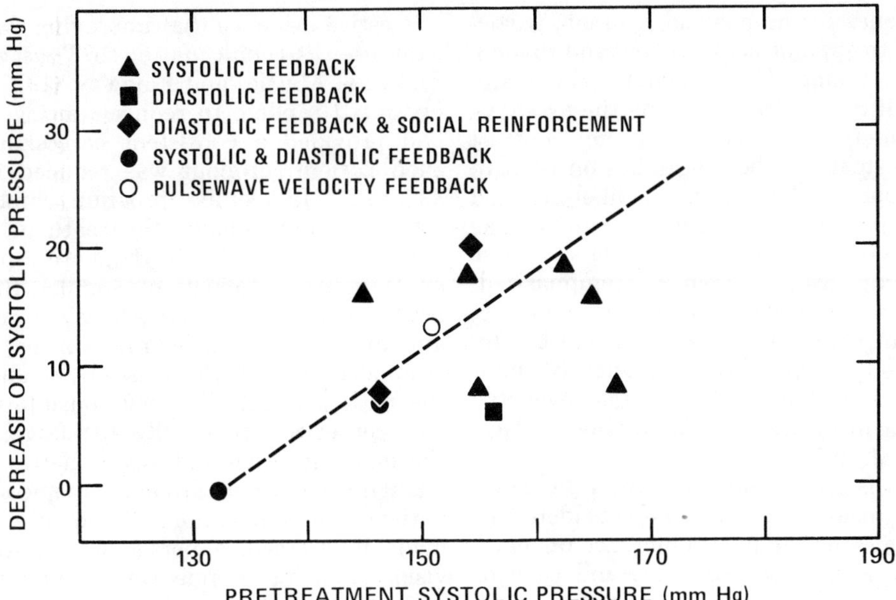

Figure 9.4. Results on systolic pressure of feedback of blood pressure compared with the relaxation therapy regression line.

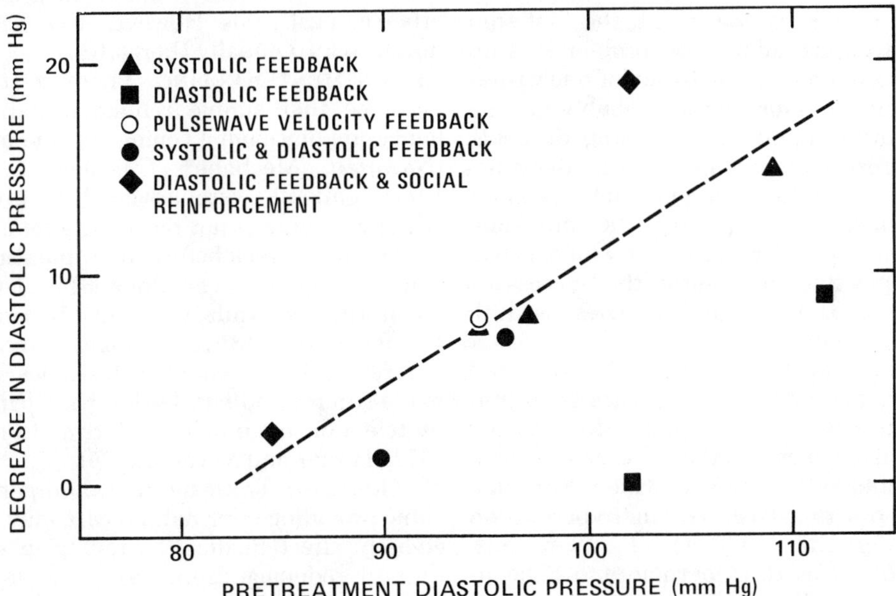

Figure 9.5. Results on diastolic pressure of blood pressure feedback compared with the relaxation therapy regression line.

relaxation regression line. Neither of these comparisons indicates superiority of biofeedback.

The overall evidence thus seems to indicate that biofeedback of blood pressure has no greater clinical effect than relaxation therapy. Thus, the extra investment in blood pressure feedback equipment would seem unwarranted unless more sophisticated and powerful methods are developed.

Methods with Indirect Effect upon Blood Pressure

As noted earlier, the treatment of hypertension can be enhanced by strengthening adherence to the medical regimen, particularly to appointment keeping and to medication taking. Unfortunately, the mammoth literature documenting the extent of the adherence problem is in some contrast to the small number of studies on what to do about it. This contrast is likely to lead to the perception that nothing can be done about poor adherence or, worse still, that the problem has been overemphasized. That the latter is not the case in the treatment of hypertension is confirmed by the repeated finding that only slightly more than half of all hypertensives take over 80% of their medication (Sackett, Gibson, Taylor, et al., 1975).

Approaches to this problem in the delivery of medical care can be considered as either preventing poor adherence or remediating adherence problems, and each of these will be considered separately.

PREVENTION OF POOR ADHERENCE

From a clinical viewpoint, the first step in preventing adherence problems is to measure aspects of the behavior one wishes to influence. This should probably include monitoring appointment keeping, dropouts from treatment, and medication taking, using a measure such as pill count. Without such information for both the individual patient and the program as a whole, it will be impossible to monitor the success or failure of the various strategies used to affect compliance.

Dropout from Treatment. The first step in ensuring adequate adherence is to prevent dropout from treatment. Maximizing the convenience of medical care has been suggested as one way to achieve this end. In one program, treatment for hypertension was offered to employees of a New York department store (Alderman and Schoenbaum, 1975). For those selecting treatment, the dropout rate at the end of 1 year was a remarkably low 3%. However, in a randomized controlled clinical trial involving 230 hypertensive Canadian steel workers, no advantage was found at the end of 6 months for those treated at work as compared with those treated by their personal physicians (Sackett et al., 1975). Dropout rate was 7% in each group.

While treatment convenience may not in itself reduce the dropout rate, there is suggestive evidence that improving the organization of a clinic may do so. Thus, when Finnerty, Mattie, and Finnerty (1973) reorganized a clinic to reduce waiting time and provided a consistent caretaker for each patient, dropout was reduced from 42% to 8%. In a similar program, emphasis was placed upon making the treatment center one of high quality, with an atmosphere encouraging participation (Stamler, Stamler, Civinelli, et al., 1975). All visits were by appointment, with little or no waiting, and, in almost all cases, the same physician saw the patient at all physician consultations. The center was physically attractive, and the staff receptive and sympathetic, with enough time per visit to allow ample staff-patient communication. Much use was made of paramedical personnel, and supervision of such personnel was accomplished through daily chart review as well as general staff case review. The dropout rate in this clinic was 20% for the 1st year, in line with the high initial dropout observed in other clinical trials. However, this was reduced to 3% annually thereafter.

Appointment Keeping. There is strong evidence that simple reminders can enhance appointment keeping. In one study (Nazarian, Mechaber, Charney, et al., 1974), patients were assigned to groups either receiving or not receiving a reminder card mailed 1 week before the appointment. Those receiving a card kept 64% of their appointments, while those in the control group kept only 48%, a clear and significant difference. Other controlled studies have made similar findings, both for mailed and for telephoned reminders (Clark and Troop, 1972; Turner and Vernon, 1976).

Medication Taking. A well-organized clinic providing personalized care may beneficially affect medication taking in addition to reducing dropouts. Thus, in the clinic described above (Stamler et al., 1975), 82% of the patients remaining in the program had diastolic blood pressure below 90 mm Hg after 2 years of treatment as compared with 67% of patients in a control group who had been referred to and treated by their own physicians. It is, of course, not clear which aspects of this program most affected adherence; indeed the results might have been due solely to different prescribing practices between the clinic and family physicians. Thus, we need to examine other studies to determine the necessary components of a program to prevent the occurrence of inaccurate medication taking.

One of the most obvious components of an adherence program to study is patient education. Educating the patient about the disease and its treatment seems so eminently sensible that it is surprising, perhaps even shocking, to find that two controlled studies showed no advantage for the educated patient.

In the previously mentioned study of Canadian steel workers, Sackett and his colleagues (1975) tested the effects of a "mastery learning" program vs. usual care. Mastery learning consisted of a slide-tape show, a booklet, and follow-up to determine recall and to remind participants of salient facts. Items covered included the facts about hypertension and its effects on life expectancy, the benefits of treatment, the need for compliance, and some simple reminders about pill taking. After 6 months of treatment, no effects of this program on either adherence, as measured by home pill count, or blood pressure were found. Even more remarkable was that in the group treated at work, education seemed to have a detrimental effect, adherence rates (as measured by pill count) were 48% vs. 62% for the usual-care group.

In another study with hypertensive patients, two different methods of conveying information were compared with routine care (Caplan, Robinson, French, et al., 1976). One group of patients received a series of lectures about the disease, its treatment, and adherence problems. A second group received and discussed similar information in small groups aimed at providing a maximum of social support, while the third group received regular clinic care. A number of indirect measures, such as self-report of adherence, knowledge of the disease, and social support, suggested that the lecture and group methods were equally beneficial, and that both were better than usual care. However, no differences were found between the three groups when blood pressure was measured, suggesting that education had no practical effect on adherence and pointing out the need to measure adherence directly and objectively, rather than by indirect self-report measures. These bewildering failures suggest that complex educational efforts do not enhance adherence, and indeed perhaps the very complexity of these programs may be the problem, for several studies (unfortunately not with hypertensives) have shown that short written instructions concerning the medical regimen enhance adherence to it (Ley, Jain, and Skilbeck, 1976; Sharpe and Mikeal, 1974).

Another approach to increasing medication taking is to take advantage of the fact that accurate feedback about the occurrence of behavior will tend to enhance performance. One way to achieve this with medication taking is through the use of medication dispensers which display the pills to be taken by date, thus conveying information about doses taken or missed. In one controlled test of such a device with 100 hypertensive patients, chlorthalidone was dispensed either in the usual bottle or in a specifically designed compliance "PAK" (Eshelman and Fitzloff, 1976). Urinalysis to detect chlorthalidone revealed that this display resulted in a compliance rate of 93% against 69% for the bottled prescription. No data for blood pressure were given. Other forms of display such as containers or pill calendars to be mounted on a wall in the kitchen or bathroom take advantage of the principle of stimulus control in addition to providing feedback about missed doses of medication. An event which is regularly associated with a behavior may come to serve as a cue for the performance of that behavior. Thus, the sight of a prominently placed pill dispenser may tend to remind patients to take their medication. Unfortunately, such devices, although promising, have not yet been adequately tested.

Another way to improve medication taking may be to simplify the dosage regimen on the supposition that the less the prescribed number of doses the better will be adherence. In a retrospective study of this issue with hypertensives, the effect of a one-tablet equivalent of three separate tablets was studied (Clark and Troop, 1972). It was found that patients shifted from the separate (three times daily) dosage to a combined dosage schedule (once daily) showed an average drop of 19 mm Hg diastolic blood pressure, the mean time on the once daily schedule being 10 months. Retrospective studies of course are fraught with error, particularly in the possibility of differential assignment of poor risk patients to one or another group, and differential retrieval of data from the record. One prospective study corrected for this difficulty and used a sequential design in which hypertensive patients were placed on placebo, followed by several times per day dosage, followed by single dose tablets, with 2 weeks spent in each phase (David, Welborn, and Pierce, 1975). Both of the latter were found superior to placebo, but no differences were found between the two regimens. However, the very short time periods used might well have obscured the longer term benefit of the simpler medication regime.

Thus, a controlled study in which 50 hypertensives were randomly allocated to either three-times-a-day or once-a-day doses of tablets and in which blood pressure was measured at the end of some 16 weeks provided one of the best tests of the effect of a simple medication regime (Schultz, 1962). Sitting blood pressures were not significantly different before randomization ($p = 0.62$ systolic; $p = 0.69$ diastolic). When we analyzed the data presented in the original paper, we found that after treatment both systolic ($p = 0.04$) and diastolic pressure ($p = 0.02$) were significantly different in favor of the combined dose. However, this difference was not found for standing blood pressures.

Thus, while the evidence for an advantage of a simple dosage regime over a complex regime is somewhat questionable, at least some evidence of superiority has been presented. Moreover, a simple regime has never been found less effective than a complex one of equal pharmacological effect. It may be, however, that in its effect upon blood pressure, the advantages and disadvantages of a single dosage regimen cancel each other out. While it may be easier to fit a single dose into one's schedule, thus enhancing the likelihood of taking medication, missing a dose results in a larger error than if medication is taken in two or three separate doses.

The final approach to preventing poor adherence to medication lies in establishing a counseling relationship specifically aimed at that result. Such a procedure was carefully explored in a recent study in which hypertensive patients were randomized into two groups, one receiving usual care from their physician, while the other received extra counseling from a pharmacist at regular visits over a 5-month period (McKenney, Slining, Henderson, et al., 1973). During visits, patients were first informed of the nature and treatment of hypertension using pamphlets followed by a discussion. At subsequent visits, lasting an average of 6 minutes each, the pharmacist

> . . . evaluated the patient's therapeutic responses to the drug and dietary management; identified and managed additional complications, reactions, and problems; evaluated the patient's understanding of the educational material; provided additional educational material; identified and managed some adverse reactions to drug therapy; referred patients to health-center personnel for specialized care; and recommended therapy changes to the physician based on the patient's therapeutic responses and compliance with prescribed therapy. . . . (pp. 1104–1111).‡

A substantial proportion of counseling time was devoted to the early identification and management of medication side effects. During 5 months of counseling, 50 suspected adverse drug reactions were identified and promptly dealt with in 24 patients. The compliant patients (those taking more than 90% of their medication) experienced a mean of 2.0 adverse reactions each, while noncompliant patients had a mean of 4.4 side effects or drug reactions.

By the end of the 5-month study, 78% of counseled patients were showing excellent (above 90%) adherence, as measured by pill count, compared with 16% of the control group. Blood pressure for the counseled group was 146/90 compared to 166/101 for the control group. Despite these promising results, one disappointing finding was reported. When counseling was stopped, the advantage shown by the counseled group vanished because their blood pressures rose to baseline levels. Preventive adherence counseling, it seems, must be a continuous process if optimal results are to be achieved.

‡ Reprinted from McKenney, J. M., Slining, J. M., Henderson, H. R., Devins, D., and Berr, M. The effect of chemical pharmacy services on patients with essential hypertension. *Circulation, 1973, 48,* 1104–1111, by permission of the American Heart Association, Inc.

ADHERENCE REMEDIATION

The old clinical saying that it is better to prevent problems occurring than to treat them is confirmed by the relatively modest results demonstrated by such treatment. The usual approach to adherence remediation is some form of counseling, which aims to identify the problem and teach the patient skills useful in coping with it. The only controlled study of this method published to date with hypertensives was a follow-up to the study of Canadian steel workers described earlier (Haynes, Gibson, Hockett, et al., 1976). Thirty-nine hypertensives who had not reached a diastolic blood pressure of 90 mm Hg or less after 6 months of treatment were allocated to one of two groups, usual care or remedial counseling. In the latter condition, patients were seen every 2 weeks by a high-school graduate counselor, were taught to measure their own blood pressure, and were asked to record both blood pressure and the amount of medication taken each day. In addition, the pattern of adherence and their life schedules were examined to identify regularly occurring events to which pill taking could be attributed. Finally, patients were praised for improvement in adherence behavior and, for each 4 mm Hg improvement in diastolic pressure, were given a $4 credit toward purchase of their sphygmomanometer.

After 6 months of treatment, a home pill count averaged 65.8% in the counseled group compared with 44.7% in the usual-care patients. Diastolic blood pressure fell by 5.4 mm Hg in the counseled group compared with 1.9 mm Hg in the usual-care group. The blood pressure changes compared between groups were not significantly different, although only the counseled group showed a significant change from the beginning to the end of the study.

Some other less well-specified remediation procedures have been used which might prove useful with some individuals or subpopulations of a clinic. Wilber and Barrow (1969) found that 88 of 220 individuals (40%) were willing to participate in a program involving regular home visits by a public health nurse. During these visits, the nurse checked the patient's blood pressure, emphasized the importance of taking medication, and made sure that patients were seeing a physician and had a supply of medication. Before the visiting nurse program began, only 15% of the patients were well controlled (diastolic blood pressure at 95 mm Hg or less). After participating for 2 years, 80% of the patients showed good control as determined by blood pressure measurements, compared with 34% of the nonvolunteer group. These differences might have been due to factors other than the home visits, since volunteers may not be comparable to non-volunteers on many dimensions. Moreover, 2 years after the program was stopped only 29% of patients showed good control.

Even though remediation has shown some promising results, a larger yield might lie in prevention. Thus, increasing participation in the treatment by minimizing dropouts may make a larger contribution to the management of hypertension than providing remedial counseling. Moreover, it seems likely that by establishing a preventive approach to counseling such as that of McKenney and his colleagues described earlier, many adherence problems can be prevented, and that adherence can be maintained as long as the counseling is continued. Obviously, some remediation may be called for, but, in our view, most time and effort should be devoted to preventing the onset of poor adherence.

Overview

We have examined two areas in which progress has been made toward enhancing the treatment of essential hypertension by means of behavior change procedures. In both areas some general conclusions can be drawn. Thus, relaxation training seems to be at least as effective as blood pressure biofeedback in reducing blood pressure. Since relaxation training is a simpler procedure and does not require costly and complicated equipment, then, for the moment, it should be preferred for clinical use. Developments in biofeedback technology such as improvements in the measurement of blood pressure may alter this state of affairs, and research into both relaxation and biofeedback procedures must, of course, continue. Among the important residual questions concerning these procedures is whether a behavior change procedure will lead to blood pressure lowering over 24 hours or whether the effects are limited to the time spent practicing the procedure. A further question concerns the long-term outcome of these procedures, particularly outcome over years rather than months.

Turning to adherence, we find a less well-developed area of much promise. More needs to be known about the phenomenon of adherence, particularly in identifying modifiable environmental factors which impinge upon medication taking. Moreover, given the problems encountered in remediating poor adherence, attention needs to be directed toward the prevention of poor adherence. Important contributions might be made by the pharmaceutical industry in packaging medication to enhance adherence and in developing longer acting agents which would then require fewer doses.

In closing, it seems well to reiterate our opening words: Several promising new behavior change approaches to the treatment of essential hypertension are emerging on stage or hovering in the wings. These include weight reduction, salt restriction, and exercise. Whether or not non-pharmacological approaches to the control of hypertension will eventually prove effective as a primary treatment, as an adjunctive treatment, or in the prevention of essential hypertension remains to be seen, but there is no doubt that a good beginning has been made and that the next decade will bring interesting developments.

Note

1. The analysis was performed in the following steps. First, treatment groups were classified into one of two sets, depending on whether or not they fulfilled the following criteria: no medication change, six or more subjects per group, report of absolute rather than percent change of blood pressure, and not selecting subjects on basis of some personal characteristic with a conceivable effect on outcome (such as age or hypnotizability). Second, a regression analysis, weighted for the number of subjects per group, was performed for the systolic and diastolic pressures of each set (Dunn and Clark, 1974, pp. 236–237). Third, the results for the two sets (fulfilling vs. not fulfilling criteria) were compared, and the differences between the residual variances, regression coefficients (slopes), and intercepts were tested for statistical significance, using the 0.05 significance level (two-tailed). If there was a significant difference, the analysis was stopped and the analysis of only the set of studies fulfilling the criteria was used as the result. If there was no difference, a second analysis was performed on the pooled data of the two sets. The regression line resulting from the analysis was inserted in Figures 9.2 and 9.3 and also was used to estimate the expected treatment effect ($-\hat{\Delta}_R$) entered in Table 9.1. For systolic pressure, the residual variance for studies fulfilling the criteria was significantly larger than for studies not fulfilling the criteria. Therefore, the regression line in Figure 9.2 is based on the former set of studies (open symbols). For diastolic pressure in Figure 9.3, the analysis could be based on pooled data.

References

Alderman, M. H., and Schoenbaum, E. E. Detection and treatment of hypertension at the work site. *N. Engl. J. Med.,* 1975, *293,* 65–68.

Apter, N., Halstead, W., and Heimburger, R. Impaired cerebral functions in essential hypertension. *Am. J. Psychiatry,* 1951, *107,* 808–813.

Bachmann, K., Zerzwy, R., Riess, P.-J., Zölch, K. A. Blutdruckstelemetrie. *Deut. Med. Wochenschr.,* 1970, *95,* 741–747.

Bech, K., and Hilden, T. The frequency of secondary hypertension. *Acta Med. Scand.,* 1975, *197,* 65–69.

Benson, H., Kotch, J. B., and Crasweller, K. D. The relaxation response: A bridge between psychiatry and medicine. *Med. Clin. N. Am.,* 1977, *61,* 929–937.

Benson, H., Rosner, B. A., Marzetta, B. R., and Klemchuk, H. M. Decreased blood pressure in borderline hypertensive subjects who practiced meditation. *J. Chronic Dis.,* 1974a, *27,* 163–169.

Benson, H., Rosner, B. A., Marzetta, B. R., and Klemchuk, H. M. Decreased blood pressure in pharmacologically treated hypertensive patients who regularly elicited the relaxation response. *Lancet,* 1974b, *1,* 289–291.

Benson, H., Shapiro, D., Tursky, B., and Schwartz, G. E. Decreased systolic blood pressure through operant conditioning techniques in patients with essential hypertension. *Science,* 1971, *173,* 740–741.

Bernstein, D. A., and Borkovec, T. D. *Progressive relaxation training: A manual for the helping professions.* Champaign, Ill.: Research Press, 1973.

Blackwell, B., Haneson, I., Bloomfield, S., Magenheim, H., Gartside, P., Nidich, S., Robinson, A., and Zigler, R. Transcendental meditation in hypertension: Individual response patterns. *Lancet,* 1976, *1,* 223–226.

Blanchard, E. B., Young, L. D., and Haynes, M. R. A simple feedback system for the treatment of elevated blood pressure. *Behav. Ther.,* 1975, *6,* 241–245.

Boyer, J. L., and Kasch, F. W. Exercise therapy in hypertensive men. *J.A.M.A.,* 1970, *211,* 1668–1671.

Brady, J. P., Luborsky, L., and Kron, R. E. Blood pressure reduction in patients with essential hypertension through metronome-conditioned relaxation: A preliminary report. *Behav. Ther.,* 1974, *5,* 203–209.

Brauer, A., Horlick, L., Nelson, E., Farquhar, J. F., and Agras, W. S. Relaxation therapy for essential hypertension: A VA outpatient study. Unpublished manuscript, Stanford University, 1978.

Caplan, R. D., Robinson, E. A. R., French, J. R. P.,

Caldwell, J. R., and Shinn, M. *Adhering to medical regimens: Pilot experiments in patient education and social support.* Ann Arbor: University of Michigan, 1976.

Caron, H. S., and Roth, H. P. Patients cooperation with a medical regimen: Difficulties in identifying the noncooperator. *J.A.M.A.*, 1968, *203,* 120–124.

Clark, G. M., and Troop, R. One tablet combination drug therapy in the treatment of hypertension. *J. Chronic Dis.*, 1972, *25,* 57–64.

Datey, K. K., Deshmukh, S. N., Dalvi, C. P., and Vinekar, S. L. "Shavasan": A yogic exercise in the management of hypertension. *Angiology,* 1969, *20,* 325–333.

David, N. A., Welborn, W. S., and Pierce, H. I. Comparison of multiple and combination tablet drug therapy in hypertension. *Cur. Ther. Res.*, 1975, *18,* 741–754.

Deabler, H. L., Fidel, E., Dillenkoffer, R. L., and Elder, S. T. The use of relaxation and hypnosis in lowering high blood pressure. *Am. J. Clin. Hypn.*, 1973, *16,* 75–83.

Dowdall, S. A. Breathing techniques that help reduce hypertension. *RN,* 1977, *40,* 73–74.

Dunn, O. J., and Clark, V. A. *Applied statistics: Analysis of variance and regression.* New York: Wiley, 1974.

Elder, S. T., and Eustis, N. K. Instrumental blood pressure conditioning in outpatient hypertensives. *Behav. Res. Ther.*, 1975, *13,* 185–188.

Elder, S. T., Leftwich, D. A., and Wilkerson, L. A. The role of systolic- versus diastolic-contingent feedback in blood pressure conditioning. *Psychol. Rec.*, 1974, *24,* 171–176.

Elder, S. T., Ruiz, Z. B., Deabler, H. L., and Dillenkoffer, R. L. Instrumental conditioning of diastolic blood pressure in essential hypertensive patients. *J. Appl. Behav. Anal.*, 1973, *6,* 377–382.

Engelman, K., and Braunwald, E. Hypotension and the shock syndrome. In G. W. Thorn, R. D. Adams, E. Braunwald, K. J. Isselbacher, and R. G. Petersdorf, (Eds.), *Harrison's principles of internal medicine,* 8th ed. New York: McGraw-Hill, 1977.

Eshelman, F. N., and Fitzloff, J. Effect of packaging on patient compliance with an antihypertensive medication. *Ther. Res.*, 1976, *20,* 215–219.

Finnerty, F. A., Mattie, E. C., and Finnerty, F. A. Hypertension in the inner city. 1. Analysis of clinic drop-outs. *Circulation,* 1973, *47,* 73–75.

Freis, E. D. Salt, volume, and the prevention of hypertension. *Circulation,* 1976, *53,* 509–594.

French, A. P., Schmid, A. C., and Ingalls, E. Transcendental meditation, altered reality testing and behavioral change: A case report. *J. Nerv. Ment. Dis.*, 1975, *161,* 55–58.

Friedman, H., and Taub, H. A. The use of hypnosis and biofeedback procedures for essential hypertension. *Int. J. Clin. Exp. Hypn.* 1977, *25,* 335–347.

Garrow, J. S. Zero muddler for unprejudiced sphygmomanometry. *Lancet,* 1963, *2,* 1205.

Goldman, H., Kleinman, K., Snow, M., Bidus, D., and Korol, B. Correlation of diastolic blood pressure and cognitive dysfunction in essential hypertension. *Dis. Nerv. Syst.*, 1974, *35,* 571–572.

Goldman, H., Kleinman, K., Snow, M. Bidus, D., and Korol, B. Relationship between essential hypertension and cognitive functioning: Effects of biofeedback. *Psychophysiology,* 1975, *12,* 569–573.

Goldring, W., Chasis, H., Schreiner, G. E., and Smith, H. W. Reassurance in the management of benign hypertensive disease. *Circulation,* 6, *14,* 260–264.

Grenfell, R. F., Briggs, A. H., and Holland, W. C. Antihypertensive drugs: A controlled evaluation. *J. Miss. State Med. Assoc.*, 1962, *3,* 93–98.

Haynes, R. B., Gibson, E. S., Hockett, B. C., Sackett, D. L., Taylor, D. W., Roberts, R. S., and Johnson, A. L. Improvement of medication compliance in uncontrolled hypertension. *Lancet,* 1976, 1265–1268.

Hersen, M., and Barlow, D. H. *Single case experimental designs: Strategies for studying behavior change.* New York: Pergamon Press, 1976.

Hinman, A. T., Engel, B. T., and Bickford, A. F. Portable blood pressure recorder: Accuracy and preliminary evaluating intradaily variations in pressure. *Am. Heart J.*, 1962, *63,* 663–668.

Jacob, R. G., Kraemer, H. C., and Agras, W. S. Relaxation therapy in the treatment of hypertension: A review. *Arch. Gen. Psychiatry,* 1977, *34,* 1417–1427.

Jacobsen, E. Variation of blood pressure with skeletal muscle tension and relaxation. *Ann. Intern. Med.*, 1939, *12,* 1194–1212.

Joyce, C. R. B. Patient cooperation and the sensitivity of clinical trials. *J. Chronic Dis.*, 1962, *15,* 1025–1036.

Julius, S. Borderline hypertension: An overview. *Med. Clin. N. Am.*, 1977, *61,* 496–511.

Kennedy, R. B. Self-induced depersonalization syndrome. *Am. J. Psychiatry* 1976, *133,* 1326–1328.

Kleinman, K. M., Goldman, H., Snow, M. Y., and Korol, B. Relationship between essential hypertension and cognitive function. II: Effects of biofeedback training generalize to non-laboratory environment. *Psychophysiology,* 1977, *14,* 192–197.

Knust, U., and Richter-Heinrich, E. Blutdrucksenkung durch instrumentelle konditionierung bei arteriellen essentiellen hypertonikern. *Deut. Gesundheitswes.*, 1975, *30,* 1014–1018.

Kristt, D. A., and Engel, B. T. Learned control of blood pressure in patients with high blood pressure. *Circulation,* 1975, *51,* 370–378.

Ley, P., Jain, V. K., and Skilbeck, C. E. A method for decreasing patients medication errors. *Psychol. Med.*, 1976, *6,* 599–601.

Littler, W. A., Honour, A. J., Sleight, P., and Stott, F. D. Continuous recording of direct arterial pressure and electrocardiogram in unrestricted man. *Br. Med. J.*, 1972, *3,* 76–78.

Luthe, W., and Schultz, J. H. *Autogenic therapy: II. Medical application.* New York: Grune & Stratton, 1969.

Maddock, R. K. Patient cooperation in taking medicines. *J.A.M.A.*, 1967, *199,* 137–172.

Masi, M., Moore, R., and Weston, A. A skeptical look at EMG training in the reduction of blood pressure in essential hypertensives. Paper presented at the Seventh Annual Meeting of the Biofeedback Research Society, Colorado Springs, Colo., February, 1976.

McKenney, J. M., Slining, J. M., Henderson, H. R., Devins, D., and Berr, M. The effect of clinical pharmacy services on patients with essential hypertension. *Circulation,* 1973, *48,* 1104–1111.

Miller, N. E. Postscript. In D. Singh, C. T. Morgan, (Eds.), *Current status of physiological psychology: Readings.* Monterey, Calif.: Brooks/Cole, 1972.

Moser, M. Report of the Joint National Committee on

Detection, Evaluation, and Treatment of High Blood Pressure; a cooperative study. *J.A.M.A.*, 1977, *237,* 255-261.

Nazarian, L. F., Mechaber, J., Charney, F., and Coulter, M. P. Effect of a mailed appointment reminder on appointment keeping. *Pediatrics,* 1974, *53,* 349-352.

Page, I. H., and Dustan, H. P. Editorial: Persistence of normal blood pressure after discontinuing treatment in hypertensive patients. *Circulation,* 1962, *25,* 433-436.

Park, L. C., and Lipman, R. S. A comparison of patient dosage deviation reports with pill counts. *Psychopharmacologia,* 1964, *6,* 299-302.

Patel, C. H. Yoga and bio-feedback in the management of hypertension. *Lancet,* 1973, *2,* 1053-1055.

Patel, C. H. Twelve-month follow-up of yoga and biofeedback in the management of hypertension. *Lancet,* 1975a, *2,* 62-64.

Patel, C. H. Yoga and biofeedback in the management of 'stress' in hypertensive patients. *Clin. Sci. Mol. Med.,* 1975b (Suppl. 48), 171s-174s.

Patel, C. H. Biofeedback-aided relaxation and meditation in the management of hypertension. *Biofeedback Self-regulation,* 1977, *2,* 1-41.

Patel, C., and Carruthers, M. Coronary risk factor reduction through biofeedback-aided relaxation and meditation. *J. R. Coll. Gen. Prac.,* 1977, *27,* 401-405.

Patel, C. H., and North, W. R. S. Randomized controlled trial of yoga and biofeedback in management of hypertension. *Lancet,* July 19, 1975, 93-95.

Peters, K. R., Benson, H., and Peters, J. M. Daily relaxation response breaks in a working population. II. Effects on blood pressure. *Am. J. Public Health,* 1977, *67,* 954-959.

Pickering, T. Yoga and biofeedback in hypertension (Letter to the editor). *Lancet,* 1973, *2,* 1440.

Pickering, T. G., Brucker, B., Frankel, H. L., Mathias, C. J., Dworkin, B. R., and Miller, N. E. Mechanisms of learned voluntary control of blood pressure patients with generalized bodily paralysis. In B. Jackson, and L. Heiner (Eds.), *Biofeedback and behavior.* New York: Plenum, 1977.

Pollack, A. A., Weber, M. A., Case, D. B., and Larogh, J. H. Limitations of transcendental meditation in the treatment of essential hypertension. *Lancet,* 1977, *2,* 71-73.

Redmond, D. P., Gaylor, M. S., McDonald, R. H., Jr., and Shapiro, A. P. Blood pressure and heart-rate response to verbal instruction and relaxation in hypertension. *Psychosom. Med.,* 1974, *36,* 285-297.

Reisen, E., Abel, R., Modan, M., Silverberg, D. S., Eliahou, H. E., and Modan, B. Effect of weight loss without salt restriction on the reduction of blood pressure in overweight hypertensive patients. *N. Engl. J. Med.,* 1978, *298,* 1-6.

Reitan, R. Intellectual and affective changes in essential hypertension. *Am. J. Psychiatry,* 1954, *110,* 817-828.

Richter-Heinrich, E., Knust, U., and Lori, M. Drop of blood pressure in patients with essential arterial hypertension by means of instrumental conditioned reflexes with a feedback connection. *Zh. Vysshei Nerv. Deiatel'nosti,* 1977, *27,* 401-404.

Richter-Heinrich, E., Knust, U., Lori, M., and Sprung, H. Zur Blutdruckkontrolle durch Biofeedback bei arteriellen essentiellen Hypertonikern. *Z. Psychol.,* 1976, *184,* 538-550.

Richter-Heinrich, E., Knust, U., Muller, W., Schmidt, K. H., and Sprung, H. Psychophysiological investigations in essential hypertensives. *J. Psychosom. Res.,* 1975, *19,* 251-258.

Sackett, D. L., Gibson, E. S., Taylor, D. W., Haynes, R. B., Hockett, B. C., Roberts, R. R., and Johnson, A. L. Randomized clinical trial of strategies for improving medication compliance in primary hypertension. *Lancet,* 1975, 1205-1207.

Schultz, F. B. The evaluation of hypertensive drugs. *J. Med. Assoc. Ala.,* 1962, *32,* 105-111.

Schwartz, G. E., and Shapiro, D. Biofeedback and essential hypertension: Current findings and theoretical concerns. In L. Birk (Ed.), *Biofeedback: Behavioral medicine.* New York: Grune & Stratton, 1973.

Sharpe, T. R., and Mikeal, R. Patient compliance with antibiotic regimens. *Am. J. Hosp. Pharm.,* 1974, *31,* 479-484.

Shoemaker, J. E., and Tasto, D. L. The effects of muscle relaxation on blood pressure of essential hypertensives. *Behav. Res. Ther.,* 1975, *13,* 29-41.

Smith, W. M. Epidemiology of hypertension. *Med. Clin. N. Am.,* 1977a, *61,* 467-486.

Smith, W. M. Treatment of mild hypertension: Results of a ten-year intervention trial. *Circ. Res.,* 1977b, *40*(Suppl. 1), 98-105.

Stamler, R., Stamler, J., Civinelli, J., Pritchard, D., Gosch, F. C., Ticho, S., Restivo, B., and Fine, D. Adherence and blood pressure response to hypertension treatment. *Lancet,* 1975, 1227-1230.

Stone, R. A., and DeLeo, J. Psychotherapeutic control of hypertension. *N. Engl. J. Med.,* 1976, *294,* 80-84.

Taylor, C. B., Farquhar, J. W., Nelson, E., and Agras, S. W. The effects of relaxation therapy upon high blood pressure. *Arch. Gen. Psychiatry,* 1977, *34,* 339-342.

Thurm, R. H., and Smith, W. M. On resetting of "barostats" in hypertensive patients. *J.A.M.A.,* 1967, *201,* 301-304.

Turner, A. J., and Vernon, J. C. Prompts to increase attendance in a community mental health center. *J. Appl. Behav. Anal.,* 1976, *9,* 141-145.

Veterans Administration Cooperative Study Group on Anti-hypertensive Agents. Effects of treatment on morbidity in hypertension. *J.A.M.A.,* 1967, *202,* 1028-1034.

Veterans Administration Cooperative Study Group on Anti-hypertensive Agents. II. Results in patients with diastolic blood pressure averaging 90 through 114 mm Hg. *J.A.M.A.,* 1970, *213,* 1143-1152.

Veterans Administration Cooperative Study Group. Effect of treatment on morbidity in hypertension. III. Influence of age, diastolic pressure and prior cardiovascular disease. *Circulation,* 1972, *45,* 991-1004.

Walsh, P., Dale, A., and Anderson, D. E. Comparison of biofeedback pulse wave velocity and progressive relaxation in essential hypertensives. *Percept. Motor Skills,* 1977, *44,* 839-843.

Wilber, J. A., and Barrow, T. G. Reducing elevated blood pressure: Experience found in a community. *Minn. Med.,* 1969, 1303-1306.

Smoking

DOUGLAS A. BERNSTEIN, PH.D.
Professor of Psychology
Department of Psychology
University of Illinois
Champaign, Illinois

RUSSELL E. GLASGOW, PH.D.
Assistant Professor of Psychology
Department of Psychology
North Dakota State University
Fargo, North Dakota

10

The Modification of Smoking Behavior

Medical evidence concerning the deleterious health consequences of habitual cigarette smoking has been accumulating since the early 1960's. Historically, concern about the possible effects of cigarette smoking on health began with a focus on lung cancer; cigarette smoking has been identified as the major risk factor for this disease (United States Public Health Service, 1975). The most important single cause of excess mortality among cigarette smokers is the development of coronary heart disease (American Heart Association, 1970; United States Public Health Service, 1975). Compared to nonsmokers, cigarette smokers also have an increased incidence of respiratory diseases, which are the major causes of both permanent and temporary disability in the United States (United States Public Health Service, 1975). It is also apparent that the risk of developing many serious diseases is reduced by the cessation of smoking (Hammond and Garfinkel, 1969; United States Public Health Service, 1975). These data, as well as figures concerning work days missed and the possible effects of smoking on unborn children, have led the World Health Organization (1975) to conclude that smoking-related diseases are the major cause of disability and premature death in developed countries and that the control of smoking could do more to prolong life and improve health than any other single action in the whole field of preventive medicine. The problem is not that the public is unaware of this information (Gallup, 1974), but that the great majority of smokers wishing to quit are unable to do so (Guilford, 1966).

This state of affairs has attracted the attention of psychologists and other behavioral scientists over the last 20 years because, on the practical side, it highlights the need for an appropriate and effective self-control technology for use with smokers desirous of quitting (National Clearinghouse for Smoking and Health, 1968, 1970, 1974). Further, smoking is of considerable interest *as behavior* and has prompted the development of a variety of theories and models which seek to account for its development, maintenance, and modification (Borgatta and Evans, 1968; Hunt, 1970; Zagona, 1967). Theories of smoking focusing primarily on affective (Ikard and Tomkins, 1973; Tomkins, 1966, 1968), behavioral (Hunt and Matarazzo, 1970; Logan, 1973), motivational (Solomon and Corbit, 1973), personality (Eysenck, 1973), and pharmacological (Jarvik, 1970; Russell, 1974; Schachter, Silverstein, Kozlowski, et al., 1977) factors as well as models attempting to integrate various of these influences (Glad, Tyre, and Adesso, 1976; Leventhal and Cleary, 1977; Mausner, 1973; Mausner and Platt, 1971) have been developed.

In the present chapter, we shall not attempt to review exhaustively the theoretical or applied literature on smoking behavior. Our purposes instead are to (a) summarize the status of research relating to the modification of smoking behavior, (b) point out approaches which do or do not seem promising, and (c) make some suggestions about the directions which future work might most profitably take. This has, of course, been done before and the conclusions of previous reviews of smoking modification efforts (Bernstein, 1969; Epstein and McCoy, 1975; Hunt and Bespalec, 1974; Keutzer, Lichtenstein, and Mees, 1968; Lichtenstein, 1971; Lichtenstein and Danaher, 1976; Lichtenstein and Keutzer, 1971; Raw, 1976a,b; Schwartz, 1969) shall provide our point of departure. In particular, a review by Bernstein and McAlister (1976) will be drawn upon heavily in this chapter.

These reviews tell us, first, that the range of approaches and techniques employed in the context of attempts to modify cigarette smoking has been wide and includes "remote control" tactics such as antismoking legislation and advertising as well as more personalized interventions involving nicotinomimetic drugs, individual and group clinics (which may or may not incorporate drugs), hypnosis, individual psychotherapy, role-playing, systematic desensitization and various other forms of overt and covert respondent and operant conditioning (e.g., contract management, stimulus control), and the like. The reviews also indicate that the results of these smoking cessation procedures contain, to borrow an old joke, both good news and bad news. The good news is that almost any intervention can be effective in eliminating or drastically reducing smoking behavior. The bad news is that these changes tend to be relatively short-lived; data from the vast majority of controlled smoking modification research have presented an all-too-familiar pattern of immediate and dramatic reduction in cigarette consumption by most subjects (exposed to nearly any treatment), followed by a relapse to or near pretreatment rates in the great majority of cases within a 12-month period (Bernstein, 1969; Hunt and Matarazzo, 1973; Hunt and Bespalec, 1974; Keutzer et al., 1968; Lichtenstein, 1971; McFall and Hammen, 1971; Schwartz, 1969). As shown in Figure 10.1, only around 20–30% of subjects who were abstinent at post-treatment are likely to be nonsmokers a year later.

Thus, in considering the results of more recent controlled experiments in smoking modification, it will be important not only to focus upon the immediate effects of various treatments and their status relative to control conditions, but also upon their long-term consequences and success rates in relation to the "standard" pictured in Figure 10.1.

CRUCIAL PROBLEMS IN SMOKING MODIFICATION RESEARCH

In the past, accumulation of unambiguously interpretable data on smoking modi-

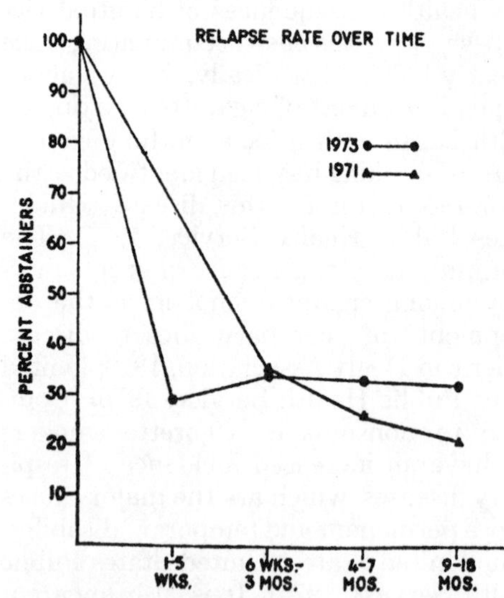

Figure 10.1. Relapse rates for subjects abstinent at treatment termination for studies appearing before 1971 and from 1971–1973. (Reproduced by permission from Hunt, W. A., and Bespalec, D. A. An evaluation of current methods of modifying smoking behavior. *J. Clin. Psychol.*, 1974, *30*, 431, © 1974 Clinical Psychology Publishing Company, Inc.)

fication has been hampered primarily by the use of relatively unsophisticated research methodology aimed at answering inappropriate research questions. Specific design problems have included omission of relevant control groups, confounding of independent variables, lack of baseline smoking data, failure to equate groups on important environmental, subject, or task variables, experimenter bias, and use of unreliable outcome data sources (Bernstein, 1969). The more subtle problem regarding the nature of investigators' research questions is represented in Figure 10.1 and has been summarized as follows:

> The basic problem in the modification of smoking behavior revolves about long-term maintenance of nonsmoking, not about production of immediate, short-term behavior change.... Efforts should be focussed upon the distillation of techniques which, regardless of their specificity ... will reliably bring about initial behavior change. At the same time, attention must be directed to development of procedures designed to maintain nonsmoking on a long-term basis. Ideally, such procedures would be a natural outgrowth of or actually incorporated in the short-term behavior change techniques. (Bernstein, 1969, pp. 435–436).*

Similar conclusions have also been reported elsewhere by reviewers who, in addition to recognizing the need for "tighter" designs and long-term treatment effectiveness, have called for investigation and use of individualized and multicomponent initial abstinence programs administered in the context of efforts to develop adaptive alternatives to smoking (Bernstein, 1974; Bernstein and McAlister, 1976; Epstein and McCoy, 1975; Hunt and Matarazzo, 1973; Lichtenstein and Danaher, 1976; Mausner, 1971; Schwartz, 1969). In the sections to follow we shall examine the degree to which these recommendations have been implemented.

CLINICS

Beginning with the pioneering work of Ejrup (1963, 1964), the smoking cessation clinic has become a popular means through which smoking reduction is attempted. Specific treatment techniques, number and length of meetings, and other factors vary considerably across clinics, but most of them involve groups of smokers coming together to receive help (and help each other) in quitting from clinic organizers who usually provide some combination of health information, encouragement, group therapy, moral support, social pressure, and suggestions for resisting temptation to smoke (Cruikshank, 1963; Delarue, 1973; Hoffstaedt, 1964; Kanzler, Jaffe, and Zeidenberg, 1976; Kanzler, Zeidenberg, and Jaffe, 1976; Lawton, 1967; Mausner, 1966; McFarland, 1965; Ross, 1967; Schlegel and Kunetsky, 1977; Schwartz and Dubitzky, 1967; Shewchuk, 1976; Shewchuk, Dubren, Burton, et al., 1977; West, Graham, Swanson, et al., 1977).

The effects of the information/encouragement type of clinics have not generally been evaluated in the context of controlled research (Bernstein, 1969; Keutzer, et al., 1968), but evidence from studies where at least some controls were employed (Delarue, 1973; Guilford, 1966, 1972; Jenks, Schwartz, and Dubitzky, 1969; Lawton, 1967; Mausner, 1966; Schwartz and Dubitzky, 1967; Thompson and Wilson, 1966; Weir, Dubitzky, and Schwartz, 1969) generally suggests that smoking reduction tends to be temporary and/or not clearly different from that accomplished through subjects' unaided efforts (Note 1). Thus, Bernstein's (1969, p. 431) conclusion that, except for the small proportion (usually about 20%) of subjects whose smoking behavior is eliminated over at least a 1-year period, "most clinics represent a great deal of wasted time and effort" still appears valid. In fact, subsequent research (Bernstein, 1970; Lichtenstein, Harris, Birchler, et al., 1973; McFall and Hammen, 1971; Sipich, Russell, and Tobias, 1974) has confirmed the fact that deliberate and isolated use of the nonspecific treatment factors contained in clinic settings (e.g., suggestion, positive expectations, placebo effects) produce post-treatment results comparable to those of clinics which carefully program specific content.

This is not to say, of course, that the clinic format is useless; the social context it

* Reprinted by permission from Berstein, D. A. Modification of smoking behavior: An evaluative review. *Psychol. Bull.*, 1969, *71*, 418–440. Copyright 1969 by the American Psychological Association.

can provide for efforts at smoking abstinence may prove to be a valuable adjunct to more specifically effective treatment procedures. In light of the negative outcome evidence accumulated to date, however, research which seeks to explore potentially important process variables such as intersubject contact (Janis and Hoffman, 1971) or therapist style (Weir et al., 1969) appears premature (Bernstein, 1969; Lichtenstein, 1971).

DRUGS

Because of the role thought to be played by nicotine in the maintenance of cigarette smoking (Jarvik, 1970, 1973; Russell, 1974) a variety of antismoking drugs have been prescribed for would-be quitters which either mimic the effects of nicotine (to reduce the smoker's craving) or mitigate the physical and psychological consequences of smoking cessation. The most widely tested nicotinomimetic agent, lobeline sulfate, has been administered in compounds such as Bantron either alone or in combination with tranquilizers, stimulants, amphetamines, and anticholinergics. Research on the effects of these agents has shown them to be relatively weak, temporary, and primarily a function of placebo and other nonspecific effects associated with receiving medication rather than of specific drug characteristics (Bernstein, 1969; Davison and Rosen, 1972; Schwartz, 1969).

No new evidence is available which challenges this conclusion with respect to nicotinomimetics or the other withdrawal medications mentioned above, but it should be noted that the possibility of using nicotine itself as an aid to smoking cessation is currently being investigated. Based upon evidence that oral or intravenous administration of nicotine tends to reduce subsequent cigarette consumption (Lucchesi, Schuster, and Emley, 1967; Jarvik, Glick, and Nakamura, 1970), a peppermint-flavored nicotine-bearing chewing gum has been developed (Ferno, Lichtneckert, and Lundgren, 1973) which provides release of nicotine for periods ranging from 15 to 30 minutes (total dose: about 4 mg). The idea, of course, is to provide nicotine while eliminating the "tar," carbon monoxide, and other harmful consequences associated with inhalation of tobacco smoke.

Evaluations of this approach in the context of abstinence attempts are just beginning to appear. In a preliminary double-blind trial during which smokers were asked to substitute nicotine or placebo gum for cigarettes "as much as possible" (Brantmark, Ohlin, and Westling, 1973), use of the nicotine-bearing gum was associated with greater reported reductions in smoking, especially among heavier (i.e., 20/day) smokers. Schneider, Popek, Jarvik, et al. (1977) described similar benefits in three cases. However, Russell, Wilson, Feyerabend, et al. (1976) did not find a 2 mg nicotine chewing gum to be more effective than a placebo gum in producing abstinence in a double-blind crossover trial. It would be premature to draw conclusions regarding the ultimate usefulness, safety (Hartelius and Tribbling, 1976), or long-term effects (Westling, 1976) of nicotine in smoking deterrence. However, to the extent that smoking is maintained by the reinforcing effects of nicotine, continued attention to the problems of (a) providing nicotine in relatively safe, palatable form, (b) maximizing the efficiency with which it is metabolized (Kozlowski, 1974), and/or (c) blocking its reinforcing properties (Schuster, 1970) may result in the development of vital adjuncts to treatment techniques which focus upon altering the nonpharmacologically based components of smoking behavior.

An alcoholic extract of oats (*Avena sativa*) has been employed as a smoking deterrent in a multiple case study design without notable success (Bye, Fowle, Letley, et al., 1974).

HYPNOSIS

For at least the last 30 years, hypnotic techniques have been used as part of antismoking interventions (Johnston and Donoghue, 1971), either to provide various kinds of direct suggestions or to uncover personality conflicts presumed to cause smoking behavior (Bryan, 1964). Hypnotic suggestions are used mainly to give cigarettes an aversive taste or smell, to associate smoking with aversive events, to associate positive events with nonsmoking and, in general, to increase subjects' motivation for gradual smoking reduction, self-monitoring, stimulus control, response chain disruption, and a variety of other learning-oriented self-control techniques. Several studies employing hypnotic procedures for smoking cessation have been reported recently (Barkley, Hastings, and Jackson, 1977; Hall and Crasilneck, 1970; Kline, 1970; Nuland and Field, 1970; Orr, 1970; Pederson, Scrimgeour, and Lefcoe, 1975; Perry and Mullen, 1975; Spiegel, 1970; Watkins, 1976), but do not significantly alter the conclusions reached by earlier reviews (Bernstein, 1969; Johnston and Donoghue, 1971). There are reports of impressive treatment success (Crasilneck and Hall, 1975; Hall and Crasilneck, 1970; Kline, 1970; Nuland and Field, 1970), but these tend to be uncontrolled multiple case reports subject to a number of methodological deficiencies, such as subject selection bias and failure to report on the typically large number of subjects lost to follow-up. Even if cause-effect data on hypnosis were available, the complexity of the treatment package in which it is usually embedded would make it difficult to separate the role of hypnosis per se from that of unsystematically applied social-learning techniques. At present, it must be concluded that, alone or as an adjunct to other approaches, hypnosis has not been demonstrated to be effective in the modification of smoking behavior.

SENSORY DEPRIVATION

Attempts to alter smoking through various types of persuasive communications (usually related to health hazards) have generally tended to influence subjects' verbal behavior more than their status as smokers (Gallup, 1974; Janis and Mann, 1965; Leventhal, 1968; Lichtenstein, Keutzer and Himes, 1969; Mann and Janis, 1968; Platt, Krassen, and Mausner, 1969; Streltzer and Koch, 1968), but evidence that exposure to sensory deprivation increases the degree to which persons are susceptible to such communications (Suedfeld, 1969) has revived some interest in the persuasion approach. The results of several recent experiments (Suedfeld, 1973; Suedfeld and Best, 1977; Suedfeld and Ikard, 1973, 1974; Suedfeld, Landon, Pargament, et al., 1972) in which a variety of antismoking and pro-nonsmoking messages were presented during 24 hours of sensory deprivation indicated that reports of substantial reductions in cigarette smoking over periods as long as 2 years have occurred (even for older, heavier smokers). However, abstinence rates, although initially as high as 100%, appear to be comparable in the long run to those attainable through other interventions, and it is of interest that inclusion of smoking-relevant messages during deprivation does not appear to be critical to treatment effectiveness. This raises the question of what is producing the changes. Obviously, the sensory deprivation approach must be evaluated against credible placebo "treatments," subjects' unaided efforts, and other interventions before conclusions about the magnitude or mechanism of its effects can be drawn, but the technique does seem to provide a powerful, nonaversive means of producing initial behavior change and thus warrants further investigation aimed at its refinement and/or incorporation into broader treatment packages.

Social-Learning Approaches

While acknowledging the generally discouraging results of any attempts to permanently modify smoking behavior, some reviewers concluded that learning theory approaches to the problem seem to be the most promising (Bernstein, 1969; Keutzer et al., 1968; Lichtenstein and Keutzer, 1971). This view was not based upon data demonstrating the superiority of social-learning techniques (such data did not exist), but upon the belief that research procedures which emphasize operational definitions and well controlled hypothesis testing experimentation on laboratory-based behavior modification techniques would ultimately provide valuable practical and theoretical knowledge about smoking, just as it has with respect to other human behaviors (Bandura, 1969; Leitenberg, 1976; Rimm and Masters, 1974). Social-learning approaches to the problem have focused either upon (a) reducing the probability of smoking behavior or (b) increasing the probability of alternative (sometimes incompatible) nonsmoking responses. Until about 1970, efforts in the former category (i.e., systematic desensitization, stimulus control, punishment, and aversive conditioning) almost totally overshadowed those in the latter (i.e., contingency contracting, positive reinforcement, nonsmoking skill training) and reports of combined approaches were relatively rare. The current status of each of the major social-learning techniques is considered below.

SELF-MONITORING

Self-monitoring of number of cigarettes smoked and, often, recording information about the situation in which smoking occurs is part of almost every social learning treatment program. Self-monitoring has usually been considered an assessment technique which is not in itself sufficient to produce behavior change. However, there have been suggestions from studies on smokers not necessarily trying to change their smoking rates that monitoring cigarette consumption may produce at least short-term reduction under some conditions (Karoly and Doyle, 1975; Leventhal and Avis, 1976; McFall, 1970). Most smoking modification studies also find that subjects' self-monitored baseline consumption rates are somewhat lower than their initial estimates of smoking frequency.

Few investigations of the treatment potential of self-monitoring have appeared in the smoking literature. Euler (1973) found self-monitoring to produce more smoking reduction than nonmonitoring or no treatment groups, but the changes were not remarkable. Two other studies evaluated positive monitoring (recording resisted urges to smoke) vs. negative monitoring (recording capitulation to smoking urges). Both reported temporary reductions in smoking but failed to demonstrate differences between conditions (McFall and Hammen, 1971; Kantorowitz, Walters, and Pezdek, 1977). A case study on the timing of self-monitoring found recording prior to smoking each cigarette to be more effective in reducing smoking than monitoring occurring after smoking (Rozensky, 1974).

SYSTEMATIC DESENSITIZATION AND RELAXATION

In the hope of either reducing stress which causes smoking and/or eliminating the stress attendant upon quitting, several investigators have employed systematic desensitization (Paul and Bernstein, 1973; Wolpe, 1958, 1969) in smoking modification interventions. Multiple case demonstrations (Kraft and Al-Issa, 1967; Morganstern and Ratliff, 1969) suggested the usefulness of the procedure in dealing with smoking behavior, but five controlled experiments (Engeln, 1969; Koenig and Masters, 1965; Levenberg and Wagner, 1976; Pyke, Agnew, and Kopperud, 1966; Wagner and Bragg, 1970) have failed to support its effectiveness (Note 2).

Three reports have appeared in which progressive relaxation was used as a coping procedure (Goldfried and Trier, 1974) to counteract urges to smoke. Two controlled studies (Sutherland, Amit, Golden, et al., 1975; Stern, Sherman, Greenberg, et al., 1975) and a multiple case report (Ravensborg, 1976) have found the technique to offer some promise, but the absolute level of results has not been impressive.

Relaxation associated with transcendental meditation has resulted in multiple case reports of long-term reductions in smoking (Benson, Greenwood, and Klemchuk, 1975), but a more controlled investigation (Ottens, 1975) failed to establish the superiority of transcendental meditation over less exotic alternatives.

PUNISHMENT AND AVERSIVE CONDITIONING (NOTE 3)

The most common social-learning-based approach to reducing the probability of smoking behavior has been to use aversive stimuli such as electric shock, noise, warm smoky air, or the consequences of rapid smoking, either following or in association with actual or imagined smoking.

Reviews of the initial and long-term effectiveness of the array of aversive control procedures described through 1970 (Bernstein, 1969; Keutzer et al., 1968; Lichtenstein and Keutzer, 1971) revealed a mixed picture. Although some success was reported, aversive control applied in a laboratory or in the natural environment appeared for the most part to be only temporarily helpful and not clearly superior to nonaversive alternatives. Rather than abandoning the approach, however, researchers have been actively engaged in refining aversive techniques and incorporating them into more elaborate interventions. Consideration of research on combined approaches will be delayed for the moment; let us first examine recent work on various aversive control procedures as applied to smoking in relative isolation.

Electrical Aversion. In spite of case reports of long-term success (Roy and Swillinger, 1971; Russell, 1970), no evidence for the permanent or differential effectiveness of electric shock as contingent punishment for smoking behavior (in the laboratory or in the natural environment) was found in early controlled experiments (Andrews, 1970; Best and Steffy, 1971; Ober, 1968; Powell and Azrin, 1968; Whitman, 1969).

Recent studies on electrical aversion have produced mixed results. Gendreau and Dodwell (1968) and Levine (1974) found contingent shock superior to control conditions on a short-term basis, but resulting in only minimal treatment effects (no follow-up data were reported). More recently, a very comprehensive study by Russell, Armstrong, and Patel (1976) failed to find contingent shock more effective than a variety of component control groups. However, a multiple baseline component analysis (Dericco, Brigham, and Garlington, 1977) found a shock condition to be superior to comparison treatments and effective in producing both short and longer term (6 month) behavior change. The authors suggested that the discrepancy between their findings and those of other investigators may be attributable to the longer program and more intense shock employed in their study. In a multiple case study, Russell (1976) found that the use of electrical aversion with highly motivated chest patients resulted in a 1-year abstinence rate of 43% overall and 66% for those completing treatment. A multiple case evaluation of a portable shock apparatus (Pope and Mount, 1975) produced 1-year reports of abstinence by nearly 70% of subjects completing all aspects of treatment.

The generally unfavorable results of experimental research in this area have been attributed to the fact that "standard" punishment procedures for smoking deal with overt responses (e.g., lighting and inhaling a cigarette) but not with the covert (i.e., cognitive) behaviors which precede, accompany, and follow those responses (Premack, 1970). Accordingly, some investigators have attempted to use electric shock to punish both the motoric and cognitive components of smoking, using varying techniques and achieving variable results. Steffy, Meichenbaum, and Best (1970) found that shocking verbalizations about smoking, accompanied or unaccompanied by actual smoking behavior, were no more effective than group discussion and eventually led to relapse. Somewhat better results occurred for subjects shocked for *thinking* about smoking while actually doing so. The absolute level of results was not impressive and the lack of long term follow-up makes these data difficult to interpret, however. Berecz (1972) had smokers self-administer shocks contingent upon imagined smoking. While this procedure was more effective than shock for actual smoking or placebo "treatment" for males classified as heavy smokers (17 cigarettes/day), no data on frequency of abstinence or long-term follow-up were presented and no between-group effects were found for females or moderately smoking males. More recently, Berecz (1976) reported a potentially valuable procedure in which smokers shocked themselves while imagining having an *urge* to smoke, thus punishing early components of the total cognitive-motoric smoking response chain. Although data on only three subjects dealt with in this way are presented, all of them were apparently abstinent 2 years after treatment (three others, shocked for imagining smoking behavior itself, initially abstained but ultimately resumed smoking). Interestingly, this technique proved ineffective with three female smokers. Controlled evaluative research on this approach is clearly warranted and must, of course, precede any conclusions about its usefulness.

Taste Aversion. Several attempts have been made to reduce smoking by associating it with strong, unpleasant tastes. The aversive stimuli have been produced as part of laboratory conditioning paradigms (Marston and McFall, 1971; Whitman, 1972) or in the natural environment through the use of special chewing gum which makes tobacco smoke taste bad (Rosenberg, 1977). None of these procedures has produced extraordinary effects on smoking. A lozenge containing a substance which creates a garlic odor and aversive taste in combination with smoking was reported to have produced an 82% abstinence rate at 4-year follow-up in a multiple case report (Seltzer, 1975), but no experimental evaluations of the material are available as yet.

COVERT AVERSION. Cognitive processes are employed to provide both smoking stimuli *and* aversive concomitants or consequences when covert sensitization (Cautela, 1967) is applied to smoking. The would-be quitter vividly imagines extreme nausea or other unpleasant stimulation while visualizing various components of smoking behavior and usually, pleasant affect accompanying imagined termination of smoking (Cautela, 1970). Again, case studies have shown promising results (Cautela, 1970; Tooley and Pratt, 1967), but evaluative data on the procedure generated by experimental studies employing varying degrees of control (Gerson and Lanyon, 1972; Lawson and May, 1970; Sachs, Bean, and Morrow, 1970; Sipich et al., 1974; Wagner and Bragg, 1970; Wisocki and Rooney, 1974) fail to support its long-term effectiveness or clear superiority to placebo procedures or subjects' unaided efforts. Although a study by Goguen (1974) indicated that relapse following covert sensitization may be retarded by additional treatment, his design could not provide evidence that factors specific to the sensitization procedure were responsible for the effect.

CIGARETTE SMOKE. The principles of extinction, negative practice, and aversive conditioning are combined in another "family" of social-learning treatments for smoking which employ stimuli from cigarettes themselves as the aversive component. These procedures are based upon two assumptions: (a) that the reinforcing aspects of almost any stimulus are reduced (and may actually become aversive) if that stimulus is presented at sufficiently elevated frequency and/or intensity and (b) that aversion based upon stimuli intrinsic to the to-be-eliminated response (smoking) is more salient and generalized than that stemming from artificial sources such as electricity (Lublin, 1969; Wilson and Davison, 1969). Three main versions of this approach have appeared: satiation (i.e., doubling or tripling smoking rate) prior to abstinence and punishment/aversive conditioning of smoking through either experimenter-controlled warm, smoky air or rapid smoking.

Early research on the satiation technique by Resnick (1968a,b) produced promising short-term results (63% abstinent after 4 months) which, although not entirely unambiguous (Lichtenstein and Keutzer, 1971; Marston and McFall, 1971) stimulated several additional evaluative experiments. Resnick's (1968b) short-term data were replicated in one instance (Marrone, Merksamer, and Salzberg, 1970), but subsequent research on the technique failed to show long-term effects or differential efficacy relative to placebo, unaided efforts, or other temporarily effective treatments (Claiborn, Lewis, and Humble, 1972; Lando, 1975b; Lando and Davison, 1975; Marston and McFall, 1971; Sushinsky, 1972). More recently, Best and Steffy (1975) failed to show a significant overall treatment effect for satiation, but did find the procedure relatively useful (44% abstinent at 4-month follow-up) for smokers characterized by internal locus of control (Rotter, 1966). Best, Owen, and Trentadue (1977) reported moderately impressive long-term results (40% abstinent at 6-month follow-up), but their satiation procedure was supplemented by other self-control procedures.

When first introduced, the use of artificially produced, warm, smoky air in contingent punishment and/or aversive conditioning of smoking was not found to produce long-term abstinence (Franks, Fried, and Ashem, 1966; Grimaldi and Lichtenstein, 1969; Wilde, 1964, 1965). Results were improved somewhat in an experiment where warm, smoky air was used in association with rapid smoking (inhaling every 6 seconds while focusing on the negative sensations produced) during laboratory treatment sessions (Lublin and Josyln, 1968), but the 12-month abstinence figure (19%) for subjects receiving this treatment was not much better than that found in studies represented in Figure 10.1. Nevertheless, the potential value of punishment/aversive conditioning (via warm, smoky air) of rapid as opposed to normal smoking has been actively explored in recent years.

Two experiments have shown that after about seven sessions of this combination of techniques almost all treated subjects report total abstinence and that about 60% of them continue such reports after 6 months (Lichtenstein et al., 1973; Schmahl, Lichtenstein, and Harris, 1972).

The research of Lichtenstein and his colleagues has also revealed that combination of warm, smoky air and rapid smoking is no more effective initially than a placebo or either component alone (after 6 months, however, all are superior to placebo "treatment"). Thus, although increased sophistication in the technical and procedural details of punishment via warm, smoky air may have improved its effectiveness relative to early trials (Wilde, 1964), Lichtenstein et al. (1973) recommended abandonment of inconvenient smoke-blowing apparatus and concentration upon investigating the potential of rapid smoking instead.

Recent studies conducted in Lichtenstein's laboratory replicated earlier promising findings regarding the effectiveness of rapid smoking, but also indicated that the technique is much more complex than it initially appeared. Factors such as the emphasis placed on the therapist-client relationship (Harris and Lichtenstein, 1974) and the criteria for treatment termination (Weinrobe and Lichtenstein, 1975) have been found to affect outcome. A report on the long-term results of a number of rapid smoking studies conducted by Lichtenstein and associates revealed that 36–47% of subjects contacted were abstinent 2–6 years after treatment (Lichtenstein and Penner, 1977).

The many recent investigations of rapid smoking (Best, 1975; Curtis, Simpson, and Cole, 1976; Danaher, 1977; Dawley and Sardenga, 1976; Glasgow, 1977; Kopel, 1974; Lando, 1975b, 1976a,b; Levenberg and Wagner, 1976; Pechacek, 1977; Relinger, Bornstein, Bugge, et al., 1977; Satterfield, 1977; Sutherland et al., 1975) have been reviewed by Danaher (1977). The results (averaging around 30% abstinent at 6 months) have been less impressive than those reported in earlier investigations, possibly because almost all of the recent studies employed a standardized treatment involving a fixed number of sessions and/or a lack of emphasis on client-therapist relationship factors.

Because of the stressful nature of the rapid smoking procedure, there has been a good deal of recent work on its physiological effects (Danaher, Lichtenstein, and Sullivan, 1976; Dawley, Ellithorpe, and Tretola, 1976; Dawley and Dillenkoffer, 1975; Horan, Hackett, Nicholas, et al., 1977; Horan, Linberg, and Hackett, 1977; Miller, Schilling, Logan, et al., 1977). These studies demonstrate that rapid smoking does stress the cardiovascular system, producing significant increases in heart rate, blood pressure, and carboxyhemoglobin levels. Although the magnitude of such changes does not appear to be as large as some have feared, a review of these studies (Lichtenstein and Glasgow, 1977) recommended that procedural safeguards (excluding high risk subjects, requiring physician approval for participation, and limiting the duration of exposure) be employed when rapid smoking is used.

In summary, it appears that rapid smoking, when employed with proper safeguards and combined with strong therapist support and positive expectations (and when continued at least until subjects are abstinent) is one of the more powerful treatment techniques available. In the absence of these features, it is not clearly superior to other approaches. As with electrical aversion (Russell et al., 1976) conditioning explanations of the treatment's effectiveness appear inadequate.

STIMULUS CONTROL

Another social-learning approach to reduction of the probability of smoking behavior is represented by stimulus-control tactics. They are based on the assumption that smoking is associated with (and ultimately prompted by) environmental cues present when it occurs. Further, it is thought that since smoking usually takes place under a wide variety of circumstances, the number and extensiveness of these controlling cues or discriminative stimuli contribute to the intransigence of the habit. Treatment involves gradual elimination of smoking through programmed narrowing of the range of stimuli which are discriminative for it. Theoretically, total abstinence is easier once smoking occurs in only a few well-defined situations instead of throughout the smoker's environment. Stimulus-control programs vary considerably with respect to how clearly they specify which environmental stimuli are to be detached from smoking. Some involve elimination of smoking from increasing numbers of specific situations while others arrange only for nonsmoking during certain temporal periods.

Despite reports of success with individual cases (Greenberg and Altman, 1976; Nolan, 1968; Roberts, 1969) it does not appear that any version of the stimulus-control approach produces immediate or long-term effects which are superior to subjects' own efforts or the use of other active or placebo treatments (Azrin and Powell, 1968; Bakewell, 1972; Bernard and Efran, 1972; Claiborn et al., 1972; Flaxman, 1978; Gutman and Marston, 1967; Levinson, Shapiro, Schwartz, et al., 1971; Marston and McFall, 1971; Sachs et al., 1970; Shapiro, Tursky, Schwartz, et al., 1971; Upper and Meredith, 1970). Fairly high subject attrition rates appear to be common.

For most subjects, stimulus-control interventions lead to clear reductions in smoking which appear to stabilize at around 10–12 cigarettes per day and after which further reductions become unlikely. Although it has been suggested that this "floor" effect is due to the appearance of "withdrawal symptoms" which act to prevent further nicotine deprivation (Levinson et al., 1971), the ease with which subjects exposed to abrupt quitting treatments are able to abstain completely favors an alternative interpretation, namely that gradual reduction in smoking rate increases the reinforcement value of each cigarette and makes those which remain as the program progresses harder and harder to relinquish (Flaxman, 1978; Mausner, 1971; Shiffman and Jarvik, 1976).

REINFORCEMENT OF NONSMOKING

We shall now consider a group of social learning techniques which seek to eliminate smoking "indirectly" by strengthening other behaviors not involving or perhaps incompatible with it. These positive reinforcement techniques usually employ contingency contracting, coverant control, or both.

In 1965, Homme suggested that smoking could be reduced by increasing the frequency of coverants ("covert operants," or thoughts) incompatible with it (e.g., "smoking causes cancer"). To do this, he advocated use of all available reinforcers, defined as any behavior more probable than the one to be reinforced (Premack, 1970). The procedure was successfully employed in combination with positive reinforcement and aversive conditioning at the case study level (Tooley and Pratt, 1967), but three subsequent experiments involving coverant control showed it to be comparable to other (temporarily) successful treatments (Keutzer, 1968; Lawson and May, 1970; Rutner, 1967). A more recent evaluation of several versions of coverant control (Danaher and Lichtenstein, 1974) resulted in similar conclusions.

Positive social reinforcement of nonsmoking behavior has frequently been employed as part of antismoking programs (Bernstein, 1969; Lichtenstein and Keutzer, 1971; Schmahl et al., 1972), but, because of confounding with other techniques, its effects are difficult to evaluate unambiguously. Early reviewers found that contingency contracting involving administration of social and/or monetary rewards produced generally unimpressive results (Bernstein, 1969; Lichtenstein and Keutzer, 1971), but later research has shown that the approach can be effective in initiating changes in smoking behavior (Axelrod, Hall, Weis, et al., 1974; Lando, 1976a; Tighe and Elliot, 1968; Winett, 1973) and thus may be useful as a component in more elaborate treatments.

CONTINUED CONTACT AFTER TREATMENT

Reviewers of the smoking modification literature have been almost unanimous in their call for increased attention to the maintenance of nonsmoking behavior (Bernstein, 1969; Bernstein and McAlister, 1976; Hunt and Matarazzo, 1973; Lichtenstein and Danaher, 1976). One obvious approach to the problem is to provide continued therapist contact following "official" treatment termination. While there have been impressive reports of success from multicomponent treatments which included (but did not assess the incremental effects of) maintenance programs (Chapman, Smith, and Layden, 1971; Lando, 1977; Morrow, Sachs, Gmeinder et al., 1973; Pomerleau and Ciccone, 1974; Tongas, Patterson, and Goodkind, 1976; Tooley and Pratt, 1967), the overwhelming majority of controlled studies in this area have produced negative results. Studies evaluating the contribution of booster sessions (Kopel, 1974; Relinger et al., 1977), telephone contacts with therapists (Bernstein, 1970; Danaher, 1977; Relinger et al., 1977; Schmahl et al., 1972), and follow-up meetings incorporating contingency contracting procedures (Lando, 1976a; Lamb, in press) have all failed to increase the long-term effectiveness of programs. The only positive findings to date have been a case study (Lewittes and Israel, 1975), a report of mixed success (St. Pierre and Lawrence, 1975), and an interesting recorded phone message service to reinforce nonsmoking (Dubren, 1977b) which was found to improve short-term (1-month) results.

MULTICOMPONENT APPROACHES

The strong though mostly temporary impact of social learning interventions on smoking prompted literature reviewers to recommend the use of multicomponent treatment packages designed to both suppress smoking behavior and reinforce more adaptive alternatives (Bernstein, 1969; Hunt and Matarazzo, 1973; Schwartz, 1969). This multicomponent approach serves as the basis for most of the highly successful social learning programs aimed at other target problems (Bandura, 1969; Leitenberg, 1976; Rimm and Masters, 1974) and researchers have recently begun to apply it in the smoking area. In the past 5 years, more than 20 multicomponent studies have appeared. They usually combine aversive control procedures (e.g., rapid smoking; smoking-contingent electric shock or warm, smoky air) with the subjects' own (usually graduated) quitting efforts aided by self-control and nonsmoking skill training tactics such as stimulus control, coverant control, social and material reinforcement of nonsmoking, lengthening of response chains, making smoking less appealing and more effortful, programming and practicing nonsmoking behaviors, responses to tempting situations, and the like.

Results from multiple case reports (Chapman et al., 1971; Morrow et al., 1973; Tooley and Pratt, 1967), evaluations of multicomponent programs against no treatment (Pomerleau and Ciccone, 1974), and investigations of variations in the delivery of multicomponent programs (Best, Bass, and Owen, 1977) have produced impressive results (55–65% of subjects abstinent at 1-year follow-up, Note 4), but more controlled evaluations of the incremental effects of combined programs have been less encouraging.

These studies have generally found that multicomponent programs have not proven superior to individual treatment components or comparison groups at follow-up (Best, 1975; Best et al., 1977; Danaher, 1977; Lando, 1976a; Mantek and Erben, 1974), produced only minimal long-term treatment effects (Brockway, Kleinmann, Edleson, et al., in press; Sutherland et al., 1975), or both (Conway, 1977; Glasgow, 1977; Harris and Rothberg, 1972; Marston and McFall, 1971; Miller and Gimpl, 1971; Ober, 1968; Pechacek, 1977; Satterfield, 1977). Investigations by Flaxman (1978) and St. Pierre and Lawrence (1975) revealed mixed results. There have been a few notable exceptions to this trend, however (Delahunt and Curran, 1976; Lando, 1977; Tongas et al., 1976). These controlled studies have reported from 56–77% of subjects abstinent at 6 months and further refinement, evaluation, and replication of such programs is certainly warranted.

Discussion

After describing the shortcomings of smoking research published through 1968, Bernstein (1969, p. 436) expressed the hope that " . . . Future investigators will recognize the necessity of restructuring the problem and, in addition, will appreciate and attempt to fulfill the methodological requirements which are prerequisites for obtaining unambiguously interpretable answers to the questions they pose." Although the years since that statement was written have not seen the development of reliable, valid, and permanently effective methods for helping all smokers to abstain, some progress has been made in terms of treatment effects, research methodology, and the ways in which the problem is conceptualized. This progress justifies a measure of cautious optimism about the future of the field and, because the social-learning approach has resulted in the clearest increments in technical, methodological, and conceptual sophistication, about the fruitfulness of applying that model to the modification of smoking behavior. The value of a behavioral or social-learning approach had been predicted in previous reviews (Bernstein, 1969; Keutzer et al., 1968; Lichtenstein and Keutzer, 1971) and now seems even more firmly established.

METHODOLOGICAL CONSIDERATIONS

Particularly in recent years, social-learning-oriented experimenters have set methodological standards in smoking research by frequently incorporating in their designs vital procedures and controls such as careful collection of baseline smoking data, factorial or component analysis of treatment packages, use of placebo and unaided quitting groups as relevant baselines against which to assess active treatments, recruitment of informants to supplement subjects' verbal or written records of smoking behavior, collection of monetary deposits to ensure full subject participation during treatment and follow-up periods, factorial combinations of treatments and experimenters, and equation of contact time across treatment groups.

Further methodological sophistication has been brought about recently by the collection of objective physiological measures of smoking to supplement subjects' self-reports. The most commonly used procedures involve analysis of expired breath samples for carbon monoxide content (Lando, 1975a; Kopel, 1975; Vogt, Selvin, Widdowson, et al., 1977) and measurement of thiocyanate levels in the blood (Butts, Kuehneman, and Widdowson, 1974; Brockway, 1978; Vogt, et al., 1977). Carbon monoxide data provide estimates of carboxyhemoglobin levels in the blood. Chemical tests for nicotine and thiocyanate in saliva and urine, and for cotinine (a metabolite of nicotine) in blood have also been developed (Densen, Davidow, Bass, et al., 1967; Gritz and Jarvik, 1973; Horning, Horning, Carroll, et al., 1973; Russell and Feyerabend, 1975; Zeidenberg, Jaffe, Kanzler, et al., 1977) but have not yet been utilized extensively in smoking modification research. Each of these techniques is time limited (Note 5) and can be influenced by variables other than number of cigarettes smoked (e.g., ambient carbon monoxide or cigarette smoke from others and ingestion of food containing cyanide), but they provide long-needed objective indices of smoking behavior which can be compared to self-reports.

Recent work with these objective smoking measures has cast some doubt upon the validity of self-monitoring. Early reports indicate that describing objective measurement procedures to subjects before assessment (Evans, Hansen, and Mittelmark, 1977) and confronting subjects claiming abstinence with discrepant chemical findings (Brockway et al., in press; Ohlin, Lundh, and Westling, 1976) increases the accuracy of self-reported smoking rates.

These improvements have greatly facilitated evaluation of the effectiveness or, more commonly, the ineffectiveness of various smoking interventions. However, because all of the features of an adequately designed experiment do not always appear together in every study reported, problems in interpreting the magnitude and/or significance of post-treatment behavior changes described by social-learning (and other) researchers still remain.

The most important design deficiency involves omission of attention-placebo and/or unaided quitting groups and though, as just noted, this error is becoming much less common than it was 10 years ago, the conditions involved are so crucial to the meaningfulness of any experiment focussed on outcome that their inclusion must become a matter of routine. Further, it is important to employ placebo "treatments" whose credibility is sufficiently high to support their usefulness; obviously ineffective or ludicrous tactics will not provide the desired baseline. This issue has been discussed elsewhere with respect to outcome evaluation of anxiety reduction interventions (Bernstein and Paul, 1971; Borkovec and Nau, 1972; Osarchuk and Goldfried, 1975), and the concerns expressed there would seem to apply to smoking research as well.

Another important, although still often neglected design feature is collection of long-term (i.e., at least 1 year) post-treatment follow-up data. Although, as shown in Figure 10.1, most of those quitters who relapse tend to do so within 3 months of treatment termination, this does not mean that no additional subjects will return to smoking after 90 days and it certainly does not justify arbitrary restriction of follow-up periods in the context of experimental evaluations of intervention packages. In fact, it is precisely within the experimental context that extended follow-up data are most critical; once controlled research allows treatment effects to be mapped over a 1- or 2-year period, subsequent laboratory and clinical follow-up evaluations can be truncated with some degree of confidence. Until this is done, however, provision of less than 12 months post-treatment data seems ill-advised (Note 6).

TREATMENT EFFECTS AND CONCEPTS

In contrast to previous reviews, it is now possible to acknowledge the existence of two treatment packages which, through some combination of specific and nonspecific effects, appear to eliminate cigarette smoking reliably for the vast majority of subjects treated and which continue to foster abstinence rates (for periods up to 6 months) clearly superior to the previously available interventions represented in Figure 10.1. Both are complex: (a) rapid smoking within a positive social treatment context (Lichtenstein, Harris, Birchler, et al., 1973; Schmahl, Lichtenstein, and Harris, 1972) and (b) multicomponent interventions which more specifically program the teaching/reinforcement of nonsmoking behaviors along with smoking suppression tactics (Delahunt and Curran, 1976; Lando, 1977; Pomerleau and Pomerleau, 1977). In addition, sensory deprivation and contingency contracting procedures appear to produce effects which are nearly as strong, although not as durable.

Bandura (1969, 1971) has pointed out that psychological treatment procedures must address themselves to and be evaluated upon three separable dimensions: the induction of behavior change, the generalization of that change, and the maintenance of change over time. As noted earlier, however, smoking modification techniques have not typically paid much attention to the development of the behavioral alternatives to smoking which are required to assure robust, long-term effects. Instead, the primary emphasis has been upon attempts to develop smoking behavior *change* techniques whose initial effects (perhaps supplemented by "booster" treatments) are strong enough to last forever. The appearance of multicomponent interventions indicates, however, that this somewhat illogical situation is beginning to change; researchers are at last recognizing that, if they are to reach the goal of long-term maintenance of nonsmoking behavior, that point at which a person stops smoking must mark the beginning of a new intervention phase, not the onset of follow-up.

Of course, the technology for building nonsmoking skills in former smokers is still rather primitive and a great deal of work will need to be done in order to learn the dimensions of its most efficient form, the ways in which it can be individualized in light of a variety of relevant subject variables (e.g., age, sex, smoking history/topography/function), and how best to integrate it with initial change techniques. As these difficult tasks progress, nonsmoking maintenance programs may become as sophisticated as those now available to alter smoking behavior, and we shall cease to place subjects in the familiar bind where, while being helped in various ways to *not* smoke, they are left almost entirely on their own with respect to the development of alternatives for dealing with the multitude of life situations which serve as eliciting or as discriminative stimuli for smoking.

DIRECTIONS FOR FUTURE RESEARCH

The remarkable similarity observed among the results of diverse treatments for smoking cessation tends to mask the enormous amount of intersubject variability observed in almost all anti-smoking programs. This variability suggests the need for determining which treatments are effective for individuals who vary on relevant subject dimensions. A number of studies have searched for general predictors of treatment outcome (Dubitzky and Schwartz, 1968; Raw, 1976a,b; Pomerleau, Adkins, and Pertschuk, 1978; Schwartz and Dubitzky, 1969). While the results have not always been consistent, individuals who are male, have a shorter smoking history, smoke relatively few cigarettes per day, comply with therapeutic instructions, and do not rely on cigarettes to reduce tension tend to be more likely to succeed in quitting or remain nonsmokers once they have quit. There have been only a few attempts to match treatments to clients and most of this work has focused on subjects' locus of control (Rotter, 1966). This approach has produced some moderate success (Best, 1975; Best and Steffy, 1975) and at least two failures (Best and Steffy, 1971; Burton, 1977). Attempts to tailor treatments to "negative affect" or high anxious smokers have also produced mixed results (Krietler, Shahar, and Krietler, 1976; Pechacek, 1976). While it is difficult to evaluate the long range contributions of the tailoring approach, it would appear that careful exploration of objective and valid subject variables as possible guides to custom-designing smoking cessation programs is a worthwhile target for future research.

Another potential means of developing effective treatment programs is to survey individuals who have been successful at modifying their smoking behavior on their own to determine what methods they used. An early report in this area (Perri, Richards, and Schultheis, 1977) found that successful smoking reducers used a greater number of techniques more frequently and longer than did unsuccessful subjects. They were also more apt to employ self-reward and behavioral problem solving procedures.

The scope of the public health problems associated with cigarette smoking (United States Public Health Service, 1975) makes it important that researchers investigate ways of efficiently disseminating effective treatment programs when they are developed. Increased emphasis should be placed on evaluating self-help (Mantek and Erben, 1974; Pomerleau and Pomerleau, 1977) and media (Dubren, 1977a; McAlister, Meyer, and Maccoby, 1976; Pomerleau, Pomerleau, and Weinstein, 1976) presentations which are economical in terms of therapist and client time (Note 7). Cost-effectiveness in research is also relevant given the current stage of knowledge. Demonstration of the potential of a treatment via single case designs (Frederiksen, 1976; Epstein and McCoy, 1975) and controlled pilot work should precede large scale factorial outcome evaluations.

Finally, despite our best efforts to eliminate smoking behavior, it may be that a substantial segment of the smoking population is either unwilling or unable to stop smoking on a long-term basis. If this is indeed the case, the development of a technology for teaching smokers to control their intake such that health risks are reduced (Frederiksen and Peterson, 1976; Frederiksen, Miller, and Peterson, 1977) may become an important goal. Research in this area is just beginning (Frederiksen and Peterson, 1976; McGrath and Hall, 1975).

In summary, progress has been made in the modification of smoking behavior, but a multitude of problems still remain. Our brief outline of each of these dimensions was designed to describe the "state of the art" and to acknowledge the fact that, " ... the cycle of relatively meaningless, though self-perpetuating experimentation ... " (Bernstein, 1969, p. 435) has been cracked if not broken. Better research and new concepts make it possible to be more hopeful about the future of smoking modification than has been reasonable at any time in the past.

Notes

1. The general public may have reached this conclusion as well. A recent poll (Gallup, 1974) indicated that only 34% of smokers wishing to quit are interested in attending a clinic. The majority seem to prefer a "do-it-yourself" program (Schwartz and Dubitzky, 1968).
2. Desensitization was employed in an additional study (Gerson and Lanyon, 1972), but its effects as distinct from other treatment variables could not be determined.
3. In practice, these procedures usually tend to overlap (Bandura, 1969) such that punishment produces some aversive conditioning and vice versa. It is also important to note that, while aversive control techniques have often been applied simply as a means of suppressing smoking behavior (Powell and Azrin, 1968), they have also been combined with aversion relief (escape or avoidance conditioning) paradigms which provide negative reinforcement for alternative, nonsmoking behavior (Wilde, 1964).
4. These results are particularly impressive since, in most cases, the subjects were long-term, heavy (≥ 30/day) smokers.
5. For example, the half-life of serum thiocyanate is about 14 days, but carbon monoxide and serum cotinine measures deteriorate to half their initial level after only 4–30 hours, respectively, in the absence of smoking (Butts et al., 1974; Vogt et al., 1977; Zeidenberg et al., 1977).
6. This suggestion need not preclude early publication of data on the immediate and short-term effects of various treatment packages and components; rather, it simply highlights the importance of gath-

ering long-term data and reporting them in short supplementary notes. To date, these have been almost nonexistent (Lichtenstein and Penner, 1977; Mann and Janis, 1968; Wilde, 1965).

7. Prevention of smoking onset through mass audience appeals is also of utmost importance and promising new techniques in this vital area are now beginning to appear (Evans, Rozelle, Mittelmark, et al., in press).

References

American Heart Association. *Report of Inter-Society Commission for Heart Disease Resources,* 1970, Vol. XLII.

Andrews, D. A. *Aversive treatment procedures in the modification of smoking.* Unpublished doctoral dissertation, Queens University, Canada, 1970.

Axelrod, S., Hall, R. V., Weis, L., and Rohrer, S. Use of self-imposed contingencies to reduce the frequency of smoking behavior. In M. J. Mahoney and C. E. Thoresen (Eds.), *Self-control: Power to the person.* Monterey, Calif.: Brooks/Cole, 1974.

Azrin, N. H., and Powell, J. Behavioral engineering: The reduction of smoking behavior by a conditioning apparatus and procedure. *J. Appl. Behav. Anal.,* 1968, *1,* 193–200.

Bakewell, H. The relevance of goal setting in a smoking reduction program. Paper presented at the annual meeting of the Western Psychological Association, Portland, April, 1972.

Bandura, A. *Principles of behavior modification.* New York: Holt-Rinehart-Winston, 1969.

Bandura, A. Psychotherapy based upon modeling principles. In A. E. Bergin and S. L. Garfield (Eds.), *Handbook of psychotherapy and behavior change: An empirical analysis.* New York: Wiley, 1971.

Barkley, R. A., Hastings, J. E., and Jackson, T. L. The effects of rapid smoking and hypnosis in the treatment of smoking behavior. *Int. J. Clin. Exp. Hypn.,* 1977, *25,* 7–17.

Benson, H., Greenwood, M. M., and Klemchuk, H. The relaxation response: Psychophysiologic aspects and clinical applications. *Int. J. Psychiatry Med.,* 1975, *6,* 87–98.

Berecz, J. Modification of smoking behavior through self-administered punishment of imagined behavior: A new approach to aversive therapy. *J. Consult. Clin. Psychol.,* 1972, *38,* 244–250.

Berecz, J. Treatment of smoking with cognitive conditioning therapy: A self-administered aversion technique. *Behav. Ther.,* 1976, *7,* 641–648.

Bernard, H. S., and Efran, J. S. Eliminating versus reducing smoking using pocket timers. *Behav. Res. Ther.,* 1972, *10,* 399–401.

Bernstein, D. A. Modification of smoking behavior: An evaluative review. *Psychol. Bull.,* 1969, *71,* 418–440.

Bernstein, D. A. The modification of smoking behavior: A search for effective variables. *Behav. Res. Ther.,* 1970, *8,* 133–146.

Bernstein, D. A. The modification of smoking behavior: Some suggestions for programmed "symptom substitution". Paper presented at the annual meeting of the Association for the Advancement of Behavior Therapy, Chicago, November, 1974.

Bernstein, D. A. and McAlister, A. The modification of smoking behavior: Progress and problems. *Addict. Behav.,* 1976, *1,* 89–102.

Bernstein, D. A., and Paul, G. Some comments on psychotherapy analogue research on small animal "phobia." *J. Behav. Ther. Exp. Psychiatry,* 1971, *2,* 225–237.

Best, J. A. Tailoring smoking withdrawal procedures to personality and motivational differences. *J. Consult. Clin. Psychol.,* 1975, *43,* 1–8.

Best, J. A., Bass, F., and Owen, L. E. Mode of service delivery in a smoking cessation programme for public health. *Can. J. Public Health,* 1977, *68,* 469–473.

Best, J. A., Owen, L. E., and Trentadue, L. Comparison of satiation and rapid smoking in self-managed smoking cessation. *Addict. Behav.,* 1978, *3,* 71–78.

Best, J. A., and Steffy, R. A. Smoking modification procedures tailored to subject characteristics. *Behav. Ther.,* 1971, *2,* 177–191.

Best, J. A., and Steffy, R. A. Smoking modification procedures for internal and external locus of control clients. *Can. J. Behav. Sci.,* 1975, *7,* 155–165.

Borgatta, E. F., and Evans, R. R. (Eds.), *Smoking, health, and behavior.* Chicago: Aldine, 1968.

Borkovec, T. D., and Nau, S. D. Credibility of analogue therapy rationales. *J. Behav. Ther. Exp. Psychiatry,* 1972, *3,* 257–260.

Brantmark, B., Ohlin, P., and Westling, H. Nicotine-containing chewing gum as an anti-smoking aid. *Psychopharmacologia,* 1973, *31,* 191–200.

Brockway, B. S. Chemical validation of self-reported smoking rates. *Behav. Ther.,* 1978, *9,* 685–686.

Brockway, B. S., Kleinmann, G., Edleson, J., and Gruenwald, K. Non-aversive procedures and their effect on cigarette smoking: A clinical group study. *Addict. Behav.,* in press.

Bryan, W. J. Hypnosis and smoking. *J. Am. Inst. Hypn.,* 1964, *5,* 17–37.

Burton, D. Consistency versus internality as initiators of behavior change. *Int. J. Addict.,* 1977, *12,* 553–563.

Butts, W. C., Kuehneman, M., and Widdowson, G. M. Automated method for determining serum thiocyanate to distinguish smokers from nonsmokers. *Clin. Chem.,* 1974, *20,* 1344–1346.

Bye, C., Fowle, A. S. E., Letley, E., and Wilkinson, S. Lack of effect of *Avena sativa* on cigarette smoking. *Nature,* 1974, *252,* 580–581.

Cautela, J. R. Covert sensitization. *Psychol. Rep.,* 1967, *20,* 459–468.

Cautela, J. R. Treatment of smoking by covert sensitization. *Psychol. Rep.,* 1970, *26,* 415–420.

Chapman, R. F., Smith, J. W., and Layden, T. A. Elimination of cigarette smoking by punishment and self-management training. *Behav. Res. Ther.,* 1971, *9,* 255–264.

Claiborn, W. I., Lewis, P., and Humble, S. Stimulus satiation and smoking: A revisit. *J. Clin. Psychol.,* 1972, *28,* 416–419.

Conway, J. B. Behavioral self-control of smoking through aversive conditioning and self-management. *J. Consult. Clin. Psychol.,* 1977, *45,* 348–357.

Crasilneck, H. B., and Hall, J. A. Hypnosis in the control of smoking. In H. B. Crasilneck and J. A. Hall (Eds.), *Clinical hypnosis: Principles and applications.* New York: Grune & Stratton, 1975, pp. 167–175.

Cruickshank, A. The anti-smoking clinic. *Lancet,* 1963, *2,* 353–354.

Curtis, B., Simpson, D. D., and Cole, S. G. Rapid puffing as a treatment component of a community smoking program. *J. Community Psychol.,* 1976, *4,* 186–193.

Danaher, B. G. Rapid smoking and self-control in the modification of smoking behavior. *J. Consult. Clin. Psychol.,* 1977, *45,* 1068–1075.

Danaher, B. G. Research on rapid smoking: Interim summary and recommendations. *Addict. Behav.,* 1977, *2,* 151–166.

Danaher, B. G., and Lichtenstein, E. An experimental analysis of coverant control: Cuing and consequation. Paper presented to the annual meeting of the Western Psychological Association, San Francisco, April 1974.

Danaher, B. G., Lichtenstein, E., and Sullivan, J. M. Comparative effects of rapid and normal smoking on heart rate and carboxyhemoglobin. *J. Consult. Clin. Psychol.,* 1976, *44,* 556–563.

Davison, G. C., and Rosen, R. C. Lobeline and reduction of cigarette smoking. *Psychol. Rep.,* 1972, *31,* 443–456.

Dawley, H. H., Jr., and Dillenkoffer, R. L. Minimizing risks involved in rapid smoking treatment. *J. Behav. Ther. Exp. Psychiatry,* 1975, *6,* 174.

Dawley, H. H., Jr., Ellithorpe, D. B., and Tretola, R. Carboxyhemoglobin levels before and after rapid smoking. *J. Behav. Ther. Exp. Psychiatry,* 1976, *7,* 13–16.

Dawley, H. H., Jr., and Sardenga, P. B. Results of smoking cessation program employing aversive cigarette smoking. *Newsletter Res. Ment. Health Behav. Sci.,* 1976, *18,* 12–17.

Delahunt, J., and Curran, J. P. The effectiveness of negative practice and self-control techniques in the reduction of smoking behavior. *J. Consult. Clin. Psychol.,* 1976, *44,* 1002–1007.

Delarue, N. C. A study in smoking withdrawal—the Toronto smoking withdrawal study centre—description of activities. *Can. J. Public Health,* 1973, *64,* S5–S19.

Densen, P. M., Davidow, B., Bass, H. E., and Jones, E. W. A chemical test for smoking exposure. *Arch. Environ. Health.,* 1967, *14,* 865–874.

Dericco, D. A., Brigham, T. A., and Garlington, W. K. Development and evaluation of treatment paradigms for the suppression of smoking behavior. *J. Appl. Behav. Anal.,* 1977, *10,* 173–181.

Dubitzky, M., and Schwartz, J. L. Ego-resiliency, ego-control, and smoking cessation. *J. Psychol.,* 1968, *70,* 27–33.

Dubren, R. Evaluation of a televised stop-smoking clinic. *Public Health Rep.,* 1977a, *92,* 358–360.

Dubren, R. Self-reinforcement by recorded telephone messages to maintain non-smoking behavior. *J. Consult. Clin. Psychol.,* 1977b, *45,* 358–360.

Ejrup, B. A proposed medical regimen to stop smoking: The follow-up results. *Swedish Cancer Soc. Yearbook,* 1963, *3,* 468–473.

Ejrup, B. Treatment of tobacco addiction: Experiences in tobacco withdrawal clinics. In *Can we help them stop?* Chicago: American Cancer Society, Illinois Division, 1964.

Engeln, R. G. *A comparison of desensitization and aversive conditioning as treatment methods to reduce cigarette smoking.* Unpublished doctoral dissertation, Washington State University, 1969.

Epstein, L. H., and McCoy, J. F. Issues in smoking control. *Addict. Behav.,* 1975, *1,* 65–72.

Euler, H. A. Reduction of cigarette smoking by self monitoring. *Z. Klin. Psychol. Psychother.,* 1973, *21,* 271–282.

Evans, R. I., Hansen, W. B., and Mittelmark, M. B. Increasing the validity of self-reports of behavior in a smoking in children investigation. *J. Appl. Psychol.,* 1977, *62,* 521–523.

Evans, R. I., Rozelle, R. M., Mittelmark, M. B., Hansen, W. B., Bane, A. L., and Havis, J. G. Deterring the onset of smoking in children: Knowledge of immediate physiological effects and coping with peer pressure, media pressure, and parent modeling. *J. Appl. Soc. Psychol.,* in press.

Eysenck, H. J. Personality and the maintenance of the smoking habit. In W. L. Dunn (Ed.), *Smoking behavior: Motives and incentives.* Washington, D.C.: Winston & Sons, 1973.

Ferno, O., Lichtneckert, S. J. A., and Lundgren, C. E. G. A substitute for tobacco smoking. *Psychopharmacologia,* 1973, *31,* 201–204.

Flaxman, J. Quitting smoking now or later: Gradual, abrupt, immediate, and delayed quitting. *Behav. Ther.,* 1978, *9,* 260–270.

Franks, C. M., Fried, R., and Ashem, B. An improved apparatus for the aversive conditioning of cigarette smokers. *Behav. Res. Ther.,* 1966, *4,* 301–308.

Frederiksen, L. W. Single-case designs in the modification of smoking. *Addict. Behav.,* 1976, *1,* 311–319.

Frederiksen, L. W., Miller, P. M., and Peterson, G. L. Topographical components of smoking behavior. *Addict. Behav.,* 1977, *2,* 55–61.

Frederiksen, L. W., and Peterson, G. L. Controlled smoking: Development and maintenance. *Addict. Behav.,* 1976, *1,* 193–196.

Gallup Opinion Index Report #108, pp. 20–21, June, 1974.

Gendreau, P. E., and Dodwell, P. C. An aversive treatment for addicted cigarette smokers: Preliminary report. *Can. Psychol.,* 1968, *9,* 28–34.

Gerson, P., and Lanyon, R. I. Modification of smoking behavior with an aversion-desensitization procedure. *J. Consult. Clin. Psychol.,* 1972, *38,* 399–402.

Glad, W. R., Tyre, T. E., and Adesso, V. J. A multidimensional model of cigarette smoking. *Am. J. Clin. Hypn.,* 1976, *19,* 82–89.

Glasgow, R. E. *The effects of a self-control manual and amount of therapist contact in the modification of smoking behavior.* Unpublished doctoral dissertation, University of Oregon, 1977.

Goguen, L. J. Overlearning of covert conditioning as a variable in the permanent modification of smoking behavior. Paper presented at the annual meeting of the Association for the Advancement of Behavior Therapy, Chicago, November, 1974.

Goldfried, M. R., and Trier, C. S. Effectiveness of relaxation as an active coping skill. *J. Abnorm. Psychol.,* 1974, *83,* 348–355.

Greenberg, I., and Altman, J. L. Modifying smoking behavior through stimulus control: A case study. *J. Behav. Ther. Exp. Psychiat.,* 1976, *1,* 97–99.

Grimaldi, K. E., and Lichtenstein, E. Hot, smoky air as an aversive stimulus in the treatment of smoking. *Behav. Res. Ther.,* 1969, *7,* 275–282.

Gritz, E., and Jarvik, M. Preliminary study: Forty-eight hours of abstinence from smoking. *Proc. Am. Psychol. Assoc.*, 1973.

Guilford, J. *Factors related to successful abstinence from smoking: Final report.* Los Angeles: American Institutes for Research, 1966.

Guilford, J. Group treatment versus individual initiative in the cessation of smoking. *J. Appl. Psychol.*, 1972, *56,* 162–167.

Gutmann, M., and Marston, A. Problems of *S*'s motivation in a behavioral program for reduction of cigarette smoking. *Psychol. Rep.*, 1967, *20,* 1107–1114.

Hall, J. A., and Crasilneck, H. B. Development of a hypnotic technique for treatment chronic cigarette smoking. *Int. J. Clin. Exp. Hypn.*, 1970, *18,* 283–289.

Hammond, E. C., and Garfinkel, L. Coronary heart disease, stroke and aortic aneurysm. *Arch. Environm. Health.*, 1969, *10,* 167–182.

Harris, D. E., and Lichtenstein, E. The contribution of nonspecific social variables to a successful behavioral treatment of smoking. Unpublished manuscript, University of Oregon, 1974.

Harris, M. B., and Rothberg, C. A self-control approach to reduced smoking. *Psychol. Rep.*, 1972, *31,* 165–166.

Hartelius, J., and Tibbling, L. Abuse and intoxication potential of nicotine chewing gum. *Br. Med. J.*, 1976, *2,* 812.

Hoffstaedt, E. G. W. Anti-smoking campaign. *Med. Officer,* 1964, *111,* 59–60.

Homme, L. E. Control of coverants, the operants of the mind. *Psychol. Rep.*, 1965, *15,* 501–511.

Horan, J. J., Hackett, G., Nicholas, W. C., Linberg, S. E., Stone, C. I., and Lukoski, H. C. Rapid smoking: A cautionary note. *J. Consult. Clin. Psychol.*, 1977, *45,* 341–343.

Horan, J. J., Linberg, S. E., and Hackett, G. Nicotine poisoning and rapid smoking. *J. Consult. Clin. Psychol.*, 1977, *45,* 344–347.

Horning, E. E., Horning, M. G., Carroll, D. I., Stillwell, R. N., and Dzidic, I. Nicotine in smokers, non-smokers, and room air. *Life Sci.*, 1973, *13,* 1331–1346.

Hunt, W. A. (Ed.). *Learning mechanisms in smoking.* Chicago: Aldine, 1970.

Hunt, W. A., and Bespalec, D. A. An evaluation of current methods of modifying smoking behavior. *J. Clin. Psychol.*, 1974, *30,* 431–438.

Hunt, W. A., and Matarazzo, J. D. Habit mechanisms in smoking. In W. A. Hunt (Ed.), *Learning mechanisms in smoking.* Chicago: Aldine, 1970.

Hunt, W. A., and Matarazzo, J. D. Three years later: Recent developments in the experimental modification of smoking behavior. *J. Abnorm. Psychol.*, 1973, *81,* 107–114.

Ikard, F. F., and Tomkins, S. The experience of affect as a determinant of smoking behavior: A series of validity studies. *J. Abnorm. Psychol.*, 1973, *81,* 172–181.

Janis, I. L., and Hoffman, D. Facilitating effects of daily contact between partners who make a decision to cut down on smoking. *J. Pers. Soc. Psychol.*, 1971, *17,* 25–35.

Janis, I. L., and Mann, L. Effectiveness of emotional role-playing in modifying smoking habits and attitudes. *J. Exp. Res. Pers.*, 1965, *1,* 84–90.

Jarvik, M. E. The role of nicotine in the smoking habit. In W. A. Hunt (Ed.), *Learning mechanisms in smoking.* Chicago: Aldine, 1970.

Jarvik, M. E. Further observations on nicotine as the reinforcing agent in smoking. In W. L. Dunn, Jr. (Ed.), *Smoking behavior: Motives and incentives.* Washington, D.C.: Winston & Sons, 1973.

Jarvik, M. E., Glick, S. D., and Nakamura, R. K. Inhibition of cigarette smoking by orally administered nicotine. *Clin. Pharmacol. Ther.*, 1970, *11,* 574–576.

Jenks, R., Schwartz, J. L., and Dubitzky, M. Effect of the counselor's approach to changing smoking behavior. *J. Counsel. Psychol.*, 1969, *16,* 215–222.

Johnston, E., and Donoghue, J. R. Hypnosis and smoking: A review of the literature. *Am. J. Clin. Hypn.*, 1971, *13,* 265–272.

Kantoritz, D. A., Walters, J., and Pezdek, K. Positive vs negative self-monitoring in the self control of smoking. Manuscript submitted for publication, 1977.

Kanzler, M., Jaffe, J. H., and Zeidenberg, P. Long and short term effects of a large scale proprietary smoking cessation program: A 4 yr. follow-up of Smokenders participants. *J. Clin. Psychol.*, 1976, *32,* 661–669.

Kanzler, M., Zeidenberg, R., and Jaffe, J. H. Response of medical personnel to an on-site smoking cessation program. *J. Clin. Psychol.*, 1976, *32,* 670–674.

Karoly, P., and Doyle, W. W. Effects of outcome expectancy and timing of self-monitoring on cigarette smoking. *J. Clin. Psychol.*, 1975, *31,* 351–355.

Keutzer, C. S. Behavior modification of smoking: The experimental investigation of diverse techniques. *Behav. Res. Ther.*, 1968, *6,* 137–157.

Keutzer, C. S., Lichtenstein, E., and Mees, H. L. Modification of smoking behavior: A review. *Psychol. Bull.*, 1968, *70,* 520–533.

Kline, M. V. The use of extended group hypnotherapy sessions in controlling cigarette habituation. *Int. J. Clin. Exp. Hypn.*, 1970, *18,* 270–282.

Koenig, K. P., and Masters, J. Experimental treatment of habitual smoking. *Behav. Res. Ther.*, 1965, *3,* 235–243.

Kopel, S. A. *The effects of self-control, booster sessions, and cognitive factors on the maintenance of smoking reduction.* Unpublished doctoral dissertation, University of Oregon, 1974.

Kopel, S. A. Carbon monoxide monitoring: Clinical and research utility for smoking reduction. Paper presented at annual meeting of the Association for the Advancement of Behavior Therapy, San Francisco, December, 1975.

Kozlowski, L. T. Urinary pH, nicotine, and the psychology of cigarette smoking. Paper presented at the annual meeting of the Association for the Advancement of Behavior Therapy, Chicago, November, 1974.

Kraft, T., and Al-Issa, I. Desensitization and reduction in cigarette consumption. *J. Psychol.*, 1967, *67,* 323–329.

Krietler, S., Shahar, A., and Krietler, H. Cognitive orientation, type of smoker, and behavior therapy of smoking. *Br. J. Med. Psychol.*, 1976, *49,* 167–175.

Lando, H. A. An objective check upon self-reported smoking levels: A preliminary report. *Behav. Ther.*, 1975a, *6,* 547–549.

Lando, H. A. A comparison of excessive and rapid

smoking in the modification of chronic smoking behavior. *J. Consult. Clin. Psychol.*, 1975b, *43*, 350–355.

Lando, H. A. Aversive conditioning and contingency management in the treatment of smoking. *J. Consult. Clin. Psychol.*, 1976a, *44*, 312.

Lando, H. A. Self-pacing in eliminating chronic smoking: Serendipity revisited? *Behav. Ther.*, 1976b, *7*, 634–640.

Lando, H. A. Successful treatment of smokers with a broad-spectrum behavioral approach. *J. Consult. Clin. Psychol.*, 1977, *45*, 361–366.

Lando, H. A. Stimulus control, rapid smoking, and contractual management in the maintenance of nonsmoking. *Behav. Ther.*, in press.

Lando, H. A., and Davison, G. C. Cognitive dissonance as a modifier of chronic smoking behavior: A serendipitous finding. *J. Consult. Clin. Psychol.*, 1975, *43*, 750.

Lawson, D. M., and May, R. B. Three procedures for the extinction of smoking behavior. *Psychol. Rec.*, 1970, *20*, 151–157.

Lawton, M. P. Group methods in smoking withdrawal. *Arch. Environ. Health*, 1967, *14*, 258–265.

Leitenberg, H. (Ed.). *Handbook of behavior modification and behavior therapy.* Englewood Cliffs, N.J.: Prentice-Hall, 1976.

Levenberg, S. B., and Wagner, M. K. Smoking cessation: Long-term irrelevance of mode of treatment. *J. Behav. Ther. Exp. Psychiatry*, 1976, *7*, 93–95.

Leventhal, H. Experimental studies of anti-smoking communications. In E. F. Borgatta and R. R. Evans (Eds.), *Smoking, health, and behavior.* Chicago: Aldine, 1968.

Leventhal, H., and Avis, N. Pleasure, addiction, and habit: Factors in verbal report on factors in smoking behavior. *J. Abnorm. Psychol.*, 1976, *85*, 478–488.

Leventhal, H. A., and Cleary, P. D. The smoking problem: A review of the research, theory, and research policies in behavioral risk modification. Report for Center for Medical Sociology and Health Services Research, Madison, Wisconsin, 1977.

Levine, B. A. Effectiveness of contingent and noncontingent electric shock in reducing cigarette smoking. *Psychol. Rep.*, 1974, *34*, 223–226.

Levinson, B. L., Shapiro, D., Schwartz, G. E., and Tursky, B. Smoking elimination by gradual reduction. *Behav. Ther.*, 1971, *2*, 477–487.

Lewittes, D., and Israel, A. C. Responsibility contracting for the maintenance of reduced smoking: A technique innovation. *Behav. Ther.*, 1975, *6*, 696–698.

Lichtenstein, E. Modification of smoking behavior: Good designs—Ineffective treatments. *J. Consult. Clin. Psychol.*, 1971, *36*, 163–166.

Lichtenstein, E., and Danaher, B. G. Modification of smoking behavior: A critical analysis of theory, research, and practice. In M. Hersen, R. M. Eisler, and P. M. Miller (Eds.), *Progress in behavior modification,* Vol. 3. New York: Academic Press, 1976, pp. 70–132.

Lichtenstein, E., and Glasgow, R. E. Rapid smoking: Side effects and safeguards. *J. Consult. Clin. Psychol.*, 1977, *45*, 815–821.

Lichtenstein, E., Harris, D. E., Birchler, G. R., Wahl, J. M., and Schmahl, D. P. Comparison of rapid smoking, warm smoky air, and attention placebo in the modification of smoking behavior. *J. Consult. Clin. Psychol.*, 1973, *40*, 92–98.

Lichtenstein, E., and Keutzer, C. S. Modification of smoking behavior: A later look. In R. D. Rubin, H., Fensterheim, A. A. Lazarus, and C. M. Franks (Eds.), *Advances in behavior therapy.* New York: Academic Press, 1971.

Lichtenstein, E., Keutzer, C. S., and Himes, K. H. Emotional role-playing and changes in smoking attitudes and behavior. *Psychol. Rep.*, 1969, *25*, 379–387.

Lichtenstein, E., and Penner, M. P. Long-term effects of rapid smoking treatment for dependent cigarette smokers. *Addict. Behav.*, 1977, *2*, 109–112.

Logan, F. A. Self-control as habit, drive, and incentive. *J. Abnorm. Psychol.*, 1973, *81*, 127–136.

Lublin, I. Principles governing the choice of unconditioned stimuli in aversive conditioning. In R. D. Rubin and C. M. Franks (Eds.), *Advances in behavior therapy.* New York: Academic Press, 1969.

Lublin, I., and Joslyn, L. Aversive conditioning of cigarette addiction. Paper read at the meeting of the American Psychological Association, Los Angeles, September, 1968.

Lucchesi, B. R., Schuster, C. R., and Emley, G. S. The role of nicotine as a determinant of cigarette smoking frequency in man with observations of certain cardiovascular effects associated with tobacco alkaloid. *Clin. Pharmacol. Ther.*, 1967, *8*, 789–796.

Mann, L., and Janis, I. L. A follow-up study on the long term effects of emotional role playing. *J. Pers. Soc. Psychol.*, 1968, *8*, 339–342.

Mantek, M., and Erben, R. Behavior therapy: New approaches towards smoking cessation. *Int. J. Health Educ.*, 1974, *17*, 1–7.

Marrone, R. L., Marksamer, M. A., and Salzberg, P. M. A short duration group treatment of smoking behavior by stimulus saturation. *Behav. Res. Ther.*, 1970, *8*, 347–352.

Marston, A. R., and McFall, R. M. Comparison of behavior modification approaches to smoking reduction. *J. Consult. Clin. Psychol.*, 1971, *36*, 153–162.

Mausner, B. Report on a smoking clinic. *Am. Psychol.*, 1966, *21*, 251–255.

Mausner, B. Some comments on the failure of behavior therapy as a technique for modifying cigarette smoking. *J. Consult. Clin. Psychol.*, 1971, *36*, 167–170.

Mausner, B. An ecological view of cigarette smoking behavior. *J. Abnorm. Psychol.*, 1973, *81*, 115–126.

Mausner, B., and Platt, E. S. *Smoking: A behavioral analysis.* New York: Pergamon Press, 1971.

McAlister, A., Meyer, A., and Maccoby, N. Long-term results of education to reduce smoking: Stanford three community study. Paper presented at American Heart Association Scientific Sessions, Miami, November, 1976.

McFall, R. M. Effects of self-monitoring on normal smoking behavior. *J. Consult. Clin. Psychol.*, 1970, *35*, 135–142.

McFall, R. M., and Hammen, C. L. Motivation, structure and self-monitoring: The role of nonspecific factors in smoking reduction. *J. Consult. Clin. Psychol.*, 1971, *37*, 80–86.

McFarland, J. W. Physical measures used in breaking

the smoking habit. *Arch. Phys. Med. Rehabil.*, 1965, *64*, 323–327.

McGrath, M., and Hall, S. M. The self-management treatment of smoking behavior. Paper presented at the annual meeting of the Western Psychological Association, Sacramento, California, April, 1975.

Miller, A., and Gimpl, M. Operant conditioning and self-control of smoking and studying. *J. Genet. Psychol.*, 1971, *119*, 181–186.

Miller, L. C., Schilling, H. F., Logan, D. L., and Johnson, R. L. Potential hazards of rapid smoking as aversion therapy. *N. Engl. J. Med.*, 1977, *297*, 590–592.

Morganstern, K. P., and Ratliff, R. G. Systematic desensitization as a technique for treating smoking behavior: A preliminary report. *Behav. Res. Ther.*, 1969, *7*, 397–398.

Morrow, J., Sachs, L., Gmeinder, S., and Burgess, H. Elimination of cigarette smoking behavior by stimulus satiation, self-control techniques, and group therapy. Paper presented at the annual meeting of the Western Psychological Association, Los Angeles, April, 1973.

National Clearinghouse for Smoking and Health. *Directory of on-going research in smoking and health.* Arlington, Va.: United States Public Health Service, 1968.

National Clearinghouse for Smoking and Health. *Directory of on-going research in smoking and health.* Arlington, Va.: United States Public Health Service, 1970.

National Clearinghouse for Smoking and Health. *Directory of on-going research in smoking and health.* Arlington, Va.: United States Public Health Service, 1974.

Nolan, J. D. Self-control procedures in the modification of smoking behavior. *J. Consult. Clin. Psychol.*, 1968, *32*, 92–93.

Nuland, W., and Field, P. B. Smoking and hypnosis: A systematic clinic approach. *Int. J. Clin. Exp. Hypn.*, 1970, *18*, 290–306.

Ober, D. C. Modification of smoking behavior. *J. Consult. Clin. Psychol.*, 1968, *32*, 543–549.

Ohlin, P., Lundh, B., and Westling, H. Carbon monoxide blood levels and reported cessation of smoking. *Psychopharmacology*, 1976, *49*, 263–265.

Orr, R. G. Hypnosis helps reluctant smokers. *Practitioner*, 1970, *205*, 204–208.

Osarchuk, M., and Goldfried, M. R. A further examination of the credibility of therapy rationales. *Behav. Ther.*, 1975, *6*, 694–695.

Ottens, A. J. The effect of transcendental meditation upon modifying the cigarette smoking habit. *J. School Health*, 1975, *45*, 577–583.

Paul, G., and Bernstein, D. A. *Anxiety and behavior: Treatment by systematic desensitization and related techniques.* New York: General Learning Press, 1973.

Pechacek, T. F. Specialized treatments for high anxious smokers. Paper presented at the annual meeting of the Association for the Advancement of Behavior Therapy, New York, 1976.

Pechacek, T. F. *An evaluation of cessation and maintenance strategies in the modification of smoking behavior.* Unpublished doctoral dissertation, University of Texas at Austin, 1977.

Pederson, L. L., Scrimgeour, W. G., and Lefcoe, N. M. Comparison of hypnosis plus counseling, counseling alone, and hypnosis alone in a community service smoking withdrawal program. *J. Consult. Clin. Psychol.*, 1975, *43*, 920.

Perri, M. G., Richards, C. S., and Schultheis, K. R. Behavioral self-control and smoking reduction: A study of self-initiated attempts to reduce smoking. *Behav. Ther.*, 1977, *8*, 360–365.

Perry, C., and Mullen, G. The effect of hypnotic susceptibility on reducing smoking behavior treated by an hypnotic technique. *J. Clin. Psychol.*, 1975, *31*, 387–390.

Platt, E. S., Krassen, E., and Mausner, B. Individual variation in behavioral change following role playing. *Psychol. Rep.*, 1969, *24*, 155–170.

Pomerleau, O. F., Adkins, D., and Pertschuk, M. Predictors of outcome and recidivism in smoking cessation treatment. *Addict. Behav.*, 1978, *3*, 65–70.

Pomerleau, O. F., and Ciccone, P. Preliminary results of a treatment program for smoking cessation using multiple behavior modification techniques. Paper presented at the annual Meeting of the Association for the Advancement of Behavior Therapy, Chicago, November, 1974.

Pomerleau, O. F., and Pomerleau, C. S. *Break the smoking habit: A behavioral program for giving up cigarettes.* Champaign, Ill.: Research Press, 1977.

Pomerleau, O. F., Pomerleau, C. S., and Weinstein, H. S. Success Over Smoking (SOS): A professionally supervised self-help smoking-cessation program. Washington: Educational Services, Inc., 1976.

Pope, J. W., and Mount, G. R. The control of cigarette smoking through the application of a portable electronic device designed to dispense an aversive stimulus in relation to subjects' smoking frequency. *Behav. Eng.*, 1975, *2*, 52–56.

Powell, J., and Azrin, N. The effects of shock as a punisher for cigarette smoking. *J. Appl. Behav. Anal.*, 1968, *1*, 63–71.

Premack, D. L. Mechanisms of self-control. In W. A. Hunt (Ed.), *Learning mechanisms in smoking.* Chicago: Aldine, 1970.

Pyke, S., Agnew, N. McK., and Kopperud, J. Modification of an overlearned maladaptive response through a relearning program: A pilot study on smoking. *Behav. Res. Ther.*, 1966, *4*, 197–203.

Ravensborg, M. R. Relaxation as therapy for addictive smoking. *Psychol. Rep.*, 1976, *39*, 894.

Raw, M. Persuading people to stop smoking. *Behav. Res. Ther.*, 1976a, *14*, 97–101.

Raw, M. The psychological modification of smoking. In S. Rachman (Ed.), *Advances in medical psychology.* London: Pergamon Press, 1976b.

Relinger, H., Bornstein, P. H., Bugge, I. D., Carmody, T. P., and Zohn, C. J. Utilization of adverse rapid smoking in groups: Efficacy of treatment and maintenance procedures. *J. Consult. Clin. Psychol.*, 1977, *45*, 245–249.

Resnick, J. H. The control of smoking behavior by stimulus satiation. *Behav. Res. Ther.*, 1968a, *6*, 113–114.

Resnick, J. H. Effects of stimulus satiation on the overlearned maladaptive response of cigarette smoking. *J. Consult. Clin. Psychol.*, 1968b, *32*, 500–505.

Rimm, D. C., and Masters, J. C. *Behavior therapy.* New York: Academic Press, 1974.

Roberts, A. H. Self-control procedures in modification of smoking behavior: Replication. *Psychol. Rep.*, 1969, *24*, 675–676.

Rosenberg, A. An investigation into the effect on cigarette smoking of a new antismoking chewing gum. *J. Int. Med. Res.*, 1977, *5*, 68–70.

Ross, C. A. Smoking withdrawal research clinics. *Am. J. Public Health*, 1967, *57*, 677–681.

Rotter, J. B. Generalized expectancies for internal versus external control of reinforcement. *Psychol. Monogr.*, 1966, *80* (Whole No. 609).

Roy, I., and Swillinger, E. Application of learning theory principles to eliminate a cigarette smoking habit: A case study. *Psychiat. Forum*, 1971, *2*, 27–31.

Rozensky, R. H. The effect of timing of self-monitoring on reducing cigarette consumption. *J. Behav. Ther. Exp. Psychiatry*, 1974, *5*, 301–303.

Russell, M. A. H. Effect of electric aversion on cigarette smoking. *Br. Med. J.*, 1970, *1*, 82–86.

Russell, M. A. H. Realistic goals for smoking and health: A case for safer smoking. *Lancet*, 1974, *1*, 254–257.

Russell, M. A. H. Effects of electric aversion on cigarette smoking. In G. Edwards, M. A. H. Russell, D. Hawks, and M. MacCafferty (Eds.), *Alcohol dependence and smoking behavior*. London: Saxon House/Lexington Books, 1976, pp. 168–171.

Russell, M. A. H., Armstrong, E., and Patel, U. A. The role of temporal contiguity in electric aversion therapy for cigarette smoking: Analysis of behavior changes. *Behav. Res. Ther.*, 1976, *14*, 103–123.

Russell, M. A. H., and Feyerabend, C. Blood and urinary nicotine in non-smokers. *Lancet*, 1975, 179–181.

Russell, M. A. H., Wilson, C., Feyerabend, C., and Cole, P. V. Effect of nicotine chewing gum on smoking behavior and as an aid to cigarette withdrawal. *Br. Med. J.*, 1976, *2*, 391–393.

Rutner, I. T. *The modification of smoking behavior through techniques of self-control.* Unpublished master's thesis, Wichita State University, 1967.

Sachs, L. B., Bean, H., and Morrow, J. E. Comparison of smoking treatments. *Behav. Ther.*, 1970, *1*, 465–472.

Satterfield, H. D. *Efficacy of self-instructions as a treatment component in smoking cessation.* Unpublished doctoral dissertation, Stanford University, 1977.

Schachter, S., Silverstein, B., Kozlowski, L. T., Perlick, D., Herman, C. P., and Liebling, S. Studies of the interaction of psychosocial and pharmacological determinants of smoking. *J. Exp. Psychol. Gen.*, 1977, *106*, 3–40.

Schlegel, R. P., and Kunetsky, M. Immediate and delayed effects of the "five-day plan to stop smoking" including factors affecting recidivism. *Prev. Med.*, 1977, *6*, 454–461.

Schmahl, D. P., Lichtenstein, E., and Harris, D. E. Successful treatment of habitual smokers with warm, smoky air, and rapid smoking. *J. Consult. Clin. Psychol.*, 1972, *38*, 105–111.

Schneider, N. G., Popek, P. Jarvik, M. E., and Gritz, E. R. The use of nicotine gum during cessation of smoking. *Am. J. Psychiatry*, 1977, *134*, 439–440.

Schuster, C. R. Comments on paper by Jarvik. In W. A. Hunt (Ed.), *Learning mechanisms in smoking.* Chicago: Aldine, 1970.

Schwartz, J. L. A critical review and evaluation of smoking control methods. *Public Health Rep.*, 1969, *84*, 489–506.

Schwartz, J. L., and Dubitzky, M. The results of helping people fight cigarettes. *Calif. Health*, 1967, *24*, 78–83.

Schwartz, J. L., and Dubitzky, M. *Psychosocial factors involved in cigarette smoking and cessation.* Berkeley, Calif.: Institute for Health Research, 1968.

Schwartz, J. L., and Dubitzky, M. Maximizing success in smoking cessation methods. *Am. J. Public Health*, 1969, *59*, 1392–1399.

Seltzer, A. P. Anti-smoking lozenge. *J. Natl. Med. Assoc.*, 1975, *67*, 311–313.

Shapiro, D., Tursky, B., Schwartz, G. E., and Schnidman, S. R. Smoking on cue: A behavioral approach to smoking reduction. *J. Health Soc. Behav.*, 1971, *12*, 108–113.

Shewchuk, L. A. Smoking cessation programs of the American Health Foundation. *Prev. Med.*, 1976, *5*, 454–474.

Shewchuk, L. A., Dubren, R., Burton, D., Forman, M., Clark, R. R., and Jaffin, A. P. Preliminary observations on an intervention program for heavy smokers. *Int. J. Addict.*, 1977, *12*, 323–336.

Shiffman, S. M., and Jarvik, M. E. Smoking withdrawal symptoms in two weeks of abstinence. *Psychopharmacology*, 1976, *50*, 35–39.

Sipich, J. F., Russell, R. K., and Tobias, L. A comparison of covert sensitization and "nonspecific" treatment in the modification of smoking behavior. *J. Behav. Ther. Exp. Psychiatry*, 1974, *5*, 201–203.

Solomon, R. L., and Corbit, J. D. An opponent process theory of motivation. II. Cigarette addiction. *J. Abnorm. Psychol.*, 1973, *81*, 158–171.

Spiegel, H. A single-treatment method to stop smoking using ancillary self-hypnosis. *Int. J. Clin. Exp. Hypn.*, 1970, *18*, 235–250.

St. Pierre, R., and Lawrence, P. S. Reducing smoking using positive self-management. *J. School Health*, 1975, *45*, 7–9.

Steffy, R. A., Meichenbaum, D., and Best, J. A. Aversive and cognitive factors in the modification of smoking behavior. *Behav. Res. Ther.*, 1970, *8*, 115–125.

Stern, N., Sherman, M., Greenberg, D., Bobbit, M., and Reiter, S. Self-control training for the modification of smoking. Unpublished manuscript, Syracuse University, 1975.

Streltzer, N. E., and Koch, G. V. Influence of emotional role-playing on smoking habits and attitudes. *Psychol. Rep.*, 1968, *22*, 817–820.

Suedfeld, P. Changes in intellectual performance and in susceptibility to influence. In J. P. Zubek (Ed.), *Sensory deprivation: Fifteen years of research.* New York: Appleton-Century-Crofts, 1969.

Suedfeld, P. Sensory deprivation used in the reduction of cigarette smoking: Attitude change experiments in an applied context. *J. Appl. Soc. Psychol.*, 1973, *3*, 30–38.

Suedfeld, P., and Best, J. A. Satiation and sensory deprivation combined: Some case studies and unexpected side effects. *Int. J. Addict.*, 1977, *12*, 337–359.

Suedfeld, P., and Ikard, F. Attitude manipulation in restricted environments: IV. Psychologically addicted smokers treated in sensory deprivation. *Br. J. Addict.*, 1973, *68*, 170–176.

Suedfeld, P., and Ikard, F. Use of sensory deprivation in facilitating the reduction of cigarette smoking. *J. Consult. Clin. Psychol.,* 1974, *42,* 888–895.

Suedfeld, P., Landon, P. B., Pargament, R., and Epstein, Y. M. An experimental attack on smoking. *Int. J. Addict.,* 1972, *7,* 721–733.

Sushinsky, L. W. Expectation of future treatment, stimulus satiation, and smoking. *J. Consult. Clin. Psychol.,* 1972, *39,* 343.

Sutherland, A., Amit, Z., Golden, M., and Roseberger, Z. Comparison of three behavioral techniques in the modification of smoking behavior. *J. Consult. Clin. Psychol.,* 1975, *43,* 443–447.

Thompson, D. S., and Wilson, T. R. Discontinuance of cigarette smoking: "Natural" and with "therapy." *J.A.M.A.,* 1966, *196,* 1048–1052.

Tighe, T. J., and Elliott, R. Breaking the cigarette habit: Effects of a technique involving threatened loss of money. *Psychol. Rec.,* 1968, *18,* 503–513.

Tomkins, S. S. Psychological model for smoking behavior. *Am. J. Public Health,* 1966, *56,* 17–20.

Tomkins, S. S. A modified model of smoking behavior. In E. Borgatta and R. Evans (Eds.), *Smoking, health and behavior.* Chicago: Aldine, 1968.

Tongas, P. N., Patterson, J., and Goodkind, S. Cessation of smoking through behavior modification. Paper presented at annual meeting of the Association for the Advancement of Behavior Therapy, New York, December, 1976.

Tooley, J. T., and Pratt, S. An experimental procedure for the extinction of smoking behavior. *Psychol. Rec.,* 1967, *17,* 209–218.

United States Public Health Service. *Health consequences of smoking.* Washington, D.C.: United States Government Printing Office, 1975.

Upper, D., and Meredith, L. A stimulus control approach to the modification of smoking behavior. *Proc. 71st Annual Convention Am. Psychol. Assoc.,* 1970, *5,* 739–740.

Vogt, T. M., Selvin, S., Widdowson, G., and Halley, S. B. Expired air carbon monoxide and serum thiocyanate as objective measures of cigarette exposure. *Am. J. Public Health,* 1977, *67,* 545–549.

Wagner, J. K., and Bragg, R. A. Comparing behavior modification approaches to habit decrement—smoking. *J. Consult. Clin. Psychol.,* 1970, *34,* 258–263.

Watkins, H. R. Hypnosis and smoking: A five session approach. *Int. J. Clin. Exp. Hypn.,* 1976, *24,* 381–390.

Weinrobe, P. A., and Lichtenstein, E. The use of urges as termination criterion in a rapid smoking treatment program for habitual smokers. Paper presented at the annual meeting of the Western Psychological Association, Sacramento, California, April, 1975.

Weir, J. M., Dubitzky, M., and Schwartz, J. L. Counselor style and group effectiveness in a smoking withdrawal study. *J. Psychother.,* 1969, *23,* 106–118.

West, D. W., Graham, S., Swanson, M., and Wilkinson, G. Five year follow-up of a smoking withdrawal clinic population. *Am. J. Public Health,* 1977, *67,* 536–544.

Westling, H. Experience of nicotine chewing gum in antismoking treatment. *Lakartidningin,* 1976, *73,* 2549–2552.

Whitman, T. L. Modification of chronic smoking behavior: A comparison of three approaches. *Behav. Res. Ther.,* 1969, *7,* 257–263.

Whitman, T. L. Aversive control of smoking behavior in a group context. *Behav. Res. Ther.,* 1972, *10,* 97–104.

Wilde, G. J. S. Behavior therapy for addicted cigarette smokers. *Behav. Res. Ther.,* 1964, *2,* 107–110.

Wilde, G. J. S. Letter to the editor. *Behav. Res. Ther.,* 1965, *2,* 313.

Wilson, T. G., and Davison, G. C. Aversion techniques in behavior therapy: Some theoretical and metatheoretical considerations. *J. Consult. Clin. Psychol.,* 1969, *33,* 327–329.

Winett, R. A. Parameters of deposit contracts in the modification of smoking. *Psychol. Rec.,* 1973, *23,* 49–60.

Wisocki, P., and Rooney, E. J. A comparison of thought-stopping and covert sensitization techniques in the treatment of smoking. *Psychol. Rec.,* 1974, *24,* 191–192.

Wolpe, J. *Psychotherapy by reciprocal inhibition.* Stanford: Stanford University Press, 1958.

Wolpe, J. *The practice of behavior therapy.* New York: Pergamon Press, 1969.

World Health Organization. *Smoking and its effects on health.* Report of a WHO expert committee, Geneva, Switzerland, 1975.

Zagona, S. V. (Ed.). *Studies and issues in smoking behavior.* Tucson: The University of Arizona Press, 1967.

Zeidenberg, P., Jaffe, J. H., Kanzler, M., Levitt, M. D., Langone, J. J., and Van Vunakis, H. Nicotine:cotinine levels in blood during cessation of smoking. *Compr. Psychiatry,* 1977, *18,* 93–101.

Problem Drinking and Alcoholism*

PETER E. NATHAN, PH.D.

Professor and Chairman
Department of Clinical Psychology
Rutgers University
New Brunswick, New Jersey

MARK S. GOLDMAN, PH.D.

Associate Professor
Department of Psychology
Wayne State University
Detroit, Michigan

11

Alcoholism is a behavioral disorder. It can be readily described by reference to such distinguishing behavioral characteristics as frequency, rate, and amount of ethanol consumption as well as by the associated behavioral dysfunctions which invariably accompany excessive alcohol consumption. However, alcohol also affects diverse organ systems. With prolonged, excessive alcohol use, its physiological effects include addiction, tolerance, and, ultimately, organ and tissue damage. Because of the potent physiological effects of alcohol—and because its abuse often appears to be beyond the alcoholic's control—many workers in the field have come to attribute the disorder largely to biological factors. However, a strong case can be made, instead, for the crucial role played by behavioral factors in both the etiology and treatment of alcoholism. To enable this demonstration, this chapter first reviews the conceptual and empirical bases of a behavioral approach to alcohol abuse. The remainder of the chapter is then given over to a review of the encouraging efforts of those who have developed behaviorally-based treatment programs to combat the Nation's number one public health problem.

* Preparation of this chapter was facilitated by NIAAA Research Grants AA00259 (to P.E.N.) and AA02898 (to M.S.G.).

Behavioral Perspectives on Problem Drinking and Alcoholism

PERSONALITY FACTORS AS EXPLANATORY VARIABLES

Earliest psychological efforts to trace the etiology of alcoholism were predominantly derived from psychodynamic theory. Consequently, they emphasized relationships between personality traits and types and development of the disorders. Overseers of this early work, however, were generally forced to conclude that these data were conflicting and, overall, that they revealed no specific personality trait or type as a consistent predictor of alcoholism (Armstrong, 1959; Sutherland, Schroeder, and Tordella, 1950; Syme, 1957). More recently, additional researchers (Cahalan and Room, 1972) have reached similar negative conclusions, while others have investigated the role of newly defined personality traits in this continuing quest. For example, McClelland, Davis, Kalin, et al. (1972) have suggested that individuals with power needs are particularly vulnerable to alcohol excess because alcohol can provide temporary satisfaction for such needs. Methodological deficiencies (for example, reliance on projective personality tests, which have been shown to have limited reliability and validity) weaken these claims, however. More promising are studies using sophisticated factor analytic techniques to identify a number of personality types associated with alcoholism (Nerviano, 1976; Skinner, Jackson, and Hoffman, 1974).

The utility of personality terms remains limited, however, due both to their imprecision and their inability to identify specific controlling variables and targets for intervention. Further use of such constructs encourages reification of intervening variables and diminishes the potency of situational factors shown to be highly predictive of a variety of behaviors (Mischel, 1968, 1973). Behavioral researchers, as a consequence, have tended to avoid use of such terms. Emphasized, instead, is the view that alcohol use and alcoholism may be most profitably conceptualized as acquired behaviors.

TENSION REDUCTION HYPOTHESIS: THE FIRST BEHAVIORAL EXPLANATION

The first—and still most influential—behavioral explanation of the etiology of alcoholism is the "tension-reduction" hypothesis. This hypothesis is based upon the common observation that alcohol appears to reduce anxiety. This being so, alcohol is presumed to reinforce drinking by alcoholics, many of whom are assumed to maintain high prevailing levels of anxiety. Formal, empirical support for the hypothesis derived from early (Conger, 1951, 1956; Masserman and Yum, 1946) and more recent studies of experimentally induced conflict in animals (Freed, 1967; Smart, 1965). The tension-reduction hypothesis has not, however, received universal support. Cappell and Herman (1972), for example, extensively reviewed a variety of (animal) analog studies of the tension-reduction hypothesis from the vantage points of avoidance and escape learning, conflict and experimental neurosis, conditioned suppression, extinction and partial reinforcement, stress and behavioral disruption, psychophysiological studies, and human self-report and risk-taking. Despite the magnitude of this effort, the conclusion was simple: the only studies providing consistent empirical support for the hypothesis were those exploring conflict situations. Brown and Cutter (1977), in a subsequent analysis of conflict studies, concluded that even they do not support a tension-reduction hypothesis, since closer approach to a bivalent goal after alcohol administration may actually increase conflict (because of increased strength of both approach and avoidance tendencies closer to the goal). Reviews of tension reduction research with human subjects also suggest the inadequacy of the simple tension-reduction view of alcohol effects (Cappell, 1974; Marlatt, 1975; Mello, 1972). In this context, Cappell and Herman (1972) observed that even if tension reduction is one of the reinforcing consequences of alcohol, it does not necessarily represent every individual's prime motivation to drink.

However, the recent research on alcohol and expectancy reviewed below suggests that the tension-reduction hypothesis may have viability for humans, although its impact in this regard may be far more complex than originally anticipated.

The failure of the tension-reduction hypothesis to achieve empirical support leads us to conclude that no simple behavioral mechanism suffices to explain the development and maintenance of excessive drinking. Both the pharmacological effects of alcohol itself and numerous intero- and exteroceptive cues and reinforcers not directly a function of these effects must also be considered in this context. The task that remains is the explication of these mechanisms. Although the task has just begun, real progress now appears to be in the making.

EXPECTANCY AND THE PHARMACOLOGICAL EFFECTS OF ALCOHOL

Recent research has, for the first time, explored the pharmacological effects of alcohol independently of alcohol expectancy (placebo) effects in a methodologically sophisticated fashion. This work suggests that a complex interaction of factors determines what many have long considered to be simply the pharmacological effects of alcohol. These factors include the actions of the drug on physiological functioning, the individual's expectancy of what the effects of the drug will be, his/her prior history of drug use, and the environment in which the ingestion takes place.

Marlatt, Demming, and Reid (1973), building on work by Engle and Williams (1972), first showed clearly the potency of alcohol expectancy effects by demonstrating that alcoholic subjects' drinking was determined by the *belief* that they were drinking alcohol rather than by the pharmacological effects of that consumption. First "priming" alcoholics with a single dose of beverage and then, under the guise of a "taste-testing" experiment, allowing subjects to regulate their own beverage consumption for 15 minutes, Marlatt and his colleagues orthogonally manipulated the actual beverage consumed (alcohol or tonic-placebo) with what subjects were told (i.e., that they were being given alcohol or that they were being given plain tonic) in a 2×2 design. Results were clear: actual consumption was determined by subjects' expectations, not by actual alcohol content. In the same context, at about the same time, it is also significant that Ludwig, Wikler, and Stark (1974) found that craving by alcoholics may be as sensitive to expectancy effects as is consumption itself.

As intriguing was the demonstration by Pliner and Cappell (1974) that the capacity of alcohol to serve as a euphoriant is determined in part by situational cues. Administering alcohol (to a blood alcohol level of 0.05%) or placebo to nonalcoholic subjects, these investigators then required subjects to complete a "creativity" task in small groups or alone. Subjects in groups revealed more positive affect on both self-report and observational measures when they had consumed alcohol. By contrast, subjects who completed the task alone showed no significant differences in self-reported affect between the alcohol and placebo conditions. For self-reported physical symptoms, the effect was reversed; solitary subjects reported more such symptoms while drinking alcohol, while subjects in groups reported no differences in symptoms between alcohol and placebo conditions. Following Schachter's (1964) two-factor model of drug effects, Pliner and Cappell (1974) concluded that alcohol induces behavioral "plasticity" such that actual behavioral effects depend on situational and cognitive—rather than strictly pharmacological—factors.

Other recent work has also demonstrated similar complex interactions vis-à-vis the effects of alcohol on anxiety. Specific to this question are the results of a series of studies using a variant of Marlatt's 2×2 design by Polivy and her associates. In this research, nonalcoholic subjects were told they were receiving alcohol (whether or not they actually did) or vitamin C (whether or not they did). In an initial study (Polivy, Schueneman, and Carlson, 1976), anxiety was induced by threatening subjects with electric shock. Although alcohol reduced consequent anxiety more than did placebo, those subjects who believed they had received alcohol were more anxious than those who believed they had received vitamin C. A second study (Polivy and Herman, 1976) investigating the effects of alcohol on eating also reported that when subjects thought they were consuming alcohol, they experienced more subjective anxiety than when they thought they had received vitamin C (even though they had actually received an equivalent alcohol dose). This study also suggested that the belief that alcohol had been consumed disinhibited normally restrained eating behavior—but inhibited normally unrestrained eating behavior! From these two sets of results, Polivy and her colleagues concluded that, independent of the influence of expectancy effects, alcohol acts as a sedative; with expectancy effects operating, however, alcohol may actually induce dysphoria in certain situations, including the laboratory setting. This conclusion is consistent with the findings of Steffen, Nathan and Taylor (1974), who monitored both self-ratings and electromyographs of alcoholics every 2 hours over 12 days of laboratory drinking by four alcoholics. They found that although muscle activity decreased as blood alcohol level (BAL) increased, subjective distress increased with BAL. Thus, even though alcohol itself appeared to act as a physiological tension-reducer, subjective and behavioral effects actually reflect tension increase.

The effects of alcohol on aggressive behavior appear to be as complex—and as subject to expectancy effects, despite the long-standing popular belief that alcohol always increases aggressivity. This complexity was portended by conflicting findings from a number of studies indicating that alcohol induces aggression (Boyatzis, 1974; Shuntich and Taylor, 1972), does not induce aggression (Bennett, Buss, and Carpenter, 1969; Smith, Parker, and Noble, 1975), or can either induce or inhibit depending on dose (Taylor and Gammon, 1975). An initial study attempting to determine the role of expectancy in the effect of alcohol on aggression (Lang, Goeckner, Adesso, et al., 1975) employed both a placebo disguised as alcohol and alcohol disguised as a nonalcoholic beverage. Aggressive behavior was found to be largely a function of expectancy, even at the substantial 0.10% BAL used in this study: subjects who thought they had consumed alcohol betrayed aggression regardless of whether or not they had actually done so while those who thought they had consumed tonic water did not emit aggressive behavior regardless of actual beverage consumed.

Expectancy factors also influence the impact of alcohol on both subjective and objective measures of sexual arousal. To this end, Wilson and Lawson (1976a,b) reported that both men and women experienced higher levels of sexual arousal when they believed they had consumed alcohol (whether or not they had actually done so) than when they thought they had consumed tonic water; at the same time, both Wilson and Lawson (1976b) and Briddell and Wilson (1976) observed that alcohol actually decreases both penile and vaginal responses to erotic atimuli. Once again, subjective alcohol effects have been shown to be relatively independent of physiologically induced alcohol effects.

Another instance of the complexity of factors influencing the behavioral effects of alcohol is provided by recent research relating alcohol and pain. In one of the most telling of these studies, Cutter, Maloof, Kurtz, et al. (1976) subjected both alcoholics and nonalcoholics to a cold pressor (pain-inducing) test before administration of 0.326 ml/kg of alcohol, 30 minutes after alcohol administration, and 30 minutes later, after a second dose double the first. Alcoholic subjects experienced a subjective decrease in pain that accelerated with dosage while nonalcoholics reported no decrease in pain. Since the groups did not differ in physiological responsivity to pain, the subjective pain reduction the alcoholics experienced must have been a function of expectancy factors interacting with the interoceptive cues of the increased dosage. Brown and Cutter (1977) then went on to test nonalcoholics' pain responses to finger pressure and cold pressor tests before and after administration of a low (0.32 g/kg) or high (0.63 g/kg) alcohol dose or a placebo. Subjects also completed a questionnaire asking about their customary drinking habits. Results showed that alcohol effects were strongly influenced by prior drinking habits. For example, while superior pain reduction was generally associated with the higher alcohol dose in solitary drinkers, that dose actually *increased* the pain experienced by subjects who usually drank at home with family or friends. In other words, alcohol expectancies were mediated by prior drinking patterns, as well as by interoceptive cues associated with differing dosages.

That interoceptive cues produced by different dosages influence expectancies has been confirmed recently by Williams and Goldman (1978). These two researchers reported that subjects showed fewer signs of intoxication on a variety of self-report and psychomotor tests at BAL's of 0.06% when they thought they had ingested alcohol than when they were led to believe they had consumed only tonic. This effect was not present at BAL's of 0.03%, at which alcohol expectancies impaired performance.

In sum, the behavioral effects of alcohol clearly result from a complex interaction of factors. Among those factors are the expectancies one holds about alcohol's effects on behavior. Although we know that these expectancies influence the behavioral effects of alcohol, there remains the question of whether expectancies only produce effects when they interact with alcohol (Pliner and Cappell, 1974) or whether they can produce certain effects in the absence of alcohol (Lang et al., 1975). Expectancy itself is as complex; it is related to belief systems, prior drinking experience, the immediate physical and social setting of drinking, dosage levels, and the rise and fall of the BAL curve. Such complexity suggests that the potential reinforcing capabilities of alcohol, manifold indeed, still remain to be clarified.

"TRADITIONAL" AND CONTEMPORARY SOCIAL LEARNING CONCEPTIONS OF ALCOHOLISM

There is also considerable evidence that alcohol use is both cued and reinforced by factors other than the real or anticipated effects of alcohol itself. To this end, the work of Jessor and his associates (Jessor, Collins, and Jessor, 1972; Jessor and Jessor, 1975) confirms that introduction to alcohol use is an integral and important part of adolescent peer-group interactions. O'Leary, O'Leary, and Donovan (1976) have even suggested, for that matter, that prealcoholics can be identified by their deficits in social skills during adolescence. A number of laboratory studies of drinking by alcoholics have also implicated a wide range of social stimuli as both cues and reinforcers for drinking (cf. Nathan, 1976; Nathan and Briddell, 1977) while, in the natural environment, Miller, Hersen, Eisler, et al. (1974) have shown that when alcoholics are subjected to the interpersonal stress of having to make assertive responses, they are more likely to turn to alcohol than are social drinkers. Similarly, imitation of a role model has also been shown to increase drinking in male social drinkers (Caudill and Marlatt, 1975).

Perhaps the most thorough and articulate explication of the "traditional" social learning view of alcoholism—the position which sees the disorder as a function of classical and operant conditioning mechanisms, the basic modes of learning—is summarized in the following excerpt from a longer position paper:

> Within a social-learning framework alcohol and drug abuse are viewed as socially acquired, learned behavior patterns maintained by numerous antecedent cues (classical conditioning) and consequent reinforcers (operant conditioning) that may be of a psychological, sociological, or physiologic nature. Such factors as reduction in anxiety, increased social recognition and peer approval, enhanced ability to exhibit more varied, spontaneous social behavior, or the avoidance of physiological withdrawal symptoms may maintain substance abuse (Miller and Eisler, 1975, p. 5).†

More recently, social learning theorists and researchers have modified their views on etiology and treatment to encompass cognitive variables. This alteration in theory and practice reflects emerging data, much of it generated by alcohol researchers, suggesting the power of expectations—cognitions—about the effects of alcohol on behavior and the effects of behavior change procedures on maintenance of treatment gains. The point these writers (Marlatt, 1978; Wilson, 1978) make most convincingly and eloquently is the following: what the alcoholic or prealcoholic tells himself or herself alcohol will do for him or her may be as important as what it actually does in determining whether or not he or she drinks to excess. And, by the same token, what the alcoholic thinks about his or her own capacity to utilize a particular treatment approach may determine more than the specifics of the intervention itself: the extent to which it will enable the alcoholic to moderate his or her drinking. Deceptively simple when reduced in this way, the impact of cognitions on behavior remains a focal point of behavioral research within and beyond alcoholism and drug abuse.

THE ROLE OF BEHAVIORAL PSYCHOLOGY—CONCLUSION

The bottom line of this review is that behavioral factors can definitely be ruled *in* in the etiology of alcoholism, although the controlling variables are far from completely understood. As a guide for future research, Goldman (1977) has suggested that four questions remain to be answered in the quest for understanding alcohol use and alcoholism: (1) Why do humans initiate drinking? (2) How is drinking maintained past the first drink? (3) How does drinking accelerate in some individuals? (4) What

† From Miller, P. M., and Eisler, R. M. Alcohol and drug abuse. In W. E. Craighead, A. E. Kazdin, and M. J. Mahoney (Eds.), *Behavior modification principles, issues, and application.* Boston: Houghton Mifflin, 1975. Copyright © 1975 by Houghton Mifflin Co. Reprinted by permission.

leads certain individuals to consume alcohol in patterns that may be associated with physical and social deterioration?

If behavioral theorists do not have all the answers to these important questions, that they can pose them—and have some research strategies and tactics for addressing them—is clearly a step in the right direction.

Behavioral Treatment of Problem Drinking and Alcoholism

TREATMENT GOALS

Until very recently, virtually everyone who treated alcoholics believed in only one goal for that treatment—total, complete, and permanent abstinence. This almost universal agreement reflected the widespread conviction that alcoholism is a physical disease which is characterized by craving for alcohol during periods of sobriety and loss of control over drinking during periods of intoxication, as well as neurological, gastrointestinal, cardiac, and hematologic disorders secondary to the excessive consumption.

Besides the life-threatening consequences of continued alcohol consumption, there are several other good reasons for choosing abstinence as the sole goal of treatment for alcoholism. The disease model of alcoholism—which posits that alcoholism is a physical disease—justifies the abstinence criterion because one cannot, obviously, allow a sick person access to the agent which causes the sickness. As important, abstinence is an exquisitely simple treatment goal to define and monitor. One is either abstinent or one is not; there are no degrees of abstinence. As well, abstinence is appropriate for all alcoholics; one would certainly not want one's alcoholic taxi driver, airplane pilot, surgeon, or accountant to strive for anything else. Finally, for those alcoholics whose alcoholism is accompanied by serious physical sequelae, a treatment goal that does not aim for abstinence is life-threatening—and, hence, unethical.

Given the impressive weight of these arguments, why has controlled social drinking engendered so much recent interest? In our judgment, controlled social drinking as an alternative goal of alcoholism treatment is viable for the following compelling reasons:

1) Some alcoholics drink normally—in controlled fashion—for substantial periods of time either spontaneously or following treatment.

2) Successful treatment for alcoholism, apparently, does not always have to be oriented toward abstinence.

3) Some alcoholics experience far greater personal distress during periods of abstinence than when they are drinking.

4) The disease model of alcoholism, built on its corollaries, loss of control and craving, does not seem to have firm basis in empirical fact.

A substantial literature, for the most part appearing during the last 10 years, now suggests that some alcoholics—precisely how many is uncertain—adopt patterns of controlled social drinking either spontaneously or following treatment (Miller and Caddy, 1977; Sobell, 1978). While many alcoholics maintain such a pattern for only a brief time before lapsing into uncontrolled consumption (Chalmers, 1978; Keller, 1978), the volume of reports of controlled drinking by alcoholics dating from publication in 1962 of Davies' follow-up of 93 recovered "alcohol addicts" to the present (Orford, Oppenheimer, and Edwards, 1976; Pattison, Sobell, and Sobell, 1977; Sobell and Sobell, 1973a) is certainly impressive. On the other hand, recent, comprehensive critical reviews of this literature (Emrick, 1975; Hamburg, 1975; Lloyd and Salzberg, 1975; Nathan and Briddell, 1977; Nathan and Lansky, 1978; Pomerleau, Pertschuk, and Stinnett, 1976) conclude that many of these reports and studies share conceptual and methodological shortcomings, some sufficient to render their findings suspect. Among them are those caused by small sample size, inadequate follow-up, incomplete assessment of drinking behavior during the follow-up period, inaccurate initial diagnosis of alcoholism, and imprecise definition of "controlled drinking" post-treatment.

The same criticisms have been leveled at the notorious "Rand Report" (Armor, Polich, and Stambul, 1976), a national survey of approximately 14,000 clients of 44 federally funded Alcoholism Treatment Centers. The notoriety of the survey derived from neglect of its major finding—that 70% of clients who completed treatment improved their drinking status at 6- and 18-month follow-ups—in favor of the following secondary finding:

> ... the improved clients include only a relatively small number who are long-term abstainers. About one-fourth of the clients interviewed at 18 months have abstained for at least 6 months ... the majority of improved clients are either drinking moderate amounts of alcohol—but at levels far below what could be described as alcoholic drinking—or engaging in alternating periods of drinking and abstention (Armor et al., 1976, p. v.).‡

The Rand Study, as both its critics and admirers have pointed out, was imperfect. Most of its follow-up assessments were based on patients' self-reports, criticized by many as unreliable and self-serving. Further, improvements in psychological functioning, job performance, family adjustment, and drinking behavior were not assessed directly; instead, these changes were inferred from behaviors *associated with* these important measures of functioning. Finally, more emphasis was placed on the import of improvements in drinking status as a measure of therapeutic efficacy than on improvement in other areas of life functioning, a decision which can also be questioned. However, the Rand Study also had important strengths. A very large group of geographically and demographically diverse clients was surveyed. Relatively sophisticated sampling procedures designed to ensure the representativeness of the sample were employed. Survey instruments which sampled a broad range of behaviors relevant to alcoholism were developed. The study succeeded in following 2000 subjects at the 6-month mark and over 600 at 18 months. Finally, the survey planned and carried out pre- and post-treatment comparisons of subjects' functioning in a variety of spheres, in that way accounting appropriately for initial differences among subjects in level of functioning. In our judgment, the Rand survey stands as a representative model of modern survey methodology; evaluated in that context, we take its findings seriously.

‡ From Armor, D. J., Polich, J. M., and Stambul, H. B. *Alcoholism and treatment.* Santa Monica, Calif.: Rand Corporation, 1976. Reprinted by permission of John Wiley & Sons, Inc.

Three separate behavioral approaches to development of controlled drinking have been reported during the past several years. All three—blood alcohol level discrimination training, broad-spectrum behavior therapy, and contingency management—are reviewed in detail later in this chapter. As a result, we will only note here that proponents of all three approaches claim that their techniques can change uncontrolled alcoholic drinking into controlled social drinking *in some alcoholic subjects for some length of time.* Unfortunately, these enthusiasts do not answer two additional crucial questions: How many alcoholics? For how long a time?

The widespread belief that craving and loss of control invariably accompany abusive drinking, a view held by those who consider alcoholism to be a physical disease, has also been questioned on empirical grounds. For example, studies have (1) reported that alcohol given to sober alcoholics in disguised form sometimes fails to induce craving for the drug (Cutter, Schwaab, and Nathan, 1970; Marlatt et al., 1973; Merry, 1966), (2) concluded that the terms are poorly understood and poorly defined (Hodgson, Rankin, and Stockwell, 1978), and (3) demonstrated that many alcoholics can modify their drinking on receiving appropriate contingent reinforcement for doing so (Gottheil, Crawford, and Cornelison, 1973; Marlatt, 1978; Nathan and O'Brien, 1971; Strickler, Bigelow, Lawrence, et al., 1976). If craving and loss of control are not universal phenomena, the question of general validity of the physical disease model of alcoholism must be raised.

The long-held view that the alcoholic who achieves abstinence is bound to experience improvement in other areas of functioning has also been challenged recently by Miller and Caddy (1977) and Pattison (1976), among others. Both cite an impressive number of studies which show that

> ... the use of total abstinence as the outcome criterion of alcoholism treatment is misleading. It may be associated with improvement, no change, or deterioration in other critical areas of total life health (Pattison, 1976, p. 180).

We believe that the data reviewed in this section of this chapter, together with the convictions of those who hold diametrically opposed views on the question of treatment goals, necessitate the following moderate —but constructive—view of the issue of choice of treatment goals:

1) Abstinence ought to be the initial goal of treatment for alcoholism. Most of us function better when we are sober. Abstinence-oriented treatment clearly works for some patients while the success rate of controlled drinking-oriented treatment is less certain. Certain death follows the decision of many chronic alcoholics to resume or continue drinking.

2) Sober alcoholics must not be led to believe that they can ever drink in controlled fashion; present data do not support the validity of this goal.

3) Alcoholics who have repeatedly tried and failed to achieve abstinence, who despair of ever doing so, and who are nonetheless physically able to drink moderately ought to be considered candidates for controlled drinking-oriented treatment because *controlled social drinking, while less desirable than abstinence, is nonetheless more desirable than uncontrolled asocial drinking.*

4) Above all, what is required, before a rational decision on treatment goal can be made for anyone, is additional comparative research on the long-term efficacy of abstinence-oriented and controlled drinking-oriented treatment. How such research might be designed is suggested elsewhere (Briddell and Nathan, 1976; Nathan, 1976; Nathan and Briddell, 1977; Nathan and Lansky, 1978; Nathan and Lipscomb, 1979).

UNIDIMENSIONAL BEHAVIORAL TREATMENT PROCEDURES

ELECTRICAL AVERSION. Electrical aversion has been closely associated through the years with behavior therapy—and, especially, with the behavioral treatment of alcoholism—because of the apparent success of Soviet physician N. V. Kantorovich's pioneering use of it more than 50 years ago. In fact, to many nonbehavioral people, electrical aversion and behavior therapy were synonymous for many years. After pairing the sight, taste, and smell of beverage alcohol with painful electric shock, Kantorovich reported that 70% of his small group of alcoholic subjects had remained abstinent during follow-up periods ranging from 3 weeks to 20 months. Control subjects given hypnotic suggestion or medication did not do as well.

Given this history, it is ironic that electrical aversion has now proven itself, in the eyes of many, to be an ineffective treatment. Despite the promise of Kantorovich's findings, it was not until the decade of the 1960's that behavioral investigators and clinicians returned to electrical aversion as a treatment for alcoholic behavior. Although most of those using the procedure, including McGuire and Vallance (1964), Blake (1965), MacCulloch, Feldman, Orford, et al. (1966) and Sandler (1969), reported varying degrees of "success," critical evaluation of their research designs reveals small numbers of subjects, short follow-up periods, relatively small proportions of patients maintaining abstinence, and the absence of direct efforts to assess development of actual conditioned aversion to ethanol. Further, and in some ways most important, none of these studies incorporated a control group that was offered a "standard" comparative treatment.

During the late 1960's and early 1970's, more sophisticated research designs were used by those studying electrical aversion. Control groups were employed, more subjects were studied, and better measures of outcome were used. Studies completed from this perspective included those by Vogler and his colleagues (1970, 1971), who reported encouraging short-term abstinence data but disproportionate losses of subjects from electrical aversion treatment groups, by Miller, Hersen, Eisler, et al. (1973), who reported no difference in posttreatment alcohol consumption by experimental and control subjects on Miller's "taste test," and by Hedberg and Campbell (1974), who compared four separate behavioral treatment approaches and reported that electrical aversion, unlike behavioral family counseling, systematic desensitization, and covert sensitization, had no apparent impact on drinking by alcoholic subjects.

Vogler and his colleagues have since investigated the efficacy of four different multifaceted treatment packages, one including electrical aversion, with alcoholics (Vogler, Compton, and Weissbach, 1975) and problem drinkers (Vogler, Weissbach, Compton, et al., 1977b). They report equivocal results: the short-term positive changes in drinking rate they observed across groups could not be attributed to any single component of the treatment package, including electrical aversion.

A convincing demonstration of the apparent ineffectiveness of electrical aversion as a treatment for alcoholism was Wilson, Leaf, and Nathan's (1975) direct test of the widespread presumption that electrical aversion conditioning establishes a conditioned aversion to ethanol. On receiving a large number of aversion conditioning trials extending over several days, their alcoholic subjects were then permitted to drink *ad libitum* in a laboratory setting which neither encouraged nor discouraged that consumption. Results? Subjects drank with undiminished enthusiasm, just as they had during a comparable *ad libitum* period pretreatment. Wilson and his co-workers concluded, predictably, that conditioned aversion had not been established by the aversion conditioning procedure.

Wilson (1978a) concluded a comprehensive review of the electrical aversion literature with a statement with which we are in full agreement: " . . . the evidence on the efficacy of electrical aversion conditioning . . . is overwhelmingly negative. Its use as a treatment modality with alcoholics should be discontinued." Continuing his discussion beyond this point, Wilson went on to question the continued use of electrical aversion on two other bases, conceptual and ethical. By conceptual Wilson referred to the naive assumption made by some that electrical aversion ought to be the treatment of choice for alcoholism because it suppresses the excessive drinking that *is* the disorder; this approach to alcoholism treatment unfortunately fails to attend to the diverse antecedent, mediational, and consequent variables—interpersonal, socioeconomic, psychological—that play crucial roles in the disorder. Wilson's ethical concerns about electrical aversion refer to the essential impossibility of obtaining truly informed consent to its use by many of the individuals to whom it has customarily been offered. Some of these persons are coerced into treatment, effectively removing all possibility of freely given consent. Moreover, even those who are not cannot be expected to weigh for themselves the conflicting data on the efficacy of electrical aversion, necessary before truly informed consent to a therapeutic procedure is possible.

Systematic Desensitization. "Treatment of choice" by many behavior therapists for neurotic behavior, systematic desensitization has rarely been employed alone as treatment for alcoholism. When it has been so used, by Kraft and Al-Issa (1967) and Kraft (1969), it was not associated with significant changes in drinking, although it did appear to reduce, at least for a time, the anxiety that often accompanies alcoholism. Systematic desensitization has also been incorporated within broad-spectrum treatment programs (Pomerleau, Pertschuk, Adkins, et al., 1978a,b) where it appears to be of value in helping patients deal with anxiety and tension. However, by itself, systematic desensitization appears to be ineffective as treatment for a disorder as multifaceted as alcoholism.

MULTIDIMENSIONAL BEHAVIORAL TREATMENT PROCEDURES

Chemical Aversion. A series of reports describing chemical aversion to treat alcoholism were published during the 1940's and 1950's by Voegtlin, Lemere and their colleagues at the Shadel Hospital in Seattle. Except for a recent report by Wiens and colleagues working at the Raleigh Hills Hospital in Portland, Oregon (1976), few additional clinical reports on chemical aversion—positive or negative—have appeared in the literature. This surprising lack of interest in a treatment as promising as chemical aversion probably derives in large part from much stronger and longer lived interest among behavioral clinicians in electric shock as a means of conditioning aversion to ethanol because of the latter's attractiveness on both theoretical and traditional grounds (Nathan and Briddell, 1977; Wilson, 1978).

Procedures followed at the Shadel Hospital were detailed by Voegtlin (1940), Lemere and Voegtlin (1950), and Lemere, Voegtlin, Broz, et al. (1946). In brief, patients were hospitalized for approximately 10 days, during which five treatment sessions were scheduled on alternate days. They took place in rooms designed to minimize distractions and maximize the salience of a large array of alcoholic beverages. To begin a conditioning session, an emetine-pilocarpine-ephedrine mixture was administered intravenously; it produced nausea within 2 to 8 minutes. At earliest signs of nausea, the patient was given a drink of his/her preferred beverage to smell and taste. Additional drinks were given over a 30-minute to 1-hour period as nausea and vomiting persisted. "Booster" reconditioning sessions were also offered to all patients at any time they felt the urge to drink subsequent to original conditioning and, routinely, at 6 and 12 months after initial treatment.

Outcome data on the first 13 years of treatment at the Shadel Hospital, based on follow-up data from 4096 of 4468 patients treated, yielded a most impressive follow-up rate of 92% of original patients successfully followed. Forty-four percent of these patients had remained totally abstinent through 2 to 13 years; an additional 7% had relapsed and then been successfully re-treated. Viewed another way, 60% of these patients had been abstinent for 1 year, 51% for 2 years, 38% for 5 years, and 23% for 10 years.

These encouraging outcome data are remarkably similar to those few reports by other facilities offering chemical aversion treatment. After 7 years of emetine conditioning treatment at the Washingtonian Hospital in Boston, Thimann (1949) reported a total success rate of 51% of patients located for follow-up, a figure identical to that of Lemere and Voegtlin. Similarly, Wiens, Montague, Manaugh, et al. (1976) reported that 63% of 261 alcoholic patients treated by emetine conditioning at Raleigh Hills Hospital in Portland were abstinent after 1 year, results strikingly similar to the 1-year figure of 60% cited by Lemere and Voegtlin. This figure is even more impressive since the Portland group considered patients who could not be located for follow-up as treatment failures.

Why are these outcome data so much better than those from other unidimensional approaches to alcoholism? And, accordingly, why haven't they precipitated a rush to establish more chemical aversion treatment facilities? Two responses to these questions come readily to mind. First, patients who chose chemical aversion programs must have substantial private financial resources or health insurance to pay for the costly inpatient treatment; as a result, most such patients are either recently or still employed. Recent or current employment, in turn, suggests that the individual retains a modicum of ability to function adequately in the world. That these patients are drawn from markedly higher educational and socioeconomic levels than alcoholics treated elsewhere also indicates their superior treatment potential. It is also clear that, to complete a chemical aversion treatment sequence, patients must be very highly motivated to change their drinking behavior since the treatment is extremely unpleasant. In short, a largely homogeneous group of highly motivated, relatively young, largely intact alcoholics has benefitted from chemical aversion. To assume, perforce, that patients widely disparate from this group would also benefit from chemical aversion is a decision clinicians treating other groups of alcoholics have apparently been unwilling to make to this time.

It is also true that chemical aversion was not the only treatment provided Shadel and Raleigh Hills patients, that the treatment provided these patients was not, in fact, unidimensional. Rehabilitation and personal counseling, family therapy, active cooperation with local Alcoholics Anonymous groups, and a warm, supportive inpatient milieu were all regular components of the therapy package offered at these facilities. This being so, it makes good sense to temper one's enthusiasm in the face of the encouraging outcome data reported by these facilities with the sobering realization that chemical aversion alone might not have been responsible for the positive outcomes attributed to it. By the same token, although definitive proof that chemically induced nausea produces a reliable aversion to alcohol in humans does not exist, it is nonetheless true that inpatient treatment facilities offering identical treatment packages except for chemical aversion have not reported equally positive outcome data. On the other hand, when Burt (1974) interviewed 34 patients who had relapsed an average of 18 months after completing the

Shadel program, only 5 of them reported nausea or fear before their first drink, suggesting that a conditioned aversion had not developed. Similarly, Voegtlin (1947) acknowledged that some of his patients did not develop alcohol aversions despite vomiting during the conditioning process.

These latter data not withstanding, we believe that chemical aversion is effective in the context of a multidimensional treatment program accompanied by adjunctive counseling and attention to social support systems and followed by booster sessions.

Blood Alcohol Level Discrimination Training. Australians Lovibond and Caddy developed a BAL discrimination training program in 1970 as a means to modify directly the uncontrolled drinking of alcoholics. The ambitious goals of their pilot treatment program were, first, to train alcoholics to discriminate a range of intoxication levels and, then, to maintain their drinking at moderate levels over extended periods of time. During an initial discrimination training phase of their pilot study, patients drank to BALs of 80 mg/100 ml while observing their subjective-visceral reactions to changing intoxication levels. Patients were required repeatedly to estimate their intoxication level at the same time, after which they were given accurate feedback on BAL. When BAL discrimination training was over, patients drank to—then beyond—a moderate BAL (65 mg/100 ml) while continuing to give BAL estimates and to receive feedback. BAL control training consisted of painful electric shock delivered to subjects whenever they drank when their BALs were in excess of 65 mg/100 ml. A control group of matched alcoholics received random, non-contingent shocks. Of 28 patients who completed their experimental treatment, 21 were drinking in "controlled fashion, exceeding 70 mg/100 ml BAL only rarely," 4 or more months after treatment.

This encouraging result must be viewed cautiously, however, for a variety of reasons. First, the follow-up was both very brief and based in large part on patients' self-reports. Second, the use of electric shock to condition a discriminated aversion to alcohol is of questionable utility in view of previously cited research pointing to the apparent ineffectiveness of shock in this context. Finally, no attempt was ever made to determine whether patients could reliably monitor BAL once accurate BAL feedback was removed. As a result, it is impossible to know whether the successful outcomes Lovibond and Caddy reported were due to the maintenance of BAL discrimination ability—as they assumed—or to the demand characteristics implicit in virtually every new treatment program.

More recently, Caddy and Lovibond (1976) undertook to examine the relative contributions of electric shock, BAL discrimination training, and "training in self-regulation" to a multidimensional treatment program. Alcoholic patients were divided into three treatment groups. The first group received BAL discrimination training, discriminated aversion conditioning, and training in self-regulation. The second group was given BAL discrimination and self-regulation training, while patients in the final group were given BAL discrimination training and discriminated aversion but not self-regulation training. Rated on their success in maintaining a controlled drinking pattern after treatment, patients in the first group ("aversion plus self regulation") were judged to be significantly more improved than either of the other two experimental groups at the 6-month mark.

Although the studies of Lovibond and Caddy suggest that short-term improvement in alcoholics' drinking is associated with treatment which includes BAL discrimination training, they do not clarify the part this training actually played in the successful outcomes observed. And, as before, their research does not prove that alcoholics can actually discriminate BAL from internal cues once the external cue of accurate feedback is removed.

Research at the Alcohol Behavior Research Laboratory, Rutgers University, has since addressed this important clinical issue by studying the processes by which both alcoholics and nonalcoholics inform themselves of their level of intoxication. In the first of these studies, Silverstein, Nathan, and Taylor (1974) looked closely at alcoholics' ability to acquire and maintain BAL discrimination accuracy. An initial baseline period revealed the four alcoholic subjects of the study to be extremely inaccurate in their untrained BAL estimations. Like the subjects of Lovibond and Caddy, however, these subjects sharpened their discrimination accuracy dramatically when external feedback on BAL was provided during the discrimination training period. When feedback was again withdrawn during a second baseline period, however, accuracy deteriorated markedly. Subjects were required to drink *ad libitum* to a target BAL of 80 mg/100 ml during the second, control training phase of this study. However, subjects could not moderate their drinking, although all had received extensive BAL discrimination training for this purpose, until feedback on BAL was again provided. When this was done, subjects monitored BAL well enough to moderate their drinking as requested. These results suggested to Nathan and his colleagues that alcoholics can only acquire and maintain BAL discrimination skills when they receive some form of occasional external feedback on BAL. Accordingly, these researchers asked whether anyone, alcoholic or not, can be trained to discriminate BAL on the basis of internal cues alone.

Huber, Karlin, and Nathan (1976) directly addressed this issue by comparing the effectiveness of internal and external BAL discrimination training provided a group of 36 male social drinkers. All subjects were first required to give estimates of BAL at several intervals during an initial programmed drinking sequence. They were then matched for discrimination accuracy and assigned to one of three training groups. Subjects receiving internal training completed body-function checklists and self-report instruments designed to teach them to associate a variety of internal sensations and feelings with a range of BAL's. Externally trained subjects were trained to calculate BAL's from a programmed booklet which taught dose-strength-time-metabolism relationships. Subjects receiving internal plus external training were given both kinds of training. All subjects were then retested for BAL estimation accuracy during a final test session. Unlike the alcoholic subjects studied previously by Silverstein and his co-workers, these nonalcoholic subjects did learn to estimate BAL on the basis of both internal and external cues.

Lansky, Nathan, and Lawson (1978) then undertook a direct test of this apparent difference between alcoholics and nonalcoholics by comparing the results of external and internal training provided matched groups of alcoholics. As expected, all subjects made highly inaccurate pretraining BAL estimates. However, when they were retested for estimation accuracy following training, the alcoholic subjects who had received external cue training estimated BAL's significantly more accurately than they had before training, while subjects trained to use internal cues barely improved in accuracy. These findings confirmed an hypothesis first put forth by Silverstein et al. (1974) and subsequently refined by Huber et al. (1976)—that alcoholics have a fundamental deficit in the ability to discriminate blood alcohol levels on the basis of internal cues: To explain this deficit, Nathan and his colleagues had proposed a variety of hypotheses. Alcoholics cannot utilize internal cues to BAL, he and his co-workers speculated in their early papers, because of inherited dysfunction of internal receptors, damage to them from the toxic effects of circulating ethanol, or the impact of tolerance on the receptors' sensitivity to changing level of alcohol in the blood.

All of these hypotheses were tested for the first time in a recent study by Lipscomb and Nathan (in press). Twenty-four nonalcoholic subjects selected to fall into four experimental groups on the basis of usual drinking pattern (heavy vs. light) and familial alcoholism (present in parent(s) vs. absent) received internal cue training according to the usual baseline-training-testing sequence of three experimental sessions. Following initial assessment of discrimination ability, subjects were then grouped according to body sway when intoxicated. Recognized as an extremely sensitive measure of intoxication, body sway has also been proposed recently as an accurate and reliable measure of tolerance to ethanol (Moscowitz, Daily, and Henderson, 1974). It is presumed that persons who show substantial differences in body sway during sobriety and intoxication have acquired little or no tolerance to the effects of ethanol while those who show little or no such differences have acquired at least moderate tolerance to ethanol. Results of this study by Lipscomb and Nathan were that groups differing in drinking pattern or familial alcoholism did not differ in the ability to utilize internal cues to BAL. By contrast, when subjects were grouped according to performance on the body sway tolerance measure, "low tolerance" subjects were significantly better able to employ internal cues to BAL than were "high tolerance" subjects. In other words, these results supported the hypothesis that the alcoholic's shifting tolerance levels prevent him from using internal cues to BAL which nonalcoholics can use to good effect.

The clinical significance of these findings seems clear. Therapeutic applications of BAL discrimination training should utilize an external dose-time-metabolism training method (like that developed by Huber et al., 1976, for example), in that way helping alcoholics make accurate estimates of BAL in the natural environment. Whether BAL discrimination training methods, promising at this time, ultimately prove more useful than existing or potential treatment methods, of course, remains to be determined by empirical means.

Operant Procedures Including Contingency Contracting. "Contingency contracting" is the technical term for a behavior modification procedure familiar to every parent: arriving at an agreement with a child that performance of a desired behavior, or modification or elimination of an unwanted behavior will result in a consequence that is rewarding to the child. Contingency contracting differs from the other operant behavior change methods described in this section in only one essential: contingency contracts involve formal contracts, agreed upon by patient and therapist, specifying both the behaviors to be emitted or eliminated and the reinforcing consequences to be provided for doing so. The other operant change procedures, by contrast, do not involve before-the-fact specification of expected behavior changes; instead the power of available reinforcers to effect free (operant) behavior change is anticipated even though the precise form of the change is not specified beforehand.

Both formal and informal treatment for alcoholism has always involved contingencies. The alcoholic whose spouse threatens to forsake their union if drinking continues is being subjected to a punishment contingency, as is the employee who is told that he/she will lose a job if he/she continues to drink. Young clinicians often marvel at the surprising in effectiveness of such powerful contingencies, at the fact that alcoholics continue to drink in the face of such devastating consequences. A behavioral explanation of this paradox contains these two elements: (1) What may appear to be punishing to an outside observer may actually be rewarding—or, at least, not punishing—to the alcoholic; (2) A contingency is maximally effective in clinical situations only when based on mutual agreement, carefully observed and consistently adhered to; spouses and employers rarely observe contingency contracts with the consistency necessary for full effectiveness.

"Community Reinforcement Counseling." The "community reinforcement counseling" program developed by Hunt and Azrin (1973), later modified by Azrin (1976), first provided chronic alcoholic inpatients with focused behavioral training designed to improve long-standing vocational, interpersonal, and familial problems. Role-playing, behavior rehearsal, structured practice, and cognitive restructuring (changing of attitudes and beliefs about the appropriateness and effectiveness of certain behaviors) were all employed in this intensive reeducation effort. When treatment resulted in more successful interactions with family, job, and friends, these new-found reinforcers could then be incorporated into a contingency management program by which patients, once again living outside the hospital, were allowed continued access to them contingent on sobriety. At a 6-month follow-up, eight alcoholic patients who had received community reinforcement counseling were found to have spent significantly less time drinking, unemployed, away from home, or institutionalized than eight other alcoholics provided only the hospital's standard therapy program.

Azrin's subsequent modification of the community reinforcement counseling method led to equally favorable outcome data. The following modifications were made in the basic contingency format: (1) 11 experimental clients were given Antabuse to reduce the possibility that impulsive drinking would destroy the contingency contract; (2) a regular reporting system, relying on clients, family, friends, and employers, was instituted to provide "early warning" of drinking or other problems; (3) a neighborhood "buddy," a source of continuing social support outside professional counseling, was trained for peer-advisement; (4) to reduce the amount of expensive professional time required for individual counseling, group counseling was begun; group sessions took place at intervals of about every two months.

It is generally recognized that every therapist strives to help his or her alcoholic patients function more effectively at home and at work in the belief that increased satisfaction with family and job will reduce dependence upon alcohol for all of life's pleasures. Why, then, do so few alcoholics in traditional therapy but so many in Azrin's program change their drinking patterns, given that both treatments focus on improvements in family and job functioning as requisites to successful treatment? Two factors may account for the relative success of Azrin's community reinforcement counseling: (1) Specific reeducation techniques for heightening effectiveness in family and vocational spheres were "targeted." By contrast, traditional therapy concentrates on achievement of insight into behavioral problems or on efforts to "improve communication" between family members without attending to specific and fundamental gaps in knowledge about how to behave in the family and on the job. (2) The understandable reluctance on the part of many therapists to struggle to improve family or job functioning and then to withhold access to them when the patient drinks. To do so, however, is to emphasize to the patient that functioning socially is more important—and can be more reinforcing—than alcohol.

CONTINGENCY CONTRACTING WITH "PUBLIC DRUNKENNESS OFFENDERS." Miller successfully employed contingency contracting (1975) with alcoholic men even more debilitated than those treated by Azrin and Hunt. Choosing 20 "public drunkenness offenders" from the Jackson, Mississippi, city jail, Miller agreed with 10 of these men to provide them a broad range of goods and services in exchange for "demonstrated attempts to control their drinking" on their release from jail. The other 10 men were control subjects who received the same goods and services whether or not they drank.

> Housing was arranged through an agreement with the Salvation Army. Normally, this agency will only allow sober individuals to board for two days. Under a special agreement, any of the subjects could be housed or fed, or both, at this agency for the duration of the program.... Employment was obtained primarily through Manpower and the Mississippi State Employment Service.... If a subject were in need of medical assistance, arrangements were made with either the Veterans Administration Hospital or the University Hospital to treat him.... Clothing was obtained via the Salvation Army Store, Goodwill Industry Store or donations to the program. Subjects eligible for veterans assistance could be provided with canteen booklets exchangeable for cigarettes, meals, or clothing at the Veterans Administration Hospital.... Subjects also received counseling sessions geared toward advising them on numerous practical problems in life, such as money management (Miller, 1975, p.916).§

Experimental subjects were denied access to reinforcers for 5 days whenever their blood alcohol levels, measured at unpredictable intervals "on the street," exceeded 10 mg/100 ml during the 2 months the program was in force. The 10 subjects who were given these material reinforcers contingently significantly decreased mean number of arrests and rate of drinking and significantly increased mean number of hours employed per week; the 10 control subjects showed essentially no changes in any of these behaviors.

Perhaps the most encouraging aspect of this treatment program was its ability to bring about change in alcohol-related behavior in chronic skid-row men whose alcoholism had previously proven inaccessible to modification by other techniques. Surprisingly, it was *contingent* access to goods and services which had previously been available to these men on a *noncontingent* basis that brought about the change.

CONTINGENCY CONTRACTING AND OPERANT STUDIES AT THE BALTIMORE CITY

§ From Miller, P. M. A behavioral intervention program for chronic public drunkenness offenders. *Arch. Gen. Psychiatry*, 1975, *32*, 915–918. Copyright © 1975, American Medical Association.

HOSPITALS. Extremely detailed analyses of the effects of contingent reinforcement and punishment have been consistent goals of a research program at the Baltimore City Hospitals (summarized by Griffiths, Bigelow, and Liebson, 1978). Bigelow's successful effort to induce abstinence in four Baltimore City Hospitals' employees in danger of being fired for drinking on the job was the group's first effort to use natural contingencies for therapeutic purposes (Bigelow, Liebson, and Lawrence, 1973). Required by contract to report daily to the hospital's Alcoholism Treatment Unit to receive disulfiram (Antabuse), the four agreed that failure to report would result in no work and no pay. The contingency produced marked improvements in all employees' job performance and attendance. Similarly, Bigelow, Strickler, Liebson, et al. (1976) reported that outpatient alcoholics required to report regularly to the same clinic for Antabuse in order to receive small installments of funds they had initially deposited with the clinic made substantial improvements in drinking pattern over the course of their contracts. And at the same institution, Liebson, Bigelow, and Flame (1973) drew up contracts with nine heroin addicts simultaneously abusing alcohol. The contracts specified that each man would be maintained on methadone as long as he continued to take disulfiram and, in that way, to maintain alcohol abstinence. The treatment was surprisingly successful with patients notoriously difficult to treat: patients drank on only 1.4% of days that methadone maintenance was contingent on disulfiram ingestion but on 19.2% of days that it was not.

The same group (Cohen, Faillace, Liebson, et al. 1971; Bigelow, Griffiths, and Leibson, 1974; Griffiths et al., 1978) has also demonstrated that chronic alcoholic inpatients will voluntarily moderate their alcohol intake (e.g., by drinking no more than 5–7 ounces of beverage alcohol a day when much more is available) when reinforcement is contingent on doing so and punishment or loss of reinforcement on not doing so. Among the reinforcers and punishers these researchers have explored have been enriched vs. impoverished ward living environments, weekend passes and special ward privileges vs. no passes and limited privileges, moderate alcohol on a subsequent drinking day vs. no alcohol on that day and usual socialization privileges vs. brief periods of interpersonal isolation.

EVALUATION OF CONTINGENCY CONTRACTING. Contingency contracting, almost certainly the most effective way to implement an operant behavior change program, has shown real promise as a means to manage the behavior of alcoholics in outpatient settings effectively. So long as reinforcement for continued sobriety is more powerful than alcohol itself—and a surprisingly large number of elements in the alcoholic's world seem to be—the alcoholic can be helped to moderate or terminate his/her drinking in this way.

BROAD-SPECTRUM BEHAVIORAL APPROACHES

In 1965, when virtually all behavioral approaches to alcoholism focused solely on modifying the maladaptive drinking response itself, Arnold Lazarus, then and now an influential behavior therapist, suggested instead that a "broad-spectrum" approach to alcoholism might work far better. Among the separate elements of Lazarus' revolutionary treatment package were the following: (1) medical attention to alcohol-related physical problems; (2) aversion conditioning to modify or eliminate abusive drinking; (3) behavioral assessment, to identify "specific stimulus antecedents of anxiety preparatory to systematic desensitization;" (4) assertive training, to better equip the patient to respond more appropriately to interpersonally stressful social situations; (5) behavioral rehearsal, to develop more adaptive and effective interpersonal skills; (6) hypnosis, "to countercondition anxiety-response habits;" (7) marital therapy, to help the patient's spouse modify his or her central role in the patient's alcoholism. The broad-spectrum behavior therapy packages described in this section of this chapter, developed years after Lazarus' paper, nonetheless follow his suggestions in amazing detail, even while they also permit ongoing assessment of efficacy not contemplated by Lazarus.

THE IBTA STUDY. Convinced that alcoholism, like other voluntary (operant) behaviors, is under the control of its environmental consequences, Mark Sobell and his wife Linda, both psychologists, designed a broad-spectrum behavioral treatment package called "individualized behavior therapy for alcoholics" (IBTA) in the early 1970's. The IBTA study they subsequently carried out has since become both well-known and controversial because its findings were that patients receiving IBTA drank in controlled fashion significantly more frequently than control patients 1 and 2 years post-treatment.

Elements of IBTA included the following:

All experimental treatment sessions focused directly on drinking behavior, tailoring the treatment as specifically as possible to meet each individual's needs, and emphasizing helping the subject identify the functions of excessive drinking and develop alternative, more beneficial ways of dealing with those situations.... The vast majority of IBTA treatment sessions can most accurately be termed "behavior change training sessions." The sequence of these sessions incorporated a four-stage process: (1) Problem Identification—Subjects were trained to identify the specific circumstances which had in the past and were likely in the future to result in drinking that would have adverse consequences for the individual; (2) Identification of Alternative Responses to Drinking—Subjects were assisted in generating a series of behavioral options to be used when confronted with problem situations; (3) Evaluation of Alternatives—Subjects were taught how to evaluate each of these behavioral options in terms of their short-term and, especially, long-term effects; (4) Preparation to Engage in the Best Behavioral Alternative—Subjects then practiced the alternative responses which could reasonably be expected to incur the least self-damaging long-term consequences in each instance. Various procedures and behavioral techniques, specific to each individual case, were used to accomplish this objective (Sobell, 1978, p. 158–159).‖

Initial outcome data, reported in 1973 (Sobell and Sobell, 1973b), revealed that both groups of experimental subjects (one trained for abstinence, the other for controlled drinking) achieved levels of functioning, including levels of alcohol ingestion, superior to their respective control groups at both the 6-month and 1-year marks. These data were based on follow-up information from 69 of the study's original 70 subjects, an impressive follow-up retention rate. At the end of the 2nd follow-up year, experimental subjects with the assigned treatment goal of controlled drinking were continuing to function better than their controls while the experimental, nondrinker subjects were doing better, but not significantly better, than their controls (Sobell and Sobell, 1976). A third-year, independent, double-blind follow-up of 53 of the study's original 70 subjects (Caddy, Addington, and Perkins, 1978) revealed a pattern similar to that of the 2nd-year data: comparison of the controlled drinking experimental group with its control group showed significantly better functioning of subjects in the experimental condition on both drinking and other life functioning measures; comparison of the nondrinking groups, however, revealed differences between groups only in nondrinking-related measures.

The IBTA study's experimental design, conceptual basis, and fundamental aims have been both roundly criticized and widely lauded. The study's critics have questioned the ethics of controlled drinking treatment in the absence of data attesting to its efficacy, the dual status of the lone follow-up worker (L. C. Sobell) as co-investigator, and heavy reliance on patient self-reports as principal sources of followup information. The study's advocates point to the unusually large number of alcoholic subjects selected, treated, and followed to the end of the 2-year follow-up mark, to the innovative nature of the broad-spectrum behavioral treatment program that was employed, and to the courage of two young investigators in choosing to study as controversial a subject as controlled drinking. Greater detail in criticism of this study is provided by Emrick (1975), Hamburg (1975), Nathan and Briddell (1977), and Nathan and Lansky (1978).

Integrated Behavior Change Techniques for Problem Drinkers and Alcoholics. Recent papers describe a set of "integrated behavior change techniques"

‖ From Sobell, M. B. Empirically derived components of treatment for alcohol problems: Some issues and extensions. In G. A. Marlatt and P. E. Nathan (Eds.), *Behavioral approaches to alcoholism.* (NIAAA-RUCUS Alcoholism Treatment Series, No. 2) New Brunswick, N.J.: Rutgers Center of Alcohol Studies, 1978. Reprinted by permission from Journal of Studies on Alcohol, Inc.

used with some success to treat groups of alcoholics and problem drinkers by Vogler and his colleagues (1975, 1977a,b) in the Los Angeles area. An unusual aspect of this work is that it reports on a set of therapeutic procedures first developed with inpatient alcoholics (Vogler et al., 1975), later used to modify the drinking of a group of problem drinkers who were outpatients. Of interest too is the fact that Vogler's treatment package bears strong resemblance to that developed by the Sobells for the earlier IBTA study. Since Roger Vogler and Mark Sobell worked together for a time at the Patton State Hospital, the similarity in their treatment packages is hardly surprising. More important is the support Vogler's data give to the combination of broad-spectrum treatment procedures first assembled by the Sobells. In principal, the Vogler studies make an additional important contribution: The "unpackaging" research design they chose was supposed to permit assessment of the relative contribution to treatment success of the several components of the total treatment package. In practice, however, the actual pattern of findings did not allow these planned comparisons.

Among the "integrated behavior change techniques" tested by Vogler were the following: videotaped self-confrontation of drunken behavior (to increase motivation for therapy); discrimination training for blood alcohol concentration (to enable subjects to judge with increased accuracy their level of intoxication, in order to maintain their drinking at more moderate levels); aversion training (to establish conditioned aversion to alcohol); discriminated avoidance practice, with painful electric shock given for overconsumption (to shape the initial conditioned aversion to alcohol so that it becomes specific to overconsumption); alternatives training and behavioral counseling (to help patients develop alternative incompatible responses to the setting events that previously occasioned overdrinking); and alcohol education.

Two matched groups of chronic hospitalized alcoholics were compared in the first investigation of the efficacy of this broad-spectrum treatment package (Vogler et al., 1975). One group of 23 men received the whole treatment package over approximately 45 days. A second group of 19 men, whose treatment lasted about half as long, received only alternatives training, behavioral counseling, and alcohol education. Subjects in both groups attended booster treatment sessions once a week during the month following treatment, then once a month for a year.

Number of subjects who had remained abstinent or were drinking in controlled fashion between each follow-up contact, a gross measure of outcome, failed to discriminate between the two subject groups. Sixty-five percent of patients in both groups met that criterion. A finer outcome measure, however, revealed that patients in the full-treatment group had consumed significantly less ethanol, reflected in ounces per month, than those in the partial-treatment group at the one-year follow-up period. By contrast, changes in preferred beverage or preferred locus of consumption and in number of days lost from work pre- and post-treatment failed to differentiate between the two groups. The same pattern of group differences were observed at the 18-month follow-up mark (Vogler et al., 1977a).

Four groups of problem drinkers participated in another trial of Vogler's integrated behavior change techniques (Vogler et al., 1977b). Subjects were considered problem drinkers if they had never been diagnosed alcoholic or been hospitalized for alcohol-related problems but had nonetheless consumed alcohol in sufficient quantities to produce legal, marital, and/or vocational problems. Eighty of an original pool of 409 subjects were followed to the 1-year follow-up mark. Sixty percent of the 409 either failed to meet selection criteria or were unwilling to participate in the program after an initial contact, while an additional 14% either dropped from treatment or could not be located for follow-up. Of these 80, 23 received the full complement of integrated behavior change techniques (Group 1), 19 were given blood alcohol level discrimination training, behavioral counseling, alternatives training, and alcohol education (Group 2), 21 received only alcohol education (Group 3), and 17 were provided behavioral counseling, alternatives training, and alcohol education (Group 4).

The treatment goal for all subjects was a moderation in drinking pattern; 50 of the 80 subjects completing treatment and follow-up had achieved this goal at the 1-year follow-up mark while another three subjects had maintained abstinence over the same period. Unexpectedly, treatment group membership was not associated with differential outcomes. The investigators explain these findings by pointing to variability among subjects in pretreatment drinking rates and social characteristics, to dependence upon self-reports by subjects for most of the outcome data, and to the strong learning orientation to treatment that subjects in all four groups were given, a factor that may have increased the motivation of all to change drinking patterns.

These findings call into question the value of the specialized behavioral treatment procedures provided subjects in Groups 1 and 2; if they added nothing to outcome, do they deserve to be maintained in broad-spectrum treatment regimens in view of their expense and requirement for skilled workers for their application? Nonetheless, one must also be impressed by the numbers of subjects in this study drinking more moderately at the 1-year follow-up mark, even if many or most of them would not ever have progressed to clinical alcoholism. Success in helping such individuals develop more moderate patterns of alcohol consumption is significant. It represents "secondary prevention" (Caplan, 1964) in a field that has had to settle for "tertiary prevention"—the least effective, most expensive kind—almost exclusively to this time.

Behavioral Treatment for Middle-Income Problem Drinkers. Pomerleau and his colleagues at the University of Pennsylvania School of Medicine recently provided broad-spectrum behavior therapy to a group of problem drinkers as different from those treated by Vogler and his colleagues as Vogler's subjects were from the chronic alcoholics to whom the Sobells earlier offered IBTA. Drinkers who met strict criteria which guaranteed their membership in the middle class, Pomerleau's patients were almost certainly more highly motivated for treatment, more intact intellectually, socially, and emotionally, and possessed of greater familial, vocational, and economic resources than any other group of broad-spectrum behavior therapy patients studied to this time.

Pomerleau's subjects were selected (1) after agreeing to attend regular treatment and follow-up sessions and to follow detailed treatment protocols and (2) on proving free from serious psychopathology. Thirty-two subjects participated in the first trial of the new treatment package. Eighteen of these problem drinkers were randomly assigned to behavioral treatment and 14 to "traditional" treatment. Both behavioral and traditional therapy were provided groups of three to seven problem drinkers for 90 minutes once a week for 3 months, then for five additional sessions programmed at increasing intervals for another 9 months (Pomerleau, Pertschuk, Adkins, et al., 1978a,b). Treatment included the following four overlapping phases:

Baseline. An interview designed to elicit a detailed drinking history and to provide information on the treatment program accompanied assessment of a prepaid treatment fee (on a sliding scale from $500 to $85, based on ability to pay). Up to $300 as a "commitment fee" was also requested at this time; this sum could be earned back if the subject followed all treatment instructions. Subjects were also instructed to keep a detailed record of alcohol consumption as well as to identify the circumstances which characteristically led to excessive drinking.

Reduction in Drinking. Following these treatment "preliminaries," subjects chose daily quotas for a week's worth of drinking at a time as well as final treatment goals. The treatment emphasis was placed on gradual, steady improvement rather than rapid but variable change. A treatment goal of moderate drinking rather than abstinence was allowed if a subject requested it, had shown some control over his or her drinking during the recent past, and there were no medical contraindications to his continued drinking. For such subjects, the final goal of this phase of the study was 3 days a week of abstinence and consumption of no more than 3 ounces of ethanol on days when drinking was permitted and no more than 10 ounces of ethanol a week overall (the "3-3-10 rule"). Abstinence-oriented subjects set similar interim goals but the final goal of abstinence within 2 weeks. To alter customary drinking patterns, subjects were taught stimulus control and contingency management techniques to enable them (1) to identify both appropriate and inappropriate drinking circumstances (e.g., drinking with the family at dinner rather than with co-workers at a tavern after work), (2) to delay or disrupt maladaptive drinking patterns (e.g., holding a glass filled with a soft drink at a cocktail party), (3) to increase the likelihood of not drinking in designated situations (e.g., choosing not to attend those gatherings at which heavy drinking by others will take place), and (4) to preplan (specifying consumption in advance of a scheduled event).

Behavior Therapy for Associated Behavioral Problems. During this phase of the program, identification and alteration of associated behavioral problems having the capacity to affect drinking behavior was undertaken. Assertion training, systematic desensitization, and deep muscle relaxation were among the behavioral techniques employed to deal with such associated problems as anger, anxiety, depression, and marital and vocational dysfunction. Behavior rehearsal, modeling, and family counseling were also added to this effort to confront problems associated with the patient's maladaptive drinking.

Maintenance of Therapeutic Gain. Patients were encouraged to develop interests in activities (hobbies, physical exercise, academic work) which can be pursued alcohol-free, in order to maintain therapeutic gains. New friends, rather than old drinking companions, were also to be found. Toward the end of this phase of treatment, contact with the therapist was gradually phased out in order to maintain the forward thrust of therapy for as long as possible.

Traditional treatment offered subjects in this study was designed to last as long and be as intensive as the behaviorally oriented treatment; it did not, however, require prepaid commitment fees nor were refunds made available. An introductory phase, lasting three sessions and devoted to development of a sense of group cohesion and mutual trust among group members, launched this treatment. Total abstinence was strongly encouraged; denial patterns were identified. The second, confrontation phase of therapy lasted six or seven sessions; it focused on development of insight into the nature of personal denial mechanisms. The third, resolution phase, lasting two or three sessions, was the time to channel the intense emotions generated in the preceding phase of treatment into productive, future-directed activity; during the same phase, adjunctive psychotherapy for depression, anxiety, family problems, etc., was provided. During the five remaining sessions of this treatment, supportive therapy for nondrinking continued.

Traditional and behavioral treatment were both provided by professionals experienced in the treatment mode they offered. Of 18 patients treated behaviorally, 16 remained in treatment throughout; by contrast, of 14 patients treated by traditional procedures, only eight remained to the end of the treatment. For those participants who remained in therapy, drinking rate decreased significantly from screening to the end of the follow-up year for both treatments. Significantly fewer behavioral participants dropped out of treatment. These data suggest an advantage for behavioral over traditional treatment: even though subjects in both groups who stayed in therapy decreased drinking rate, significantly more behavioral than traditional subjects stayed with treatment. On the other hand, it is impossible to identify the variables in behavioral treatment responsible for this outcome difference since the two treatments differed so completely: extratreatment factors like prepaid commitment fees and monetary penalties for dropping from treatment were not part of traditional therapy, and subjects in the traditional group could only aspire to abstinence while those in the behavioral group could aim either for abstinence or controlled drinking. It is also worth noting that the traditional treatment offered subjects in this study was undoubtedly superior to the standard hospital milieu "treatment" offered subjects in most other comparative treatment studies, making the difference in retention rates between the two treatments that much more impressive.

Behavioral Medicine, Alcoholism, and Problem Drinking: A Brief Overview

Behavioral approaches to alcoholism have generated a multitude of spoken and written words over the past decade. Some have been paeans, some, perjoratives.

The contributions of the behavioral way of viewing and treating alcoholics derive, above all, from the fundamental respect for empirical data it seeks to instill. Complementing this exaltation of objective proof is persistent effort to phrase every unanswered question in such a way that its answer can come from research conducted according to the rules of scientific evidence. Opinion, unproven hypothesis and conjecture, in short, have no place in the behavioral approach to alcoholism. Of more immediate practical value are the efforts of behavioral researchers and clinicians to intervene: development of multidimensional treatment packages, exploration of alternative treatment goals, debunking of old ways of treating alcoholics which have little or no demonstrable efficacy are all signal contributions to alcoholism treatment.

Those who have criticized behavioral approaches to alcoholism have done so largely on the basis of the latter efforts. Some of these criticisms have been apt. When most deserved, these criticisms have centered on instances in which behavior therapists have transgressed their own fundamental precept by *going beyond their data.* Behavioral clinicians who proclaim preemptively that controlled social drinking is the best goal for all alcoholics, who concentrate their behavior change efforts on maladaptive drinking because it can be readily quantified, instead of including the alcoholic's associated behavioral deficits and excesses in a treatment package, or who contrast a new behavioral procedure with an old and ineffective one, thereby proving the superiority of the former—all have forsaken a precious birthright.

The basic tenets of a behavioral approach to alcoholism remain as valid now as they were when Kantorovich undertook to evaluate his electrical aversion treatment, Voegtlin and Lemere gathered their carefully documented outcome data attesting to the power of chemical aversion, and their spiritual descendents developed novel behavioral treatment packages which they then subjected to searching evaluation. What is required now is translation of a proven strategy into an effective tactic.

References

Armor, D. J., Polich, J. M., and Stambul, H. B. *Alcoholism and treatment.* Santa Monica, Calif.: Rand Corporation, 1976.

Armstrong, J. D. The search for the alcoholic personality. *Ann. Am. Acad. Polit. Soc. Sci.*, 1959, *315*, 40–47.

Azrin, N. H. Improvements in the community reinforcement approach to alcoholism. *Behav. Res. Ther.* , 1976, *14*, 339–348.

Bennett, R. M., Buss, A., and Carpenter, J. A. Alcohol and human physical aggression. *Q. J. Stud. Alc.*, 1969, *30*, 870–876.

Bigelow, G., Liebson, I., and Lawrence, C. Prevention of alcohol abuse by reinforcement of incompatible behavior. Paper presented at the annual meeting of the Association for Advancement of Behavior Therapy, December, 1973.

Bigelow, G., Liebson, I., and Griffiths, R. R. Alcoholic drinking: Suppression by a behavioral time-out procedure. *Behav. Res. Ther.*, 1974, *12*, 107–115.

Bigelow, G., Strickler, D., Liebson, I., and Griffiths, R. Maintaining disulfiram ingestion among outpatient alcoholics: A security deposit contingency contracting procedure. *Behav. Res. Ther.*, 1976, *14*, 378–381.

Blake, B. C. The application of behavior therapy to the treatment of alcoholism. *Behav. Res. Ther.*, 1965, *3*, 78–85.

Boyatzis, R. E. The effect of alcohol consumption on the aggressive behavior of men. *Q. J. Stud. Alc.*, 1974, *35*, 959–972.

Briddell, D. W., and Nathan, P. E. Behavior assessment and modification with alcoholics: Current status and future trends. In M. Hersen, R. M. Eisler, and P. M. Miller (Eds.), *Progress in behavior modification*, Vol. 2. New York: Academic Press, 1976.

Briddell, D. W., and Wilson, G. T. The effects of alcohol and expectancy set on male sexual arousal. *J. Abnorm. Psychol.*, 1976, *85*, 225–234.

Brown, R. A. and Cutter, H. S. Alcohol, customary drinking behavior, and pain. *J. Abnorm. Psychol.*, 1977, *86*, 179–188.

Burt, D. W. Characteristics of the relapse situation of alcoholics treated with aversive conditioning. *Behav. Res. Ther.*, 1974, *12*, 121–123.

Caddy, G. R., Addington, H. J., and Perkins, D. Individualized behavior therapy for alcoholics. A third year independent double-blind follow-up. Unpublished manuscript, 1978.

Caddy, G. R., and Lovibond, S. H. Self regulation and discriminated aversive conditioning in the modification of alcoholics' drinking behavior. *Behav. Ther.*, 1976, *7*, 223–230.

Cahalan, D., and Room, R. Problem drinking among American men aged 21–59. *Am. J. Public Health*, 1972, *62*, 1473–1482.

Caplan, G. *Principles of preventive psychiatry.* New York: Basic Books, 1964.

Cappell, H. An evaluation of tension models of alcohol consumption. In Y. Israel et al. (Eds.), *Research advances in alcohol and drug problems.* New York: Wiley, 1974.

Cappell, H., and Herman, C. P. Alcohol and tension reduction—A review. *Q. J. Stud. Alc.*, 1972, *33*, 33–64.

Caudill, B. D., and Marlatt, G. A. Modelling influences in social drinking: An experimental analogue. *J. Consult. Clin. Psychol.*, 1975, *43*, 405–415.

Chalmers, D. K. The alcoholic's controlled drinking time. Unpublished manuscript, 1978.

Cohen, M., Liebson, I. A., Faillace, L. A., and Allen, R. P. Moderate drinking by chronic alcoholics. *J. Nerv.*

Ment. Dis., 1971, *153*, 434–444.
Conger, J. J. The effects of alcohol on conflict behavior in the albino rat. *Q. J. Stud. Alc.*, 1951, *12*, 1–29.
Conger, J. J. Alcoholism: Theory, problem and challenge. II. Reinforcement theory and the dynamics of alcoholism. *Q. J. Stud. Alc.*, 1956, *14*, 291–324.
Cutter, H. S. G., Maloof, B., Kurtz, N. R., and Jones, W. C. "Feeling no pain." Differential responses to pain by alcoholics and non-alcoholics before and after drinking. *J. Stud. Alc.*, 1976, *37*, 273–277.
Cutter, H. S. G., Schwab, E. L., and Nathan, P. E. Effects of alcohol on its utility for alcoholics. *Q. J. Stud. Alc.*, 1970, *30*, 369–378.
Emrick, C. D. A review of psychologically oriented treatment of alcoholism. *J. Stud. Alc.*, 1975, *36*, 88–108.
Engle, K. B., and Williams, T. K. Effect of an ounce of vodka on alcoholics' desire for alcohol. *Q. J. Stud. Alc.*, 1972, *33*, 1099–1105.
Freed, E. The effect of alcohol upon approach-avoidance conflict in the white rat. *Q. J. Stud. Alc.*, 1967, *28*, 236–254.
Goldman, M. S. *Alcohol use and abuse: A behavioral perspective.* Teaneck, N.J.: Behavioral Sciences Tape Library, 1977.
Gottheil, E., Crawford, H., and Cornelison, F. S. The alcoholic's ability to resist available alcohol. *Dis. Nerv. Syst.*, 1973, *34*, 80–84.
Griffiths, R. R., Bigelow, G. E., and Liebson, I. The relationship of social factors to ethanol self-administration in alcoholics. In P. E. Nathan, G. A. Marlatt, and T. Løberg (Eds.), *Alcoholism: New directions in behavioral research and treatment.* New York: Plenum Press, 1978, pp. 351–380.
Hamburg, S. Behavior therapy in alcoholism: A critical review of broad-spectrum approaches. *J. Stud. Alc.*, 1975, *36*, 69–87.
Hedberg, A. G., and Campbell, L. A comparison of four behavioral treatments of alcoholism. *J. Behav. Ther. Exp. Psychiatry*, 1974, *5*, 251–256.
Hodgson, R., Rankin, H., and Stockwell, T. Craving and loss of control. In P. E. Nathan, G. A. Marlatt, and T. Løberg (Eds.), *Alcoholism: New directions in behavioral research and treatment.* New York: Plenum Press, 1978, pp. 341–350.
Huber, H., Karlin, R., and Nathan, P. E. Blood alcohol level discrimination by non-alcoholics: The role of internal and external cues. *J. Stud. Alc.*, 1976, *37*, 27–39.
Hunt, G. M., and Azrin, N. H. The community-reinforcement approach to alcoholism. *Behav. Res. Ther.*, 1973, *11*, 91–104.
Jessor, R., Collins, M. I., and Jessor, S. L. On becoming a drinker: Social-psychological aspects of an adolescent transition. *Ann. N.Y. Acad. Sci.*, 1972, *197*, 199–213.
Jessor, R., and Jessor, S. L. Adolescent development and the onset of drinking; a longitudinal study. *J. Stud. Alc.*, 1975, *36*, 27–51.
Keller, M. A nonbehaviorist's view of the behavioral problem with alcoholism. In P. E. Nathan, G. A. Marlatt, and T. Løberg (Eds.), *Alcoholism: New directions in behavioral research and treatment.* New York: Plenum Press, 1978, pp. 381–397.
Kraft, T. Alcoholism treated by systematic desensitization: A follow-up of eight cases. *J. R. Coll. Gen. Prac.*, 1969, *18*, 336–340.
Kraft, T., and Al-Issa, I. Alcoholism treated by desensitization: A case study. *Behav. Res. Ther.*, 1967, *5*, 69–70.
Lang, A. R., Goeckner, D. J., Adesso, V. T., and Marlatt, G. A. The effects of alcohol on aggression in male social drinkers. *J. Abnorm. Psychol.*, 1975, *84*, 508–518.
Lansky, D., Nathan, P. E., and Lawson, D. M. Blood alcohol level discrimination by alcoholics: The role of internal and external cues. *J. Consult. Clin. Psychol.*, 1978, *46*, 953–960.
Lazarus, A. A. Towards the understanding and effective treatment of alcoholism. *S. Afr. Med. J.*, 1965, *39*, 736–741.
Lemere, F., and Voegtlin, W. L. An evaluation of the aversion treatment of alcoholism. *Q. J. Stud. Alc.*, 1950, *11*, 199–204.
Lemere, F., Voegtlin, W. L., Broz, W. R., and O'Halloren, P. Conditioned reflex treatment of alcohol addiction. V. Type of patient suitable for this treatment. *North-West. Med. Seattle*, 1946, *4*, 88–89.
Liebson, I., Bigelow, G., and Flame, R. Alcoholism among methadone patients: A specific treatment method. *Am. J. Psychiatry*, 1973, *130*, 483.
Lipscomb, T. R., and Nathan, P. E. Effect of family history of alcoholism, drinking pattern, and tolerance on blood alcohol level discrimination. *Arch. Gen. Psychiatry*, in press.
Lloyd, R. W., and Salzberg, S. C. Controlled social drinking: An alternative to abstinence as a treatment goal for some alcohol abusers. *Psychol. Bull.*, 1975, *82*, 815–842.
Lovibond, S. H., and Caddy, G. R. Discriminated aversive control in the moderation of alcoholics' drinking behavior. *Behav. Ther.*, 1970, *1*, 437–444.
Ludwig, A. M., Wikler, A., and Stark, L. H. The first drink; psychobiological aspects of craving. *Arch. Gen. Psychiatry*, 1974, *30*, 539–547.
MacCulloch, M. J., Feldman, M. P., Orford, J. F., and MacCulloch, M. L. Anticipatory avoidance learning in the treatment of alcoholism: A record of therapeutic failure. *Behav. Res. Ther.*, 1966, *4*, 187.
Marlatt, G. A. Alcohol, stress, and cognitive control. Paper read at NATO-sponsored International Conference on Dimensions of Stress and Anxiety, 1975.
Marlatt, G. A. Craving for alcohol, loss of control, and relapse: A cognitive-behavioral analysis. In P. E. Nathan, G. A. Marlatt, and T. Løberg (Eds.), *Alcoholism: New directions in behavioral research and treatment.* New York: Plenum Press, 1978, pp. 271–314.
Marlatt, G. A., Demming, B., and Reid, J. B. Loss of control drinking in alcoholics: An experimental analogue. *J. Abnorm. Psychol.*, 1973, *81*, 233–241.
Masserman, J. H., and Yum, K. S. An analysis of the influence of alcohol and experimental neurosis in cats. *Psychosom. Med.*, 1946, *8*, 36–52.
McClelland, D. C., Davis, W. N., Kalin, R., and Warner, E. *The drinking man: Alcohol and human motivation.* New York: Free Press, 1972.
McGuire, R. J., and Vallance, M. Aversion therapy by electric shock, a simple technique. *Br. Med. J.*, 1964, *1*, 151–152.
Mello, N. K. Behavioral studies of alcoholism. In B. Kissen and H. Begleiter (Eds.), *The biology of alcoholism, Physiology and Behavior*, Vol. 2. New York: Plenum Press, 1972.
Merry, J. The "loss of control" myth. *Lancet*, 1966, *1*,

1267–1268.

Miller, P. M. A behavioral intervention program for chronic public drunkenness offenders. *Arch. Gen. Psychiatry*, 1975, *32*, 915–918.

Miller, P. M., and Eisler, R. M. Alcohol and drug abuse. In W. E. Craighead, A. E. Kazdin, and M. J. Mahoney, (Eds.), *Behavior modification principles, issues, and application*. Boston: Houghton Mifflin, 1975.

Miller, P. M., Hersen, M., Eisler, R. M., and Dilsman, G. Effects of social stress on operant drinking of alcoholics and social drinkers. *Behav. Res. Ther.*, 1974, *12*, 67–72.

Miller, P. M., Hersen, M., Eisler, R., and Hemphill, D. P. Electrical aversion therapy with alcoholics: An analogue study. *Behav. Res. Ther.*, 1973, *11*, 491–497.

Miller, W. R., and Caddy, G. R. Abstinence and controlled drinking in the treatment of problem drinkers. *J. Stud. Alc.*, 1977, *38*, 986–1003.

Mischel, W. *Personality and assessment*. New York: Wiley, 1968.

Mischel, W. Toward a cognitive social learning reconceptualization of personality. *Psychol. Rev.*, 1973, *80*, 252–283.

Moscowitz, H., Daily, J., and Henderson, R. *Acute tolerance to behavioral impairment of alcohol in moderate and heavy drinkers*. Report to the Highway Research Institute, National Highway Traffic Safety Administration, Department of Transportation, Washington, D.C. 1974.

Nathan, P. E. Alcoholism. In H. Leitenberg, (Ed.), *Handbook of behavior modification*. New York: Appleton-Century-Crofts, 1976.

Nathan, P. E., and Briddell, D. W. Behavior assessment and treatment of alcoholism. In B. Kissin and H. Begleiter (Eds.), *The biology of alcoholism*, Vol. 5. New York: Plenum Press, 1977.

Nathan, P. E., and Lansky, D. Management of the chronic alcoholic: A behavioral viewpoint. In J. P. Brady and H. K. H. Brodie (Eds.), *Controversy in psychiatry*. Philadelphia: W. B. Saunders, 1978.

Nathan, P. E., and Lipscomb, T. R. Behavior therapy and behavior modification in the treatment of alcoholism. In J. H. Mendelson and N. K. Mello (Eds.), *Diagnosis and treatment of alcoholism*. New York: McGraw-Hill, 1979.

Nathan, P. E., and Lisman, S. A. Behavioral and motivational patterns of chronic alcoholics. In R. E. Tarter and A. A. Sugerman (Eds.), *Alcoholism, interdisciplinary approaches to an enduring problem*. Reading, Mass.: Addison-Wesley, 1976.

Nathan, P. E., and O'Brien, J. S. An experimental analysis of the behavior of alcoholics and nonalcoholics during prolonged experimental drinking. *Behav. Ther.*, 1971, *2*, 455–476.

Nerviano, V. J. Common personality patterns among alcoholic males: A multivariate study. *J. Consult. Clin. Psychol.*, 1976, *44*, 104–110.

O'Leary, D. E., O'Leary, M. R., and Donovan, D. M. Social skill acquisition and psychosocial development of alcoholics: A review. *Addict. Behav.*, 1976, *1*, 111–120.

Orford, J., Oppenheimer, E., and Edwards, G. Abstinence or control: The outcome for excessive drinkers two years after consultation. *Behav. Res. Ther.*, 1976, *14*, 409–418.

Pattison, E. M. A conceptual approach to alcoholism treatment goals. *Addict. Behav.*, 1976, *1*, 117–192.

Pattison, E. M., Sobell, M. B., and Sobell, L. C. (Eds.), *Emerging concepts of alcohol dependence*. New York: Springer, 1977.

Pliner, P., and Cappell, H. Modification of affective consequences of alcohol: A comparison of social and solitary drinking. *J. Abnorm. Psychol.*, 1974, *83*, 418–425.

Polivy, J., and Herman, C. P. Effects of alcohol on eating behavior: Influence of mood and perceived intoxication. *J. Abnorm. Psychol.*, 1976, *85*, 607–610.

Polivy, J., Schueneman, A. L., and Carlson, K. Alcohol and tension reduction: Cognitive and physiological effects. *J. Abnorm. Psychol.*, 1976, *85*, 595–606.

Pomerleau, O. F., Pertschuk, M., Adkins, D., and Brady, J. P. A comparison of behavioral and traditional treatment for middle income problem drinkers. *J. Behav. Med.*, 1978a, *1*, 187–200.

Pomerleau, O., Pertschuk, M., Adkins, D., and d'Aquili, E. Treatment for middle income problem drinkers. In P. E. Nathan, G. A. Marlatt, and T. Løberg (Eds.), *Alcoholism: New directions in behavioral research and treatment*. New York: Plenum Press, 1978b, pp. 143–160.

Pomerleau, O. F., Pertschuk, M., and Stinnett, J. A critical examination of some current assumptions in the treatment of alcoholism. *J. Stud. Alc.*, 1976, *37*, 849–867.

Sandler, J. Three aversive control procedures with alcoholics: A preliminary report. Paper read at the annual meeting of the Southeastern Psychological Association, April, 1969.

Schachter, S. The interaction of cognitive and physiological determinants of emotional state. In L. Berkowitz (Ed.), *Advances in experimental social psychology*. New York: Academic Press, 1964.

Shuntich, R., and Taylor, S. The effects of alcohol on human physical aggression. *J. Exp. Res. Pers.*, 1972, *6*, 34–38.

Silverstein, S. J., Nathan, P. E., and Taylor, H. A. Blood alcohol level estimation and controlled drinking by chronic alcoholics. *Behav. Ther.*, 1974, *5*, 1–15.

Skinner, H. A., Jackson, D. N., and Hoffman, H. Alcoholic personality types: Identification and correlates. *J. Abnorm. Psychol.*, 1974, *83*, 658–666.

Smart, R. G. Effects of alcohol on conflict and avoidance behavior. *Q. J. Stud. Alc.*, 1965, *26*, 187–205.

Smith, R., Parker, E., and Noble, E. Alcohol and affect in dyadic interaction. *Psychosom. Med.*, 1975, *37*, 25–40.

Sobell, M. B. Empirically derived components of treatment for alcohol problems: Some issues and extensions. In G. A. Marlatt and P. E. Nathan (Eds.), *Behavioral approaches to alcoholism*. (NIAAA-RUCUS Alcohol Treatment Series, No. 2) New Brunswick, N.J.: Rutgers Center of Alcohol Studies, 1978.

Sobell, M. B., and Sobell, L. C. Individualized behavior therapy for alcoholics. *Behav. Ther.*, 1973a, *4*, 49–72.

Sobell, M. B., and Sobell, L. C. Alcoholics treated by individualized behavior therapy: One year treatment outcome. *Behav. Res. Ther.*, 1973b, *11*, 599–618.

Sobell, M. B., and Sobell, L. C. Second-year treatment outcome of alcoholics treated by individualized behavior therapy: Results. *Behav. Res. Ther.*, 1976,

14, 195–215.

Steffen, J. J., Nathan, P. E., and Taylor, H. A. Tension-reducing effects of alcohol: Further evidence and some methodological considerations. *J. Abnorm. Psychol.*, 1974, *83*, 542–747.

Strickler, D., Bigelow, G., Lawrence, C., and Liebson, I. Moderate drinking as an alternative to alcohol abuse: A non-aversive procedure. *Behav. Res. Ther.*, 1976, *14*, 279–288.

Sutherland, E. H., Schroeder, H. G., and Tordella, C. L. Personality traits and the alcoholic. *Q. J. Stud. Alc.*, 1950, *11*, 547-561.

Syme, L. Personality characteristics of the alcoholic. *Q. J. Stud. Alc.*, 1957, *18*, 288–301.

Taylor, S., and Gammon, C. The effects of type and dose of alcohol on human aggression. *J. Pers. Soc. Psychol.*, 1975, *32*, 169–175.

Thimann, J. Conditioned reflex treatment of alcoholism, II. The risk of its application, its indications, contraindications and psychotherapeutic aspects. *N. Engl. J. Med.*, 1949, *241*, 408–410.

Voegtlin, W. L. The treatment of alcoholism by establishing a conditioned reflex. *Am. J. Med. Sci.*, 1940, *199*, 802–809.

Voegtlin, W. L. Conditioned reflex therapy of chronic alcoholism: Ten years experience with the method. *Rocky Mountain Med. J.*, 1947, *44*, 807–812.

Vogler, R. E., Compton, J. V., and Weissbach, T. A. Integrated behavior change techniques for alcoholics. *J. Consult. Clin. Psychol.*, 1975, *43*, 233–243.

Vogler, R. E., Lunde, S. E., Johnson, G. R., and Martin, P. L. Electrical aversion conditioning with chronic alcoholics. *J. Consult. Clin. Psychol.*, 1970, *34*, 302–307.

Vogler, R. E., Lunde, S. E., and Martin, P. L. Electrical aversion conditioning with chronic alcoholics: Follow-up and suggestions for research. *J. Consult. Clin. Psychol.*, 1971, *36*, 450.

Vogler, R. E., Weissbach, T. A., and Compton, J. V. Learning techniques for alcohol abuse. *Behav. Res. Ther.*, 1977a, *15*, 31-38.

Vogler, R. E., Weissbach, T. A., Compton, J. V., and Martin, G. T. Integrated behavior change techniques for problem drinkers in the community. *J. Consult. Clin. Psychol.*, 1977b, *45*, 467–479.

Wiens, A. N., Montague, J. R., Manaugh, T. S., and English, C. J. Pharmacological aversive conditioning to alcohol in a private hospital: One year follow-up. *J. Stud. Alc.*, 1976, *37*, 1320–1324.

Williams, R., and Goldman, M. S. The parameters of the alcohol expectancy effect. Unpublished manuscript, Wayne State University, 1978.

Wilson, G. T. Alcoholism and aversion therapy: Issues, ethics and evidence. In G. A. Marlatt and P. E. Nathan (Eds.), *Behavioral Assessment and Treatment of Alcoholism.* New Brunswick, N.J.: Rutgers Center of Alcohol Studies, 1978a.

Wilson, G. T. Booze, beliefs, and behavior: Cognitive processes in alcohol use and abuse. In P. E. Nathan, G. A. Marlatt, and T. Løberg (Eds.), *Alcoholism: New directions in behavioral research and treatment.* New York: Plenum Press, 1978b, pp. 315–340.

Wilson, G. T., and Lawson, D. M. Expectancies, alcohol, and sexual arousal in male social drinkers. *J. Abnorm. Psychol.*, 1976a, *85*, 587–594.

Wilson, G. T., and Lawson, D. M. Effects of alcohol on sexual arousal in women. *J. Abnorm. Psychol.*, 1976b, *85*, 489–497.

Wilson, G. T., Leaf, R., and Nathan, P. E. The aversive control of excessive drinking by chronic alcoholics in the laboratory setting. *J. Appl. Behav. Anal.*, 1975, *8*, 13–26.

Behavioral Medicine and Beyond: The Example of Obesity*

ALBERT J. STUNKARD, M.D.
Professor
Department of Psychiatry
University of Pennsylvania School of Medicine
Philadelphia, Pennsylvania

12

Obesity occupies a central position in the concerns of behavioral medicine.

Historically, behavioral control of obesity was one of the first medical concerns to be subjected to intensive behavioral analysis.

Currently, more people are receiving behavioral treatment for obesity than are receiving behavioral treatment for all other conditions combined. The behavioral treatment of obesity, furthermore, has become the most common paradigm for research in behavioral treatment.

In the future, the path travelled in the development of behavioral approaches to obesity may well serve as a guide to the development of behavioral medicine—and beyond.

These are rash propositions. Let me support them, at first briefly, and then by devoting the rest of this chapter to the past, present, and future of the behavioral control of obesity.

The Past. In 1962, long before behavioral medicine had been conceived as a field of endeavor, Ferster, Nurnberger, and Levitt carried out what may still be the most detailed applied behavioral analysis of a health-related behavior in their now classic paper, "Behavioral Control of Eating." Although their therapeutic results were never published and are said to have been modest (Stunkard, 1975), this paper has informed and inspired a generation of workers in the field. As the first operant analysis of a health-related behavior to achieve wide recognition, it served as an important counterweight to the largely classical conditioning background of behavior therapy which then dominated the field as a result of the achievements of systematic desensitization.

The Present. Treatment of obesity by commercial weight reduction programs has recently been enriched by the introduction of behavior modification into the traditional group format. As a result, every week 400,000 people receive behavioral treatment for obesity under lay auspices, a number far in excess of those being treated by behavioral measures for all other conditions combined.

Research paradigms have recently been discussed by Bandura (1978) who writes eloquently of their value in the advancement of a research field, pointing out the virtues of the treatment of snake phobias as a standardized measure for the study of behavior therapy. It is thus worthy of note that obesity has supplanted snake phobias as a paradigm for therapeutic research. Even Bandura, who did so much to develop the methodology for studying snake phobias, is finding increasing use for this new model.

The Future. Behavioral measures for the control of obesity are already in advance of those for the control of many other disor-

* Preparation of this chapter was supported in part by National Institute of Mental Health Grant MH 31050-02.

ders and what we can see of future trends suggests that obesity may increasingly serve as a guide for the development of behavioral medicine. The experience with obesity has already made clear one trend—lay auspices and lay personnel can help clients to manage problems which had heretofore required "treatment" provided by professional therapists. One aspect of this trend has been to redefine the management of at least some interventions in health-related behaviors as education rather than treatment and the agents of this change as teachers rather than therapists. Another aspect of this trend has been to make clear that, however broad its application, it is still confined to what might be called clinical interventions or what Wynder and his colleagues have termed "individual preventive medicine" (Kristein, Arnold, and Wynder, 1977). The focus of these efforts is upon what people can be taught to help them preserve their health through their own initiative. Wynder has contrasted this approach to individuals to what he calls "managerial preventive medicine" which pertains to health risks that can be controlled through environmental management rather than by personal behavior. The influence of the Swedish "Diet and Exercise" Program described below, in changing the foods served in institutional cafeterias, is an example of managerial preventive medicine which has already proven its effectiveness.

A number of the measures proposed in this chapter are examples of managerial preventive medicine. They utilize behavioral principles and are concerned with health-related behaviors. Will they be viewed by a developing behavioral medicine as a part of its domain? Or will behavioral medicine retain its still largely clinical character?

A major contribution of obesity to behavioral medicine may be in helping to define the boundaries of this new discipline.

The First Steps: Behavioral Therapy with Individuals and Small Groups

Although the origins of behavioral attention to obesity go back to the aforementioned paper by Ferster et al. in 1962, it was a report by Stuart in 1967 that introduced the current widespread interest in the behavioral control of obesity and ignited a virtual explosion of research on the topic. This research has already given rise to 50 controlled clinical trials and at least five extensive reviews (Abramson, 1973; Jordan and Levitz, 1975; Stuart, 1976; Stunkard, 1975; Stunkard and Mahoney, 1976). The reasons for the sharp impact of Stuart's report are not hard to find: it described an effective treatment.

It has been, in the past, fairly easy to assess the effectiveness of any out-patient treatment for obesity because the results of traditional treatments have been so uniformly poor and the treatments so obviously ineffective. Only 25% of persons entering conventional out-patient treatment for obesity lose more than 20 pounds and 5% more than 40 pounds (Stunkard and McLaren-Hume, 1959).

Against this background, Stuart's report on "Behavioral Control of Overeating" (Stuart, 1967) stands out, for it describes the best results obtained to that time in the out-patient treatment of obesity and constitutes a landmark in our understanding of this disorder. Even the absence of a control group does not vitiate the significance of its findings. Figures 12.1 and 12.2 show that the 8 patients who remained in treatment out of an original 10 lost large amounts of weight: six lost more than 30 pounds and three of these lost more than 40 pounds.

A comprehensive description of behavioral treatments for obesity is beyond the scope of this report and the interested reader is referred to the extended descriptions of Mahoney and Mahoney (1976a,b) and of Stunkard and Mahoney (1976) and to the detailed manual by Ferguson (1975). Nevertheless, a brief description of some of the essential elements may be useful in conveying something of the nature of this effective new intervention. The program developed at the University of Pennsylvania (Penick, Filion, Fox, et al., 1971) was based upon that used by Stuart in his original study and is representative of the first generation of behavioral programs. Some later programs have been expanded to include important cognitive considerations, increased physical activity, and systematic nutrition education, but they do not appear to have materially increased the effective-

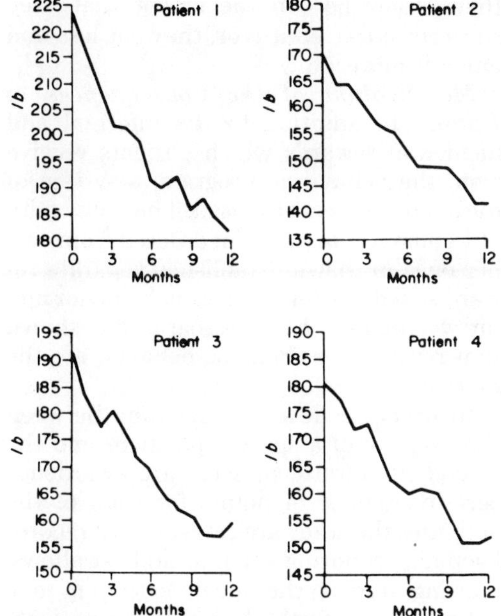

Figure 12.1. Profiles of four women undergoing behavior therapy for obesity. (Reprinted with permission from Stuart, R. B. Behavioral control of overeating. *Behav. Res. Ther.*, 1967, *5*, 357–365, © 1967, Pergamon Press, Ltd.)

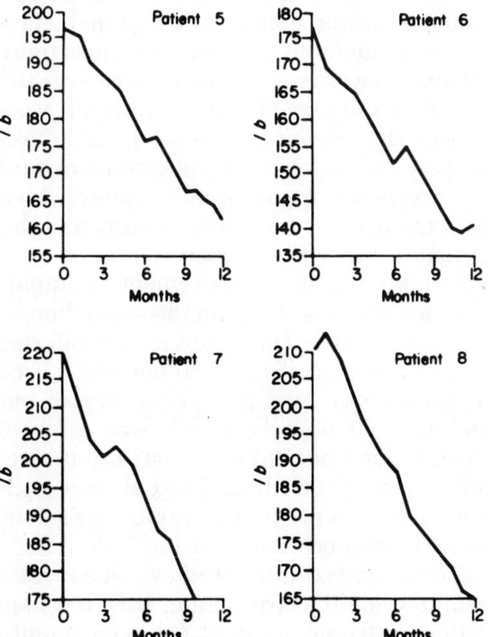

Figure 12.2. Profiles of four women undergoing behavior therapy for obesity. (Reprinted with permission from Stuart, R. B. Behavioral control of overeating. *Behav. Res. Ther.*, 1967, *5*, 357–365, © 1967, Pergamon Press, Ltd.)

ness of treatment. Thus, the description which follows contains what are still the essential ingredients of behavioral weight control programs.

The University of Pennsylvania program consisted of four elements: (1) description of the behavior to be controlled; (2) control of the stimuli which precede eating; (3) development of techniques to control the act of eating; (4) modification of the consequences of eating.

Description of the Behavior to be Controlled. Patients are asked to keep careful records of the food that they eat. Each time they eat, they write down precisely what it was, how much, at what time of day, where they were, who they were with, and how they felt. The immediate reaction of many patients to this time-consuming and inconvenient procedure was grumbling and complaints. In retrospect, such reactions occurred far more frequently when we were starting the program and may well have been due to our own uncertainty about the techniques. More recently, since we have ourselves become convinced of its effectiveness and stress its importance in a wholehearted manner, patients have responded more positively. Many have come to the view that record-keeping may be the single most important part of the behavioral program. It vastly increases patients' awareness of their eating behavior. Despite years of struggle with the problem, once patients begin to keep records they are surprised at how much they eat and the circumstances of their eating.

Control of the Stimuli Which Precede Eating. A behavioral analysis traditionally begins with a study of the events which precede the behavior to be controlled. Stimulus control of eating involves many measures which are traditional in weight-reduction programs: every effort is made to limit the amount of high-calorie food kept in the house and to limit access to food that must be kept in the house. For times when eating cannot be resisted, adequate amounts of low-calorie foods, such as celery and raw carrots, are to be available.

In addition, the behavioral program introduces new and distinctive measures. For example, most patients report that their eating takes place in a wide variety of places and at many different times during the day.

Some note that if they eat while watching television, it is not long before watching television makes them eat. The various times and places have become discriminative stimuli for eating. In an effort to decrease the number and potency of discriminative stimuli that control eating, patients are encouraged to confine all eating, including snacking, to one place. In order not to disrupt domestic routines, this place is usually the kitchen.

A parallel effort is made to develop new discriminative stimuli for appropriate eating and to increase their power. For example, patients are encouraged to use distinctive table-settings; perhaps an unusually colored place mat and napkin, and special silver. Initially, no effort is made to decrease the amount of food the patients eat, but they are encouraged to use the distinctive table settings whenever they eat, even for a small between-meals snack. (One middle-aged housewife, impressed by the importance of this measure, went so far as to take her distinctive table setting with her whenever she dined out.)

Development of Techniques to Control the Act of Eating. Specific techniques are utilized to help the patients decrease their speed of eating, to become aware of the components of the eating process, and to gain control over these components. Exercises include counting each mouthful of food eaten during a meal, or each chew, or each swallow. Patients are encouraged to practice putting down their eating utensils after every third mouthful until that mouthful is chewed and swallowed. Then, longer delays are introduced, starting with 1 minute toward the end of the meal (when it is more easily tolerated), and moving to more frequent delays, longer delays, and delays earlier in the meal.

Patients are encouraged to stop pairing their eating with activities such as reading the newspaper and watching television, and to make conscious efforts to make eating a "pure" experience. They are urged to do whatever they can to make meals a time of comfort and relaxation, and particularly to avoid old arguments and new problems at the dinner table. They are encouraged to savor the food as they eat it, to make a conscious effort to become aware of what they are chewing, and to enjoy the act of swallowing and the warmth and fullness in their stomachs. To the extent that they succeed in this endeavor, they eat less and enjoy it more.

Modification of the Consequences of Eating. In addition to the informal and incidental rewards which patients receive from the behavioral program, a system of formal rewards is also used. The University of Pennsylvania program differed from earlier ones in that it established separate reward schedules for changes in behavior and for weight loss. Later research has shown that rewards for changing behavior are the more effective.

In order to decrease the time between the exercise of a specific behavior and the attendant reward, patients are awarded a certain number of points for each of the activities that they are carrying out: record-keeping, counting chews and swallows, pausing during the meal, eating in one place, and so forth. Not only do patients receive a certain number of points for each activity, but they can earn extras, such as double the number of points, when they devise an alternative to eating in the face of strong temptation.

These points, which serve to provide immediate reinforcement for adaptive behavior, are cumulated and converted into more tangible rewards, often in concert with the spouse. Examples of popular rewards are a trip to the movies and relief from housekeeping chores. A more impersonal reward is conversion of points into money which patients bring to the next meeting and donate to some worthy cause.

Promptness of reinforcement is important for success. One middle-aged housewife said, "My husband was always offering to buy me a car if I lost 50 pounds. I used to work away at it and knock myself out and lose 30 pounds, which was a lot of weight, but what did it get me? I didn't get half a car. I got nothing. I've only lost eight pounds in this program so far and he's done all sorts of good things for me."

Three Important Studies. Soon after Stuart's landmark program, the first controlled outcome study of behavior modification of obesity reported an average weight loss of 10.5 pounds among moderately overweight women university students (Harris, 1969). Subjects in a no-treatment control group gained 3.6 pounds, a significant difference ($p < 0.01$).

A no-treatment control group, such as that used by Harris, was quite acceptable in psychotherapy research in 1969. Yet it has serious disadvantages, for refusing treatment to someone who has come seeking it is far from a neutral event. The resultant disappointment could well produce weight gains that would make the treatment condition appear to be more effective than it actually was. The problem calls for the use of a placebo control group to match the attention and interest received by patients in the active treatment program. An elaborate study by Wollersheim (1970) provided precisely such controls and opened up new vistas in research on psychological treatment.

Wollersheim's elegant factorial design contained four experimental conditions: behavioral treatment, "nonspecific therapy" based upon traditional psychiatric methods, "social pressure" modelled on lay weight control programs and, finally, a no-treatment control group. Four therapists each treated a different group of five patients in each of the three treatment conditions for 10 sessions over a 3-month period. Figure 12.3 shows that at the end of treatment, and at 8-week follow-up, subjects in the behavioral ("focal") treatment condition had lost more weight than those in the no-treatment condition. In addition, they had lost significantly more weight than those in the two placebo control conditions, who had themselves lost significantly more weight than those in the no-treatment condition. The behavioral treatment clearly contributed something to the outcome which was over and above the usual effects of psychotherapy.

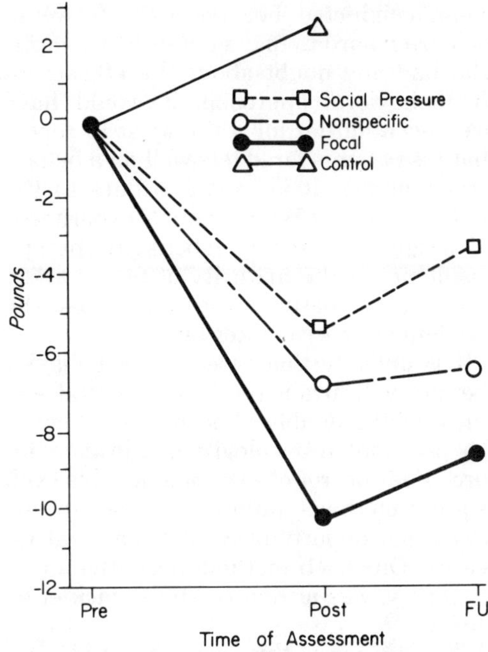

Figure 12.3. Mean weight loss of the focal (behavioral) treatment group, the two alternative treatment control groups, and the no-treatment control group. (From Wollersheim, J. P. Effectiveness of group therapy based upon learning principles in the treatment of overweight women. *J. Abnorm. Psychol.*, 1970, *76*, 462–474. Copyright © 1970 by the American Psychological Association. Reprinted by permission.)

This contribution seems to have resulted from the specific effects of the behavioral intervention. For not only did this condition produce greater weight loss, but it also produced major changes in self-reports concerning eating behaviors. Statistically significant differences between "focal" therapy and the other three conditions were found in four of the six factors assessed by the questionnaire: "emotional and uncontrolled eating," "eating in isolation," "eating as a reward," and "between-meal eating". Whatever caused the weight loss in the two placebo control conditions apparently did it without affecting these behaviors. The "focal" therapy apparently produced weight loss by means of its proposed rationale.

Wollersheim's study solved the problem of placebo controls, but, in so doing, brought psychotherapy research face-to-face with another problem that had seemed mercifully distant: the problem of experimenter bias. Although Wollersheim's placebo treatments controlled for the patient's expectations of treatment, they could not control for the therapist's. This is hardly a trivial matter. A large measure of therapeutic effectiveness may be the result of the therapist's expectations. Development of the methodology of the double-blind experiment in psychopharmacology has shown how powerful this influence can be when dealing with drugs. It is surely more powerful in the more emotional case of behavior therapy. Also, therapists' expectations of the effectiveness of behavioral approaches must have been at a peak of optimism in the behaviorally oriented department at the University of Illinois where Wollersheim conducted her research. It would have been hard to find a potential therapist who had any doubt about the efficacy of the behavioral approach; it would have been even harder for a therapist to report that his patients fared less well on a behavioral regimen. It is thus a tribute to the sophistication of Wollersheim's experimental design that research in behavior therapy has achieved the maturity of facing a key problem of mature research areas—the problem of experimenter bias.

It is unlikely that research on behavior therapy will attain the economy and elegance of the double-blind methodology of the psychopharmacologist in the near future. The control of experimenter bias will require methods tailored to the special needs and opportunities of behavioral research. One such method, deceptive in its simplicity, was introduced by Penick et al. (1971).

The essence of this ingenious study was to give up, at the start, the notion that therapists could be unbiased in the use of therapies which they favored, and disfavored. Instead, therapists were selected on the basis of their commitment either to a behavioral, or a traditional, approach to therapy. Penick further biased the outcome against the behavioral approach by selecting therapists of vastly different experience for the two conditions: for the behavioral treatment, the therapists were beginners; for the control condition, they were experts.

Therapists for the behavioral treatment were a male experimental psychologist with a strong background in learning theory but little clinical experience and a female research assistant with no previous experience in therapy. The control therapy was carried out by Penick himself, an internist, who, at the time, had had 10 years of experience in the treatment of obesity and was completing a psychiatric residency which had given him considerable additional training in group therapy. The female co-therapist was a research nurse who had worked with Penick for several years. They utilized supportive psychotherapy, instruction about nutrition and dieting, and upon request, appetite suppressants.

Each therapeutic team began with the conviction that its method was superior and sought, in a competitive way, to prove it. For, despite his curiosity about behavioral methods, Penick was convinced that inexperienced practitioners could not match his own highly accomplished performance.

In addition to its ingenious method of attempting to control for bias, Penick's study is worthy of note for the character of its patients. A great many behavior modification trials have been carried out with mildly overweight college students. By contrast, the patients in Penick's study were severely obese—78% overweight. Two cohorts, of 8 and 7 persons, respectively, were treated in weekly group meetings lasting 2 hours for a period of 3 months.

What were the results? The weight losses for each subject are plotted in Figures 12.4 and 12.5 and they show that subjects treated with behavior modification lost more weight than those treated by the full armamentarium of traditional therapy. In each cohort, the median weight loss for the behavior modification group was greater than that of the control group: 24 pounds vs. 18 pounds for the first cohort; 13 vs. 11 for the second.

The weight losses of the control group are comparable to those found in the medical literature—none lost 40 pounds and only 24% lost more than 20 pounds. By contrast, 13% of the behavior modification group lost more than 40 pounds and 53% lost more than 20 pounds. Although the differences between the experimental and control groups for these weight losses did not reach statistical significance, that for weight losses of over 30 pounds did ($p = 0.015$ by the Fisher exact probability test.)

One further point should be noted. The variability in the weight losses of the behavior modification subjects was considerably greater than that of the patients treated by traditional methods ($F = 4.38$, $p < 0.005$). The five best performers were patients in the behavior modification condition as was the single least effective patient—the only patient who actually gained weight during treatment. Greater variability in weight loss by behavioral patients has since been confirmed by other authors. Such greater variability has in other circumstances been associated with greater specificity of the treatment and this explanation of the findings seems reasonable. It would appear that for half of the patients,

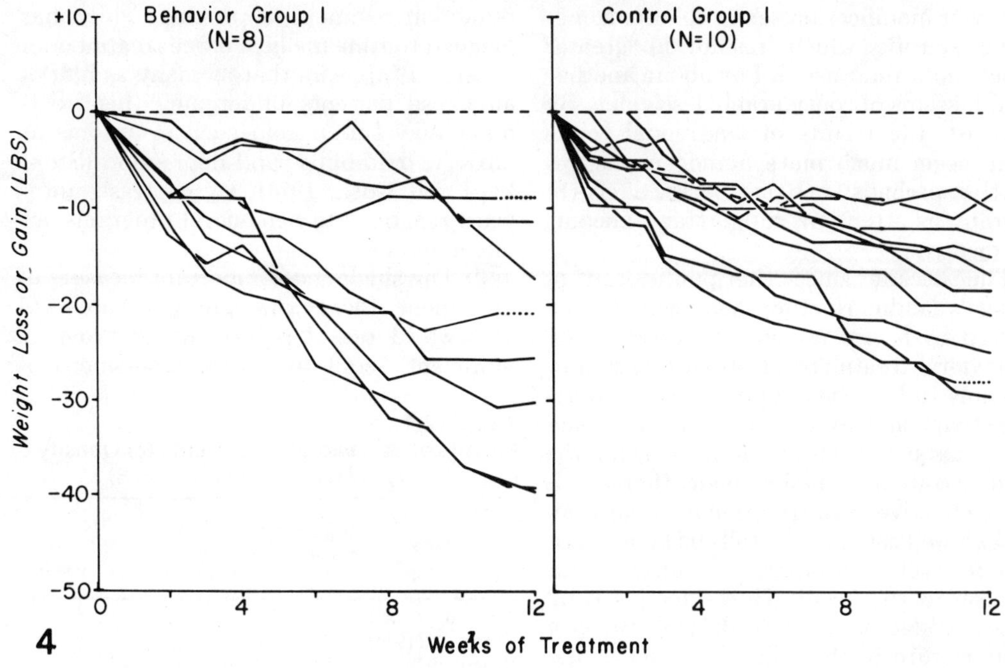

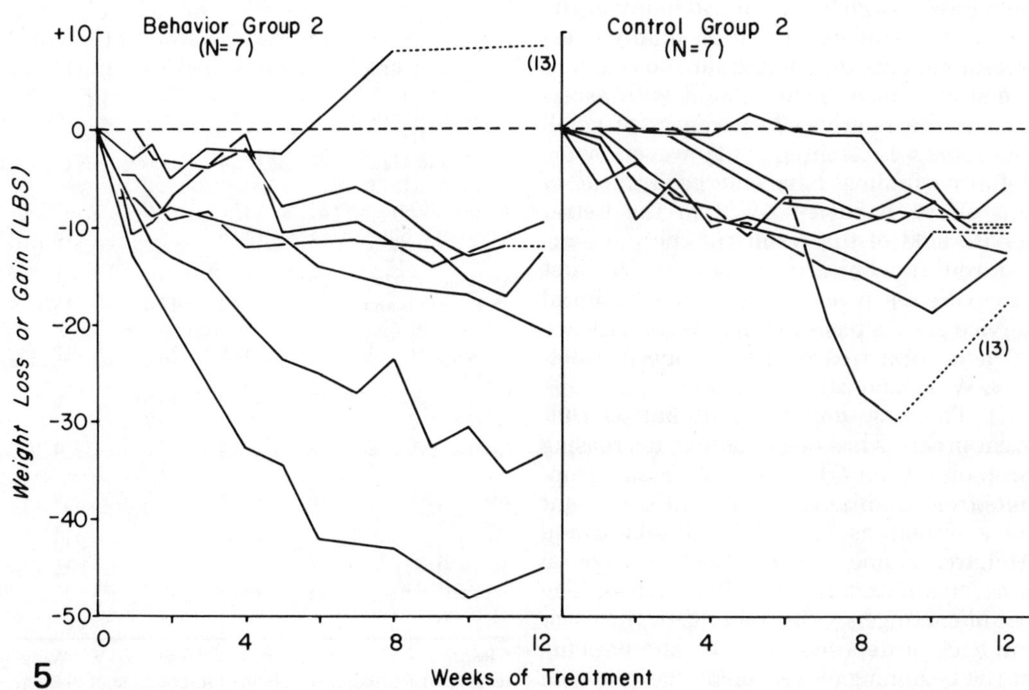

Figures 12.4 and 12.5. Weight changes of severely obese people in two cohorts. Dotted lines represent interpolated data based upon weights obtained during follow up. Note the greater weight loss of behavior modification groups and the greater variability of this weight loss as compared to the control groups. (Reprinted with permission from Penick, S. B., Fillion, R., Fox, S., and Stunkard, A. J. Behavior modification in the treatment of obesity. *Psychosom. Med.,* 1971, *33,* 49–55.)

behavior modification seems to offer something specific which results in greater weight loss than usual. For about another half, it seems of considerably less value. By contrast, the results of traditional treatment seem much more homogeneous, reflecting, perhaps, such nonspecific effects of therapy as attention, support and encouragement.

The decade since the publication of Stuart's landmark study has been characterized by a vast amount of work on the behavioral treatment of obesity. It is now possible to look back upon these 10 years of activity and to sort out what has, and what has not, been accomplished, for the demonstration that behavior therapy is more effective than traditional therapy, although well established, tells us little about its effectiveness as a practical measure for the control of obesity. How effective is it?

Several factors make it difficult to get a clear picture of the clinical impact of behavioral treatments for obesity. Sample sizes have been small, treatment has been restricted to short time periods, and follow-up data are negligible. Far too many of the subjects of studies have been mildly overweight college women and far too many of the studies have been content with ascertaining the relative effectiveness of small differences in technique. However, some definitive findings have emerged from all of this effort. A review of 21 of the better reports and of the results of the more-or-less routine clinical treatment of the first 125 patients in a well-established clinical service gives a basis for the overall efficacy of behavioral treatments for obesity (Jeffery, Wing, and Stunkard, 1978).

1) The first important finding is that great progress has been made in decreasing drop-outs from treatment. Whereas drop-outs from traditional outpatient treatment were as high as 25 to 75% (Stunkard and McLaren-Hume, 1959), most behavioral programs report rates of 10% or less. The use of contingency contracting, or the earning back of deposits made by the patients at the beginning of treatment, has played a major part in coping with the problem of drop-outs, but it appears that other aspects of the behavioral programs also play a part.

2) The second major advance has been in reducing untoward side effects of weight reduction regimens, a problem which has plagued routine medical office treatment of obesity. It appears that as many as half of all obese patients undergoing this treatment may suffer from such symptoms as anxiety, irritability, and depression (Stunkard and Rush, 1974). By contrast, untoward reactions to behavioral programs are uncommon.

3) The single most important measure of treatment efficacy is weight loss. Table 12.1 reviews 21 recent reports which provided sufficient detail to permit assessment of

Table 12.1
Results of Behavioral Treatments for Obesity*
(from Jeffery, Wing, & Stunkard, 1978)

STUDY	No. of Patients	Initial Weight (lb)	Mean Weight Loss† (lb)	Treatment Length (weeks)
Abrahms and Allen (1974)	23	182.5	11.9	9
Hagen (1974)	18	153.0	15.0	10
Hall (1972)	10	173.0	3.2	4
Hall et al. (1974)	40		11.1	10
Hall et al. (1975)	25	197.6	15.0‡	12
Hanson et al. (1976)	32	212.0	13.0‡	10
Harris (1969)	7	171.1	6.9	10
Harris and Bruner (1971)	11	164.7	7.4	12
Harris and Bruner (1971)	6	143.7	1.8	16
Harris and Hallbauer (1973)	27	165.4	8.0	12
Jeffery (1974)	34	183.8	6.0	7
Levitz and Stunkard (1974)	73	180.8	4.2	12
Mahoney (1974)	9		7.4	8
McReynolds and Lutz (1976)	41	178.4	17.4	15
Penick et al. (1971)	15	251.0	22.3	12
Romanczyk (1974)	17	175.7	10.6	6
Romanczyk et al. (1973)	18	178.8	7.0	4
Romanczyk et al. (1973)	18	173.0	8.0	4
Stuart (1967)	8	183.6	37.8	52
Stuart (1971)	6		14.0	15
Wollersheim (1970)	18	154.1	10.4	12

* Reprinted with permission from Jeffery, R. W., Wing, R. R., and Stunkard, A. J. Behavior treatment of obesity: The state of the art in 1976, Behav. Ther., 1978, 9, 189–199.

† Data describe the most effective treatment combination only. Results from control groups and partial treatments are not included.

‡ Extrapolated from weight reduction indices.

weight loss results. This assessment included assurance that the studies met such basic criteria as that the results were based upon all patients starting treatment, dropouts were included, etc. Table 12.1 shows that the weight losses of no more than half the programs exceeded 10 pounds and those of only 20% exceeded 15 pounds. There are many reasons for these limitations—most of the programs were short-term, many involved patients who were only mildly overweight, and a large number were carried out by inexperienced therapists. However, the fact remains: the results are modest and, from the perspective of clinical utility, disappointing.

These results from the research literature are not dissimilar to those which have been reported recently from a program with a primarily clinical focus. Jeffery et al. (1978) found a weight loss of no more than 11.0 pounds among the first 125 patients in a behaviorally oriented obesity treatment program.

4) There is great variability in weight changes during treatment, as first noted by Penick et al. (1971) and even greater variability following treatment. Very little is known about factors underlying this variability.

5) Prediction of the outcome of treatment for obesity has generally been unsuccessful. Recently, however, three predictors have been established. The first is the extent of weight loss early in treatment. Jeffery et al. (1978) report a correlation of 0.40 ($p < 0.01$) between weight loss during the 1st week of treatment and that during the next 20 weeks, a finding that is particularly instructive since the patients' only assignment during the 1st week had been to record their eating behavior.

The second factor predicting outcome is percentage overweight (Murray, 1975), a robust finding which has also been found in nonbehavioral treatments—intestinal bypass surgery (Mills and Stunkard, 1976) and patient self-help groups (Garb and Stunkard, 1974). Percentage overweight is closely linked to a third and even more powerful predictor of weight loss recently described by Sullivan, Bjurö, Garellick, et al. (in press). An equation incorporating measurements of fat cell number, basal metabolic rate, and cephalic insulin stimulation has been able to predict 80% of the variance in weight loss in a group of patients treated in Gothenburg, Sweden.

6) Patients with onset of obesity early in life lose as much weight as those with onset in adult life (Jeffery et al., 1978). This finding appears somewhat at variance with predictions based upon expected fat cell size and number. There is no information on possible differences in the ability to maintain weight loss by juvenile- and adult-onset obese persons.

7) Despite the fact that behavioral techniques can be adapted for use by less skilled therapists, skill of the therapist does have a positive effect upon outcome of therapy. Two studies have shown that therapist experience was positively related to weight loss (Levitz and Stunkard, 1974; Jeffery et al., 1978).

8) Clinically significant weight losses achieved by behavioral treatment for obesity are not well maintained (Stunkard, 1977; Stunkard and Penick, in press). Whether they are better maintained than weight losses achieved by other—nonsurgical—treatments is impossible to determine because of insufficient information on the long-term effects of these other treatments. This is an important, and disappointing, conclusion, for it had been hoped that the first generation of behavioral treatments might produce enduring changes in weight-related behaviors and, as a consequence, long-term weight loss.

This review suggests that the limits of effectiveness of current behavioral technologies for the control of obesity may have been reached. To go beyond these limits may require new technologies or new combinations of technologies. Two recent studies suggest that the effectiveness of behavior therapy can be increased by combining it with other measures. Lindner and Blackburn (1976) have reported a marked increase in weight loss when behavior therapy is combined with the use of the protein-sparing-modified fast (Bistrian, Blackburn, and Flatt, 1975; Bistrian, Blackburn, Flatt, et al., 1976) and Craighead, O'Brien, and Stunkard (1978) have reported similar results when it is combined with pharmacotherapy. However, such relatively small incremental advances in the improvement of clinical practice ignore what may well be the major contribution of behavioral technologies to the improvement of health care—applicability to larger groups.

One of the most important implications of the study by Penick, et al. was the promise of the greater applicability of behavior therapy, for it showed that behavior modification, devised by a team with little experience in the modality, or even any clinical experience, was more effective in the treatment of obesity than was the best alternative program devised by a highly skilled research team. In fact, the inexperienced therapists achieved a two-fold increase in weight loss over conventional measures. Lesser increases in effectiveness have brought about major changes in the management of other disorders. The questions arise: How can the advantages of behavioral weight control programs be exploited most effectively? Can they be applied to populations larger than the clinical ones for which they were developed?

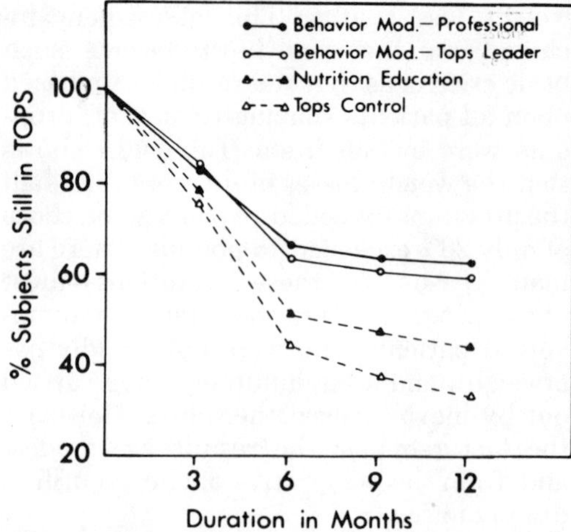

Figure 12.6. Attrition rate of TOPS subjects over a 1-year period under four experimental conditions. (From Levitz, L., and Stunkard, A. J. A therapeutic coalition for obesity: Behavior modification and patient self-help. *Am. J. Psychiatry, 1974, 131*, 423–427. Copyright © by the American Psychiatric Association. Reprinted by permission.)

Application of Behavioral Measures to Large Groups

The first controlled effort to explore the application of behavioral measures to large groups was carried out with TOPS (Take Off Pounds Sensibly), a 30-year-old self-help group for obesity that enrolls over 300,000 members in 12,000 chapters in all parts of the United States (Stunkard, Levine, and Fox, 1970; Garb and Stunkard, 1974). The study involved all 298 female members of 16 TOPS chapters situated in West Philadelphia and its adjacent suburbs (Levitz and Stunkard, 1974).

Four treatment conditions, each containing four matched TOPS chapters, were employed for a total of 12 weeks: behavior modification by psychiatrists, behavior modification by (lay) TOPS chapter leaders, nutrition education carried out by TOPS chapter leaders (who had received an amount of training in this area comparable to that provided the chapter leaders in behavioral modification) and, finally, continuation of the standard TOPS program. The most striking effects were upon attrition rate, a major problem in TOPS and, indeed, all large-scale weight control programs. Figure 12.6 shows that the attrition rate in the two behavior modification conditions was lower during treatment, and significantly lower 1 year later. At follow-up, 38 and 41% of subjects had dropped out of the chapters which had received behavior modification, compared to 55% for the nutrition education and 67% the standard TOPS programs. Despite the bias against the results of behavior modification resulting from the differential attrition rates, behavior modification produced significantly greater weight loss than did the control conditions, both at the end of treatment and at 1-year follow-up.

This program was a useful feasibility study. It taught us that behavior modification can be introduced into large populations through appropriate institutional auspices. TOPS, apparently, is not to be such an institution. It has made no effort to capitalize upon the program to which it made such an important contribution. Ironically, the chief beneficiaries are TOPS' main competitors, the commercial weight reduction organizations. They have already begun to develop strong behavioral components to programs which had traditionally been confined to inspirational lectures, nutrition education, and group pressure. It is estimated that 400,000 Americans are now exposed each week to behavioral measures for the control of obesity under commercial auspices. Controlled clinical trials of these programs are sorely needed. They represent one of the first approaches to the control of obesity which is sufficiently far-reaching to warrant description as a public health measure.

Traditional public health efforts in the field of weight control have been conspicuous for their absence until quite recently. Three nontraditional programs, however, have been carried out recently, and each has profound implications for behavioral medicine.

THE STANFORD HEART DISEASE PREVENTION PROGRAM

The first of these studies is the Stanford Heart Disease Prevention Program, which consisted of a broad spectrum intervention to reduce coronary risk factors in three towns of 14,000 each (Farquhar, Maccoby, Wood, et al., 1977). A rigorous evaluation has been added to the value of this highly innovative project.

The major intervention in the Stanford Three-Community Study was an intensive and sophisticated media campaign which contained during each of 2 years, 50 television and 100 radio spots, 3 hours of television and several hours of radio programming, columns, stories and advertisements in the local weekly newspapers, posters and billboards, printed matter sent via direct mail and other materials. The dominant characteristic of the media campaign was its organization as a total integrated information system based initially upon data gathered from preliminary surveys and later upon information collected during the course of the campaign. In one of the three towns the media campaign was supplemented by a face-to-face instruction program directed at two-thirds of the participants identified as being in the top quartile of risk of coronary heart disease. One town received no campaign and served as a control.

Although much of the program was not explicitly behavioral, it grew in large part out of research on behaviorally oriented interventions, and its results were most encouraging. By the end of the 2nd year of the campaign, risk of coronary disease had decreased by 17% in the treatment communities, as measured by the Cornfield risk index, whereas it had increased by 6% in the control community. Even more striking are the results shown in Figure 12.7: a reduction in risk factors among high-risk participants of 30%. Such a reduction in coronary risk has been compared to an increase in life expectancy at 45 of 5 years, a greater increase in life expectancy for middle-aged men than that achieved by all the medical advances which have occurred during the present century.

THE SWEDISH "DIET AND EXERCISE" PROGRAM

The second large-scale, nontraditional health promotion activity was the most broadly based program yet undertaken: the "Diet and Exercise" Program of the Swedish National Board of Health and Welfare

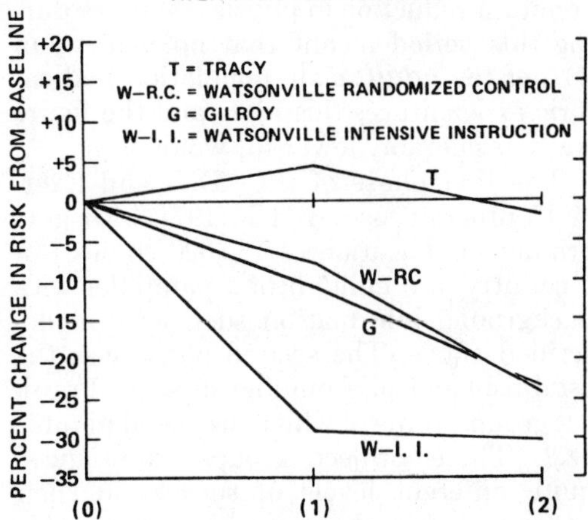

Figure 12.7. Percentage change in baseline (0) in risk of coronary heart disease after 1 and 2 years of behaviorally oriented health education programs in three communities. Tracy, the control town, shows no change in risk factors. Subjects in Gilroy, the "media only" town, show a steady decrease in risk factors over the 2 years of the program, as do Watsonville randomized control subjects, who did not receive face-to-face counselling. Watsonville intensive instruction subjects, who received both media and face-to-face counselling, show a rapid decline during the 1st year and then no further change. (Reprinted with permission from Farquhar, J. W., Maccoby, N. M., Wood, P. D., et al. Community education for cardiovascular health. *Lancet,* June 4, 1977, 1192–1195.)

(Isaksson, in press). It was stimulated by a concern of academicians—primarily nutritionists—with what was seen as a deterioration in the Swedish diet. Although this problem was serious, it was not notably greater than that of other affluent Western societies. Indeed, there had been some improvement in the Swedish diet since the turn of the century, largely in the increase in the especially low level of intake of fruits and green vegetables. However, in almost all other categories, the diet had become more unhealthful, with increasingly higher levels of caloric density and lower levels of nutrient density. For example, there had been a great increase in the consumption of fats and sugar, in high-fat dairy products such as cheese and cream, a shift toward meat with a higher fat content, and a marked decrease in the consumption of bread and cereals. Because of these dietary changes it was necessary to consume 2500 calories in order to meet daily requirements for several essential nutrients. Yet the concomitant reduction in physical activity during this period meant that no more than 20% of the *adult,* male population had caloric expenditures this high, and the figure was considerably lower for women.

The first phase of the "Diet and Exercise" program occurred in 1971 with government publication of 180,000 copies (for a country of 8 million) of a pamphlet with background information such as that described above. The second phase was the establishment of a number of special project groups, some of which are listed in table 12.2. These project groups experienced quite different levels of success in their endeavors and their experiences provide useful guidelines for such efforts in the future. One of the more successful endeavors was that of Project Group "Institutions," which carried out studies of institutional food service programs and held conferences throughout the country making dietary recommendations to people responsible for employee restaurants, old age institutions, and nurseries. The group produced special information packages to be used in the training of the staffs of institutions and distributed posters with simple texts for further instruction of both staff and guests. These efforts were widely accepted, with considerable improvement in the food served in institutions.

Table 12.2
"Diet and Exercise" (Sweden)

Project Groups	
	1. Institutions
	2. Exercise
	3. Diet and Expense
	4. Mass Media
	5. Education

Project Group "Exercise" worked with the 200,000 leaders of the sports movement, augmenting their activities and enlisting their help in promoting the dietary programs. The publishing and public relations capabilities of the sports movement are considerable and were thus obtained at no cost to the "Diet and Exercise" program. No outcome data are available on the results of this apparently effective enterprise.

Project Group "Diet and Expense" had considerable success in developing and promoting reasonably priced and nutritionally well-balanced daily menus for use by housewives. This effort was particularly important in view of the widespread belief that nutritious food is too expensive for the average person to afford.

An advisory Committee on Industrial Questions was formed some time after the original project groups, as a result of the unanticipated interest of industry in the original pamphlet which initiated the campaign. Much to the surprise of the staff, this pamphlet was voluntarily accepted by the food industry as its official guide for product development and both the food industry and other commercial organizations gave considerable backing to the program as it developed.

Two Project Groups were notable for their relative lack of success. They were the Groups devoted to "Mass Media" which tried to establish liaison with these agencies and that on "Education" which tried to introduce improved nutritional education into the schools.

A major operational activity of "Diet and Exercise" was through concentration on special themes. One of the first, derived from research showing that Swedish breakfasts were poor from a nutritional point of view, was entitled "Start Your Day in a Better Way." Recipes for simple nutritious breakfasts were widely publicized, along with a program of calisthenics. Fifty per cent of retail stores took part in the campaign by mounting attractive window displays showing appropriate breakfasts and by distributing large numbers of pamphlets which had been produced by "Diet and Exercise." Newspaper coverage reached 95%.

Another thematic program, carried out in cooperation with the Bread Institute, was designed to increase the limited consumption of bread by 25%. The theme of this program was very widely publicized —"The National Social Welfare Board wants you to eat six to eight slices of bread every day." High visibility was achieved: 81% of people reported having seen the slogan. Several months later the number who remembered it is whimsically said to have been as high as those who remembered the colors of the Swedish flag. The injunction "The National Social Welfare Board wants you to . . . " even became the starting point for bawdy jokes, an encouraging sign of observer recognition. Furthermore, the program seems to have worked. Sales of bread increased, breaking a trend of falling bread consumption of several years duration, and did this in the face of a considerable increase in cost of bread and during a time when the consumption of pastries fell by 9%.

What have been the effects of this unprecedented nationwide health promotion program? Unfortunately, evaluation has not kept pace with intervention and the results are fragmentary and, in critical areas, absent. Although rather detailed plans for evaluation had been drawn up, and an extensive baseline survey of knowledge, attitudes, and behavior of individuals had been carried out, lack of funds has prevented follow-up surveys. A major lesson of the "Diet and Exercise" program, thus, is the need for assured funding for evaluation before embarking on intervention programs.

The most effective evaluation was carried out on measures of food consumption, which reflected the goals of the campaign. Thus, there was a small but significant reduction in consumption of sugar and sugar products such as soft drinks, and the aforementioned arrest and reversal of the decline in the consumption of bread and cereals. The dairy industry developed a special low (0.5 per cent) fat milk and promoted it so successfully that it captured 25% of the market. Increasing consumption of cream and other milk products, however, meant that the total intake of fat from dairy products remained at about the same level.

The Swedish "Diet and Exercise" Program is a landmark in the mobilization of an entire nation in the interests of health promotion. We need to learn more about this program which has been reported to date only briefly and only in the Swedish literature.

THE GERMAN TELEVISION WEIGHT REDUCTION PROGRAM

The third large-scale nontraditional health promotion activity was a German exploration of the use of television in a program of weight control (Ferstl, Henrich, Richter, et al., 1977). It represented a cooperative effort of one of the two television channels of the German Federal Republic and the Max Planck Institute of Psychiatry in Munich. It consisted of seven "packages" or sections, each lasting 1 month and consisting of a major 45-minute show in prime time one Sunday evening a month together with 3-minute reminder shows on the other Sunday evenings. By virtue of its prestigious sponsors, the size of the population reached by the program was unprecedented for a health promotion program: 7.8 million people. The standard television rating system revealed that 35% of these viewers—2.8 million—were overweight, of whom 1.8 million viewed more than one of the major shows and 140,000 viewed at least five.

The content of the program consisted of most of the features of traditional behavioral programs such as self-monitoring, stimulus control, methods of changing eating habits, self-reinforcement, and contracting, with stimulus control playing a major part. In addition, considerable information was given regarding obesity and its hazards, nutrition, and training in counting calories. A sequence of 37 rules was carefully delineated, ranging from simple principles and techniques to more complicated ones. Modeling played an important part of the program and was carried out by ten obese persons, half men and half women, who demonstrated the various behavioral techniques and discussed usage and problems in implementation. The models lost unrealistically large amounts of weight for a behavioral program—from 37 to 54 pounds—probably as a result of crash dieting and other "unbehavioral" behaviors.

The investigators made an effort to evaluate the cost/effectiveness of the television program by comparing it with their extensively studied bibliotherapy program and with a combination television plus bibliotherapy program. Samples were drawn to assess the four treatment modalities; they were unusually well-matched, averaging 42% overweight (Note 1), 40 years in age, and consisting of 64% women.

Table 12.3 shows how each of the four samples of 300 persons were broken down into two subsamples, one of 250 which received the standard treatment and one of 50 which was selected for more extensive investigation. Later analyses confirmed the wisdom of this precaution, for the extensive investigation was reactive in the "television alone" condition (where subjects lost 11 pounds in the intensive study condition and only 5.5 pounds in the standard treatment condition ($p < 0.01$) but not in the other three conditions.

Another check on the quality of the data provided valuable information about the validity of self-reported weights. One week before the end of the program, a 10% sample of participants was contacted and asked if they would agree to a home visit to discuss the program. No mention was made of weight in the inquiry. At the time of the visit, the interviewer weighed the subject on scales brought to the house for this purpose. Measured weights were remarkably close to self-reported weights.

After the vast amount of effort, the results of the television treatment were disappointing. The values for the standard treatment conditions are summarized in Table 12.4.

The most striking finding is the effectiveness of bibliotherapy alone, and its far greater effectiveness than television alone. Considerable confidence can be placed in the bibliotherapy results, since they are remarkably similar to those obtained in two previous studies carried out by this same research group. Although television alone produced a weight loss which was statistically significantly greater than that in the no-treatment condition ($p < 0.01$), the difference (3.3 pounds) is of questionable clinical significance. Furthermore, the addition of television did not significantly increase the weight loss achieved by bibliotherapy alone.

Why was this effect so limited? The most likely explanation is that the density of the television programs was not great enough to achieve significant impact. Face-to-face behavioral weight reduction programs traditionally utilize weekly meetings of at least an hour and efforts that we have made to increase the length of this interval have resulted in a decrement in performance.

Table 12.3
"Television/Obesity Program" (Germany)

Evaluation Design

NEITHER			TV
250	50	50	250
LETTER	50	50	BOTH
250			250

Table 12.4
Results of the German Television Weight Reduction Program

Treatment	Drop-Out Rate (%)	Weight Loss (lb)	Success Rate (Feinstein, 1960, Criterion) (%)
Control	52	2.2	3
		* (Control vs. TV alone)	
TV alone	54	5.5	5
		** (TV alone vs. Bibliotherapy alone)	
Bibliotherapy alone	40	16.3	25
		** (TV alone vs. TV and bibliotherapy)	
TV and bibliotherapy	38	18.7	32

* $p < 0.01$.
** $p < 0.001$.

Although the effectiveness of television in changing behavior has not been systematically studied, market research suggests that frequent multiple impacts are necessary to change buying patterns even marginally. The Stanford Three-Community Study, which used such frequent, multiple impacts, exerted a cumulative effect which continued to grow for 2 full years.

Disappointing as have been its substantive effects, the Max Planck Institute study has been a valuable feasibility study and has laid the foundations for the evaluation of large-scale media efforts at changing health behaviors.

The Many Potential Influences of the Future

The developments of the very recent past make it clear that leadership in broad-scale efforts to control obesity is passing to nonmedical agencies. As we look to the future there is every reason to believe that this trend will accelerate; the most promising new methods for controlling obesity seem to lie almost entirely outside the province of the medical profession. For obesity is, in very large part, a result of the way we live, of our life styles, and the most effective means for controlling obesity today appear to lie in alternations in our life styles. Such an undertaking as altering the life styles of a nation is far beyond the capability of a profession such as medicine. It will require changes in those powerful social and economic forces which have given rise to these life styles and which sustain them.

These forces are powerful indeed. Consider just the impact upon our nutritional practices of the amount spent each year by the food industry in the United States to advertise its products—$1.2 billion! (McGovern, 1977). Efforts by physicians to treat individual patients on a one-by-one basis are puny in comparison with these forces. They might be likened to exhortations to a swimmer to persevere against a raging current. What are the possibilities of swimming *with* the current?

Changing the social and economic forces which maintain our life styles is by no means as overwhelming a task as it might at first appear. In the first place, relatively small changes in each of the institutions could, by their cumulative—and perhaps potentiating—effect bring about considerably larger changes in the end product. Second, these are not simply blind, economic forces. They involve human beings in positions of responsibility which enable them to make choices between alternatives. Within their constraints, people choose what helps over what hurts. Finally, there is the possibility of generating powerful new social forces which can change existing patterns. Interest in personal health can be precisely this kind of force. The persuasive "Perspective on the Health of Canadians" (Lalonde, 1974) and the subsequent activities of the Long-Range Planning Committee of the Canadian Department of Health and Welfare illustrate how many agencies might be mobilized in the interest of improved health and the prevention of disease. Consider first the contribution of industry.

INDUSTRY

The leadership in the control of obesity currently exercised by industry depends largely upon one type of activity: direct service to clients. But, Table 12.5 shows that such direct service to clients is only one of five approaches which would seem ideally suited to industry efforts at research and development. The other four are development of new food products, delivery of food through restaurants and catering services, provision of opportunities for exercise through health clubs, health spas, and sporting goods manufacturers and, finally, insurance incentives.

One of the most notable of the foods developed for weight reduction purposes was Metrecal, developed from the "Rockefeller Diet" of the mid-1950's. Metrecal was taken up by the public with an enthusiasm which astonished its pharmaceutical manufacturer and it broke a variety of sales

Table 12.5
Components of Industry Approaches to Weight Control

(Clinical) service delivery
Product development
Delivery system—Restaurants
Delivery systems—Health clubs and spas
Insurance incentives

records before its poorly understood decline and fall. Diet foods have become increasingly popular since Metrecal and low calorie beverages are coming to occupy an increasing part of the soft drink market. The potential for development of new products for weight control seems virtually unlimited. Two promising new areas of research are the development of nonabsorbable fats and non-nutritive sweeteners.

The third component of an integrated industry approach to weight reduction is the restaurant and food service industries. Despite the widespread concern with body weight on the part of vast numbers of persons who eat out, most find it awkward or impossible to secure satisfying, low-calorie, non-atherogenic foods in restaurants. Even when restaurants serve low-calorie dishes, all-too-frequently the choice is limited and the selection uninspired. There is great need for restaurants which serve an assortment of attractively prepared low-calorie dishes. This need could be met either by the establishment of specialty restaurants or, perhaps more promisingly, by modifying some of the items on the menus of traditional restaurants and by appropriate promotion of them. Already one pilot study has produced encouraging results. A restaurant chain in Houston, Texas has begun to list the caloric content of a few items on its menu, selected for their limited fat and calories and prepared with polyunsaturated oils (Foreyt, 1977). The initial response was an increase in consumption of these items sufficiently promising to induce the company to expand their number and to introduce a special menu to describe them.

The growth of large catering agencies which furnish complete food services for schools, businesses, and other institutions provides another important strategic opportunity for nutritional intervention. Large and increasing numbers of people eat in facilities served by these agencies and the nutritional education they receive in the process doubtless carries over to meals eaten elsewhere and to their future eating practices. Any improvement in the nutritional quality of the foods provided by these agencies would thus benefit vast numbers of people now and, hopefully, in the future. Such improvement need not await the uncertain outcome of efforts at building a market in the highly competitive restaurant business; it could flow directly from management decisions involving a small number of experts in the relevant disciplines. Indeed, the most successful of the "Diet and Exercise" efforts was that devoted to modifying the food served by large catering agencies (Isaksson, in press).

Health clubs and spas have already demonstrated their appeal to a large and growing market, even as free-standing enterprises. They might be more effective, and less costly, as part of an integrated network of weight reduction agencies which included also restaurants for eating out, food products for eating at home, and nutritional/behavioral programs of direct service to clients. Enlisting the sporting goods industry in such enterprises is an unexplored area of possibly great effectiveness.

The greatest potential for health behavior change by industry may lie in an almost totally unexplored agency—life and health insurance. Assessment of the risk of death and disability lies at the heart of the insurance industry and the industry has achieved remarkable accuracy in predicting such outcomes for population groups and in modifying predictions on the basis of changing health contingencies. It has, with rare exceptions, not attempted to alter these contingencies. In that direction may lie an unparalleled promise for the future. The insurance companies may well possess the most powerful incentives for health behavior change in our society today.

THE MEDIA

The results of the Stanford Heart Disease Prevention Program have documented the effectiveness of an integrated media campaign in changing unhealthful life styles in small populations. It has been followed by programs on at least two United States commercial television stations in which an attractive, mildly overweight newscaster has described and carried out a step-by-step description of a weight loss program over periods of 8 to 10 weeks. These programs have demonstrated conclusively that commercial television can go far beyond its traditional health behavior function of conveying information (and, to some extent, changing attitudes) and can teach health behavior skills, such as weight control, in a persuasive manner. Furthermore, by daily presentations and by the use of modeling, these efforts possess strengths that are not available to traditional clinical weight reduction programs. Unfortunately, the programs devised so far may have been quite effective but they have not been adequately evaluated. We have learned from the large-scale German study described above how to carry out such evaluation. The time is ripe for a combined effort.

EDUCATION

Schools furnish a golden opportunity to provide nutritional education and practical experience with good nutrition. The current deterioration of food quality in American schools and the failure of the "Diet and Exercise" program to influence significantly the Swedish school system are particularly regrettable and suggest the importance of informing parents and school boards of the need for vigorous advocacy of a more adequate nutritional policy in the schools.

Failures of nutrition education do not, of course, stop at the elementary school level. The low state of nutrition education in schools of medicine must also contribute to our nutritional problems, including obesity.

GOVERNMENT

The potential of government in the control of obesity is as yet almost totally unrealized. Yet, taxation could be used to effect major changes in health behavior; just as improved health behavior might lead to lowered insurance premiums, so it might also lead to tax rebates. A second area where government could have a major impact is in the improvement of the nutrition of the vast number of government employees that it feeds every day, in and out of the military. Finally, the climax of a vigorous, integrated program of obesity control could be capped by the promotional activities of prominent government figures. Franklin Roosevelt had a great impact in transforming poliomyelitis from a feared plague to a national challenge. Here is a power which can be exercised with remarkably little cost to produce a remarkably great effect.

WORK-SITE TREATMENT

A promising opportunity for changing health behavior is provided by the use of work sites for the conduct of programs of medical service. "On-the-job training" has a long and honorable history in industry. On-the-job training for improved health behavior can be as rewarding, to worker and employer alike. The potential of the work site as a locus for the provision of long-term health care has recently been demonstrated in a pilot project in a related area. Hypertension, like obesity, is rarely cured but it does respond to effective and available treatment. A large percentage of hypertensive persons, however, receive treatment which is inadequate to control their blood pressure (Wilber, 1973). Thus, in a pilot project, carried out under union auspices in New York City, less than 50% of the hypertensives in conventional treatment had achieved satisfactory results. By contrast, a specially designed work-site program achieved long-term control of blood pressure in over 80% and radically reduced days of hospitalization for cardiovascular causes (Alderman and Schoenbaum, 1975). The author has recently completed a controlled clinical trial of a work site program for obesity with this union. The results were promising: not only were they better at the work site than at a medical site, but also persons treated by union personnel outperformed those treated by professional personnel.

VOLUNTARY AGENCIES

Some religious groups inculcate an enviable series of health behaviors in their members as well as provide assistance for others outside the group. The Smoking Cessation Clinics conducted by the Seventh Day Adventists are landmarks in such endeavors. Other health promotional activities could be carried out under other religious auspices; weight control should be a prime candidate.

Fraternal organizations often take a special interest in the health of others—the Shriners in crippled children and the Lions in those with visual impairment. An enlightened membership might decide to deal with its own health problems—obesity, for example—as well as those of its beneficiaries.

Recreational organizations have traditionally had a strong interest in health behavior. The gymnasiums of the Young Men's Christian Association are among the important health facilities of many American communities; they are now being increasingly utilized in the rehabilitation of patients following myocardial infarction. Obesity control would be a logical next step.

Voluntary health agencies such as the Heart Associations in different countries occupy a special position in the health care system. They have great promise for disseminating new information about weight control and new techniques for achieving it.

Youth groups have traditionally had a major concern for health. This concern can now be more effectively translated into action by use of the newer behavioral techniques.

PERMUTATIONS AND COMBINATIONS

This paper has outlined what might be called single-factor approaches to the control of obesity. However, future approaches are not likely to be limited to such inefficient, one-by-one, forms of intervention. Combinations of different interventions seem particularly promising, for combining interventions may accomplish more than simply adding their effects—it may actually multiply them.

Summary

Behavioral medicine owes much to developments in the behavioral control of obesity. Historically, obesity was one of the first problems to be subjected to careful applied behavioral analysis and currently more people are receiving behavioral treatment for obesity than for all other conditions combined. However, the greatest importance of obesity for behavioral medicine may well lie in the future. For current developments and future trends in the behavioral control of obesity may foreshadow developments in all of behavioral medicine. Foremost among these trends is the application of behavioral measures to larger and larger populations. This application is being carried out by two instruments. The first is essentially clinical interventions by progressively less highly trained personnel. The second is the use of new methods of organization—of communities and of entire nations—and the innovative use of technologies such as television. Already, both of these instruments have achieved impressive results and the future of such applications seems bright indeed. These new behavioral measures for the control of obesity extend to the very boundaries of behavioral medicine—and even beyond.

Note

1. Percentage overweight was calculated from the Broca Index (normal weight in kilograms = height in centimeters−100). In accord with current practice in Germany, 20 percent was subtracted from the Broca-derived normal weight to yield the normal weight used in the study. These weights are less than those for comparable heights according to American height/weight tables, meaning that the extent of overweight in this study was overestimated by American standards.

References

Abrahms, J. L., and Allen, G. J. Comparative effectiveness of situational programming, financial payoffs, and group pressure in weight reduction. *Behav. Ther.,* 1974, *5,* 391–400.

Abramson, E. E. A review of behavioral approaches to weight control. *Behav. Res. Ther.,* 1973, *11,* 547–556.

Alderman, M. H., and Schoenbaum, E. E. Detection and treatment of hypertension at the work site. *N. Engl. J. Med.,* 1975, *293,* 65–68.

Bandura, A. On paradigms and recycled ideologies. *Cogn. Ther. Res.,* 1978, *2,* 79–103.

Bistrian, B. R., Blackburn, G. L., Flatt, J. P., Sizer, J., Scrimshaw, N. S., and Sherman, M. Nitrogen metabolism and insulin requirements in obese diabetic adults on a protein sparing modified fast. *Diabetes,* 1976, *25,* 494–504.

Blackburn, G. L., Bistrian, B. R., and Flatt, J. P. Role of a protein sparing fast in a comprehensive weight reduction program. In A. Howard (Ed.), *Recent advances in obesity research,* Vol. 1. London: Newman, 1975, pp. 279–281.

Craighead, L., O'Brien, R., and Stunkard, A. J. New treatments for obesity. Paper presented at the annual meeting of the American Psychiatric Association, Atlanta, May, 1978.

Farquhar, J. W., Maccoby, N. M., Wood, P. D., Alexander, J. K., Breitrose, H., Brown, B. W., Haskell, W. L., McAlister, A. L., Meyer, A. J., Nash, J. D., and Stern, M. P. Community education for cardiovascular health. *The Lancet,* June 4, 1977, 1192–1195.

Feinstein, A. R. The measurement of success in weight reduction: An analysis of methods and a new index. *J. Chronic Dis.,* 1960, *10,* 439–456.

Ferguson, J. M. *Learning to eat: Behavior modification for weight control.* Palo Alto, Calif.: Bull Pub-

lishing Co., 1975.
Ferster, C. B., Nurnberger, J., and Levitt, E. B. Behavioral control of eating. *J. Mathetics,* 1962, *1,* 87–109.
Ferstl, R., Henrich, G., Richter, M., Buhringer, G., and Brengelmann, J. C. Die Beeinflussung des Übergewichts. Abschlussbericht, The Max Planck Institute for Psychiatry, Munich, Germany, September 30, 1977.
Foreyt, J. Personal communication, 1977.
Garb, J. R., and Stunkard, A. J. A further assessment of the effectiveness of TOPS in the control of obesity. *Arch. Intern. Med.,* 1974, *134,* 716–720.
Hagen, R. L. Group therapy vs bibliotherapy in weight reduction. *Behav. Ther.,* 1974, *5,* 224–234.
Hall, S. M. Self-control and therapist control in the behavioral treatment of overweight women. *Behav. Res. Ther.,* 1972, *10,* 59–68.
Hall, S. M., Hall, R. G., Borden, B. L., and Hanson, R. W. Follow-up strategies in the treatment of overweight. *Behav. Res. Ther.,* 1975, *13,* 167–172.
Hall, S. M., Hall, R. G., Hanson, R. W., and Borden, B. L. Permanence of two self-managed treatments of overweight in university and community populations. *J. Consult. Clin. Psychol.,* 1974, *42,* 781–786.
Hanson, R. W., Borden, R. L., Hall, S. M., and Hall, R. G. Use of programmed instruction in teaching self-management skills to overweight adults. *Behav. Ther.,* 1976, *7,* 366–373.
Harris, M. B. Self-directed program for weight control: A pilot study. *J. Abnorm. Psychol.,* 1969, *74,* 263–270.
Harris, M. B., and Bruner, C. G. A comparison of a self-control and a contract procedure for weight control. *Behav. Res. Ther.,* 1971, *9,* 347–354.
Harris, M. B., and Hallbauer, E. S. Self-directed weight control through eating and exercise. *Behav. Res. Ther.,* 1973, *11,* 523–529.
Isaksson, B. Diet and exercise. Assessment of the Swedish program. In G. Bray (Ed.), *Second Fogarty International Conference on Obesity.* Washington, D.C.: United States Government Printing Office, in press.
Jeffery, D. B. A comparison of the effects of external control and self-control on the modification and maintenance of weight. *Journal of Abnormal Psychology,* 1974, *83,* 404–410.
Jeffery, R. W., Wing, R. R., and Stunkard, A. J. Behavioral treatment of obesity: The state of the art in 1976. *Behav. Ther.,* 1978, *9,* 189–199.
Jordan, H. A., and Levitz, L. S. A behavioral approach to the problem of obesity. *Obesity Bariatric Med.,* 1975, *4,* 58–69.
Kristein, M., Arnold, C., and Wynder, E. Health economics and preventive care. *Science,* 1977, *195,* 457–462.
Lalonde, M. *A new perspective on the health of Canadians.* Ottawa, Canada: Ministry of Health and Welfare, 1974.
Levitz, L., and Stunkard, A. J. A therapeutic coalition for obesity: Behavior modification and patient self-help. *Am. J. Psychiatry,* 1974, *131,* 423–427.
Lindner, P. G., and Blackburn, G. L. Multidisciplinary approach to obesity utilizing fasting modified by protein-sparing therapy. *Obesity Bariatric Med.,* 1976, *5,* 198–216.
Mahoney, M. J. Self-reward and self-monitoring techniques for weight control. *Behav. Ther.,* 1974, *5,* 48–57.
Mahoney, M. J., and Mahoney, K. Treatment of obesity: A clinical exploration. In B. J. Williams, S. Martin, and J. P. Foreyt (Eds.), *Obesity: Behavioral approaches to dietary management.* New York: Brunner/Mazel, 1976a.
Mahoney, M. J., and Mahoney, K. *Permanent weight control: A total solution to the dieter's dilemma.* New York: Norton, 1976b.
McGovern, G. Dietary goals for the United States. *Report of the select committee on nutrition and human needs of the United States Senate.* Washington, D.C.: United States Government Printing Office, 1977.
McReynolds, W. T., and Lutz, E. N. Weight loss resulting from two behavior modification procedures with nutritionists as therapists. *Behav. Ther.,* 1976, *7,* 283–291.
Mills, M. J., and Stunkard, A. J. Behavioral changes following surgery for obesity. *Am. J. Psychiatry,* 1976, *133,* 527–531.
Murray, D. C. Treatment of overweight: 1. The relationship between initial weight and weight change during behavior therapy of overweight individuals. Analysis of data from previous studies. *Psychol. Rep.,* 1975, *37,* 243–248.
Penick, S. B., Filion, R., Fox, S., and Stunkard, A. J. Behavior modification in the treatment of obesity. *Psychosom. Med.,* 1971, *33,* 49–55.
Romanczyk, R. G. Self-monitoring in the treatment of obesity: Parameters of reactivity. *Behav. Ther.,* 1974, *5,* 531–540.
Romanczyk, R. G., Tracey, D. A., Wilson, G. T., and Thorpe, G. L. Behavioral techniques in the treatment of obesity: A comparative analysis. *Behav. Res. Ther.,* 1973, *11,* 629–640.
Stuart, R. B. Behavioral control of overeating. *Behav. Res. Ther.,* 1967, *5,* 357–365.
Stuart, R. B. A three-dimensional program for the treatment of obesity. *Behav. Res. Ther.,* 1971, *9,* 177–186.
Stuart, R. B. Behavioral control of overeating: A status report. In G. A. Gray (Ed.), *Obesity in perspective.* Washington, D.C.: United States Government Printing Office, 1976.
Stunkard, A. J. From explanation to action in psychosomatic medicine: The case of obesity. *Psychosom. Med.,* 1975, *37,* 195–236.
Stunkard, A. J. Behavioral treatment for obesity: Failure to maintain weight loss. In R. B. Stuart (Ed.), *Behavioral self-control.* New York: Brunner/Mazel, 1977.
Stunkard, A. J., Levine, H., and Fox, S. The management of obesity: Patient self-help and medical treatment. *Arch. Intern. Med.,* 1970, *125,* 1067–1072.
Stunkard, A. J., and Mahoney, M. J. Behavioral treatment of the eating disorders. In H. Leitenberg (Ed.), *Handbook of behavior modification and behavior therapy.* Englewood Cliffs, N.J.: Prentice Hall, 1976, pp. 45–73.
Stunkard, A. J., and McLaren-Hume, M. The results of treatment of obesity. A review of the literature and report of a series. *Arch. Intern. Med.,* 1959, *103,* 79–85.
Stunkard, A. J., and Penick, S. B. Behavior modification in the treatment of obesity: The problem of

maintaining of weight loss. *Arch. Gen. Psychiatry,* in press.

Stunkard, A. J., and Rush, A. J. Dieting and depression reexamined: A critical review of reports of untoward responses during weight reduction for obesity. *Ann. Intern. Med.,* 1974, *81,* 526–533.

Sullivan, L., Bjurö, R., Garellick, G., Krotiewski, M., and Perrson, G. The predictive value of adipose tissue cellularity, basal metabolism rate and cephalic insulin stimulation in the treatment of obesity. *Int. J. Obesity,* in press.

Wilber, J. A. The problem of undetected and untreated hypertension in the community. *Bull. N. Y. Acad. Med.,* 1973, *49,* 510–520.

Wollersheim, J. P. Effectiveness of group therapy based upon learning principles in the treatment of overweight women. *J. Abnorm. Psychol.,* 1970, *76,* 562–574.

Index